Handbook of
Nurse Anesthesia

Claudette Dion
20 Congress St. # 3
Milford, MA 01757

Handbook of
Nurse Anesthesia

Second Edition

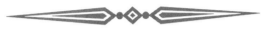

John J. Nagelhout, PhD, CRNA
Director, School of Anesthesia
Kaiser Permanente
California State University at Fullerton
Pasadena, California

Karen L. Zaglaniczny, PhD, CRNA, FAAN
Director of Perioperative Services, Education and Research
Director, Graduate Program of Nurse Anesthesia
William Beaumont Hospital
Oakland University
Royal Oak, Michigan

Valdor L. Haglund, Jr., MS, CRNA
Detroit Receiving Hospital
Assistant Professor of Anesthesia
Wayne State University
Detroit, Michigan

W.B. SAUNDERS COMPANY
An Imprint of Elsevier Science
Philadelphia London Montreal Sydney Tokyo Toronto

W.B. SAUNDERS COMPANY
An Imprint of Elsevier Science

The Curtis Center
625 Walnut Street, Suite 300
Philadelphia, PA 19106-3399

Vice-President, Nursing Editorial Director: Sally Schrefer
Senior Editor: Michael S. Ledbetter
Developmental Editor: Lisa P. Newton
Project Manager: Gayle May Morris

Second Edition

Printed in the United States of America.

International Standard Book Number: 0-7216-8624-9

03 04 SG/F 9 8 7 6 5 4

The complexity of clinical anesthesia practice continues to increase as new procedures and drugs are introduced and as our methods of conceptualizing and managing diseases evolve. Anesthetists must stay abreast of current practices in a variety of disciplines, since our patients may arrive with an array of medical problems and surgical needs. When selecting the format of this handbook, we chose not to simply produce a condensed version of our text, *Nurse Anesthesia*. We believe that there is a need for a single comprehensive source containing information on common diseases, procedures, and drugs, and that such a source, in a handbook format, would complement the larger text and provide an "in the operating room" guide for practice. This second edition of our handbook has been totally reviewed and revised to include the most up-to-date clinical information available. Today, many clinicians practice at more than one facility, and thus may be called on to provide anesthesia care in a broader spectrum of operative and diagnostic situations. A comprehensive reference guide is an essential tool for hands on management in the modern operating suite.

We compiled the *Handbook of Nurse Anesthesia* as a single source that provides:
- A thorough overview of the *common diseases* encountered in surgical patients.
- A *procedure manual* and guidelines for anesthesia management for a wide variety of diagnostic and surgical procedures.
- A convenient and comprehensive *drug reference* for clinical use.

A standardized format was designed and customized for use throughout each of the three individual sections of the *Handbook*. Several appendices at the end of the *Handbook* offer the clinician easy access to the difficult airway algorithm, ACLS Algorithms, hemodynamic formulas, guidelines for fluid and blood therapy, latex allergy guidelines, pulmonary function testing, preoperative laboratory values, AANA Standards of Practice, and much more.

John J. Nagelhout
Karen L. Zaglaniczny
Valdor L. Haglund, Jr.

NOTICE

Anesthesia is an ever-changing field. Standard safety precautions must be followed, but as new research and clinical experience broaden our knowledge, changes in treatment and drug therapy become necessary or appropriate. The editors of this work have carefully checked the generic and trade drug names and verified drug dosages to ensure that the dosage information in this work is accurate and in accord with the standards accepted at the time of publication. Readers are advised, however, to check the product information currently provided by the manufacturer of each drug to be administered to be certain that changes have not been made in the recommended dose or in the contraindications for administration. This is of particular importance in regard to new or infrequently used drugs. It is the responsibility of the treating physician, relying on experience and knowledge of the patient, to determine dosages and the best treatment for the patient. The editors cannot be responsible for misuse or misapplication of the material in this work.

THE PUBLISHER

ACKNOWLEDGMENTS FOR THE SECOND EDITION

We are especially gratified with the comments and widespread acceptance of the first edition of this handbook by the anesthesia community. Its extensive use as a clinical guide confirms our assumptions that a convenient and inclusive source such as this is essential in modern anesthesia practice. We have incorporated many of these comments in revising and updating this new edition. Each section has been thoroughly edited to include the latest information available on common diseases, procedures, and drugs encountered during daily practice.

We would like to thank the following individuals for their suggestions and review in the preparation of this second edition:

Florence Acosta, RN, BSN
Jeremy Adams, MS, CRNA
Loreto Albaran, MS, CRNA
Marina Arndt, MS, CRNA
Cheryl Baxa, MS, CRNA
Michelle Branham, MS, CRNA
Mark Campbell, RN, BSN
Anne Cloherty, RN, BSN
Ceri Fass, RN, BSN
Lori Hockenberry, MS, CRNA

Mark Hunter, MS, CRNA
Casey March-Arnett, MS, CRNA
Mary Moriconi, MS, CRNA
Joseph Nickerson, MS, CRNA
Christopher O'Hagan, RN, BSN
Shonna Parks, RN, BSN
Alisa Richardson, RN, BSN
Doug Roberts, MS, CRNA
Lisa Tyson, MS, CRNA
Denise Zeleny, MS, CRNA

We would also like to thank the following individuals who were also instrumental in the production of this book: The staff at Harcourt Health Sciences, Michael Ledbetter, Senior Editor, Lisa Newton, Developmental Editor, Victoria Legnini, Editorial Assistant, Thomas Eoyang, Former Vice President and Editor-in-Chief of Nursing Books, and Maura Connor, Former Editor; Retta Smith and Emily MacLean from Kaiser Permanente. Again we would like to thank our professional colleagues, friends, and especially our families for their support.

ACKNOWLEDGMENTS FROM THE FIRST EDITION

The production and success of this book required the collaborative efforts of many contributors. We wish to recognize each of the following contributors for his or her knowledge and expertise in the field of anesthesia and extensive review and research in each topic area:

Janet Baskin, CRNA, MS
Carol Bernicke, CRNA, MS
Michael D. Duronio, CRNA, MS
Geri Evon-Gabourie, CRNA, MS
Curt Feldhak, CRNA, MS
Nancy Fisher, CRNA, MS
Donna Funke, CRNA, MS
Carrie Hajjar, CRNA, MS
Jennifer Hourigan, CRNA, MS
Mary Jennett, CRNA, MS
Kendra Kayser, CRNA, MS
Patti S. Leupp, CRNA, MS
Cynthia Lynn, CRNA, MS

Ronald Manningham, CRNA, MS
Kellie Martin, CRNA, MS
Louise Minore, CRNA, MS
Lisa Mueller, CRNA, MS
Colette Neenan, CRNA, MS
Oscar Ong, CRNA, MS
Sally Range, CRNA, MS
Alan R. Roberts, CRNA, MS
Roxanna Robinson, CRNA, MS
Susan Vander Laan, CRNA, MS
Richard VanTuyl, CRNA, MS
Ruth I. Watts, CRNA, MS

We are also indebted to others who have facilitated the development and realization of this book. These include the staff at W.B. Saunders Company, Maura Connor, Editor, Stephanie Klein, Editorial Assistant, Frank Messina, Senior Copy Editor, Frank Polizzano, Production Manager, and Thomas Eoyang, Vice President and Editor-in-Chief of Nursing Books. We acknowledge the support of the staff at Henry Ford Hospital, Detroit Receiving Hospital, University of Detroit Mercy, and Wayne State University during our worthwhile endeavors. Finally, we would also like to thank our professional colleagues, friends, and especially our families for their patient endurance and endless encouragement.

John J. Nagelhout
Karen L. Zaglaniczny
Valdor L. Haglund, Jr.

CONTENTS

PART 1

Common Diseases 1

SECTION I
Cardiovascular System 2

A. Ischemic Heart Disease 2
B. Arrhythmias 6
C. Myocardial Infarction 6
D. Hypertension 11
E. Congestive Heart Failure 13
F. Shock 16
G. Valvular Heart Disease 18
H. Cardiomyopathy 25
I. Peripheral Vascular Disease 29
J. Pericardial Processes/Tamponade 34

SECTION II
Respiratory System 37

A. Chronic Obstructive Pulmonary Disease/Emphysema/ Obstructive Disease 37
B. Asthma 39
C. Pneumonia 40
D. Tuberculosis 42
E. Pulmonary Embolism 43
F. Cor Pulmonale 45
G. Pulmonary Hypertension 46
H. Upper Respiratory Infection 48
I. Restrictive Pulmonary Diseases 49
J. Adult Respiratory Distress Syndrome 51
K. Pneumothorax and Hemothorax 52

SECTION III
Central Nervous System 54

A. Seizures 54
B. Cerebrovascular Disease 56
C. Hydrocephalus 57
D. Parkinson's Syndrome 59
E. Guillain-Barré Syndrome 60
F. Multiple Sclerosis 61
G. Myasthenia Gravis 62
H. Myasthenic Syndrome 65
I. Intracranial Hypertension 65
J. Autonomic Dysreflexia 67
K. Spinal Cord Injury 68

SECTION IV
Musculoskeletal System   70

A.   Muscular Dystrophy   70
B.   Kyphoscoliosis   72
C.   Malignant Hyperthermia   73

SECTION V
Endocrine System   75

A.   Diabetes Mellitus   75
B.   Diabetes Insipidus   76
C.   Thyroid Disease   77
D.   Cushing's Disease   80
E.   Addison's Disease   80
F.   Acromegaly   81
G.   Pheochromocytoma   82
H.   Hypoaldosteronism   84
I.   Hyperaldosteronism   85

SECTION VI
Hepatic System   86

A.   Hepatitis   86
B.   Cirrhosis/Portal Hypertension   87
C.   Hepatic Failure   89

SECTION VII
Renal System   95

A.   Urolithiasis   95
B.   Acute Renal Failure   96
C.   Chronic Renal Failure   97

SECTION VIII
Hematologic System   100

A.   Anemia   100
B.   Sickle Cell Disease   101
C.   Polycythemia Vera   102
D.   Leukemia   103
E.   AIDS/HIV Infection   105
F.   Coagulopathies   106

SECTION IX
Gastrointestinal System   110

A.   Diaphragmatic Hernia   110
B.   Hiatal Hernia/Gastric Reflux   111
C.   Gallstone/Gallbladder Disease   112
D.   Pancreatitis   113
E.   Carcinoid Syndrome   114

SECTION X
Other Conditions   116

A.   Obesity   116
B.   Glaucoma/Open Globe   117
C.   Hypothermia   119
D.   Hyperthermia   120
E.   Systemic Lupus Erythematosus   121
F.   Immunosuppression   123
G.   Malnutrition   123
H.   Geriatrics   125
I.   Scleroderma   126

PART T

Common Procedures   127

SECTION I
Gastrointestinal System   128

A.   Cholecystectomy   128
B.   Laparoscopic Cholecystectomy   129
C.   Liver Resection   130
D.   Liver Transplant   132
E.   Pancreatectomy   135
F.   Whipple's Resection   137
G.   Splenectomy   138
H.   Gastrectomy   140
I   Gastrostomy   141
J.   Small Bowel Resection   143
K.   Appendectomy   143
L.   Colectomy   145
M.   Herniorrhaphy   146
N.   Gallbladder Lithotripsy   147
O.   Esophagoscopy/Gastroscopy   149
P.   Colonoscopy   150
Q.   Esophageal Resection   151
R.   Anal Fistulotomy/Fistulectomy   155
S.   Hemorrhoidectomy   156
T.   Adrenalectomy   157
U.   Pheochromocytoma   159

SECTION II
Genitourinary System   161

A.   Transurethral Resection of the Prostate   161
B.   Radical Prostatectomy   162
C.   Extracorporeal Shock Wave Lithotripsy (ESWL)   164
D.   Nephrectomy   166
E.   Kidney Transplant   168
F.   Cystectomy   173
G.   Cystoscopy   174
H.   Penile Procedures   175
I.   Scrotal Procedures   176

SECTION III
Neuroskeletal System   177

A.   Lumbar Laminectomy/Fusion   177
B.   Anterior Cervical Diskectomy/Fusion   178
C.   Thoracic and Lumbar Spinal Instrumentation and Fusion   180
D.   Spinal Cord Injuries   184

SECTION IV
Neurologic System   190

A.   Cerebral Aneurysm   190
B.   Posterior Fossa Procedures   195
C.   Transsphenoidal Tumor Resections   197
D.   Craniotomy   198
E.   Stereotactic Surgery   200
F.   Cranioplasty   203
G.   Pituitary Tumors   204
H.   Arteriovenous Malformation Neurosurgery   207
I.   Electroconvulsive Therapy   209
J.   Ventriculoperitoneal Shunt   210
K.   Epilepsy Surgery   211

SECTION V
Intrathoracic and Extrathoracic   214

A.   Mediastinoscopy   214
B.   Open Lung Biopsy (Wedge Resection of Lung Lesion)   216
C.   Thoracotomy   217
D.   Bronchopulmonary Lavage   218
E.   Thymectomy   219
F.   Bronchoscopy   221
G.   Lung and Heart/Lung Transplantation   224
H.   One-Lung Ventilation (OLV)   228
I.   Breast Biopsy   229
J.   Mastectomy   231

SECTION **VI**
Cardiac Surgery and Anesthesia Considerations 233

A. Coronary Artery Disease   233
B. Valvular Heart Disease   236
C. Cardiac Tamponade and Constrictive Pericarditis   239
D. Cardiopulmonary Bypass (CPB)   240
E. Cardiac Surgery Plan of Care   242
F. Supplemental Information   255

SECTION **VII**
Vascular Surgery   257

A. Abdominal Aortic Aneurysm   257
B. Peripheral Vascular Procedures   260
C. Thoracic Aortic Aneurysm   264
D. Aorto-Bifemoral Bypass Grafting   266
E. Carotid Endarterectomy   268
F. Portasystemic Shunts   270

SECTION **VIII**
Orthopedics   272

A. Hip Arthroplasty   272
B. Knee (Total Knee Replacement) Arthroplasty   275
C. Shoulder (Total Shoulder) Arthroplasty   276
D. External Fixator Placement and Open Reduction and Internal Fixation of Extremities   278
E. Pelvic Reconstruction   279
F. Hip Pinning (Open Reduction and Internal Fixation)   282
G. Open Reduction and Internal Fixation of Extremities   284
H. Arthroscopy   286

SECTION **IX**
Head and Neck   288

A. Thyroidectomy   288
B. Parathyroidectomy   290
C. Tracheotomy   291
D. Laryngectomy   293
E. Radical Neck Dissection   296
F. Maxillofacial Trauma   298
G. Tonsillectomy and Adenoidectomy   300
H. Nasal Surgery   301
I. LeFort Procedures   303
J. Uvulopalatopharyngoplasty (UPPP)   304
K. Ocular Procedures   306
L. Orbital Fractures   310
M. Rhytidectomy/Facelift   312
N. Dacryocystorhinostomy   314
O. Ptosis Surgery   315

SECTION **X**
Obstetrics and Gynecology   317

A.   Cesarean Section   317
B.   Anesthesia for Vaginal Delivery   322
C.   Gynecologic Laparoscopy   323
D.   Hysterectomy—Vaginal or Total Abdominal   324
E.   Loop Electrosurgical Excision Procedure   325
F.   In Vitro Fertilization   326
G.   Pelvic Exenteration   327
H.   Dilatation and Curettage (D & C)   328

SECTION **XI**
Pediatrics   329

A.   Anatomy and Physiology   329
B.   Pharmacology   332
C.   Fluids   334
D.   Equipment   335
E.   Myringotomy   336
F.   Tonsillectomy and Adenoidectomy   338
G.   Pediatric Intra-abdominal Procedures   339
H.   Repair of Congenital Diaphragmatic Hernia   341
I.   Pediatric Hernia Repair   344
J.   Genitourinary Procedures   345

SECTION **XII**
Anesthesia for Therapeutic/Diagnostic Procedures   347

A.   Overall Anesthetic Care Plan   347
B.   Anesthesia for CT Scan and MRI   350
C.   Nuclear Medicine   352
D.   Brachytherapy   354
E.   Cardioversion   355
F.   Automatic Implantable Cardioverter Defibrillator (AICD)   356
G.   Cardiac Radiofrequency Ablation   357
H.   Endoscopy   358

SECTION **XIII**
Other Procedures   359

A.   Burns   359
B.   Trauma   361
C.   Laser Procedures Involving the Airways   363

PART 3

Drugs: Listed Alphabetically   367

APPENDICES

1 Drugs   487
2 Pediatric Drug Doses   490
3 Guidelines for Fluid Management   491
4 Difficult Airway Algorithm   499
5 Advanced Cardiac Life Support Algorithms   500
6 Hemodynamic Formulas   511
7 Pulmonary Function Test Values   512
8 Nomogram for the Determination of Body Surface Area of
      Children and Adults   513
9 Pediatric Conversion Factors   515
10 Emergency Therapy for Malignant Hyperthermia   517
11 Anesthesia Apparatus Checkout Recommendations   519
12 Preoperative Laboratory Tests   521
13 Standards for Nurse Anesthesia Practice   523
14 Latex Allergy   524

1

Common Diseases

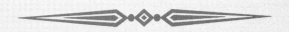

Cardiovascular System

A. Ischemic Heart Disease

DEFINITION

Ischemic heart disease (IHD) describes the condition in which atherosclerotic plaque is present in the coronary arteries, giving way to coronary artery disease (CAD).

INCIDENCE

More than ten million adults in the United States have IHD, and it is the leading cause of death (500,000 deaths/year). The first manifestation of IHD is often acute myocardial infarction resulting in sudden death.

The overall prognosis of patients with IHD is dependent upon the frequency and severity of cardiac arrhythmias, myocardial infarction, and left ventricular (LV) dysfunction. About 25 million people in the United States undergo anesthesia and operation each year—of these, 7 million are considered to be at high risk because of the presence of IHD.

ETIOLOGY

IHD is due to the presence of atherosclerotic plaque in the coronary arteries that causes narrowing and subsequently impedes blood flow. Angina pectoris is the presenting complaint of the patient experiencing a reduction in coronary artery blood flow. Dyspnea that occurs after the onset of angina indicates acute LV dysfunction, which can lead to congestive heart failure (CHF) from myocardial ischemia. The most important risk factors are advanced age and male gender. Other risk factors include hyperlipidemia, hypertension, cigarette smoking, diabetes, obesity, sedentary life style, familial history of premature development of IHD, and other psychosocial characteristics. There are three types of angina: stable, variant, and unstable (Prinzmetal's). *Stable angina* is chest pain that occurs predictably when there is an increase in cardiac work. As the heart rate increases (usually above 100 beats per minute) demand exceeds supply and angina becomes evident. *Variant angina* is due to coronary artery spasm of unknown cause that gives way to ischemia and ultimately chest pain. *Unstable angina* is a combination of stable and variant angina and usually represents an advanced degree of CAD. These patients may have angina at rest.

DIAGNOSTIC AND LABORATORY FINDINGS
Cardiac Evaluation

A complete history and physical examination, chest x-ray, and electrocardiogram (ECG) should be performed in the patient with known or suspected IHD. If the initial evaluation suggests IHD, stress testing may be indicated. An exercise ECG with or without concomitant administration of intravenous radionucleotide (i.e., thallium) is usually performed. If the stress test is suggestive of IHD, cardiac catheterization may then be indicated. In addition, transthoracic echocardiography is also available as a noninvasive means to further evaluate overall cardiac function.

History

The clinician should elicit the severity and functional limitations imposed by IHD. Evaluation of symptoms as they relate to exercise tolerance, dyspnea, angina, and peripheral edema will give a qualitative estimate of the degree of impairment. Symptoms in some individuals may not be present at rest, so the patient's response to physical activity should be elicited through careful, appropriate questioning (e.g., Can they climb a flight of stairs?). One must be able to identify borderline CHF since the stress of anesthesia and operation may elicit overt failure perioperatively.

Evaluation of LV Function

Good	Impaired
By History and Physical Examination	
Angina	Prior myocardial infarction
Essential hypertension	Evidence of CHF
No evidence of CHF	
By Cardiac Catheterization	
Ejection fraction > 0.55	Ejection fraction < 0.40
LVEDP < 12 mmHg	LVEDP > 18 mmHg
Cardiac index > 2.5 L/min/m^2	Cardiac index < 2.0 L/min/m^2
No ventricular dyskinesia	Multiple areas of ventricular dyskinesia

CLINICAL MANIFESTATIONS

Angina

Angina pectoris is substernal chest pain that often radiates to the neck, jaw, left shoulder, or left arm and is frequently precipitated by exertion. It may be relieved with rest or sublingual nitroglycerin.

	Exercise-Induced	Occurs at Rest	Night Pain	ST Segment
Stable	Yes	No (yes with emotion)	Occasionally with dream	↓ ST
Unstable	Yes	Yes	Yes	↓ or ↑ ST
Variant	Rarely	Yes	Early in A.M.	↑ ST usually— can also be depressed

TREATMENT

Treatment goals are geared toward using those measures to decrease myocardial oxygen demand and increase supply (i.e., increase coronary blood flow). This can be achieved in various ways.

General Medical Means

- Control related pathology—CHF, hypertension
- Smoking cessation
- Weight loss
- Exercise
- Stress modification
- Antithrombotic medications—low-dose aspirin may prevent reinfarction
- Avoidance of heavy meals or cold prior to exertion

Drug Therapy

- Nitrates
- β-blockers
- Calcium channel blockers
- Combined therapy

Revascularization—When Patient's Condition Is Refractory to Drug Therapy

- Coronary artery bypass graft
- Angioplasty

ANESTHETIC CONSIDERATIONS

Preoperative

The goal is to decrease anxiety and thus sympathetic stimulation, which may otherwise increase myocardial oxygen demand, causing ischemia. Benzodiazepines (e.g., midazolam) and/or narcotics may be administered for preoperative sedation and amnesia. Nitroglycerin may also be administered prophylactically to optimize coronary blood flow.

Intraoperative

Prevent intraoperative events that adversely affect the balance between myocardial oxygen supply and demand. Factors that can *decrease oxygen supply* and *increase oxygen demand* are listed below.

Decrease Oxygen Supply	Increase Oxygen Demand
1. Decreased CBF: increased heart rate, increased diastolic BP, increased $PaCO_2$	1. Sympathetic stimulation
2. Coronary artery spasm	2. Increased heart rate
3. Decreased CaO_2, anemia, PaO_2	3. Increased systolic BP
4. Increased preload	4. Increased myocardial contractility
	5. Increased afterload

The goal is to maintain heart rate and blood pressure within 20% of normal. While it is generally accepted that a heart rate above 100 bpm is more likely to cause ischemia, it has been shown that ischemia may also develop at rates below 100 bpm.

Induction

Most induction drugs are acceptable provided they are administered judiciously. Laryngoscopy and intubation time should be kept at a minimum to decrease sympathetic stimulation and its deleterious effects. If hypertension exists in the patient prior to anesthesia, the following drugs can be used to facilitate a smooth, stress-free induction.

Lidocaine   1 to 2 mg/kg IV 90 seconds prior to laryngoscopy
Nitroprusside   1 to 2 μg/kg IV 15 seconds prior to laryngoscopy
Esmolol   1 mg/kg IV before induction
Fentanyl   1 to 3 μg/kg IV during induction

Maintenance

It is imperative to maintain normal or optimize LV function. Volatile anesthetics will minimize increases in sympathetic activity and oxygen demand. Inclusion of nitrous oxide with an inhalational agent or alone as part of a nitrous oxide/opioid technique is also acceptable. A high-dose narcotic technique with the addition of a volatile anesthetic to treat undesired increases in blood pressure has also been used effectively.

Muscle Relaxation

Any of a number of nondepolarizing muscle relaxants may be used. Intermediate-acting relaxants (vecuronium, atracurium, cisatracurium) have been used successfully, as have longer-acting relaxants (doxacurium, pipecuronium, pancuronium). Choice of relaxant may be determined by its potential effect on heart rate, length of procedure, plan for emergence (i.e., will the patient be mechanically ventilated postoperatively or is "fast tracking" to be considered), and cost. Pancuronium can cause a dose-dependent increase in heart rate (which could potentially lead to myocardial ischemia), however, it can also be used to off-set the bradycardia that ensues when high-dose narcotics are used.

Reversal Agents

Anticholinesterase drugs (pyridostigmine, neostigmine) and anticholinergics (atropine, glycopyrrolate, scopolamine) are considered safe. Many clinicians prefer glycopyrrolate because of its tendency to preserve a somewhat "normal" heart rate when used in combination with an anticholinesterase.

EMERGENCE

The same considerations apply here as for induction of anesthesia (i.e., prevent increases in myocardial oxygen demand and decreases in supply). Patients with severe IHD may need treatment for hypertensive episodes during emergence from anesthesia and into the postoperative period.

POSTOPERATIVE CARE

Maintenance of normal cardiac dynamics (blood pressure and heart rate), normal PaO_2 and $PaCO_2$, and adequate pain relief are essential to prevent sympathetic stimulation and its deleterious effects on myocardial oxygen supply and demand.

PROGNOSIS

IHD is a chronic condition that requires continuous management throughout the perioperative period. Its prognosis is related to the stage of the disease process and its symptoms and limitations.

B. Arrhythmias

The current drugs of choice for common arrhythmias are listed in Table 1/I/B-1. Detailed notes about these arrhythmias and their treatments are given in Box 1/I/B-1. Several reports have indicated that when given to asymptomatic or mildly symptomatic patients, some antiarrhythmic agents may become pro-arrhythmic.

C. Myocardial Infarction

DEFINITION

Myocardial infarction (MI) or myocardial cell death occurs when a portion of heart muscle is deprived of its blood supply due to blockage, acute thrombosis, or spasm of a coronary artery.

INCIDENCE AND PREVALENCE

The clinician should first determine if the patient has a previous history of MI. The likelihood of perioperative reinfarction correlates with the time elapsed since prior MI. The average reinfarction rate is 6% if time elapsed since the first MI is 6 months. Therefore elective surgery, especially thoracic or abdominal, *should be delayed for 6 months following MI*. Even with a 6-month delay, these patients are still at greater risk than patients who have not suffered an MI. In high-risk patients, invasive hemodynamic monitoring, transesophageal echocardiography, and aggressive treatment of cardiac alterations have reduced the risk of reinfarction.

The incidence of reinfarction is also increased in patients undergoing intrathoracic or intra-abdominal operations lasting more than 3 hours. Factors increasing the potential for reinfarction include hypotension (i.e., mean arterial less than 60 mmHg) lasting longer than 10 minutes, hypertension and tachycardia, diabetes, smoking, and hyperlipidemia.

ETIOLOGY

When myocardial oxygen supply (i.e., coronary blood flow) does not meet demand (myocardial oxygen consumption), ischemia or infarction may occur. The risk for perioperative MI increases when a patient who has suffered a previous infarction comes to the operating room for anesthesia and operation.

LABORATORY TESTS

Laboratory tests as indicated by the history and physical examination may include electrolytes, complete blood count, blood urea nitrogen, creatinine, cardiac enzymes (MB bands), and a coagulation profile. Twenty-four hour Holter monitoring may be necessary if the patient is at risk for ischemic episodes or arrhythmias. Echocardiography, stress testing or cardiac catheterization may become necessary in the patient with cardiac disease. The approach must be individualized to the needs and risks of the patient.

CLINICAL MANIFESTATIONS

Many patients are asymptomatic following an MI. Common manifestations of coronary artery disease include poor exercise tolerance, angina (stable or unstable), dyspnea, congestive heart failure, and arrhythmias. These patients may be risk-stratified according to the New York Heart Association Functional Classification and the American Society of Anesthesiologists (ASA) Classification.

TREATMENT AND ANESTHETIC CONSIDERATIONS

Anesthesia care begins with a thorough history and physical examination. The history reveals risk factors for IHD, activity tolerance, determination of angina (stable or unstable), and use of coronary vasodilators (e.g., nitroglycerin). The physical examination may reveal extra heart sounds (i.e., S_3 and/or S_4), rales/rhonchi, jugular venous distention, peripheral edema, or other findings consistent with underlying cardiac disease. The anesthetist should communicate any findings with the primary physician and surgeon to weigh the risks/benefits of the proposed surgical procedure. The importance of minimizing stress (demand) and optimizing myocardial perfusion (supply) intraoperatively cannot be overemphasized. Reduction of stress begins in the preoperative area with the use of individualized sedation. Any increase in metabolic work during the perioperative period increases myocardial oxygen demand, which may result in myocardial ischemia or infarction. Myocardial oxygen supply and demand must be balanced for an optimal outcome.

Four questions must therefore be answered before the patient proceeds to anesthesia/operation. These questions are often determined by careful history-taking. The first three questions to be addressed are: *What is the extent of coronary artery disease? Is additional therapy indicated (e.g., cardiac catheterization, angioplasty, or CABG)? What is the extent of ventricular compromise?* How the clinician determines the answers to these questions will inevitably affect the administration and titration of anesthetics. Finally, the fourth question to be asked is: *Will the patient tolerate surgery?*

Standard monitoring should always be considered in these patients. In addition, ECG monitoring of lead II (inferior ischemia) and lead V_5

TABLE 1/I/B-1 Drugs of Choice for Common Arrhythmias

Arrhythmia	Drug of Choice	Alternatives	Remarks
Atrial fibrillation or flutter[1]*	Calcium antagonists (verapamil, diltiazem) or a β-blocker (esmolol) to slow ventricular response[1]	Digoxin to slow ventricular response Quinidine, procainamide, disopyramide, flecainide, propafenone, or sotalol for long-term prevention Ibutilide for termination of the arrhythmia	Digoxin, verapamil, diltiazem, and possibly β-blockers may be dangerous for patients with Accessory Pathway disturbances (e.g., Wolff-Parkinson-White syndrome). Amiodarone in low doses has also been effective for prevention. Radiofrequency catheter ablation has been used in selected patients.
Other supraventricular tachycardias[2]	Adenosine, verapamil[3], or diltiazem[3] for termination	Esmolol, another β-blocker, or digoxin for termination	DC cardioversion or atrial pacing may be effective for some patients. Radiofrequency catheter ablation may be indicated. Quinidine, procainamide, disopyramide, diltiazem, β-blockers, verapamil, flecainide, propafenone, or digoxin may be effective for long-term suppression.
Premature ventricular complexes (PVCs) or nonsustained ventricular tachycardia	No drug therapy indicated for asymptomatic patients	For symptomatic patients, a β-blocker	Sudden cardiac death may still occur, despite therapy. For post-MI patients, β-blocker therapy has decreased mortality. Treatment with flecainide or moricizine has increased mortality.

Sustained ventricular tachycardia[4,5]	Lidocaine for acute treatment[4,5]	Procainamide, bretylium, amiodarone[4,5]	β-blockers (e.g., sotalol), procainamide, quinidine, amiodarone, disopyramide, flecainide, propafenone, or mexiletine may be effective for long-term prevention.[6]
Ventricular fibrillation[7]	Lidocaine[7]	Amiodarone, procainamide, bretylium[7]	See footnote 6.
Digitalis-induced ventricular tachyarrhythmias[5,8]	Digoxin-immune Fab (digoxin antibody fragments—*Digibind*)	Lidocaine, phenytoin	Self-limited if digoxin is stopped. Phenytoin may be effective. Avoid DC cardioversion and bretylium, except for ventricular fibrillation or sustained ventricular tachycardia. A β-blocker or procainamide can make heart block worse.
Torsades de pointes (acquired)	Magnesium sulfate	Cardiac pacing, isoproterenol	Causative agents (e.g., quinidine) should be discontinued. Magnesium sulfate in a dose of 1 g IV, repeated once if necessary, may be effective even in absence of hypomagnesemia. Potassium should be used to raise serum K to between 4 and 5.5 mEq/L.[8]

* Superscript numbers refer to the numbered list in Box 1/I/B-1.
From Drugs for cardiac arrhythmias. *Med Lett.* 38:75-76, 1996.

BOX 1/I/B-1   Notes to Table 1/I/B-1

1. DC cardioversion is the safest and most effective treatment. For patients with atrial flutter, atrial pacing can also be effective. Patients with Wolff-Parkinson-White syndrome and atrial fibrillation should be treated with IV procainamide if hemodynamically stable and, if not, with DC cardioversion.
2. Vagotonic maneuvers (i.e., carotid sinus massage, gagging, the Valsalva maneuver, or increasing venous return by straight leg raising) may first be attempted.
3. Verapamil and diltiazem should be used with great care in those patients receiving IV β-blockers, quinidine, or those with congestive heart failure.
4. DC cardioversion is the safest and most effective treatment. It is preferred for sustained ventricular tachycardia causing hemodynamic compromise. Chest "thump" and/or IV lidocaine may be attempted .
5. Some ventricular tachycardias can be caused or exacerbated by bradycardia or heart block. In the presence of high-grade heart block, antiarrhythmic drugs can cause cardiac standstill. A temporary pacemaker should be inserted before using antiarrhythmic drugs in these scenarios; pacing may abolish the arrhythmia. When a drug must be used in the presence of heart block, lidocaine is least likely to increase the block.
6. Specialized techniques such as programmed stimulation of the heart may be required to select long-term therapy, and some patients may be candidates for implanted cardioverter/defibrillators (see *Med Lett.* 1994;36:86) or radiofrequency catheter ablation (see *Med Lett.* 1996;38:40).
7. Defibrillation is the treatment of choice; drugs are for prevention of recurrence.
8. KCl can be given carefully, 10 to 20 mEq/hr IV, to patients with low or normal serum potassium concentrations. Extreme care must be taken to keep serum potassium below 5.5 mEq/L. In the presence of heart block not associated with paroxysmal atrial tachycardia, potassium should be withheld if the serum concentration is greater than 4.5 mEq/L because high serum potassium may increase atrioventricular block.

(anterior ischemia), ST-segment trend analysis, esophageal ECG (to identify P waves, posterior ischemia), and/or transesophageal echocardiography can be used perioperatively. Invasive intravascular lines, such as a central venous pressure (CVP) line, a pulmonary artery (PA) catheter (to evaluate right- and left-sided heart pressures, pulmonary capillary wedge pressure, pulmonary and systemic vascular resistances, and cardiac output/index), and an arterial line for beat-to-beat evaluation of blood pressure and frequent blood specimen analyses, may need to be considered. These measures should be used to optimize anesthetic care when the patient is at risk because of clinical history and/or the surgical procedure.

Recognition and aggressive treatment of ischemia is vital. Careful, vigilant monitoring perioperatively will allow rapid intervention in the patient at risk for cardiac complications. Likewise, interpretation of data and prompt initiation of treatment have been shown to improve outcome.

Fluid management in these patients should be individualized to the length/type of operation and the degree of left ventricular compromise. A CVP or PA catheter can offer useful information in these high-risk patients. Intraoperative overhydration (i.e., fluid overload) may lead to postoperative hypertension and congestive heart failure.

Urine output should be closely monitored in the cardiac patient (approximately 0.5 to 1.0 mL/kg/hr). It is believed to be a reflection of renal perfusion and thus cardiac output, provided renal function is normal. Urine output may also be an indicator of overall patient volume status.

Choice of anesthetic in these patients should be individualized to the patient and the proposed procedure. General, regional, and local anesthetic techniques have all been used successfully. Is is important for the clinician to understand that patient outcome is based on *how* the agents are administered, rather than the specific technique used.

General and spinal anesthesia are similar when the risk of perioperative MI and death is considered. A combined general-epidural technique for vascular surgery has been suggested to lower cardiac complications. The incidence and risk of congestive heart failure are higher with general anesthesia in patients with severe coronary artery disease.

Emergence from anesthesia should be smooth and stress-free, with special efforts made to maintain cardiac hemodynamics (myocardial oxygen supply and demand). Time of extubation may need to be delayed until cardiovascular stability is established.

Ongoing postoperative observation of high-risk patients is essential to identify and aggressively treat cardiac complications. Shivering, fever, pain, wide swings in blood pressure, tachycardia, arrhythmias, and congestive heart failure may alter cardiac dynamics, leading to ischemia (and MI). Careful fluid management may also minimize the potential for postoperative ischemic events and improve outcome.

Recognizing the importance of complications and mortality related to anesthesia and surgery is the first step toward prevention. Patients at risk for perioperative cardiac complications can be risk-stratified, and the information used to plan the safest anesthetic and intraoperative monitoring.

D. Hypertension

DEFINITION

Hypertension (HTN) is a systolic blood pressure (SBP) greater than 160 mm Hg or diastolic blood pressure (DBP) greater than 90 mm Hg or both. Mortality and morbidity increase with increasing levels of either SBP or DBP.

INCIDENCE

Hypertension (HTN) is the most common circulatory derangement, affecting more than 60 million Americans. The prevalence of HTN increases with age, and approximately half of those over 65 years of age have systolic or diastolic HTN.

ETIOLOGY

Blood pressure (BP) is regulated by baroreceptors and secretion of vasoactive hormones (renin, angiotensin, aldosterone, and catecholamines). Any abnormality in this system can lead to HTN. *Essential* HTN has no identifiable cause and accounts for more than 90% of HTN. *Secondary* HTN is caused by renal disease, coarctation, Cushing's syndrome, pheochromocytoma, primary aldosteronism, or pharmacologic agents.

DIAGNOSIS AND LABORATORY FINDINGS

Persistent elevation of SBP greater than 160 mm Hg and/or DBP greater than 90 mm Hg is seen. Renal disease, coarctation, hyperadrenocorticism, and pheochromocytoma are common secondary causes. Organ system involvement is determined through diagnostic testing.

TREATMENT

When DBP is greater than 90 mm Hg, drug treatment is usually employed, although isolated systolic HTN may respond to diet modification and weight loss. Patients with borderline HTN can decrease their BP with exercise and weight loss. If DBP exceeds 105 mm Hg, aggressive treatment is needed to decrease morbidity and mortality from myocardial infarction, congestive heart failure, cerebrovascular accident, and renal failure.

Drugs used to treat HTN include diuretics, angiotensin-converting enzyme (ACE) inhibitors, calcium antagonists, β-blockers, and vasodilators. Initial treatment is usually with a diuretic, angiotensin-converting enzyme inhibitor, or a β-blocker. A combination of two antihypertensives are often used to minimize the undesirable physiologic responses of any one particular drug (such as a compensatory increase in renin activity). Serum potassium levels should be monitored, as hypokalemia or hyperkalemia may be a side effect.

ANESTHETIC CONSIDERATIONS

Preoperative

Reviewing the patient's medication and determining adequacy of BP control is essential. Associated organ dysfunction should be evaluated, looking particularly for orthostatic hypotension, ischemic heart disease, cerebrovascular disease, peripheral vascular disease, and renal dysfunction. Anti-HTN medications should be continued preoperatively. If emergency surgery is imminent, the patient with uncontrolled HTN should have their BP maintained at or near 140/90, provided no evidence of cerebral ischemia or renal dysfunction is present.

Ideally, patients should be normotensive prior to surgery. During anesthesia/operation in the hypertensive patient, BP is more likely to decrease precipitously. Chronic HTN is frequently associated with hypovolemia and ischemic heart disease, therefore a decrease in BP is more likely to result in myocardial ischemia.

Induction

During induction of anesthesia, the clinician should expect exaggerated changes in BP and hypotension due to drug-induced vasodilation in the presence of a decrease in intravascular fluid volume. Laryngoscopy and intubation may cause exaggerated rises in BP and should be performed as smoothly as possible. Methods used to attenuate hypertension and tachycardia during induction of anesthesia include deepening anesthesia by including a volatile anesthetic, opioids, lidocaine, and β-blockers.

Maintenance

Intraoperatively, the goal is to minimize wide swings in BP and tachycardia. A volatile anesthetic is ideal for allowing rapid adjustment of anesthetic depth in response to changes in BP. Increases in BP in response to surgical stimulation is the most common intraoperative change. Volatile agents produce a dose-dependent decrease in BP. A nitrous oxide/opioid technique may also be used, however, a volatile anesthetic may be needed to control undesirable increases in BP. Vasoactive agents can be used intraoperatively to treat HTN or hypotension.

Monitors include routine use of electrocardiographic monitoring leads II and V_5 to best detect cardiac ischemia. Direct arterial pressure monitoring may be warranted.

Postoperative

HTN in the postoperative period is common because of pain and an exaggerated sympathetic response. Hypovolemia related to intraoperative fluid management may also contribute to HTN seen postoperatively. Prompt assessment/treatment of postoperative HTN is necessary to decrease the potential for myocardial ischemia, arrhythmia, congestive heart failure, cerebrovascular accident, and bleeding. If HTN continues despite adequate analgesia, labetalol (0.1 to 0.25 mg/kg IV every 10 minutes), esmolol (0.5 to 1.0 mg/kg), or other β-blockers may be given. Hydralazine (2.5 to 10 mg IV every 10 to 20 minutes) may be considered, however, its potential to increase heart rate should be considered. In extreme cases of unmanageable hypertension postoperatively, sodium nitroprusside or nitroglycerin may need to be considered.

E. Congestive Heart Failure

DEFINITION

Congestive heart failure (CHF) is the failure of the myocardium to function properly, causing pulmonary congestion and ultimately pulmonary edema. CHF may involve one or both sides of the heart.

ETIOLOGY

CHF is usually caused by impaired myocardial contractility (secondary to ischemic heart disease or cardiomyopathy), cardiac valve abnormalities, systemic hypertension, or pulmonary hypertension (*cor pulmonale*). CHF in the preoperative period is the most important contributor to postoperative cardiac morbidity and mortality. Normal adaptive cardiac mechanisms that allow the heart to maintain cardiac output (CO) are the Frank-Starling relation (i.e., an increase in stroke volume accompanies an increase in end-diastolic pressure), inotropic state, afterload, heart rate, myocardial hypertrophy and dilation, sympathetic nervous system activity, and humoral-mediated responses.

DIAGNOSTIC AND LABORATORY FINDINGS

1. Cardiac index is less than 2.5 L/min in severe CHF.
2. Ejection fraction is often less than 0.50 (50%).
3. Left ventricular end-diastolic pressure (LVEDP) parallels the end-diastolic volume and is increased in the presence of CHF. Left ventricular end-diastolic pressure is normally less than 12 mm Hg, and right ventricular end-diastolic pressure is normally less than 5 mm Hg.

CLINICAL MANIFESTATIONS
Left Ventricular Failure
- Fatigue
- Dyspnea due to interstitial pulmonary edema
- Orthopnea
- Paroxysmal nocturnal dyspnea
- Acute pulmonary edema
- Tachypnea and rales
- Tachycardia and peripheral vasoconstriction
- Oliguria
- Pleural effusion

Right Ventricular Failure
- Systemic venous congestion—jugular venous distention
- Hepatomegaly
- Ascites
- Peripheral edema—dependent and pitting edema

TREATMENT
Treatment of CHF includes the use of digitalis, diuretics, vasodilators, and/or inotropes.

Digitalis
Digitalis is the only orally effective positive inotropic agent currently in use. Digoxin is excreted mainly by the kidneys and its elimination parallels creatinine clearance. In the perioperative period, sensitivity to digoxin can be increased if there are decreases in renal function or hypokalemia. Prophylaxis with digitalis is controversial in those patients with CHF undergoing elective surgery. Elderly patients undergoing thoracic surgery, however, may benefit. Digitalis may be continued in the preoperative period, especially if it is used to control heart rate. Toxicity should be suspected if the patient complains of nausea and vomiting, cardiac arrhythmias are present, and the serum digitalis level is greater than 3 mg/mL. Treatment of digitalis toxicity includes correction of hypokalemia, treatment of arrhythmias, and insertion of a temporary pacemaker if complete heart block ensues. If surgery cannot be delayed in the patient with digitalis toxicity, it is important to avoid sympathomimetics (ketamine) and hyperventilation (leading to hypokalemia).

Diuretics

Loop diuretics (e.g., furosemide) are often given to patients with CHF. Chronic administration of these drugs can lead to hypovolemia, orthostatic hypotension, and hypokalemia. Monitoring serum electrolytes (i.e., potassium) is essential, especially if the patient is treated with digitalis preparations.

Vasodilators

Vasodilators are the mainstay in the treatment of CHF as they decrease the impedance against which the left ventricle must work. Hypotension can result, however, and is a limiting factor in treating CHF with these drugs. Invasive monitoring (arterial and PA catheters) may become necessary when information regarding cardiac output, filling pressures, and systemic, pulmonary, and peripheral vascular resistances is needed to treat these patients effectively. Commonly used vasodilators include the following drugs.

> Nitroglycerin   0.5 to 5 mg/kg/min IV
> Hydralazine   25 to 100 mg PO
> Nitroprusside   0.5 to 5 mg/kg/min IV
> Prazosin   1 to 5 mg PO
> Captopril   25 to 75 mg PO
> Enalapril   5 to 40 mg PO

Inotropes

Intravenous dopamine and dobutamine are frequently used perioperatively to improve myocardial contractility. The combination of these two drugs administered together provides beneficial renal effects (from dopamine) and beta effects (from dobutamine) at doses that are unlikely to increase afterload. A PA catheter should be used to monitor the effects of these drugs on CO/CI and filling pressures.

ANESTHETIC CONSIDERATIONS

If surgery is absolutely necessary, the goal is to optimize CO. Ketamine, etomidate, and midazolam, given slowly and sparingly, have all been used successfully to induce anesthesia in the patient with CHF. Volatile anesthetics must be used with caution because of their propensity to cause myocardial depression. Severe CHF requires careful titration of all anesthetic agents for maintenance. Positive-pressure ventilation may help by decreasing pulmonary congestion and improving arterial oxygenation but may also reduce venous return and lower blood pressure. Therefore invasive monitoring should strongly be considered in these patients. CO can be supported with dopamine, dobutamine, or both as needed. Regional anesthesia may be used for extremity surgery in the patient with CHF. Anesthetic technique and agents should be individualized for each patient, with consideration of the medical history and surgical procedure.

F. Shock

HEMORRHAGIC SHOCK

DEFINITION

Hemorrhagic shock is a complication that arises from acute blood loss, also referred to as hemodynamic or vascular collapse. There is a decreased intravascular fluid volume that leads to a decreased venous return and cardiac output, and subsequently leads to inadequate organ/tissue perfusion.

ETIOLOGY

Hemorrhagic shock is a result of acute blood loss, frequently owing to trauma. Along with a decrease in intravascular fluid volume, sympathetic nervous system activity is increased, redirecting blood flow to the brain and heart. If this condition persists, a detrimental decrease in renal and hepatic blood flow occurs. Anaerobic metabolism is increased (lactate production) and metabolic (lactic) acidosis is manifested.

TREATMENT

Blood replacement therapy typically includes administration of whole blood or packed red cells. Crystalloids (balanced salt solutions) are also used because fluid shifts accompany hemorrhage but controversy exists whether colloids (albumin, dextran, hetastarch) are a better resuscitive fluid medium. Invasive monitoring, including arterial BP, CVP, and urinary drainage system to guide volume replacement, may become necessary. A pulmonary arterial catheter is helpful to determine CO, filling pressures, systemic and pulmonary vascular resistances, and oxygen extraction and delivery to the tissues. Dopamine may be useful in some cases, especially if the goals are a mild inotropic effect and an increase in renal blood flow. Vasopressors may be necessary as well to preserve cerebral and cardiac perfusion until intravascular fluid volume can be replaced. Other blood component therapy may need to be considered as more banked blood is given (e.g., fresh frozen plasma and platelets).

ANESTHETIC CONSIDERATIONS

Induction (if possible) and maintenance typically require invasive monitoring of blood pressure. Ketamine is used to induce anesthesia because it stimulates the sympathetic nervous system. Additional anesthetic agents must be carefully titrated to the patient's hemodynamic status. Treatment of hemorrhagic shock includes control of bleeding and replacement of intravascular volume (with whole blood and/or packed red blood cells) while maintaining adequate perfusion pressures to the vital organs.

SEPTIC SHOCK

DEFINITION
Septic shock is shock due to the presence of pathogenic organisms or their toxins in the blood.

ETIOLOGY
Early Phase
The early phase is characterized by hypotension due to a decrease in systemic vascular resistance. An increase in CO, elevated temperature, and hyperventilation also manifest themselves. Vasodilation is probably caused by endotoxins from bacterial cell walls that release vasoactive substances (i.e., histamine) and can last up to 24 hours.

Late Phase
CO may also be increased in this phase. Dilation of peripheral vessels gives over to the shunting of blood away from vital organs and lactic acidosis develops as a result of impaired tissue oxygenation. Intravascular fluid volume may fall because of damaged muscle. Oliguria is often present. Coagulation defects are common.

DIAGNOSIS AND LABORATORY FINDINGS
Septic shock is suggested by the development of hypotension in the presence of perioperative oliguria.

TREATMENT
Treatment includes intravenous antibiotics and restoration of intravascular fluid volume. Antibiotics should be started immediately. Typically, two antibiotics are used to cover both gram-positive (clindamycin) and gram-negative bacteria (gentamicin). Fluid replacement should be guided by PA catheter measurements of cardiac filling pressures and urine output. Intravenous dopamine is effective when supportive function is needed.

ANESTHETIC CONSIDERATIONS
No specific anesthetic drug has been proven ideal in the presence of septic shock. The anesthetic management should be individualized to each patient.

G. Valvular Heart Disease
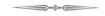

DEFINITION

Valvular heart disease is characterized by abnormalities that alter the normal flow of blood through the heart and may eventually effect cardiac loading conditions. The most frequently encountered cardiac valve lesions produce *pressure* overload (mitral stenosis, aortic stenosis) or *volume* overload (mitral regurgitation, aortic regurgitation) on the left atrium or left ventricle.

AORTIC STENOSIS

INCIDENCE AND PREVALENCE

Two types of aortic stenosis (AS) are commonly identified: *congenital* and *acquired*. Provided there are no other cardiac lesions, congenital AS is the most common cardiac valvular abnormality, with rheumatic disease responsible for less than 5% of these cases. AS can also be acquired, where calcific disease is the most common form. Valvular aortic stenosis without accompanying mitral valve disease is more common in men.

ETIOLOGY AND PATHOLOGY
Congenital

The congenital (non-rheumatic) form of AS results from progressive calcification and tightening of a congenitally abnormal bicuspid valve. These stenotic valves may have unicuspid, bicuspid, or tricuspid leaflet morphology, but the bicuspid variety is the most common (greater than 50%). Aortic stenosis due to rheumatic fever almost always occurs in association with mitral valve disease.

Acquired

The most common form of acquired aortic stenosis is calcific aortic stenosis, where degeneration of the valve apparatus increases with age. Calcium deposits build up on normal cusps, preventing them from opening and closing completely.

The anatomic obstruction to left ventricular outflow produces an increase in left ventricular pressure to maintain stroke volume. A pressure gradient across the stenotic valve develops and there is an increased workload on the ventricle. Increased wall tension contributes to LV hypertrophy. Cardiac output is maintained by the hypertrophied ventricle, which may sustain a large pressure gradient across the LV outflow tract for years without evidence of clinical symptoms. Over time, diastolic function is reduced so that small changes in volume give way to large changes in LV filling pressures.

Significant aortic stenosis is associated with a peak systolic transvalvular pressure gradient exceeding 50 mm Hg and an aortic valve orifice area of less than 1 cm^2 (normal area: 2.6 to 3.5 cm^2). The atrial contribution to ventricular filling may be as high as 40% in patients with aortic stenosis (about 20% normally). Left ventricle end-diastolic pressures (LVEDP) are often elevated, causing symptoms of pulmonary congestion despite normal left ventricular contractility. LVEDP values that are normal may in fact represent a patient who is hypovolemic.

DIAGNOSIS

As mentioned, a long latency period exists (approximately 40 to 50 years) during which obstruction increases gradually and the pressure load on the myocardium increases while the patient remains asymptomatic. Patients with advanced AS may begin to have angina, syncope, and signs of congestive heart failure. They also have a characteristic systolic murmur, best heard in the second right intercostal space, which transmits sound to the neck. Cardiac catheterization will give vital information about intracavitary pressures, the gradient across the aortic valve, and contractility. In patients with calcific AS, echocardiography often shows thickening and calcification of the aortic valve and decreased mobility of the valve leaflets. The incidence of arrhythmias leading to severe hypoperfusion accounts for syncope and the increased incidence of sudden death in patients with AS.

TREATMENT

When significant symptoms develop, most patients die without surgical treatment within 2 to 5 years. Percutaneous transluminal valvuloplasty may be an alternative to surgery, but restenosis usually occurs within 6 to 12 months.

ANESTHETIC CONSIDERATIONS

- Maintain normal sinus rhythm
- Avoid tachycardia and hypotension (myocardial depression)
- Avoid sudden increases or decreases in systemic vascular resistance
- Optimize intravascular fluid volume to maintain venous return and left ventricular filling

Regional anesthesia in the patient with AS should be limited to peripheral-type procedures. If conduction anesthesia is used (i.e, spinal or epidural), the sensory level of blockade should be limited to lower levels so that profound hypotension (due to sympathectomy) does not occur. Treatment in this case would be to use a vasoconstricting drug.

PROGNOSIS

The 5-year survival rate for adults with aortic valve replacement is approximately 85%.

AORTIC REGURGITATION

INCIDENCE AND PREVALENCE

Rheumatic fever is a common cause of disease of the aortic valve that inevitably leads to valve incompetence (regurgitation). Other causes of regurgitation include infective endocarditis, trauma, congenital bicuspid valve, and diseases of connective tissue.

ETIOLOGY AND PATHOLOGY

Aortic regurgitation may be caused by disease of the aortic valve leaflets, the wall of the aortic root, or both.

The fundamental problem is that part of the LV stroke volume is allowed to flow backward into the ventricle after being ejected during systole (i.e., regurgitation). In *chronic* aortic regurgitation, the LV progressively dilates and becomes hypertrophied eccentrically. End-diastolic volume increases to maintain an effective stroke volume. Ventricular compliance increases initially, and LVEDP is usually normal or only slightly elevated.

In *acute* aortic regurgitation, the regurgitant volume fills a ventricle of normal size that cannot accommodate both the regurgitant volume and the left atrial inflow volume. The sudden rise in LVEDP is transmitted back to the pulmonary circulation, causing acute pulmonary congestion.

DIAGNOSIS

Most patients with chronic aortic regurgitation remain asymptomatic for 10 to 20 years. When symptoms develop, exertional dyspnea, orthopnea, and paroxysmal nocturnal dyspnea are the principal complaints.

In acute aortic regurgitation, patients develop sudden clinical manifestations of cardiovascular collapse, weakness, severe dyspnea, and hypotension. Chronic aortic regurgitation is recognized by its characteristic diastolic murmur (best heard in the second intercostal space, right sternal border), widened pulse pressure, decreased diastolic pressure, and bounding peripheral pulses.

TREATMENT

Arterial blood pressure should be decreased to reduce the diastolic gradient for regurgitation using afterload reduction via arterial vasodilators and angiotensin-converting enzyme (ACE) inhibitors. Early surgery is indicated for patients with acute aortic regurgitation because medical management is associated with a high mortality rate. Patients with chronic aortic regurgitation should undergo surgery before irreversible ventricular dysfunction occurs.

ANESTHETIC CONSIDERATIONS

- Avoid sudden decreases in heart rate
- Avoid sudden increases in systemic vascular resistance
- Minimize drug-induced myocardial depression

Most patients tolerate spinal and epidural anesthesia provided intravascular volume is maintained.

PROGNOSIS

Favorable clinical responses to valve replacement have been reported in patients with evidence of relatively severe preoperative ventricular dysfunction. Aortic valve replacement significantly improves left ventricular performance in most patients with chronic aortic regurgitation.

MITRAL STENOSIS

INCIDENCE AND PREVALENCE

Pure mitral stenosis (MS) occurs in 25% of patients; MS and mitral regurgitation (MR) occur in 40% of patients.

ETIOLOGY AND PATHOLOGY

The predominant cause of MS is rheumatic fever, which occurs about four times more frequently in women. Less common etiologies are congenital MS (in children) and complications associated with carcinoid syndrome, systemic lupus erythematosus, and rheumatic arthritis.

After the initial episode of acute rheumatic fever, stenosis of the mitral valve takes about 2 years to develop. Symptomology appears after 20 to 30 years, when they mitral valve orifice is reduced from its normal 4 to 6 cm^2 to less than 2 cm^2. In MS, the anterior and posterior valve cusps fuse at their edges, followed by shortening of the chordae as they thicken, producing obstruction to flow into the LV. The narrowed valvular orifice causes an increase in left atrial volume and pressure. LV filling and stroke volume in the presence of mild MS are usually maintained at rest by increased left atrial pressure. LV stroke volume may decrease when effective atrial contraction is lost or with tachycardia. Acute increases in left atrial pressure that subsequently result are transmitted to the pulmonary capillaries.

Pulmonary hypertension occurs from rearward transmission of the elevated left atrial pressure and irreversible increases in pulmonary vascular resistance. Chronic increases in pulmonary capillary wedge pressure (PCWP) are partially compensated by increases in pulmonary lymph flow; however, any acute increase in PCWP may result in pulmonary edema. Transudation of fluid into the pulmonary interstitial space, decreased pulmonary compliance, and increased work of breathing lead to dyspnea on exertion.

DIAGNOSIS

About 50% of MS patients present with an acute onset of congestive heart failure, that is often associated with paroxysmal attacks of atrial fibrillation (this arrhythmia occurs in 40% of patients with MS). Stasis of blood in the left atrium predisposes to thrombus formation. The predominate symptom of MS is dyspnea from the reduced compliance of the lungs. Rupture of pulmonary-bronchial venous communications causes hemoptysis.

Cardiac catheterization allows quantification of the mitral valve orifice and transmitral gradients. Angiography will be important in those patients with angina. Two-dimensional echocardiography can also provide information about orifice size. MS is recognized during auscultation by an opening snap that occurs early in diastole and by a rumbling diastolic heart murmur best heard at the cardiac apex. The chest x-ray may show left atrial enlargement and evidence of pulmonary edema.

TREATMENT

Medical management is primarily supportive and includes limitation of physical activity, diuretics, and sodium restriction. Digoxin is useful in patients with atrial fibrillation, and β-blockers may control heart rate in some patients. Anticoagulation therapy is used in patients with a history of emboli and in those at high risk (i.e., those older than 40 years of age with a large atrium and chronic atrial fibrillation). Surgical correction is undertaken once significant symptoms develop. Recurrent MS following valvuloplasty is usually managed with valve replacement. Catheter-balloon valvuloplasty using a percutaneous venous introduction and a trans-septal approach to the mitral valve may be used to decrease the degree of MS in selected patients.

ANESTHETIC CONSIDERATIONS

- Avoid sinus tachycardia or rapid (uncontrolled) atrial fibrillation
- Avoid marked increases in central blood volume associated with overtransfusion or Trendelenburg position
- Avoid drug-induced decreases in systemic vascular resistance
- Avoid events that may exacerbate pulmonary hypertension and evoke right ventricular failure, such as arterial hypoxemia and hypoventilation

If hypotension occurs, fluid administration may benefit these often fluid-depleted patients. Vasoconstrictors should be avoided and early use of positive inotropes (e.g., epinephrine, dopamine, dobutamine) may be helpful.

Regional anesthesia is acceptable in the patient with MS, provided higher levels of sensory/sympathetic blockade are avoided during conduction blockade (resulting hypotension may be difficult to treat based on the pathophysiology of MS).

PROGNOSIS

When MS produces total incapacity, 20% of patients die within 6 months without surgical correction.

MITRAL REGURGITATION

INCIDENCE AND PREVALENCE

Severe mitral regurgitation requiring surgical repair occurs in about 5% of men and less than 1.5% of women.

ETIOLOGY AND PATHOLOGY

Abnormalities of the mitral annulus, leaflets, chordae tendineae, and papillary muscles may cause mitral regurgitation. *Chronic* mitral regurgitation is usually the result of rheumatic fever; congenital abnormalities; or dilatation, destruction, or calcification of the mitral annulus. *Acute* mitral regurgitation is most often the result of myocardial ischemia or infarction, infective endocarditis, or chest trauma.

The mitral valve orifice lies adjacent to the aortic valve. At the onset of ventricular contraction, about half the regurgitant volume is ejected into the left atrium prior aortic valve opening. The total volume of regurgitant flow into the left atrium depends on the systemic vascular resistance and forward stroke volume. Effective cardiac output will be effectively diminished in symptomatic patients, whereas "total" left ventricular output (forward and regurgitant) is usually elevated.

Interestingly, there is typically little enlargement of the left atrial cavity, however there is a significant rise in mean atrial pressure that leads to pulmonary congestion. The degree of atrial compliance will determine the clinical manifestations. Patients with normal or reduced atrial compliance (e.g., acute mitral regurgitation) will demonstrate pulmonary congestion and edema. Those with increased atrial compliance (i.e., chronic mitral regurgitation with a large, dilated atrium) will demonstrate signs of decreased cardiac output. Most patients fall between these two extremes and exhibit symptoms of both pulmonary congestion and low cardiac output.

DIAGNOSIS

Symptoms of mitral regurgitation can take up to 20 years to develop. Chronic weakness and fatigue secondary to low cardiac output are prominent features. On auscultation, the cardinal feature of mitral regurgitation is a blowing pansystolic murmur, best heard at the cardiac apex and often radiating to the left axilla. The regurgitant flow is responsible for the "v" wave present on the recording of the pulmonary artery occlusion pressure. The size of the v wave correlates with the magnitude of the regurgitant flow.

TREATMENT

Medical treatment typically includes digoxin, diuretics, and vasodilators. Reduction of afterload increases the forward stroke volume and decreases the regurgitant volume. Surgical treatment is usually reserved for patients with moderate to severe symptoms.

ANESTHETIC CONSIDERATIONS

- Avoid sudden decreases in heart rate
- Avoid sudden increases in systemic vascular resistance
- Minimize drug-induced myocardial depression
- Monitor the size of the v wave as a reflection of regurgitant flow

Prophylactic antibiotics are recommended. Spinal and epidural anesthesia are tolerated well, provided bradycardia is avoided.

PROGNOSIS

In most patients with mitral regurgitation, the clinical course and the quality of life improve following valve replacement. The original cause of mitral regurgitation that warranted the operation is also important to the outcome following surgical treatment. In patients in whom mitral dysfunction is secondary to ischemic heart disease, the 5-year survival rate is approximately 30%; in rheumatic mitral regurgitation, the 5-year survival rate is approximately 70%.

TRICUSPID REGURGITATION

ETIOLOGY AND PATHOLOGY

Tricuspid regurgitation is commonly a result of right ventricular enlargement secondary to pulmonary hypertension. Pulmonary hypertension may itself be indirectly due to chronic left ventricular failure, since chronic left ventricular failure often leads to sustained increases in pulmonary vascular pressures. This chronic increase in afterload causes the right ventricle to progressively dilate, and excessive dilation of the tricuspid annulus eventually results in tricuspid incompetency or regurgitation. Tricuspid regurgitation can also be secondary to infective endocarditis, rheumatic fever, carcinoid syndrome, chest trauma, or congenital malformations. Fortunately, the right atrium and vena cavae are compliant and accommodate the volume overload with a minimal increase in right atrial pressure.

DIAGNOSIS

Patients with isolated tricuspid regurgitation are often totally asymptomatic for many years (greater than 20 years). Some physical signs may be present early, such as pulsatile neck veins and systolic heart murmurs heard throughout the cardiac cycle. Other complaints that the patient may give are fatigue, weakness, and a feeling of fullness in the abdomen, probably due to congestion in the liver (positive hepatojugular reflex). Some patients report cyanosis, which may result from blood flow from the right to the left atrium in those with a patent foramen ovale.

TREATMENT

Tricuspid regurgitation is generally well tolerated, and some degree of regurgitation has been reported in many normal individuals during echocardiography. Even surgical removal of the tricuspid valve is usually well tolerated. Treatment of the underlying disease process will be more important than the tricuspid regurgitation itself.

ANESTHETIC CONSIDERATIONS

Many patients with clinically significant tricuspid regurgitation who undergo surgery/anesthesia will also have pulmonary hypertension and possibly mitral or aortic valve disease.
- Maintain intravascular fluid volume and central venous pressure in the high-normal range
- Avoid increases in pulmonary vascular resistance
- Avoid PEEP and high mean airway pressures because they reduce venous return and increase right ventricular afterload
- Most patients tolerate spinal and epidural anesthesia well
- Prophylactic antibiotics are recommended

PROGNOSIS

Excellent results have been reported with the use of tricuspid annuloplasty in patients with moderate tricuspid regurgitation. Management of severe tricuspid regurgitation entails annuloplasty or valve replacement. Durability of more than 10 years has been established with valvular prostheses.

H. Cardiomyopathy

DEFINITION

Cardiomyopathies are acute or chronic diseases of the myocardium that may also involve the endocardium and pericardium. They are characterized by myocardial dysfunction unrelated to coronary artery disease, valvular abnormalities, or hypertension. They ultimately affect contractile function, and life-threatening congestive heart failure (CHF) is common to all cardiomyopathies.

ETIOLOGY

Cardiomyopathies can be classified according to their associated hemodynamics and morphologies: dilated, restrictive, hypertrophic, and obliterative.

DILATED CARDIOMYOPATHY

While the etiology of dilated cardiomyopathies is usually idiopathic, other causes are attributed to nutritional deficits or alcohol abuse. In some patients in whom febrile illness occurs prior to the onset of cardiac dysfunction, a virus may be the cause. Dilated cardiomyopathies can be acute or chronic and lead to a decrease in myocardial contractility, often involving both ventricles. This leads to decreased cardiac output (CO) and increased filling pressures. Mitral and tricuspid insufficiency may occur if dilation becomes severe. The ECG may reveal LVH, ST and T-wave abnormalities, first-degree heart block, or bundle branch block. Arrhythmias can also be seen, such as PVCs and atrial fibrillation. Chest x-ray may show cardiac enlargement and interstitial pulmonary edema. Diagnosis by echocardiography requires an ejection fraction of less than 0.40, a dilated and hyperkinetic left ventricle, and mild to moderate regurgitation. Mural thrombi often form (typically in the left atrium), and systemic embolization is common.

TREATMENT

Patients with dilated cardiomyopathy must avoid unnecessary physical activity and exhibit total abstinence from alcohol. CHF is treated with digoxin and diuretics. Vasodilator treatment or an inotrope with vasodilator properties (amrinone or milrinone) may also be helpful. Ventricular arrhythmias are treated with procainamide or quinidine. Because of the increased risk of pulmonary embolism, these patients may be treated with anticoagulants (not proven to be of benefit). Patients with associated collagen vascular disease, sarcoidosis, or inflammation on endocardial biopsy are treated with corticosteroids preoperatively. Tachyarrhythmias can be treated with β-blockers. Patients with coronary artery disease and dilated cardiomyopathy may benefit from coronary revascularization to improve left ventricular (LV) function. With advanced CHF, these patients may be candidates for heart transplant, provided pulmonary hypertension does not exist.

ANESTHETIC CONSIDERATIONS

- Avoid drug-induced myocardial depression (i.e., avoid inhalational agents, if possible)
- Maintain normovolemia
- Prevent increases in afterload
- Invasive monitoring may be necessary if manipulation of pulmonary and systemic vascular resistances is needed

Excess cardiovascular depression on induction in patients with a history of alcohol abuse may reflect undiagnosed dilated cardiomyopathy; however, failure of this expected response to intravenous induction agents may reflect a slow circulation time. During maintenance, myocardial depression produced by volatile agents must be considered. Opiates exhibit benign effects on cardiac contractility but may not produce unconsciousness. Also, an opioid, nitrous, benzodiazepine technique may cause unexpected cardiac depression. Increases in heart rate associated with surgical stimulation may be treated with β-blockers. Nondepolarizing muscle relaxants that exhibit few cardiovascular effects are advised. Intravenous fluids should be guided by cardiac filling pressures; therefore a pulmonary artery catheter aids early recognition of the need for inotropes or vasodilators. Prominent "*a*" waves reflect mitral or tricuspid regurgitation. Intraoperative hypotension is treated with ephedrine. Phenylephrine could adversely affect afterload due to increased systemic vascular resistance (SVR).

Regional anesthesia may be used in selected patients, although caution is indicated in avoiding abrupt sympathetic blockade as seen in spinal or epidural anesthesia.

PROGNOSIS

Prognosis of dilated cardiomyopathy is poor, with a 5-year survival rate of 25% to 40%. The cause of death in 75% of these patients is CHF. Pulmonary embolism or sudden death from arrhythmia is found in over 50% of these patients on autopsy.

RESTRICTIVE CARDIOMYOPATHY

This condition manifests as impaired diastolic filling that produces increased filling pressures and decreased CO mimicking constrictive pericarditis. Restrictive cardiomyopathy causes a greater impairment of LV than right ventricular (RV) filling. LV filling pressures are usually greater than RV filling pressures, and the left ventricle becomes less compliant. There is no effective treatment for this disease, and death is often the result of cardiac arrhythmia or intractable CHF. Anesthetic management follows the same principles used in cardiac tamponade.

HYPERTROPHIC CARDIOMYOPATHY

This disease is an autosomal dominant hereditary condition. The peak incidence is in patients 50 to 70 years of age. Most elderly patients diagnosed with this condition are female.

The genetic defect involves increased density of calcium channels, thus affecting the contractile process of the heart. The disease manifests as unexplained myocardial hypertrophy, often with greater thickening of the interventricular septum compared with the wall of the left ventricle. Echocardiography reveals a large variation in the location and extent of the hypertrophy. The disease is therefore often referred to as *hypertrophic cardiomyopathy with or without LV outflow obstruction.* These patients should not participate in sports because of the risk of sudden death. There is hypertrophy of the left ventricle, which becomes slitlike and elongated. The ejection fraction is often greater than 0.80, reflecting the hypercontractile condition of the heart even with severe LV outflow obstruction. Mitral regurgitation may be present and indicates interference with movement of the septal leaflet of the mitral valve (systolic anterior motion—SAM) by the hypertrophied septum. The degree of ventricular outflow obstruction is influenced by contractility, preload, and afterload.

CLINICAL MANIFESTATIONS

The major symptoms include angina, syncope, tachyarrhythmias, and CHF. Angina that is relieved by placing the patient in the recumbent position is pathognomonic for this disease, because the increase in LV size in recumbency decreases the outflow obstruction. These patients are especially susceptible to coronary ischemia due to the marked LV hypertrophy, particularly when subendocardial blood flow is decreased from excessive pressure in the left ventricle.

To maintain CO, adequate atrial contribution to CO is necessary; therefore atrial fibrillation is poorly tolerated. In addition, tachyarrhythmias impair diastolic filling time, which also decreases CO. These patients are prone to systemic embolization, and even asymptomatic patients are at risk for sudden unexpected death from LV outflow obstruction or ventricular tachycardia.

Cardiac murmurs may indicate LV outflow obstruction or mitral regurgitation in patients with hypertrophic cardiomyopathy. These murmurs are characterized by their marked variation with different maneuvers. Valsalva's maneuver decreases LV size, which increases the outflow obstruction; LV systolic pressures increase, causing the murmur of mitral regurgitation to intensify as well. Nitroglycerin and the standing position also intensify the murmur. Chest x-ray and ECG reveal LV hypertrophy, which may be the only sign in an asymptomatic patient. Abnormal Q waves may be seen in leads II, III, AVF, or V_4 to V_6, mimicking a pseudoinfarction pattern. This diagnosis should be considered in any young patient with an ECG suggestive of myocardial infarction. Cardiac catheterization will suggest mitral regurgitation or increased LV end-diastolic pressure. Decreased LV compliance causes increases in the height of the "*a*" wave to over 30 mm Hg. If LV outflow obstruction exists, there will be a pressure gradient across the aortic valve.

TREATMENT

The goal of treatment in these patients is to relieve the obstruction to LV outflow. This is often achieved with β-blockers to lower the heart rate and decrease contractility. Calcium channel antagonists may also help. Caution should be taken to prevent drug-induced hypotension and negative inotropic effects; therefore nitroglycerin should be avoided in these patients who present with angina. Should CHF also exist, treatment becomes more difficult. Diuretics can lead to hypovolemia and digoxin can increase cardiac contractility; both of which may worsen the obstruction. Cardioversion may be necessary to maintain normal sinus rhythm. Patients with atrial fibrillation require anticoagulant treatment to prevent embolization. These patients are at risk for infective endocarditis and should receive prophylactic antibiotic treatment for dental or surgical procedures. Myotomy or myomectomy under cardiac bypass may be needed in 10% to 15% of patients. Mitral valve replacement may also be needed.

ANESTHETIC CONSIDERATIONS

Anesthetic management is directed at minimizing LV outflow obstruction. Any drug or event that decreases cardiac contractility or increases preload or afterload will decrease the LV outflow obstruction.

Preoperative

Preoperative medications should minimize anxiety. Expansion of intravascular fluid volume will help to maintain intraoperative stroke volume and lessen the adverse effects of positive-pressure ventilation.

Induction

Intravenous induction is acceptable provided sudden decreases in SVR are avoided. Some degree of myocardial depression can be tolerated. Ketamine is not a good choice because the increased myocardial contractility will enhance LV outflow obstruction and decrease the stroke volume. Laryngoscopy should be smooth and stress-free, and responses may be blunted by using a volatile anesthetic, opioid, or β-blocker before laryngoscopy.

Maintenance

During maintenance, mild cardiac depression while maintaining intravascular fluid volume and SVR is desirable. Opiates alone are not the best choice since they do not provide cardiac depression and can decrease SVR. Opiates combined with nitrous oxide, however, may be helpful in providing myocardial depression and a slight increase in SVR. Care should be used if spinal or epidural anesthesia is used because of the hemodynamic changes that may occur with sympathectomy (it may increase the LV outflow obstruction). Nondepolarizing muscle relaxants with little effect on the circulation are best for skeletal muscle paralysis. Tachycardia associated with pancuronium is not desirable in these patients.

Invasive monitors, such as a pulmonary artery catheter, as well as transesophageal echocardiography may be useful. Intraoperative hypotension in response to decreased preload or afterload can be treated with an α-agonist (phenylephrine, 50 to 100 μg IV). β-agonists, such as ephedrine, dopamine, or dobutamine, should be avoided because an increase in cardiac contractility or heart rate can worsen outflow obstruction. Most important in maintaining blood pressure is prompt replacement of blood loss and titration of fluids to the cardiac filling pressures. Persistent hypertension can be treated with titration of a volatile anesthetic. Vasodilators (sodium nitroprusside or nitroglycerin) should be used with caution since they decrease SVR and may worsen the problem. Maintenance of normal sinus rhythm is vital to optimize the atrial component to ventricular filling. β-blockers may be needed to slow a persistently increased heart rate.

OBLITERATIVE CARDIOMYOPATHY

Obliterative cardiomyopathy is considered a variant of restrictive cardiomyopathy and is characterized by a marked decrease in ventricular compliance. This condition may occur in association with hypereosinophilic syndromes. Cardiac arrhythmias, conduction disturbances, systemic embolization, and valvular inefficiency are common. Treatment may include steroids.

I. Peripheral Vascular Disease

DEFINITION
Peripheral vascular disease (PVD) is an inflammation or disease of the peripheral vasculature.

ETIOLOGY
Peripheral vascular disease may manifest as systemic vasculitis or arterial occlusive disease; there are several types of PVD.

TAKAYASU'S ARTERITIS

Takayasu's arteritis is a chronic inflammation of the aorta and its major branches. It causes multiple organ dysfunction.

MANAGEMENT OF ANESTHESIA
Corticosteroid supplementation may be needed in patients already treated with these drugs. These patients also may be taking anticoagulants, therefore regional anesthesia may be controversial. Blood pressure may be difficult to measure noninvasively in the upper extremities, so an arterial line line may be necessary. Preoperatively, it is wise to evaluate range of motion of the cervical spine since hyperextension of the head during laryngoscopy may compromise cerebral blood flow (the carotid arteries are shortened as a result of the vascular inflammatory process). Finally, a major anesthetic goal intraoperatively is maintenance of an adequate perfusion pressure.

THROMBOANGITIS OBLITERANS

DEFINITION
Thromboangitis obliterans is an inflammatory process of the wall and connective tissue surrounding the arteries and veins, especially in the extremities. It is often associated with the thrombosis and occlusion that commonly results in gangrene. Jewish males between the ages of 20 to 40 years seem to have a higher incidence.

MANAGEMENT OF ANESTHESIA

Prevention of cold-induced vasospasm is a major concern. Increasing the ambient room temperature and using convective warming devices (e.g., warming blankets, fluid warmers) will help maintain body temperature. Noninvasive blood pressure monitoring is preferable over invasive (arterial) monitoring in this patient population. Regional anesthesia is acceptable; however, the concomitant use of vasoconstrictors should be avoided (i.e., epinephrine).

PROGNOSIS

The prognosis depends on the progression of the associated underlying disease. Raynaud's phenomenon (i.e., spasm of the digital arteries) is often associated with a period of "remission."

CHRONIC PERIPHERAL ARTERIO-OCCLUSIVE DISEASE

DEFINITION

Chronic peripheral arterio-occlusive disease is typically the result of peripheral atherosclerosis and often occurs in association with coronary or cerebral atherosclerosis.

ETIOLOGY AND CLINICAL MANIFESTATIONS

Occlusion of the distal abdominal aorta or the iliac arteries frequently presents as claudication of the hips and buttocks. Elderly individuals often present with occlusion of the common femoral or superficial femoral arteries. This produces a syndrome of claudication from the calf area of the lower extremity.

TREATMENT

Treatment includes revascularization, such as femoral-femoral bypass or any of a number of different femoral-to-distal bypass procedures.

ANESTHETIC CONSIDERATIONS

The major risk for operative revascularization is associated ischemic heart disease. While these procedures can be performed under general anesthesia, regional (i.e., epidural) anesthesia prior to anticoagulant therapy has not been associated with untoward events. Infrarenal cross-clamping of the distal aorta in the patient with PVD is associated with minimal hemodynamic derangements. Typically, monitoring of right-sided heart pressures (i.e., CVP) is sufficient unless left-sided heart disease requires the use of a pulmonary artery catheter. Thromboembolic complications, particularly in the kidneys, usually reflect dislodgement of atherosclerotic debris. Spinal cord damage is unlikely, and special monitoring is not mandatory.

SUBCLAVIAN STEAL SYNDROME

Occlusion of the subclavian or innominate artery by an atherosclerotic plaque proximal to the origin of the vertebral artery may result in reversal of blood flow from the brain, leading to syncopal episodes. The pulse in the ipsilateral arm is usually absent or diminished (10 mm Hg lower).

CORONARY-SUBCLAVIAN STEAL SYNDROME

This syndrome occurs when incomplete stenosis of the left subclavian artery leads to reversal of blood flow. The patient typically presents with angina and a decreased systolic blood pressure (at least 20 mm Hg lower) in the ipsilateral arm. Bilateral brachial artery blood pressure measurement is helpful in the differential diagnosis and may be helpful in the preoperative assessment in patients with an internal mammary to coronary artery bypass.

ANEURYSMS OF THE THORACIC AND ABDOMINAL AORTA

DEFINITION
Diseases of the aorta are frequently aneurysmal, whereas occlusive disease is most likely to affect the peripheral arteries.

ETIOLOGY
The primary event in aortic dissection is a tear in the intimal wall through which blood surges and creates a false lumen. The adventitia then separates up and/or down the aorta for various distances. Associated conditions include hypertension (which is present in 80% of these patients), Marfan's syndrome, blunt chest trauma, pregnancy, and iatrogenic surgical injury (e.g., resulting from aortic cannulation during cardiopulmonary bypass). Aortic dissections involving the ascending aorta are considered *Type A,* and those involving the descending aorta (i.e., beyond the origin of the left subclavian artery) are considered *Type B.* Aneurysms can also be classified as saccular, fusiform, or dissecting.

CLINICAL MANIFESTATIONS
Signs and symptoms include: excruciating chest pain; a decrease or absence of peripheral pulses, stroke, paraplegia, and ischemia of extremities; vasoconstriction and hypertension; myocardial infarction; and cardiac tamponade.

TREATMENT
Early, short-term treatment includes the use of β-blockers or other cardioactive agents that decrease systolic blood pressure (to approximately 100 mm Hg) and aids in decreasing myocardial contractility and vascular resistance. Ultimately, surgical intervention is often necessary.

ANESTHETIC CONSIDERATIONS
Abdominal Aortic Aneurysm
History and physical examination with special focus on cardiac function is essential. Hypertension and diabetes mellitus may also be present. Preoperative analysis of important laboratory work should include hematology, chemistry, and coagulation profiles. Serum glucose levels should be kept below 200 mg/dL.

Monitors
Routine monitors should be employed including leads II and V_5 of the electrocardiogram. In addition, blood pressure should be invasively monitored with an arterial catheter. This allows intraoperative monitoring of arterial

blood gases, serum potassium, glucose, hemoglobin and hematocrit, and coagulation parameters. Transesophageal echocardiography and/or a pulmonary artery catheter may be used to enhance hemodynamic monitoring.

Induction

Most intravenous induction agents are acceptable provided they are used judiciously in conjunction with a nondepolarizing muscle relaxant. A nasogastric tube and urinary drainage catheter can be placed. Positioning for surgery is usually supine or lateral, depending on the location of the incision.

Maintenance

General anesthesia or a combined technique (i.e., general and epidural) has been used successfully. Selection of appropriate agents will depend on the patient's physical status.

Intravenous Fluids

Surgically, an abdominal approach will typically require 10 to 15 mL/kg/hr. of crystalloid (i.e., balanced salt solutions), and a retroperitoneal approach will require only 10 mL/kg/hr. NOTE: *Adequate fluid replacement is the major factor in preventing renal failure.* It is important to monitor the hemodynamic parameters and urine output. Systemic blood pressure should be maintained 10 to 15 mmHg above normal during aortic cross-clamping. Mannitol (25 g) and heparin (5000 to 10,000 units) are administered prior to cross-clamping. Activated coagulation times (ACT) are monitored (i.e., baseline before and then 5 minutes after heparin administration). The therapeutic goal is an ACT that is two to three times normal. Protamine may be given to reverse this effect.

Hemodynamics

Should opioid anesthesia prove ineffective in controlling blood pressure intraoperatively, the addition of nitroprusside or nitroglycerin may be considered. Blood pressure is maintained slightly below normal before aortic cross-clamping. If the aorta is clamped *below* the renal arteries, elevations in blood pressure are minimal. If the aorta is clamped *above* the renal arteries, a greater increase in blood pressure will be observed. Should the aorta be clamped above the supraceliac artery, an even greater increase in blood pressure can be expected. Patients with aorto-occlusive disease will not exhibit the significant rises in blood pressure observed in those with aneurysmal disease.

Blood Loss

Surgical blood loss may be replaced with autologous blood, packed red blood cells, or colloid therapy such as hetastarch. Administration of fresh-frozen plasma and platelets depends on coagulation values and the number of packed red blood cells transfused.

Unclamping

1. Lighten the depth of anesthesia prior to unclamping, allowing the blood pressure to climb 30 to 40 mm Hg.
2. Be prepared to transfuse 1 unit of blood.

3. Should systemic blood pressure drop precipitously, the surgeon may reclamp until acceptable blood pressure is restored.
4. Use vasopressors as necessary.

Emergence

Consider the patient's preoperative physical status, the amount of intraoperative fluid administered, blood loss, the length of procedure, and the presence or absence of any untoward intraoperative events. The patient may require postoperative ventilation for a period of time to limit wide swings in hemodynamic parameters.

Complications

Complications include bleeding, infection, coagulation abnormalities, renal failure, and ischemia distal to the site of repair (visceral or spinal cord).

Thoracic Aortic Aneurysm

Note: Systemic blood pressure should be monitored above the aneurysm (right or left radial artery depending on the site at the arch). This will allow assessment of cerebral perfusion pressure as well as the perfusion pressure to the kidneys. During aortic resection, mean arterial pressure should be maintained at 100 mm Hg in the upper body and above 50 mm Hg distal to the aneurysm. Frequently, an endobronchial tube is required to facilitate surgical exposure.

These procedures are usually done with profound hypothermia, total circulatory arrest, or cardiopulmonary bypass. Large bore venous access is necessitated to allow large volumes of blood/fluid to be replaced rapidly. Eight to 10 units of blood should be available. Heart rate and blood pressure should be maintained at below normal levels. The most common surgical approach is via a thoracotomy incision.

Prior to initiation of cardiopulmonary bypass, the aorta is cross-clamped proximal to the level of the left subclavian artery and distal to the aortic lesion. Doing so produces a mechanical decompression with the oxygenator. If cross-clamping is done without the benefit of a surgical bypass shunt, vasodilator therapy will be needed to control left ventricular afterload. A pulmonary artery catheter is typically used. The risk of spinal cord ischemia/damage increases as the cross-clamp period extends beyond 30 minutes. Postoperative complications are similar to those for abdominal aortic aneurysm. These patients are at greater risk of renal failure, and visceral and spinal cord ischemia.

J. Pericardial Processes/Tamponade

PERICARDITIS

DEFINITION
Pericarditis is an inflammatory process of the pericardium.

ETIOLOGY
Pericarditis is typically the result of a viral infection.

CLINICAL MANIFESTATIONS
There is a sudden onset of severe chest pain. Auscultation reveals a friction rub, which is "leathery" in quality and increases in intensity on exhalation. Sinus tachycardia and a low-grade fever are also common.

TREATMENT
Treatment is symptomatic with analgesics and corticosteroids. Acute pericarditis in the absence of pericardial effusion does not alter cardiac function.

PERICARDIAL EFFUSION

DEFINITION
Pericardial effusion is the accumulation of fluid in the pericardial space that is often associated with pericarditis.

ETIOLOGY
The pericardial space normally contains 20 to 25 mL of pericardial fluid; pressure here is subatmospheric, decreasing on inspiration and increasing on exhalation. Clinical effects depend on whether the fluid is creating a tamponade effect. If the fluid in the pericardium accumulates slowly, the pericardium can stretch to accommodate the increased volume without a concomitant increase in pressure. When the fluid volume increases rapidly, tamponade is possible.

DIAGNOSTIC AND LABORATORY FINDINGS
While echocardiography is best at detecting pericardial effusion, CT scans can also be beneficial.

CHRONIC CONSTRICTIVE PERICARDITIS

DEFINITION
Chronic constrictive pericarditis resembles cardiac tamponade. Venous pressure is increased and stroke volume is decreased. Chronic constrictive pericarditis can interfere with filling of the heart during diastole.

ETIOLOGY

Most cases of chronic constrictive pericarditis are idiopathic, however, chronic renal failure, radiation, rheumatoid arthritis, and cardiac surgery are all possible contributing factors. There is fibrous scarring and adhesion of both pericardial layers, which leads to a somewhat rigid shell around the heart.

DIAGNOSTIC AND LABORATORY FINDINGS

Diagnosis depends on a history and physical examination that recognizes the increase in venous pressure despite no other signs of cardiac disease. Although both sides of the heart may be involved, the primary manifestations are those related to right ventricular failure with venous congestion, hepatosplenomegaly, and ascites. Atrial arrhythmias are common. Kussmaul's sign (i.e., exaggerated neck vein distention on inspiration) is also common, whereas pulsus paradoxus is more typical of cardiac tamponade. Chest x-ray reveals a normal to small heart with calcium evident in the pericardium. ECG reveals low-voltage QRS complexes, inverted T-waves, and notched P-waves. CT scan and echocardiography will effectively reveal pericardial thickening.

TREATMENT

Treatment involves surgical removal of the constricting pericardium, which can result in bleeding from the epicardium. Cardiopulmonary bypass may be needed, especially if bleeding is difficult to control. Surgical correction is not immediately followed by decreases in right atrial pressure or increased cardiac output. Right atrial pressure normalizes within 3 months after surgery. Generally, myocardial function is normal.

ANESTHETIC CONSIDERATIONS

Provided hypotension does not exist as a result of pericardial tamponade, anesthetics used should not depress myocardial contractility, cause hypotension, lower the heart rate, or impede venous return. Maintenance is best accomplished by using a combination of benzodiazepines, opioids, and nitrous oxide, with or without a low concentration of volatile agent. Nondepolarizing muscle relaxants with minimal circulatory effects are best; however, the modest increase in heart rate with pancuronium is usually tolerated. Preoperative optimization of the patient's fluid status is important. If hemodynamic changes occur secondary to pericardial tamponade, an appropriate change in anesthetic management should follow.

A pulmonary artery catheter may provide beneficial information during the recovery period that is associated with wide swings in blood pressure and cardiac output. Arrhythmias are common during the procedure, and antiarrhythmic drugs, as well as a mechanical defibrillator, should be available. Patients may require postoperative ventilatory support; patients should be monitored for arrhythmias and low cardiac output, which may necessitate treatment.

CARDIAC TAMPONADE

DEFINITION

Cardiac tamponade is the accumulation of fluid in the pericardial space that elevates intrapericardial pressure.

INCIDENCE/ETIOLOGY

The incidence varies and cardiac tamponade may be characterized as acute or chronic. It is most commonly the result of trauma, infection, or neoplastic disease states. It can present following cardiac surgery.

DIAGNOSTIC AND LABORATORY FINDINGS

Echocardiography is the best method to detect pericardial fluid. Chest x-rays do not reveal a change in the cardiac silhouette until 250 mL of fluid have accumulated.

CLINICAL MANIFESTATIONS

As pressure in the pericardial space rises, CVP also rises. Right atrial pressure may be monitored to determine whether tamponade is present. Other signs and symptoms include activation of the sympathetic nervous system (as manifested by sinus tachycardia), equalization of atrial and left ventricular filling pressures, decreased voltage and electrical alternans on ECG, paradoxical pulse, hypotension, and muffled heart sounds (Beck's triad).

TREATMENT

Pericardiocentesis under local anesthesia may be used to surgically release the tamponade. Pericardiotomy under local or general anesthesia is recommended when tamponade develops from trauma or cardiac surgery and becomes symptomatic. Temporary measures to maintain stroke volume include administration of intravenous fluids, inotropes to increase contractility, and correction of metabolic acidosis if needed.

ANESTHETIC CONSIDERATIONS

If the intrapericardial pressure contributing to tamponade is not relieved before induction of anesthesia, the goal is to maintain cardiac output. A primary goal is to avoid decreases in contractility, systemic vascular resistance, and heart rate. Ketamine is a suitable choice for induction and maintenance. While pancuronium is a logical choice for muscle relaxant because it maintains heart rate, other nondepolarizing muscle relaxants may be used as long as they do not contribute to decreasing the heart rate or systemic vascular resistance. Positive-pressure ventilation can also decrease venous return. Continuous CVP and invasive blood pressure monitoring can be instituted prior to anesthesia if the patient's condition permits. Maintenance of CVP with IV fluids should be used to maintain venous return. The surgeon should be prepared for emergency pericardiocentesis in the event of circulatory collapse after induction of anesthesia.

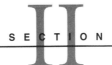

Respiratory System

A. Chronic Obstructive Pulmonary Disease/Emphysema/ Obstructive Disease

DEFINITION

Chronic obstructive pulmonary disease (COPD) is a term used to describe a variety of airway-related disease processes, such as: emphysema, asthma, chronic bronchitis, bronchiectasis, and cystic fibrosis. These conditions cause an increase in resistance to flow of gases in the airway that often result in acute and chronic disease states that are reversible or irreversible.

INCIDENCE AND PREVALENCE

In the United States, COPD is most common in males over 50 years of age. It remains the second most common cause of mortality.

ETIOLOGY

The primary predisposing factor is a history of smoking. COPD results from three major pathophysiologic occurrences: chronic infection due to irritation of the bronchi from inhaling smoke or other irritating substances; chronic obstruction of small airways due to excess mucus production, infection, and airway edema; and entrapment of air in alveoli, resulting in abnormal enlargement of alveolar airspaces. Exacerbations may be precipitated by infection, congestive heart failure, oxygen therapy that blunts hypoxic drive, and pulmonary thromboembolism.

LABORATORY RESULTS

Chest x-rays often show hyperinflation and diaphragmatic flattening, right ventricular hypertrophy, a dilated proximal pulmonary artery, and attenuated pulmonary vasculature in the presence of associated pulmonary vascular disease. Pulmonary function tests will show a decreased FEV_1/FVC ratio. Emphysematous patients have increased respiratory volume and total lung capacity but decreased diffusing capacity for carbon monoxide. The partial pressure of both oxygen (PaO_2) and carbon dioxide ($PaCO_2$) are generally not affected until the later stages of COPD. The ECG may exhibit right ventricular hypertrophy when right-sided heart failure is present. With the chronic respiratory acidosis that often accompanies COPD, $PaCO_2$ is elevated, and pH is low or normal. Acute exacerbations often result in an elevated $PaCO_2$ and an acidic pH. Hematocrit may be elevated in both the acute and chronic disease states.

CLINICAL MANIFESTATIONS

Patient History

Chronic bronchitis is often manifested by a chronic productive cough, exertional dyspnea, and wheezing. Emphysema is primarily manifested by exertional dyspnea that is progressive in nature with or without a productive cough or wheezing.

Physical Examination

Patients with COPD often have an increased anteroposterior chest diameter ("barrel chest"), hyper-resonance to percussion, and wheezing or rhonchi on auscultation of the chest. Accessory muscles for breathing are used; these patients have a prolonged expiratory phase of respiration and use "pursed lip" breathing; clubbing of the fingers also may occur.

TREATMENT

Conservative management includes low-flow oxygen via nasal cannula or Venturi mask, bronchodilators, β_2-adrenergic agonists, ipratropium bromide, theophylline, and anti-inflammatory agents (e.g., cromolyn sodium and adrenocortical steroids). Aggressive therapy includes subcutaneous injection of epinephrine or terbutaline sulfate, inhaled bronchodilators, aminophylline, adrenocortical steroids, and intubation and mechanical ventilation in cases not responsive to other therapies.

ANESTHETIC CONSIDERATIONS

Both general and regional anesthesia have been proven acceptable, but these patients are susceptible to postoperative respiratory failure. When sedation is given as during a regional technique, great care should be taken since these patients are extremely sensitive to the respiratory depressant effects of these drugs. Blockade above a sensory level of T-6 may decrease expiratory reserve volume (ERV) so that there is an ineffective cough and thus poor clearance of secretions. With general anesthesia, the clinician should attempt to avoid cold, dry inspired gases. Volatile agents may produce bronchodilation. Nitrous oxide can cause enlargement and rupture of pulmonary bullae, leading to pneumothorax. Opioids may be used but can be associated with preoperative and postoperative ventilatory depression. Controlled ventilation with high tidal volume (10 to 15 mL/kg) and slow inspiratory rates optimize PaO_2, minimize airflow turbulence, and optimize V/Q matching. During spontaneous ventilation with volatile agents, a greater degree of respiratory depression can be seen in patients with COPD. Perioperative ABGs should be monitored.

PROGNOSIS

The overall long-term prognosis is good for hospitalized patients with acute exacerbations and those with COPD who are stable with therapy. Right ventricular hypertrophy with associated failure is a poor prognostic sign.

B. Asthma

DEFINITION

Asthma is a respiratory condition that encompasses periodic attacks of bronchospasm associated with dyspnea, cough, and wheezing. Many factors (e.g. autonomic, endocrine, infectious, immunologic) play a role in this disorder. Bronchospastic episodes are typically short-lived and reversible, and patients respond to therapy with complete recovery between episodes.

INCIDENCE AND PREVALENCE

Asthma affects 3% to 5% of the population, with 65% of patients developing symptoms before age 5. Males are affected twice as often as females.

ETIOLOGY

Environmental factors such as dust, cold, fumes, animal dander, pollen, chemicals, or stress (emotional/physical) can precipitate a bronchospastic episode. An overreactive parasympathetic nervous system allows the release of mediators causing the bronchiolar hyperreactivity. Vagal afferents in the bronchial tree are sensitive to these stimuli and, when stimulated, cause bronchoconstriction to occur. Airway obstruction develops as airway passages constrict, become edematous (producing mucus), that inevitably leads to inspiratory/expiratory resistance to air flow. Hyperinflation distal to airway obstruction, altered pulmonary mechanics, and an increase in the work of breathing occur secondary to impaired expiration. Respiratory alkalosis occurs as a result of the alteration in the V/Q relationships. Resultant hypoxemia occurs without hypercapnia and hyperventilation. Worsening obstruction invariably leads to hypercapnia and respiratory acidosis.

LABORATORY RESULTS

Chest x-ray may be normal or exhibit overinflation as well as other causes/complications of asthma (e.g., pulmonary edema, pneumonia, or pulmonary hypertension). Arterial blood gases in the early phase of an asthma attack reveal mild hypoxemia, hypocarbia, and respiratory alkalosis. As the attack intensifies, hypoxemia worsens, and hypercarbia and respiratory acidosis develop. PFTs show a decrease in FEV_1 and FVC; FRC and total lung capacity are increased. ECG may show PVCs, RBBB, or right atrial/ventricular compromise. The eosinophil count is typically elevated.

CLINICAL MANIFESTATIONS

During remission, patients are asymptomatic (i.e., pulmonary function is normal). Dyspnea, inspiratory/expiratory wheezing, a nonproductive cough, prolonged expiration, tachycardia, and tachypnea characterize a typical attack. In addition, patients may complain of chest tightness and use accessory muscles for respiration.

TREATMENT

Treatment includes bronchodilators, β_2-adrenergic agonists, ipratropium bromide and theophylline, oxygen therapy, anti-inflammatory agents (cromolyn sodium or hydrocortisone, methylprednisolone or prednisone), and fluid therapy.

ANESTHETIC CONSIDERATIONS

A complete preoperative evaluation should be performed and include history of the disease and current status, auscultation of lung sounds, and prescribed medication. Active wheezing may predispose the patient to a life-threatening event in the perioperative period. Those prone to frequent episodes of bronchospasm should be taking therapeutic doses of theophylline, bronchodilating inhalers, and in some cases glucocorticoids, and their compliance should be verified. Sedatives (e.g., benzodiazepines) should be administered carefully to avoid respiratory depression and apnea. Use care when opioids are administered, especially those associated with histamine release, which may lead to bronchospasm. The use of regional anesthetic techniques may help in avoidance of airway manipulation and the concomitant threat of inducing bronchospasm. Therefore any patient with bronchospastic disease undergoing general anesthesia (i.e., endotracheal intubation) may predispose to bronchospasm; the patient should be deeply anesthetized prior to intubation. IV lidocaine given approximately 3 minutes before laryngoscopy/intubation may blunt untoward airway responses. All volatile inhalational agents possess bronchodilating properties, however, isoflurane and desflurane can also cause airway irritation. When muscle relaxation is required, those drugs that have a potential to release histamine (e.g., d-tubocurarine, atracurium) should be used with caution. If possible, warm and humidify inspired gases, and if intraoperative bronchospasm occurs, inhaled bronchodilators, subcutaneous terbutaline, aminophylline, and/or volatile agents may be used for treatment. Intraoperative bronchospasm may be detected by noting changes in lung sounds, rising airway pressures, and difficulty in ventilation. Reversal agents (i.e., anticholinesterase plus anticholinergics) are typically administered together to reverse the effects of nondepolarizing muscle relaxants. Anticholinesterase drugs may themselves precipitate bronchospasm. To prevent the likelihood of this occurring, it has been suggested that the anticholinergic drug be given prior to the anticholinesterase agent (i.e., given separately). "Deep" extubation to decrease the likelihood of bronchospasm on emergence has been recommended for those not at risk for aspiration.

PROGNOSIS

An acute asthmatic attack during the perioperative period is associated with an increase in mortality/morbidity. Asthma by itself results in approximately 5000 deaths in the United States each year.

C. Pneumonia

DEFINITION

Pneumonia is an acute infection of the lung parenchyma caused by bacteria or viruses.

INCIDENCE AND PREVALENCE

More than 1 million cases of pneumonia are diagnosed each year with a majority of these occurring in winter months. The onset of pneumonia is also associated with a number of risk factors, namely: a history of recent URI; age, with infants and elderly persons at increased risk; immunosuppression; COPD; sepsis; smoking; mechanical ventilation; airway obstruction by tumors, secretions, or a foreign body; and neurologic impairment.

ETIOLOGY

Microorganisms that contribute to pneumonia may enter the respiratory tract in several ways (e.g., exhaled by others or from contaminated respiratory equipment). A commonly inhaled microorganism is influenza virus. Pulmonary aspiration of oropharyngeal secretions may contain grampositive or negative microorganisms. Gram-negative bacteria and *Staphylococcus* are typically transmitted in blood; the pathogen multiplies, releasing toxins and stimulating inflammatory and immune responses. An antigen-antibody reaction, along with endotoxins from microorganisms, damage alveolo-capillary and bronchial membranes. Infectious debris/exudate secondary to inflammation/edema fill terminal bronchioles. V/Q alterations develop. *Staphylococcus* or gram-negative bacteria may cause necrosis of lung parenchyma.

LABORATORY RESULTS

ABGs may reveal hypoxemia secondary to shunting and respiratory alkalosis. In cases of severe lung impairment or impaired tissue oxygenation, ABGs may show hypercarbia and metabolic acidosis. Blood and sputum cultures/gram stains are used to identify the offending organism. Leukocytosis is common. Dehydration may mask patterns of lobar, segmental, or diffuse patterns of infiltration on chest x-ray. The ECG may reveal arrhythmias (e.g., tachycardia, PVCs) or patterns of myocardial ischemia (i.e., ST-T wave inversion).

CLINICAL MANIFESTATIONS

Fever, chills, productive or nonproductive cough, malaise, pleural pain, dyspnea, and hemoptysis may be present. Symptoms may be minimal or masked in the elderly, debilitated, or neutropenic patient.

TREATMENT

Bacterial pneumonia is treated with antibiotics based on the causative organism. *Viral* pneumonia is treated with supportive therapy alone. Fundamental treatment for all types of pneumonia include: adequate hydration; good pulmonary hygiene, including deep breathing, coughing, and chest percussion; rest; and oxygen. In severe cases, ventilatory support with supplemental oxygen may be required to maintain adequate gas exchange.

ANESTHETIC CONSIDERATIONS

The patient should be evaluated prior to anesthesia/operation by ensuring adequate antibiotic coverage and pulmonary toilet to improve V/Q mismatch. As an example, individuals with existing cardiopulmonary disease will be less likely to tolerate hypoxemia and the increase in work of breathing associated with pneumonia. Perioperative IV drugs should be administered gradually. Regional anesthesia may be desirable when appropriate since it reduces the risk of postoperative pulmonary dysfunction. Because they decrease the normal ventilatory response to hypercarbia, volatile anesthetics in residual concentrations may reduce respiratory drive, especially after prolonged procedures. General anesthesia interferes with mucociliary clearance; therefore inspired gases should be warmed by using either a humidifier or an "artificial nose" (i.e., heat moisture exchanger), and the patient should be suctioned during surgery when necessary. Patients with marginal pulmonary function or those with upper abdominal/chest incisions may require postoperative mechanical ventilation following general anesthesia.

PROGNOSIS
In most cases, full recovery is likely with early and adequate treatment.

D. Tuberculosis

DEFINITION
Tuberculosis is a chronic granulomatous disease that is spread primarily by aerosol transmission.

INCIDENCE AND PREVALENCE
In the past and prior to specific antimicrobial therapy, tuberculosis was a significant cause of death and disability in North America. It presently affects approximately 28,000 individuals in North America. The elderly, debilitated, malnourished, and those immunosuppressed and living in crowded conditions are most often affected.

ETIOLOGY
Tuberculosis is caused by the acid-fast bacillus *Mycobacterium tuberculosis.* Once inspired, the bacilli multiply, causing nonspecific pneumonitis. Some bacilli migrate to the lymph nodes, encounter lymphocytes, and precipitate the immune response. Phagocytes engulf colonies of bacilli in the lung, isolating them and forming granulomatous tubercules. Infected tissues inside the tubercles create caseation necrosis (a cheese-like material). Isolation of the bacilli is completed by formation of scar tissue around the tubercle. After approximately 10 days, the immune response is complete and further bacilli multiplication is prevented. After isolation of bacilli and development of immunity, tuberculosis can remain dormant for life. Reactivation may occur if live bacilli escape into bronchi or in states of decreased immunity. Patients with laryngeal tuberculosis or lung cavitation have the highest infectivity rate.

LABORATORY RESULTS
Diagnosis is made by positive tuberculin skin (PPD) testing, chest x-ray, and positive sputum culture. A positive skin test alone may indicate only expo-

sure to the tuberculin bacteria and is not by itself evidence of active disease. Chest x-ray findings consistent with tuberculosis in the presence of acquired immunodeficiency syndrome (AIDS) may be atypical.

CLINICAL MANIFESTATIONS

Many patients are asymptomatic. Common manifestations include low-grade fever, fatigue, weight loss, anorexia, lethargy, and a worsening cough (i.e., purulent sputum). Some patients occasionally develop pleural effusions, meningitis, bone or joint disease, genitourinary abscesses, or peritonitis. Chest pain, dyspnea, and hemoptysis are not common.

TREATMENT

Drugs of choice for treatment include isoniazid, rifampin, streptomycin, or ethambutol.

ANESTHETIC CONSIDERATIONS

The patient is placed in "Respiratory Isolation" until such time/therapy that they are no longer transmitters of the disease. Whenever possible, disposable equipment (i.e., filters and anesthesia circuits) should be used. Nondisposable equipment must be thoroughly sterilized. Postpone elective surgery in actively infected individuals until adequate chemotherapy has been administered (usually 3 weeks of treatment) and verified by a negative sputum sample. Consider the implications of organ dysfunction that may be secondary to the disease or its treatment. While the pulmonary system is most commonly affected by the disease, chemotherapeutic agents used for treatment may lead to organ toxicity (i.e., liver, kidneys, or peripheral nervous system).

PROGNOSIS

After 10 weeks of appropriate therapy 75% of patients have organism-free sputum. Length of therapy ranges from 9 to 18 months. Bacilli are usually rendered inactive after 3 weeks of chemotherapy.

E. Pulmonary Embolism

DEFINITION

Pulmonary embolism is an occlusion of the pulmonary vascular bed by an embolus. It may be due to blood clots, fats, tissue fragments, tumor cells, air, amniotic fluid, or foreign objects.

INCIDENCE AND PREVALENCE

Pulmonary embolism is a leading cause of morbidity and mortality in the United States and is responsible for approximately 50,000 deaths per year. It is the most common cause of acute pulmonary disease in hospitalized patients.

ETIOLOGY

Pulmonary embolism is due primarily to venous stasis, alterations or abnormalities in the blood vessel wall, and hypercoagulation. Most of these emboli arise from thromboses in vessels of the pelvis or lower extremities. The emboli can result in massive occlusion/blockage of a major branch of the pulmonary circulation; embolus with infarction of a portion of lung tissue; embolus without infarction (i.e., not severe enough to cause permanent lung injury); or multiple pulmonary emboli, either chronic or recurrent. The pattern of occurrence and severity determine the degree of hypoxic vasoconstriction, pulmonary edema, atelectasis, vagal stimulation, and release of neurohumoral substances such as histamine. Pulmonary emboli may also cause systemic hypotension, pulmonary hypertension, decreased cardiac output, and shock.

LABORATORY RESULTS

Pulmonary angiography is the most definitive diagnostic tool. Chest x-ray may be normal or show only subtle changes. A V/Q scan may reveal an embolus if a perfusion defect exists in an area of normal ventilation. ABGs may be normal but typically reveal hypoxemia, respiratory alkalosis, and hypocapnia. ECG may show tachycardia or signs of right-sided ventricular failure (e.g., R > S in V_1), including tall, peaked T-waves, right-axis deviation, or right bundle branch block.

CLINICAL MANIFESTATIONS

Clinical manifestations may range from tachypnea, tachycardia, dyspnea, and anxiety to pleural pain, pleural friction rub, pleural effusion, hemoptysis, fever, leukocytosis, severe pulmonary hypertension, and shock. Physical examination reveals wheezing, rales, or pleural friction rub on chest auscultation, and tachycardia, splitting of the second heart sound, or systolic ejection murmur over the pulmonic valve.

TREATMENT

Prevention is primary. Low-dose heparin therapy, Coumadin, aspirin, dextran, pneumatic leg compression, elastic compression stockings, and early ambulation can serve as prophylaxes. Intravenous heparin is the initial treatment once a pulmonary embolus has been diagnosed. Thrombolytic therapy is indicated in cases of massive pulmonary embolism or circulatory collapse.

ANESTHETIC CONSIDERATIONS

Patients who undergo a surgical procedure are at risk for deep venous thrombosis (DVT) and pulmonary embolus. Subcutaneous heparin, dextran, and pneumatic leg compression devices may help prevent perioperative DVT. Regional anesthesia may decrease the incidence of DVT and subsequent pulmonary embolism for some surgical procedures. Patients with a history of pulmonary embolism or DVT may already be on anticoagulant therapy, so one must check prothrombin time (PT) and partial thromboplastin time (PTT). The clinician should avoid regional anesthesia in the presence of a prolonged bleeding time or residual anticoagulation. Vena cava umbrella filters can be placed under local anesthesia with sedation. Hypotension may occur during placement of the apparatus because of decreased venous return. Sudden unexplained hypotension, bronchospasm, decreased $PetCO_2$, elevated CVP, and elevated PAP may indicate intraoperative pulmonary embolism.

PROGNOSIS

Statistics on prognosis are presently unavailable.

F. Cor Pulmonale

DEFINITION

Cor pulmonale is right ventricular hypertrophy that eventually leads to right-sided heart failure.

INCIDENCE AND PREVALENCE

Cor pulmonale is noted in 10% to 30% of patients admitted to the hospital with congestive heart failure. It occurs in males 5 times more often than in females.

ETIOLOGY

Cor pulmonale usually is caused by left-sided heart failure and is often due to pulmonary disease and elevated pulmonary vascular resistance.

LABORATORY RESULTS

Chest x-ray reveals evidence of COPD, RVH, dilation of the main pulmonary artery, and decreased markings of peripheral pulmonary vasculature. ECG may reveal signs of right atrial enlargement (peaked P-waves in the limb leads) and/or right ventricular hypertrophy (R > S in V_1, right axis deviation), atrial fibrillation, or right bundle branch block (rSR' in V_1). PFTs will generally exhibit those changes consistent with the primary pulmonary disease.

CLINICAL MANIFESTATIONS

In cor pulmonale, clinical manifestations are difficult to detect and may resemble those of many different respiratory disorders. Fatigue, retrosternal chest discomfort, dyspnea, cough, activity-induced weakness, or syncope may occur. Physical assessment may reveal distended neck veins, right ventricular gallop, pulmonic and tricuspid valve murmurs, split S_2 heart sound, JVD, pulsus paradoxus, hepatosplenomegaly, and dependent peripheral edema.

TREATMENT

Treatment centers on treating the underlying right-sided heart failure or pulmonary disease. The goal is to reduce pulmonary hypertension and normalize PaO_2, $PaCO_2$, and pH if pulmonary vasoconstriction is reversible. Rest, supplemental oxygen, antibiotics, digitalis, diuretics, and bronchodilators can provide effective treatment.

ANESTHETIC CONSIDERATIONS

Avoid elective surgery until reversible components of pulmonary disease are corrected. Administration of anesthetics to those individuals with pulmonary infection should also be avoided. Bronchospasm should be absent or have been treated. The patient should be appropriately hydrated with intravenous fluids and blood work for serum electrolytes should be within normal limits. Sedatives and narcotics effects are potentiated and may cause respiratory depression; therefore judicious dosing and monitoring is essential. Anticholinergics may increase the heart rate and physiologic dead space, so their use should be individualized. Monitoring should include ECG, noninvasive blood pressure (arterial monitoring may be necessary), urinary drainage catheter, and PA catheter if necessary. Regional anesthesia may be appropriate if high sensory levels are not required. Intermittent positive-pressure ventilation may improve arterial oxygenation. Significant decreases in $PaCO_2$ may lead to metabolic alkalosis and hypokalemia.

PROGNOSIS

The prognosis is best in COPD patients who have near-normal arterial oxygenation and is worst in patients with intrinsic vascular disease or pulmonary fibrosis.

G. Pulmonary Hypertension

DEFINITION

Pulmonary hypertension is an increase in pulmonary artery pressure of 5 to 10 mm Hg above normal (i.e., 15 to 18 mm Hg).

INCIDENCE AND PREVALENCE

Primary pulmonary hypertension is rare and generally affects women 20 to 40 years of age. *Secondary* pulmonary hypertension is more common. It can occur after cardiovascular or respiratory disorders that increase the volume/pressure of blood entering the pulmonary arteries or that narrow/obstruct the pulmonary arteries.

ETIOLOGY

Pulmonary hypertension is characterized by an increase in pulmonary vasculature resistance that is caused by an anatomic or vasomotor defect.

Primary Pulmonary Hypertension

In this type of pulmonary hypertension, the pulmonary arterioles become narrowed because of vascular smooth muscle hypertrophy and formation of fibrous lesions around the vessels. As vessels narrow, resistance increases and pulmonary hypertension begins. High pressures may be generated to the right ventricle, leading to failure or cor pulmonale. Death usually ensues within 5 years of diagnosis secondary to cor pulmonale.

Secondary Pulmonary Hypertension

There are four causes of secondary hypertension: increased LV filling pressures (as seen in coronary artery disease and mitral valve disease); increased pulmonary blood flow (L-to-R shunting occurs as in VSD/PDA); obliteration and/or obstruction of the pulmonary vascular bed by chronic obstructive airway disease, pulmonary embolism, pulmonary vasculitis, or pulmonary fibrosis; and pulmonary vasoconstriction secondary to hypoxemia, acidosis, or both. Secondary hypertension is reversible if the underlying cause is resolved.

LABORATORY RESULTS

Diagnosis is confirmed with cardiac catheterization when other possible causes have been excluded. Chest x-rays may show an enlarged border of the right side of the heart. ECG may reveal signs of right ventricular hypertrophy (i.e., R > S in V_1).

CLINICAL MANIFESTATIONS

Signs and symptoms are often masked by primary pulmonary or cardiovascular disease. Pulmonary hypertension may not be evidenced until pulmonary artery pressure equals systemic pressure. Resting pulmonary artery pressure generally does not rise until the effective cross-sectional area of the vascular bed is decreased by 50% or more. Patients may complain of fatigue, chest discomfort, and dyspnea, especially with exertion and tachypnea.

TREATMENT

Primary Pulmonary Hypertension

No curative treatment is available. Oxygen, cardiac glycosides, diuretics, fluid control, and bronchodilators may be used as palliative treatments.

Secondary Pulmonary Hypertension

Treatment of the underlying disorder is most effective. Oxygen may reverse hypoxic vasoconstriction. Digitalis and diuretics may be used for right ventricular failure.

ANESTHETIC CONSIDERATIONS

Reversible coexisting disease should be corrected preoperatively, and baseline ABGs should be obtained. Preoperative sedation may depress ventilation. Anticholinergics may depress mucociliary activity and impair clearance of secretions. Bronchospasm and increases in pulmonary and systemic pressures may be avoided during intubation if the depth of anesthesia is adequate. Regional anesthesia may be appropriate for cases not requiring high sensory levels of blockade. Nitrous oxide may increase pulmonary vascular resistance when high doses of opioids are given. Monitoring requirements depend on the severity of disease and type of surgery.

PROGNOSIS

The prognosis is poor; most individuals die within 5 years of the initial diagnosis. The prognosis is better with secondary pulmonary hypertension and when the underlying cause can be reversed.

H. Upper Respiratory Infection

DEFINITION

Upper respiratory infection is a viral or bacterial infection of the upper respiratory tract.

INCIDENCE AND PREVALENCE

Statistics are unavailable.

ETIOLOGY

Bacterial upper respiratory tract infections often are secondary to impairment of normal host defense mechanisms (e.g., mucociliary transport, cough reflexes). Viral respiratory infections impair normal respiratory defense mechanisms.

Types of Upper Respiratory Infection

- *Sinusitis:* Sinusitis of the frontal/maxillary sinuses is more common in adults; sinusitis of the ethmoid sinus is more common in children. Sinusitis may lead to intracranial infection.
- *Otitis media:* A middle ear infection caused by bacteria that migrate from the nasopharynx; most frequently caused by pneumococci or *Haemophilus influenzae.*
- *Pharyngitis:* Pharyngitis is usually viral; 20% of all bacterial cases are caused by group A streptococci.
- *Peritonsillar abscess:* Occurs secondary to streptococcal tonsillitis.
- *Retropharyngeal infection:* Caused by the retropharyngeal spread of infection; most cases occur in children.
- *Ludwig's angina:* Cellulitis of the submandibular, sublingual, and submental areas; usually caused by streptococci.
- *Epiglottitis:* Infection of the epiglottis that is due to *H. influenzae,* type B. Progresses rapidly and may be potentially lethal because inflamed tissue leads to obstruction.

LABORATORY RESULTS

Sinusitis: Based on signs and symptoms
Otitis media: Based on evaluation of signs and symptoms concerning the tympanic membrane
Pharyngitis: Based on throat culture to identify causative organism
Peritonsillar abscess: Based on signs and symptoms
Retropharyngeal infections: Based on signs and symptoms
Ludwig's angina: Based on signs and symptoms
Epiglottitis: Based on signs and symptoms

CLINICAL MANIFESTATIONS

Sinusitis is manifested by pain and tenderness over the affected sinuses, nasal drainage, fever, and facial or forehead discomfort. Purulent otitis media results in bulging tympanic membranes and obscured bony landmarks. Serous otitis media results in retracted tympanic membranes and no alteration in bony landmarks. Chronic otitis media may result in tympanic membrane perforation and hearing loss. Acute mastoiditis is a rare complication. Pharyngitis usually is manifested by throat pain and fever; dysphagia often occurs. Peritonsillar abscess is manifested by fever, chills, dysphagia with drooling, and a muffled voice. Trismus may also be present. The manifestations of retropharyngeal infections are similar to those of pharyngitis and peritonsillar abscess. Ludwig's angina manifests as edema of the anterior neck and floor of the mouth, fever, and dysphagia secondary to elevation of the tongue. Upper airway obstruction can occur. Epiglottitis is manifested by rapid progression of fever, inspiratory stridor, drooling and dysphagia, and severe respiratory distress.

TREATMENT

Sinusitis: Decongestants and analgesics. If intracranial spread ensues, high-dose antibiotics and surgical drainage may be required.

Otitis media: Analgesics, antibiotics, decongestants, and, in case of progressive hearing loss, myringotomy.

Pharyngitis: Analgesics; antibiotics for bacterial pharyngitis.

Peritonsillar abscess: Surgical drainage and antibiotics.

Retropharyngeal infections: Surgical drainage and antibiotics, as necessary.

Ludwig's angina: Analgesics and antibiotics. Airway compromise may mandate intubation, however intubation of the trachea may be impossible, necessitating tracheostomy.

Epiglottitis: Early airway management (i.e., intubation or tracheostomy) and antibiotics

ANESTHETIC CONSIDERATIONS

Anesthetic considerations are based on the specific type and severity of upper respiratory infection. In the presence of active upper airway infection, risks of delaying surgery must be weighed against risks of proceeding with anesthesia. If surgery is not an emergency, it is safest to delay the procedure in the presence of fever and/or an elevated WBC count, when the surgery is on the thorax or abdomen, or when surgery is expected to last longer than 1 hour.

PROGNOSIS

Complete recovery is likely for most upper respiratory infections, especially with appropriate treatment. Some upper respiratory infections, such as epiglottitis, are associated with higher mortality.

I. Restrictive Pulmonary Diseases

DEFINITION

Restrictive pulmonary diseases are diseases that cause pulmonary dysfunction secondary to decreased lung elasticity, resulting in poor lung compliance and increased work of breathing. They may be *extrinsic* or of an *acute/chronic intrinsic* type.

INCIDENCE AND PREVALENCE

Statistics are unavailable.

ETIOLOGY

Acute Intrinsic Restrictive

Acute intrinsic restrictive pulmonary disease is usually a result of intravascular fluid leakage into the interstitium and alveoli secondary to capillary endothelial damage or increased pulmonary vascular pressures.

Some of these disorders include adult respiratory distress syndrome (ARDS), aspiration pneumonitis, neurogenic pulmonary edema, high-altitude pulmonary edema, and opiate-induced pulmonary edema.

Chronic Intrinsic Restrictive

Chronic intrinsic restrictive pulmonary disease is generally a progressive pulmonary fibrosis that gives way to vascular destruction and can lead to pulmonary hypertension, cor pulmonale, and pneumothorax.

These disorders include hypersensitivity pneumonitis, sarcoidosis, eosinophilic granuloma, and alveolar proteinosis.

Chronic Extrinsic Restrictive

Chronic extrinsic restrictive pulmonary disease is due to other disorders that hamper expansion of the lungs (e.g., pleural, thoracic cage, or diaphragmatic disorders). Physical lung compression leads to decreased lung volumes that cause increased airway resistance. Mechanical changes of the chest increase the work of breathing; as pulmonary vascular resistance increases secondary to compression, a concomitant decrease in productive cough leads to recurrent pulmonary infections and eventually obstructive pulmonary disease.

Chronic extrinsic restrictive pulmonary diseases/conditions include fibrosis, effusion, kyphoscoliosis, pectus excavatum, obesity, ascites, and pregnancy.

CLINICAL MANIFESTATIONS

Clinical manifestations depend on the disorder but may include include tachypnea, dyspnea, cough, bronchospasm, pulmonary vascular vasoconstriction, pulmonary hypertension, cor pulmonale, and arterial hypoxemia.

TREATMENT

Treatment also depends on the specific restrictive disorder and may include oxygen therapy, bronchodilators, corticosteroids, and mechanical ventilation with positive end-expiratory pressure.

ANESTHETIC CONSIDERATIONS

- Restrictive pulmonary disease does not dictate drug choices for induction and maintenance of general anesthesia.
- Select and administer drugs to avoid postoperative ventilatory depression.
- Regional anesthesia may be acceptable, but sensory levels of blockade above T-10 may impair respiratory muscle function.
- Controlled ventilation may maximize oxygenation and ventilation.

- Poorly compliant lungs may require high inflation pressures.
- Postoperative mechanical ventilation may be necessary.
- Extubation should be done only when patients clearly meet the criteria.
- Decreased lung volumes may impair cough and interfere with postoperative secretion removal.

J. Adult Respiratory Distress Syndrome

DEFINITION

Adult respiratory distress syndrome (ARDS) is a term that refers to a variety of infiltrative lung pathologies resulting from diffuse alveolocapillary injury and resulting in a significant increase in capillary alveolar permeability. Increased lung water and high concentrations of proteins in the lung parenchyma and alveoli often result in acute respiratory failure and death.

INCIDENCE AND PREVALENCE

Approximately 150,000 to 200,000 new cases of ARDS are diagnosed yearly in the United States. ARDS is precipitated by a number of conditions and frequently affects young people who were previously in excellent health.

ETIOLOGY

Alveolocapillary damage may occur secondary to aspiration or inhalation injuries or indirectly from the activation/aggregation of neutrophils and the release of inflammatory mediators (leukocytes and macrophages) in response to sepsis, trauma, shock, activation of complement, the coagulation cascade, and other causes. Specific causative mechanisms are not known.

Initial alveolocapillary damage results in increased permeability, pulmonary edema, inactivation of surfactant, impaired gas exchange, and decreased lung compliance with decreased ventilation and shunting of pulmonary blood flow. If the syndrome does not begin to resolve following the initial phase, it leads to fibrotic changes. Collagen formation results with progressive obliteration of alveoli, respiratory bronchioli, and interstitium; a decrease in lung compliance; decreased V/Q; and eventually respiratory failure.

LABORATORY RESULTS

Chest x-ray may initially be clear or exhibit bilateral diffuse infiltrates. Later, infiltrates will become extensive and progress to complete opacification. In early stages, ABGs may show hyperventilation-induced respiratory alkalosis and mild hypoxemia that improves with the administration of supplemental oxygen. In the later stages of ARDS, hypoxemia is not improved by oxygen administration, and hypercarbia develops because of increased dead space ventilation.

CLINICAL MANIFESTATIONS

Classically, patients with ARDS have rapid shallow respirations, respiratory alkalosis, marked dyspnea, diffuse decreased chest wall compliance, and hypoxemia unresponsive to oxygen therapy. In late stages, metabolic acidosis, hypotension, decreased cardiac output, and death may occur.

TREATMENT

Early recognition and treatment with supportive therapy and prevention of complications afford the best chance of recovery from ARDS. Therapy may include fluid management, oxygen administration, mechanical ventilation with use of PEEP, inspiratory hold or reverse inspiratory/expiratory ratio, steroid administration, and cardiac drugs. Extracorporeal membrane oxygenation is sometimes used in the most severe cases, but it is associated with complications and has not been proven to improve survival.

ANESTHETIC CONSIDERATIONS

The goal is to provide adequate anesthesia while maintaining a physiologic state that is often precarious. Regional anesthesia may be acceptable, if it is not contraindicated by hemodynamic instability, coagulopathy, or sepsis. Ventilation with high fractional inspired oxygen and PEEP are often necessary and make patient transport technically difficult. High PEEP levels may cause hemodynamic instability. An arterial line, CVP, and PA catheters are typically required. An altered volume of distribution and rate of drug metabolism, as well as altered liver and kidney function, require more gradual and decreased dosing of benzodiazepines, narcotics, muscle relaxants, induction agents, and inhalation agents. The use of dinitrogen monoxide is rarely possible because of high fractional inspired oxygen requirements.

PROGNOSIS

Even with therapy, 52% of these patients die.

K. Pneumothorax and Hemothorax

DEFINITION

Pneumothorax is the presence of air or gas in the pleural space. Hemothorax is the presence of blood in the pleural space.

INCIDENCE AND PREVALENCE

Spontaneous pneumothorax occurs unexpectedly in healthy persons; most often in males 20 to 40 years of age. Secondary pneumothorax and hemopneumothorax are generally the result of trauma.

ETIOLOGY

Spontaneous pneumothorax is caused by the rupture of blebs on the visceral pleura. The cause of this bleb formation is unknown. Secondary pneumothorax is caused by rib fractures and by the rupture of a bleb or bulla as seen in chronic obstructive pulmonary disease or secondary to mechanical ventilation, especially if PEEP is used. Hemothorax is secondary to trauma.

LABORATORY RESULTS

Chest x-ray usually shows subcutaneous emphysema, pneumomediastinum, and pneumopericardium. Free fluid, as with hemothorax, may be best seen on a cross-table lateral film.

CLINICAL MANIFESTATIONS

Pneumothorax

Onset is with sudden pleural (i.e., inspiratory) chest pain, tachypnea, and mild dyspnea. With a large or tension pneumothorax, mediastinal shift may occur. Chest excursion becomes asymmetric. Breath sounds are absent over the affected area. Hypoxemia, hypotension, and severe dyspnea may occur.

Hemothorax

Symptoms are similar to those of pneumothorax and, in the case of significant chest trauma, may include signs of hypovolemia.

TREATMENT

Unless the pneumothorax is small and not expanding, a chest tube must be inserted to decompress the chest. If a chest tube is not immediately available in the presence of tension pneumothorax, a large-bore needle can be inserted into the anterior second intercostal space for immediate decompression of the affected side. Tension pneumothorax is a life-threatening emergency. Hemothorax is also treated with a chest tube on the affected side and, if blood loss is significant, may also require fluid or blood replacement.

ANESTHETIC CONSIDERATIONS

Pneumothorax or hemothorax can significantly interfere with oxygenation and ventilation. Decreased cardiac output, as with tension pneumothorax, can exacerbate intrapulmonary shunting. Cyanosis indicates both cardiac and pulmonary involvement. Nitrous oxide can quickly expand the size of a pneumothorax if a chest tube is not in place. In the case of a ventilator-related pneumothorax, mortality is significantly reduced if a chest tube is placed in less than 30 minutes. Development of tension pneumothorax during general anesthesia is manifested by sudden hypotension, loss of pulmonary compliance, or decreased ventilating volume. Patients with significant trauma may require fluid resuscitation and cardiovascular support. Agents chosen should have minimal cardiac depressant effects.

PROGNOSIS

Prognosis depends on the severity of the chest trauma that is associated with pneumothorax or hemothorax.

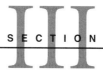

Central Nervous System

A. Seizures

DEFINITION
Seizures are the result of abnormal electrical discharges in the brain.

INCIDENCE AND PREVALENCE
Seizures affect approximately 0.5% to 1% of the population in the United States. Numerous types of seizures exist, but most are generalized tonic-clonic seizures. The likelihood of a recurrent seizure after a single seizure is approximately 50% in the following 3 years, with the greatest incidence during the first 6 months.

ETIOLOGY
Most seizures are idiopathic. Idiopathic seizure disorders usually begin in childhood. Seizure onset in adults may indicate an expanding intracranial hematoma, tumor, intracranial hemorrhage, metabolic disturbance, infection, trauma, alcohol or addictive drug withdrawal, eclampsia (in pregnant women), previous trauma causing an irritative phenomenon in the brain, and local anesthesia toxicity.

DIAGNOSTIC AND LABORATORY FINDINGS
Seizures can be detected with electroencephalography (signals can be augmented with methohexital, etomidate, or ketamine), electrolyte abnormalities, and examination of the cerebrospinal fluid for infection. Magnetic resonance imaging (MRI) is better than computed tomography (CT scan) in detecting focal intracranial lesions.

CLINICAL MANIFESTATIONS
Clinical manifestations include focal or generalized tonic-clonic seizures and an increase in the cerebral metabolic rate of oxygen ($CMRO_2$).

TREATMENT
The first priority is to protect and secure the airway, oxygenate, and ventilate. Supportive care and treatment of the underlying problem are needed.

Grand Mal Seizures
Appropriate drug therapy for grand mal seizures includes midazolam 1 mg/min IVP until seizures stop or a total of 10 mg. Diphenylhydantoin or phenytoin (Dilantin) with an intravenous load of 15 mg/kg over 20 minutes is also used. No more than 50 mg/min are infused, and then followed by daily maintenance doses of 300 to 500 mg orally or IV for adults. The

therapeutic serum level is 10 to 20 mg/mL. Phenobarbital can also be used to control seizures with an IV dose of 100 mg/min IV up to a total of 20 mg/kg. The therapeutic serum level is 20 to 40 mg/mL.

Eclamptic Seizures

Magnesium sulfate, a mild CNS depressant and vasodilator, is used for eclamptic seizures. An initial IV loading dose is 2 to 4 g administered over 15 minutes followed by a continuous infusion of 1 to 3 g/hr. The therapeutic serum level is 4 to 8 mEq/L.

Local Anesthesia Toxicity

Thiopental (50 to 100 mg), midazolam (1 to 5 mg), or diazepam (5 to 20 mg IV push) are used to treat local anesthesia toxicity.

ANESTHETIC CONSIDERATIONS

Electrolytes, cultures, and serum drug levels should be obtained preoperatively. All current medications should be considered, and particular attention paid to any anticonvulsant drugs being taken and their possible cardiopulmonary effects and interactions with anesthetics. When phenytoin (Dilantin) is administered IV, particular care should be taken to infuse and flush with normal saline; infusion should be no faster than 50 mg/min. Arrhythmias, hypotension, and arrest can occur if administration is too rapid. The intraoperative requirement for nondepolarizing muscle relaxants (NDMRs) may be increased. Other anticonvulsant medications used are phenobarbital, primidone, carbamazepine (increases requirement for NDMRs), valproic acid, and ethosuximide. Metrizamide, a water-soluble contrast agent, can produce seizures if allowed to enter the intracranial compartment in a high concentration.

Patients on antiepileptic drugs build a resistance to the effects of neuromuscular blocking agents and opioids because of changes in the number of receptors, altered drug metabolism, and interaction with endogenous neurotransmitters. A "paralyzing" dose of muscle relaxant stops peripheral but not CNS manifestations of seizure activity.

Methohexital can activate epileptic foci, and ketamine can potentially lower seizure threshold. Atracurium possesses a laudanosine metabolite that is a CNS stimulant. Enflurane in concentrations greater than 2.5% that produces hypocarbia (i.e., pCO_2 less than 25 mm Hg) may produce seizures. Magnesium sulfate may increase sensitivity to all muscle relaxants. Hyperventilation of the lungs decreases delivery of additional local anesthesia to the brain; respiratory alkalosis and hyperkalemia result in hyperpolarization of nerve membranes.

PROGNOSIS

Seizures (convulsions) are a chronic condition managed for life. Seizures due to eclampsia typically resolve after delivery. Some individuals with a history of seizures may undergo surgery to locate the foci by electrophysiologically "mapping" different areas of the brain. This usually requires a cooperative patient since craniotomy is performed under local anesthesia with minimal IV sedation. Otherwise, general anesthesia is used for these procedures.

PART 1   **Common Diseases**

B. Cerebrovascular Disease

DEFINITION
Cerebrovascular disease is any of a collection of disorders that affect the vasculature of the brain; the primary disorder being cerebrovascular accident (CVA or "stroke") as a result of hemorrhage and ischemia.

INCIDENCE AND PREVALENCE
Cerebrovascular disease is the third leading cause of death in the United States.

ETIOLOGY
The major risk factors for the development of cerebrovascular disease are hypertension and diabetes. Other risk factors include atherosclerosis, inflammatory processes, dissecting aneurysm, disorders affecting the myocardium, CHF, polycythemia, cigarette-smoking, use of oral contraceptives, and postpartum infection. The different classifications of cerebrovascular disease can manifest as the following, listed below.

- *Transient ischemic attack (TIA):* A temporary, focal episode of neurologic dysfunction that develops suddenly and lasts a few minutes to hours, but usually never more than 24 hours. Approximately 41% of these individuals may eventually suffer a stroke.
- *Reversible ischemic neurologic deficit (RIND):* Neurologic symptoms that persist up to 6 to 8 weeks before resolving.
- *Progressive stroke:* A stroke in progress. Neurologic symptoms and deficits develop slowly and are not reversible.
- *Complete stroke:* Neurologic deficits are predominant.
- *Amaurosis fugax:* A sudden, temporary or fleeting blindness caused by a decrease in cerebral perfusion to the retina.

DIAGNOSTIC AND LABORATORY FINDINGS
CT scan, MRI, cerebral angiography, and clinical examination are useful.

CLINICAL MANIFESTATIONS
Clinical manifestations involve numerous neurologic deficits. See the classification of symptoms under Etiology.

TREATMENT
Treatment includes risk-factor reduction (i.e., controlling hypertension, avoiding a high-fat diet, smoking cessation, and decreasing obesity). In addition, carotid artery surgery (endarterectomy) may be indicated (over 100,000 are performed yearly).

ANESTHETIC CONSIDERATIONS
Preoperative evaluation should include a careful analysis of cardiovascular, neurologic, and pulmonary systems, as well as laboratory results and current medications. If the patient is scheduled for carotid endarterectomy, consider the benefits and risks associated with regional versus general anesthesia. Selection of anesthetic agents is based on the patient's need and the

surgeon's desires. The goal is to ensure a smooth induction, maintenance, and emergence, with avoidance of wide swings in blood pressure. Moreover, an awake, extubated patient is the desired outcome so that immediate neurologic assessment can be performed. Cardioactive agents such as sodium nitroprusside, nitroglycerin, and Neo-Synephrine should be readily available.

PROGNOSIS

Mortality from an acute CVA ranges from 15% to 30%. The leading cause of death in victims of stroke is a subsequent stroke. The risk of recurrent stroke is approximately 9% each year. About 45% of individuals who suffer a stroke will have another stroke within 5 years.

C. Hydrocephalus

DEFINITION

Hydrocephalus is an abnormal accumulation of cerebrospinal fluid (CSF) due either to an excessive production or decreased absorption that leads to an increase in pressure in the ventricles of the brain. The rise in intraventricular pressure causes adjacent brain tissue compression and progressive enlargement of the cranium.

INCIDENCE AND PREVALENCE

Hydrocephalus in newborns occurs in 3 of every 1000 births and is usually secondary to meningomyelocele. Hydrocephalus is common after subarachnoid hemorrhage because of impaired CSF circulation through the basal cistern. It is often a complication of a ruptured brain aneurysm. Hydrocephalus may occur in neonates due to obstruction of CSF circulation within the brain's ventricular system or at a site of reabsorption.

ETIOLOGY

Hydrocephalus can be divided into two main types: *Obstructive* and *Nonobstructive.*

> *Obstructive:* Results from obstruction to CSF flow; depending on the site, can be further divided into *communicating* or *noncommunicating.*

> *Communicating obstructive (Extraventricular hydrocephalus):* Results from obstruction to CSF absorption by the arachnoid villi, usually from remote inflammatory disease or traumatic subarachnoid hemorrhage.

> *Noncommunicating obstructive (Extraventricular hydrocephalus):* Secondary to obstruction to CSF flow between the lateral and fourth ventricules (ventricles dilate proximal but not distal to the obstruction).

Obstructive hydrocephalus results from congenital malformation scar tissue, fibrin deposits following intraventricular hemorrhage or infection, tumors, or cysts. Nonobstructive hydrocephalus results from excessive CSF production by the choroid plexus. Choroid plexus papillomas or benign tumors of the glomus of the lateral ventricles are common etiologies.

DIAGNOSTIC AND LABORATORY FINDINGS

Hydrocephalus can be diagnosed by CT scan, MRI, and by signs of increased intracranial pressure.

CLINICAL MANIFESTATIONS

Early signs and symptoms: Apnea, bradycardia, vomiting, increasing head circumference, headaches, mentation changes

Late signs and symptoms: Bulging fontanelle, "setting sun" eyes, CN VI palsy, limb spasticity, decreased level of consciousness leading to nonresponsiveness

ANESTHETIC CONSIDERATIONS

With hydrocephalus, intracranial pressure is elevated and the stomach is full. Hypoventilation, hypoxia, and hypertension are to be avoided. Intravenous induction should be rapid and smooth. There should be minimal to no premedication or cricoid pressure and the baseline neurologic status must be established. Once the airway is secure, hyperventilate the patient until ventricles are decompressed. The patient is maintained on N_2O/O_2 and increments of thiopental if needed until intracranial pressure is reduced, then an inhalation agent or opioid can be added. Sudden removal of large CSF volumes may lead to bradycardia and hypotension; this can be prevented by rapid replacement with saline and/or gradual removal of CSF. Although heat is lost due to surgical exposure, some degree of hypothermia may be appropriate in these patients. Narcotics are given in small amounts (or not given at all) to enable rapid neurologic assessment upon awakening from anesthesia.

TREATMENT

A bypass shunt is inserted to allow CSF to flow from the lateral ventricles to the peritoneal cavity (ventriculoperitoneal shunt). This type of shunt is preferable because of the lower incidence of complications and need for revision with growth. Ventriculoatrial and ventriculopleural shunts are less popular because of the risk of infection, microemboli, and hydrothorax. The lumboperitoneal shunt (between the lumbar subarachnoid space and the peritoneal space) may be used.

PROGNOSIS

Hydrocephalus is a chronic condition and requires continual monitoring for shunt patency, signs and symptoms of infection, and neurological changes (i.e., changes in the level of consciousness). Any type of shunt may require revisions.

D. Parkinson's Syndrome

DEFINITION

Parkinson's syndrome is also known as paralysis agitans. It is characterized by onset of degenerative disease of the CNS (specifically the extrapyramidal system) where there is loss of dopamine cell bodies in the substantia nigra in the brain. The dopamine deficiency causes the clinical signs and symptoms.

INCIDENCE AND PREVALENCE

Parkinson's syndrome occurs generally between 60 and 80 years of age. Distribution in males and females is equal.

ETIOLOGY

The exact cause is unknown. There is no hereditary component. The syndrome has been observed to develop after encephalitis, intoxication with carbon monoxide, and chronic ingestion of antipsychotic drugs.

DIAGNOSTIC AND LABORATORY FINDINGS

None presently.

CLINICAL MANIFESTATIONS

Clinical manifestations include slow resting tremors, bradykinesia, rigidity, a slow shuffling gait, and an expressionless face. The patient may present with a unilateral tremor or rigidity of an upper extremity.

TREATMENT

The goal is to increase the activity of the remaining dopaminergic cells in the substantia nigra. This can be accomplished in three ways.

1. Administer L-dopa orally (a dopamine precursor that crosses the blood-brain barrier), thereby increasing the concentration of dopamine in the substantia nigra.
2. Administer an oral medication such as bromocriptine, which increases the dopamine receptor activity in the substantia nigra. Other similar medications used occasionally are trihexyphenidyl hydrochloride (Artane) and amantadine, but these are less effective.
3. Administer selegline (Deprenyl) orally, which works by inhibiting the enzymes that break down dopamine in the substantia nigra.

ANESTHETIC CONSIDERATIONS

Those patients being treated with L-dopa should continue to receive their medication throughout the perioperative period, including the usual morning dose the day of operation. Because of the short elimination half-life of L-dopa and dopamine, interruption in therapy for greater than 6 to 12 hours can result in a loss of therapeutic effect. Abrupt withdrawal of L-dopa may lead to skeletal muscle rigidity that interferes with ventilation. L-Dopa also sensitizes the cardiovascular system and may predispose the patient to perioperative arrhythmias. Long-term L-dopa therapy can cause blood pressure fluctuations because of autonomic instability; therefore invasive blood pressure monitoring may be necessary. L-Dopa therapy causes an increase in renal blood flow and Na^+ excretion. It also causes a concomitant decrease in renin release, intravascular fluid volume, and systemic blood pressure during induction of anesthesia. These swings in blood pressure often require aggressive fluid administration with either crystalloid and colloids. Drugs that block dopamine uptake (e.g., phenothiazines, butyrophenones) may exacerbate symptoms and should therefore be avoided. Ketamine may provoke exaggerated sympathetic nervous system response and its use is questionable.

PROGNOSIS

Symptoms are treated with medication, but patients may still have ambulation problems secondary to rigidity and bradykinesia.

E. Guillain-Barré Syndrome

DEFINITION

Guillain-Barré syndrome is an acute form of idiopathic polyneuritis characterized by a sudden onset of weakness or paralysis. Typically seen first in the lower extremities, it spreads cephalad the next few days to involve skeletal muscles of the arms, trunk, and head.

INCIDENCE

Guillain-Barré syndrome occurs in 1 to 2 individuals per 100,000 individuals.

ETIOLOGY

CNS bulbar involvement is most frequently manifested as bilateral facial paralysis. The most common symptoms are difficult swallowing due to pharyngeal muscle weakness and impaired ventilation due to intercostal muscle paralysis. Lower motor neuron involvement gives way to flaccid paralysis, and corresponding tendon reflexes are diminished. Sensory disturbances occur as paresthesias in the distal extremities and generally precede the onset of paralysis. Pain occurs in different forms, such as headache, backache, or tenderness to deep pressure. Wide fluctuations in blood pressure (orthostatic), abnormalities on ECG (e.g., conduction disturbances, tachycardia), diaphoresis, peripheral vasoconstriction and thromboembolism may be seen as a result of autonomic nervous system dysfunction. Complete recovery can occur within weeks when "segmental" demyelination in the CNS is the primary pathologic change. A mortality rate of 3% to 8% is due to sepsis, respiratory distress syndrome, and pulmonary embolism.

DIAGNOSIS

Diagnosis is based on clinical findings of progressive bilateral weakness in the extremities. Examination of CSF by lumbar puncture will reveal increased levels of protein although cell counts remain normal. A viral etiology is supported by the observation that this syndrome develops after a respiratory or gastrointestinal infection in about half of all cases.

TREATMENT

Treatment is symptomatic. Monitor vital capacity; if it is less than 15 mL/kg, ventilatory support may be necessary. Corticosteroid therapy is not considered useful in these patients. Plasma exchange or infusion of gamma globulin may be of some benefit.

ANESTHETIC CONSIDERATIONS

As a result of the lower motor neuron and subsequent autonomic nervous system dysfunction, these patients may have an exaggerated response to noxious stimuli during operation/anesthesia. Regurgitation/aspiration during induction of anesthesia is a very real concern, however, succinylcholine should also be avoided (i.e., use of a nondepolarizing muscle relaxant). Blood pressure should be monitored invasively (arterial line) because of compensatory cardiovascular responses to changes in posture, blood loss, or positive pressure. Postoperative mechanical ventilatory support may be needed. The presence of any neurologic deficits prior to surgery should be documented appropriately on the pre-anesthetic evaluation.

PROGNOSIS

The prognosis varies by individual.

F. Multiple Sclerosis

DEFINITION

Multiple sclerosis (MS) is a demyelinating, acquired disease of the CNS characterized by random and multiple sites of demyelination of the corticospinal-tract neurons in the brain and spinal cord.

ETIOLOGY

Although the exact cause is unknown, the major pathologic change consists of a loss of myelin covering axons in the form of demyelinative plaques. Multiple sclerosis (MS) does not affect the peripheral nervous system.

INCIDENCE AND PREVALENCE

There seems to be an increased risk of developing MS (1:1000) in those individuals living in northern temperate zones such as North America, Europe, and southern portions of New Zealand/Australia. The incidence is greater among inner city dwellers and affluent socioeconomic groups. Evidence for a genetic factor is demonstrated by a 12- to 15-fold increase among first-degree relatives. MS is a disease of young adults. Females have a 2:1 greater incidence than males, and females tend to develop MS at a younger age. The development of symptoms later in life (after 35) is associated with a slower progression of symptoms. There may be a viral or inflammatory component. A transmissible agent has not been identified.

DIAGNOSTIC AND LABORATORY TESTS

Visual, brainstem, auditory, and somatosensory evoked potentials can be used to elicit the slow nerve conduction that occurs as a result of demyelination in specific areas. CT scan and MRI may demonstrate demyelinative plaques.

CLINICAL MANIFESTATIONS

Clinical manifestations reflect the site of demyelination in the CNS and spinal cord. "Ascending" spastic paresis of skeletal muscle is often prominent. Presenting symptoms may include unilateral vision impairment. Of all patients with demyelination, 10% to 15% develop full blown MS. Symptoms develop over the course of a few days, remain stable for a few weeks, then improve. The incidence of seizure disorders increases, and the course of MS is characterized by exacerbations and remissions of symptoms at unpredictable intervals over a period of several years. Residual symptoms persist during remission.

TREATMENT

There is no cure for MS and treatment is symptomatic. Corticosteroids are used to shorten the durations of attack, and skeletal muscle spasticity is treated with baclofen (Lioresal), dantrolene, and benzodiazepines (Valium). Immunosuppressive therapy and plasmapheresis may benefit some patients. Patients should avoid stress and fatigue.

ANESTHETIC CONSIDERATIONS

A baseline neurologic examination must first be documented. The impact of surgical stress on the natural progression of MS should also be considered. Any postoperative increase in body temperature may be more likely than drugs to be responsible for exacerbation of MS. Spinal anesthesia has been implicated in postoperative exacerbation of MS, whereas epidural or peripheral nerve block has not. General anesthesia is most often chosen. The use of succinylcholine should be avoided, due to the possible exaggerated release of potassium. The response to nondepolarizing muscle relaxants (NDMRs) may be prolonged because of coexisting muscle weakness and decreased muscle mass.

PROGNOSIS

The course of MS is unpredictable. Exacerbations and remissions are common. In the late-onset type, the course is generally progressive.

G. Myasthenia Gravis

DEFINITION

Myasthenia gravis (MG) is a chronic autoimmune disease involving the neuromuscular junction in skeletal muscle.

INCIDENCE AND PREVALENCE

Myasthenia gravis occurs in 1:20,000 adults. Females between 20 and 30 years of age are most often affected. Males are often older than 60 years when the disease manifests. Females are affected more often than males.

ETIOLOGY

There is a decrease in the total number of available receptors (due to inactivation or destruction by antibodies) for acetylcholine at the postsynaptic neuromuscular junction that results in skeletal muscle weakness and progression to early exhaustion. An estimated 70% to 80% of functional acetylcholine receptors are lost, explaining the early exhaustion seen in individuals as well as the marked sensitivity to nondepolarizing muscle relaxants. The origin of the autoimmune response is unknown but the thymus is thought to play a role, since hyperplasia of the gland is found in over 70% of individuals (10% to 15% have thymomas). Approximately 75% of patients undergo remission after surgical removal of the thymus.

LABORATORY RESULTS

Patients suspected to have the disease should undergo clinical evaluation, including a Tensilon (edrophonium) test and electromyography (EMG).

CLINICAL MANIFESTATIONS

MG is classified on the basis of the skeletal muscles involved and the severity of the symptoms.

Type I   Limited to extraocular muscles in 10% of patients.

Type IIA   Slowly progressive; a mild form of skeletal muscle weakness; spares the respiratory muscles; responds to anticholinesterase well.

Type IIB   More severe; does not respond well to drugs; respiratory muscles may be involved.

Type III   Acute onset; rapid deterioration of skeletal muscle strength (within 6 months).

Type IV   Severe form; results from type I or II.

The hallmark symptom of MG is weakness and rapid exhaustion of voluntary skeletal muscles with repetitive use followed by partial recovery with rest. Skeletal muscles innervated by the cranial nerves are especially vulnerable, as reflected by ptosis and diplopia, which may be the initial symptoms of the disease.

Signs and Symptoms

The clinical course of MG is marked by periods of exacerbation and remission. EMG shows decreased voltage with repetitive stimulation. Initially, the most common complaints are ptosis and diplopia from weakness in extraocular movement. Weakness of pharyngeal and laryngeal muscles (bulbar muscles) results in dysphagia, dysarthria, and difficulty in handling oral secretions. Skeletal muscle strength may be normal in well-rested patients, but exercise leads to rapid weakness. Arm, leg, or trunk weakness can occur in any combination and is usually distributed asymmetrically. These patients may be at an increased risk for regurgitation and aspiration of gastric contents. MG may also be associated with cardiomyopathy. Other autoimmune diseases may be present (thyroid, rheumatoid arthritis, systemic lupus erythematosus, pernicious anemia). Pregnancy, emotional stress, and surgery may precipitate skeletal muscle weakness.

TREATMENT

- *Anticholinesterase drugs:* These drugs inhibit the enzyme responsible for hydrolysis of acetylcholine, thereby increasing the amount of neurotransmitter available at the neuromuscular junction. Neostigmine can be used (15 mg oral dose equals 1.5 mg IM dose equals 0.5 mg IV dose). Pyridostigmine lasts longer (3 to 6 hours) and produces fewer muscarinic side effects (60 mg orally equals 2 mg IV or IM dose). Phospholine iodine is extremely potent and is reserved for severe MG. Interestingly, excessive anticholinesterase drugs may in themselves result in skeletal muscle weakness, referred to as "*cholinergic crisis.*"
- *Corticosteroids*: Prednisone (50 to 100 mg orally every day) interferes with the production of antibodies that are believed to be responsible for degradation of cholinergic receptors.
- *Plasmapheresis:* This process removes circulating antibodies to acetylcholine, resulting in improved skeletal muscle strength.
- *Thymectomy:* This is recommended for patients with drug-resistant MG. About 75% of these patients demonstrate a marked improvement in skeletal muscle strength; drug therapy is no longer required or the dosage can be decreased.

ANESTHETIC CONSIDERATIONS

Preoperative opioids should be used with caution. Explain to the patient that postoperative intubation and mechanical ventilation may be necessary. The likelihood for postoperative ventilation after thymectomy is based on the following criteria:
- Duration of MG for more than 6 years
- Chronic obstructive pulmonary disease related to MG
- Dose of pyridostigmine greater than 750 mg/day during the 48 hours preceding surgery
- Preoperative vital capacity of less than 2.9 L is less likely to require postoperative ventilatory support with the transcervical approach

Because the response to neuromuscular blocking agents is difficult to predict, a peripheral nerve stimulator is recommended. Sensitivity to NDMR and to succinylcholine may increase. For induction, use short-acting intravenous agents, short-acting NDMRs, or succinylcholine to facilitate intubation, also realizing that some patients may be intubated without the use of a muscle relaxant. Maintenance of anesthesia can be accomplished with oxygen, nitrous oxide, and a volatile anesthetic agent. If an NDMR is used, the initial dose should be reduced by $1/3$ to $1/2$. Narcotics may have a prolonged effect. The patient may require postoperative ventilatory support.

PROGNOSIS

MG is a chronic, lifelong disease.

H. Myasthenic Syndrome

DEFINITION
Also called Eaton-Lambert syndrome, myasthenic syndrome is a rare disorder of neuromuscular transmission resembling myasthenia gravis.

CLINICAL MANIFESTATIONS
Clinical manifestations include skeletal muscle weakness in patients with small cell carcinoma of the lung.

ETIOLOGY
Myasthenic syndrome is an autoimmune disease where immunoglobulin-G antibodies are produced in response to presynaptic calcium channels.

TREATMENT
Anticholinesterase drugs that are effective in treating myasthenia gravis are *not* effective with this syndrome. 4-Aminopyridine, which stimulates the presynaptic release of acetylcholine, may improve skeletal muscle strength.

ANESTHETIC CONSIDERATIONS
Patients are sensitive to depolarizing and NDMR. (Decrease dose.)

I. Intracranial Hypertension

DEFINITION
The cranial cavity has three intracranial constituents: blood, brain tissue, and cerebrospinal fluid. Intracranial elastance is reduced when one of these three constituents are affected. As a result, intracranial pressure (ICP) rises so that an ICP of 20 to 25 mm Hg is the threshold for intracranial hypertension. Intervention should then be instituted. The rigid, bony skull allows little room for the brain, cerebrospinal fluid, or the cerebral blood volume to expand. Since these constituents are essentially incompressible, a volume change in any singular compartment requires a reciprocal change in the volume of one or both of the remaining compartments if the ICP is to remain normal.

ETIOLOGY
Head injury, stroke, intracranial hemorrhage, infection, tumor formation, post-ischemia or post-hypoxic states, hydrocephalus, osmolar imbalances, and pulmonary disease can all cause increases in ICP. As ICP progressively increases, cerebral perfusion pressure (CPP) is diminished, and focal ischemia occurs. If ICP is already high, even small increases in intracranial volumes result in marked intracranial hypertension and global ischemia. When space-occupying lesions are present, intracranial tissue shifts and localized pressure gradients develop, causing vascular compression and regional ischemia.

LABORATORY RESULTS

MRI and CT scan are the two most prominent tests to evaluate tumors, hemorrhage, stroke, and areas of ischemia. Lumbar puncture is used to diagnose infections and hydrocephalus.

CLINICAL MANIFESTATIONS

Symptoms of increased ICP include headache, nausea and vomiting, mental changes, and disturbances in consciousness and vision. During the early stages of intracranial hypertension, symptoms are most common in the early morning hours. Increased $PaCO_2$ and the associated cerebral vasodilation that occurs during sleep may produce an increase in intracranial contents that exceeds the limits of compensation, and ICP increases. Progressive increases in ICP eventually result in unexplained fatigue and drowsiness. Papilledema may be seen, which is accompanied by visual disturbances. A first-time seizure in an adult with no apparent cause should arouse suspicion of increased ICP. Systemic blood pressure may be elevated in order to maintain cerebral perfusion pressure in the presence of intracranial hypertension (i.e., CPP = MAP – ICP where *cerebral perfusion pressure = mean arterial pressure* to *intracranial pressure*).

TREATMENT

Patients with intracranial hypertension or reduced intracranial elastance can be managed using various interventions. All are based on the concept that ICP can be reduced or intracranial elastance can be improved by reducing one of the three intracranial constituents. See specific interventions below, under Anesthetic Considerations.

ANESTHETIC CONSIDERATIONS

Cerebral blood volume can be manipulated in various ways. Endotracheal intubation will allow prompt management of those conditions that might increase cerebral blood flow (CBF) and consequently increase ICP, related to hypoxemia and hypercarbia. Neuromuscular blockade will often prevent increases in cerebral venous volume (and ICP) that result from coughing, straining, or actively exhaling. Cerebral venous drainage is facilitated by elevating the head of the bed, however, this maneuver may also decrease venous return, and cardiac output (i.e., mean arterial blood pressure), thereby reducing cerebral perfusion pressure. Appropriate analgesia and sedation prevent increases in the cerebral metabolic rate of oxygen ($CMRO_2$) and any increases in CBF. Hyperventilation acutely reduces CBF, although CBF usually returns to its original level even with prolonged hyperventilation. Barbiturates in sufficient doses suppress both the $CMRO_2$ and CBF in association with profound EEG suppression. Caution should be used when barbiturate therapy is implemented because of concomitant vasodilation and myocardial depression. Brain tissue volume is usually reduced by diuresis. Osmotic diuresis with mannitol reduces brain water. Mannitol can be used as a continuous infusion or as treatment for acute episodes of increased ICP. Maximum reduction of ICP is accomplished with large doses of mannitol administered rapidly, then followed by furosemide. When a patient emerges from anesthesia, increased ICP caused by any coughing or bucking (especially on the endotracheal tube) must be considered.

Extubation while the patient is still anesthetized and/or the concomitant use of IV lidocaine are possible ways to ameliorate these potential problems.

PROGNOSIS

Quick and appropriate management to reduce ICP leads to a full recovery for most patients.

J. Autonomic Dysreflexia

DEFINITION

Autonomic dysreflexia (or autonomic hyperreflexia) is a disorder that appears after resolution of spinal shock.

INCIDENCE AND PREVALENCE

The incidence and prevalence depend on the level of spinal cord transection. About 85% of patients with spinal cord transection above T6 may exhibit this syndrome. Autonomic dysreflexia is unlikely to be associated with a cord transection below T10. The stimulation of a surgical procedure; however, is a potent trigger of autonomic dysreflexia, even in patients with no previous history of this response.

ETIOLOGY

Autonomic dysreflexia can be initiated by cutaneous or visceral stimulation below the level of spinal cord transection. Distention of a hollow viscus (bladder or rectum) is a common stimulus. This stimulus initiates afferent impulses that enter the spinal cord below that level. These impulses elicit reflex sympathetic activity over the splanchnic outflow tract. This outflow is isolated from inhibitory impulses such that generalized vasoconstriction persists below the level of injury. Vasoconstriction results in increased blood pressure, which is then perceived by the carotid sinus. Subsequent activation of the carotid sinus results in decreased efferent outflow from the sympathetic nervous system. Activity from the CNS is manifested as a predominance of parasympathetic nervous system activity at the heart and peripheral vasculature. This predominance cannot be produced below the level of spinal cord transection (this part of the body remains neurologically isolated). Therefore vasoconstriction persists below the level of spinal cord transection. If spinal cord transection is above the level of splanchnic outflow (T4 to T6), vasodilation in the neurologically intact portion of the body is insufficient to offset the effects of vasoconstriction (reflected by persistent hypertension).

LABORATORY RESULTS

None.

CLINICAL MANIFESTATIONS

The hallmark symptoms of autonomic dysreflexia are hypertension and bradycardia, which result from stimulation of the carotid sinus and cutaneous vasodilation above the level of spinal cord transection. Hypertension persists because vasodilation cannot occur below the level of injury. Nasal stuffiness reflects vasodilation. Other symptoms may include headache, blurred vision (due to hypertension), increased operative blood loss, loss of consciousness, seizures, cardiac arrhythmias, and pulmonary edema.

TREATMENT

Treatment includes ganglionic blockers (trimethaphan, pentolinium), alpha-adrenergic antagonists (phentolamine, phenoxybenzamine), and direct-acting vasodilators (nitroprusside). General or regional anesthesia can be used. Drugs that lower blood pressure by central action alone are not predictably effective.

ANESTHETIC CONSIDERATIONS

Airway control and ventilation with large tidal volumes (10 to 15 mL/kg) are necessary to avoid hypercarbia and atelectasis. Special care should be taken when moving patients with chronic spinal cord injury. Preoperative hydration helps prevent hypotension during induction and aids in maintenance of anesthesia. Prevention of autonomic hyperreflexia is key in the treatment of autonomic dysreflexia. Use NDMR to facilitate intubation and prevent reflex skeletal muscle spasms. Avoid using succinylcholine. Have nitroprusside and other cardioactive agents readily available to treat precipitous hypertension.

PROGNOSIS

Autonomic dysreflexia is a chronic, lifelong potential condition of spinal cord transection patients.

K. Spinal Cord Injury

DEFINITION

The spinal cord is vulnerable to trauma, compression by intradural or extradural tumors, and vascular injuries.

INCIDENCE AND PREVALENCE

Approximately 10,000 persons suffer acute spinal cord injuries each year that result in paraplegia and quadriplegia. Two thirds are male, and 70% to 80% are ages 11 to 30. The mortality rate before reaching the hospital is 30% to 40%; the mortality rate during the first year decreases to 10%.

ETIOLOGY

Spinal cord injuries result from motor vehicle accidents, falls, sport injuries (especially diving), and penetrating injuries (especially gunshot wounds). The spinal cord itself is not usually severed but is injured by compression from bone, foreign body, hematoma, edema, and ischemia.

DIAGNOSTIC AND LABORATORY RESULTS

A clinical examination is needed.

CLINICAL MANIFESTATIONS

Clinical manifestations include changes in cardiopulmonary responses, fluids and electrolytes, temperature control function, and abnormal responses to drugs. Injuries at levels T2 to T12 cause paraplegia but leave the upper extremities and diaphragm intact. Injuries at levels C5 to T1 cause varying degrees of upper-extremity paralysis as well.

TREATMENT

For acute injury, the ABCs of resuscitation are used (i.e., A = airway, B = breathing, C = circulation). Avoid neck motion and subsequent further cord damage. Maintain spinal cord perfusion with volume and vasoactive drugs. If the spinal cord is compressed by bone or hematoma, decompression is necessary.

ANESTHETIC CONSIDERATIONS

Cervical ("halo") traction sometimes necessitates fundamental changes in airway management of the patient with a cervical spine injury. An assistant may be needed to help maintain neck immobility during laryngoscopy/intubation. Alternative techniques for securing the airway (e.g., fiberoptic intubation) are sometimes necessary. Nasal intubation is contraindicated in the presence of basilar skull fracture. Be prepared for emergent cricothyroidotomy, if necessary. Use anticholinergic agents to reduce secretions. Ventilate the patient with large tidal volumes (10 to 15 mL/kg) to avoid hypercarbia and atelectasis. Move the patient carefully to prevent injury to the limbs and trunk. Check pressure areas to prevent breakdown. Some cardioacceleration and vasoconstrictor tone is lost as a result of cord injuries that involve levels T1 to T4. Spinal cord shock is present. Respiratory compromise is possible, depending on the level of spinal injury. Maintain spinal cord perfusion with volume and vasoactive agents.

PROGNOSIS

Spinal cord injury is a chronic condition that will require management for life.

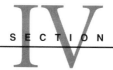

Musculoskeletal System

A. Muscular Dystrophy

DEFINITION

Muscular dystrophy is a hereditary disease characterized by painless degeneration and atrophy of skeletal muscles. There is progressive, symmetric skeletal muscle weakness and wasting but no clinical evidence of muscle denervation, as reflexes and sensations remain intact. Mental retardation is often present. Increased permeability of skeletal muscle membranes precedes clinical evidence of the disease. The most common and severe form of the disease is categorized as pseudohypertrophic (Duchenne's) muscular dystrophy. Other less common forms include limb-girdle, facioscapulohumeral (Landouzy-Dejerine), nemaline rod myopathy, and oculopharyngeal dystrophy.

ETIOLOGY

Pseudohypertrophic muscular dystrophy occurs in 3 of every 10,000 births. It is caused by an X-linked recessive gene and becomes apparent in males aged 2 to 5 years.

CLINICAL MANIFESTATIONS

Initially, symptoms such as waddling gait, frequent falling, and difficulty climbing stairs reflect involvement of the proximal skeletal groups of the pelvis. Affected skeletal muscle may become larger as a result of fatty infiltration, accounting for the designation of this disorder as pseudohypertrophic. Steady deterioration of skeletal muscle strength results in confinement to a wheelchair by 8 to 11 years of age. Kyphoscoliosis may develop, which reflects the unopposed actions of the antagonists of the dystrophic muscles. Skeletal muscle atrophy can predispose to long bone fractures from trauma. Degeneration of cardiac muscle invariably accompanies muscular dystrophy, and thus congestive heart failure is common. Characteristic ECG findings include a tall R wave in lead V_1, a deep Q wave in limb leads, a short P-R interval, and sinus tachycardia. Mitral regurgitation may be due to papillary muscle dysfunction and decreased myocardial contractility.

Chronic weakness of inspiratory respiratory muscles and a decreased ability to cough can result in loss of pulmonary reserve and an accumulation of secretions, predisposing to pneumonia. Respiratory insufficiency often remains covert because impaired skeletal muscle function prevents patients from exceeding their limited breathing capacity. With further progression of the disease, kyphoscoliosis can contribute further to a restrictive pattern of lung disease. Sleep apnea is possible and may contribute to pulmonary hypertension.

LABORATORY RESULTS

Laboratory findings include a serum creatine kinase level that is 30 to 300 times normal, even early in the disease, reflecting skeletal muscle necrosis and the increased permeability of skeletal muscle membranes. Creatine kinase concentration is elevated in approximately 70% of female carriers. Skeletal muscle biopsy early in the course of the disease may demonstrate necrosis and phagocytosis of muscle fibers.

ANESTHETIC CONSIDERATIONS

Anesthetic considerations for the patient with pseudohypertrophic muscular dystrophy must account for the increased permeability of skeletal muscle membranes and decreased cardiopulmonary reserve. Succinylcholine may be associated with exaggerated potassium release, leading to life-threatening cardiac arrhythmias. Ventricular fibrillation occurring after induction of anesthesia with succinylcholine has been observed in patients later discovered to have pseudohypertrophic muscular dystrophy. Responses to nondepolarizing muscle relaxants usually are normal, but the possibility of a prolonged response should be considered when coexisting skeletal muscle weakness is prominent. Dantrolene sodium (Dantrium) should be available because of the increased incidence of malignant hyperthermia in these patients. Malignant hyperthermia has been observed after only a brief period of halothane administration alone, although most cases were triggered by succinylcholine or with prolonged inhalation of halothane. Hypomotility of the gastrointestinal tract may delay gastric emptying, which in the presence of weak laryngeal reflexes, increases the risk of regurgitation and aspiration. Depressant effects of volatile anesthetics on myocardial contractility can be exaggerated. Cardiac arrest after induction of anesthesia has been reported in afflicted patients. Monitoring should be directed at early detection of malignant hyperthermia (capnography, temperature) and cardiac depression. Postoperative pulmonary dysfunction must be anticipated and clearance of secretions must be facilitated. Delayed pulmonary insufficiency may occur up to 36 hours postoperatively, despite apparent recovery to the preoperative level of skeletal muscle strength.

TREATMENT

Regional anesthesia avoids many of the unique risks of general anesthesia in these patients; during the postoperative period it provides analgesia, which may facilitate chest physiotherapy.

PROGNOSIS

Muscular dystrophy requires chronic, life-long management.

PART 1 **Common Diseases**

B. Kyphoscoliosis

DEFINITION

Kyphoscoliosis is a deformity of the costovertebral skeletal structures that is characterized by anterior flexion (kyphosis) and lateral curvature (scoliosis) of the vertebral column.

ETIOLOGY

The incidence of idiopathic kyphoscoliosis is about 4 in 1000. The disease seems to have a familial predisposition, with females being affected about 4 times more often than males.

A vertebral column curve of greater than 40 degrees is considered severe and is most likely associated with physiologic alterations in cardiopulmonary function. Restrictive lung disease and pulmonary hypertension progressing to cor pulmonale are the principal causes of mortality in patients with kyphoscoliosis. As the scoliotic curve worsens, more lung tissue is compressed, resulting in decreased vital capacity and dyspnea with mild exertion. Work of breathing is increased by abnormal mechanical properties of the thorax and by increased airway resistance resulting from small lung volumes. The alveolar to arteriolar difference for oxygen is increased. The arterial carbon dioxide pressure ($PaCO_2$) is usually normal, but relatively minor insults such as bacterial or viral upper respiratory tract infections may result in acute respiratory failure. A poor cough reflex contributes to frequent pulmonary infections. Pulmonary hypertension reflects increased pulmonary vascular resistance due to compression of lung vasculature by the curve in the spine and the pulmonary vascular response to arterial hypoxemia.

ANESTHETIC CONSIDERATIONS

Anesthetic management of these patients should begin with a thorough preoperative assessment of the physiologic derangements produced by the skeletal deformity. Pulmonary function tests (PFT), specifically vital capacity and FEV_1, will reflect the magnitude of restrictive lung disease. ABGs are helpful in detecting unrecognized arterial hypoxemia or acidosis that could be contributing to pulmonary hypertension. These patients may enter the preoperative period with pneumonia due to chronic aspiration of gastric fluid. Any reversible components of pulmonary dysfunction, such as infections or bronchospasm, should be corrected before elective surgery is performed. Preoperative medication should be administered judiciously because of the narrow margin of safety in these patients (decreased ventilatory reserve) and the adverse effects on the pulmonary vascular resistance that would occur with respiratory acidosis from hypoventilation. Intraoperatively, controlled ventilation will facilitate adequate arterial oxygenation and elimination of CO_2. N_2O should be used with caution because it may increase pulmonary vascular resistance. Arterial oxygen saturation should be monitored continuously to ensure adequacy of oxygenation/ventilation. CVP measurements may provide an early warning of increased pulmonary vascular resistance produced by nitrous oxide. It has been suggested that these patients have an increased incidence of malignant hyperthermia, so vigilant monitoring of end-tidal carbon dioxide and temperature is recommended.

C. Malignant Hyperthermia

DEFINITION

Malignant hyperthermia is a hypermetabolic disorder of the skeletal muscle that is triggered by anesthetic agents.

INCIDENCE AND PREVALENCE

This disorder is relatively rare, affecting approximately 1 in 50,000 adults and 1 in 15,000 children. A genetic component seems to be related to the incidence of malignant hyperthermia. The incidence increases when succinylcholine (itself a triggering agent) is used with other triggering agents. Thus, triggering agents include succinylcholine, all inhalational anesthetic agents (except nitrous oxide), and potassium salts. Additional agents that may trigger malignant hyperthermia are curare and phenothiazine. Malignant hyperthermia has been found to be associated with other muscle disorders, such as Duchenne's muscular dystrophy.

ETIOLOGY

The precise etiology of malignant hyperthermia is not well understood; however, it is thought that a defect in calcium metabolism in the sarcoplasm leads to high concentrations. The high concentration of calcium allows for sustained muscle contraction. Accelerated metabolism associated with the sustained contractions is accompanied by acidosis and heat production. There is a depletion of adenosine triphosphate, acidosis, cell membrane destruction, and cell death.

LABORATORY RESULTS

The definitive diagnosis of malignant hyperthermia is made by muscle biopsy and in vitro isometric contracture testing in the presence of caffeine, halothane, or both. Although not definitive, creatinine kinase tests should be performed on patients considered susceptible to malignant hyperthermia. Elevated resting levels of creatine kinase are found in about 70% of patients susceptible to malignant hyperthermia. Other laboratory findings consistent with malignant hyperthermia crisis are carbon dioxide partial pressure (PCO_2) greater than 46 mm Hg; elevated lactate, potassium, and creatine phosphokinase levels; and pH less than 7.28.

CLINICAL MANIFESTATIONS

Clinical findings related to hypermetabolism may vary. Common findings are hypercarbia, tachycardia, hypoxemia, metabolic and respiratory acidosis, tachypnea, hyperkalemia, arrhythmias, hypotension, flushing, cyanosis, mottling, extreme increases in body temperature, sweating, tea-colored urine, and muscle rigidity. The earliest clinical sign is increased end-tidal carbon dioxide, followed by tachycardia. If untreated, malignant hyperthermia produces late signs of renal failure, disseminated intravascular coagulation, pulmonary edema, blindness, seizures, paralysis, and coma.

TREATMENT

A treatment protocol for malignant hyperthermia is outlined below:

1. Inform the surgeon and request termination of the surgery, if possible.
2. Discontinue administration of all inhalation anesthetics and succinylcholine; hyperventilate the patient with 100% oxygen at high flow rates; monitor end-tidal carbon dioxide.
3. Enlist the help of additional anesthesia and operating room staff; have a malignant hyperthermia cart brought to the operating room.
4. Reconstitute dantrolene sodium with sterile water; administer IV dantrolene sodium in 2.5 mg/kg boluses until signs of malignant hyperthermia abate.
5. Draw arterial blood gases; treat acidosis with sodium bicarbonate, with dose increases in 1 to 2 mEq/kg increments, or as guided by ABGs. Draw serum for electrolytes, creatine kinase, myoglobin, glucose, and coagulation studies.
6. Treat hyperkalemia with an infusion of 10 units of regular insulin in 50 mL of 50% glucose.
7. Insert a three-way Foley catheter and obtain urine samples for myoglobin level determination; attempt to maintain a urine output of greater than 2 mL/kg/hr by giving intravenous fluids, mannitol, and/or furosemide.
8. Initiate aggressive cooling as indicated by the patient's core temperature.
9. Treat persistent or life-threatening arrhythmias with standard antiarrhythmic agents; Ca^{2+} channel blockers should not be used.
10. After the malignant hyperthermia event, the patient should be monitored for at least 24 hours in an intensive care unit.

The Malignant Hyperthermia Association of the United States (MHAUS) Malignant Hyperthermia Hotline consultant may be contacted for expert medical advice. The malignant hyperthermia event should be reported to the North American Malignant Hyperthermia Registry.

ANESTHETIC CONSIDERATIONS

A detailed anesthesia history is imperative. If the patient or family has a history of malignant hyperthermia, all triggering agents should be avoided. The anesthesia machine vaporizers should be removed and the circuit and carbon dioxide absorber canisters should be changed. The machine should be flushed with oxygen (10 L/min) for 10 to 20 minutes prior to surgery. The patient should be well sedated. Consider administering dantrium preoperatively (do not use phenothiazine). If malignant hyperthermia is diagnosed, patient and family counseling and education is necessary.

PROGNOSIS

The overall mortality rate is 10%. Without the use of dantrium, the mortality rate climbs to 70%. Early treatment may decrease the mortality rate to approximately 5%.

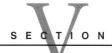

S E C T I O N

Endocrine System

A. Diabetes Mellitus

DEFINITION

Diabetes mellitus is a chronic systemic disease characterized by a broad array of abnormalities, the most notable of which is disturbed glucose metabolism, resulting in inappropriate hyperglycemia.

ETIOLOGY

About 5.5 million people in the United States have diabetes mellitus. Diabetes is divided into two categories, insulin-dependent diabetes mellitus (IDDM) and non-insulin-dependent diabetes mellitus (NIDDM).

IDDM typically develops before the age of 16 and evidence points to a genetic predisposition to the disease. Resulting from autoimmune destruction of pancreatic beta cells, IDDM may be precipitated by a viral infection. About 15% of these individuals have other autoimmune diseases such as hypothyroidism, Graves' disease, Addison's disease, or myasthenia gravis. The genetic predisposition is more of a reflection of susceptibility to the disease, rather than its inheritance. These patients depend on exogenous insulin to prevent ketoacidosis.

The other form of diabetes, NIDDM (or adult-onset diabetes), most often develops after the age of 35 and evidence suggests a genetic predisposition. The prevalence increases with age, particularly among black females. While many of these individuals may require insulin therapy, they are not usually prone to ketoacidosis. Nevertheless, NIDDM may progress to the extent that insulin is needed to prevent ketoacidosis. Patients with NIDDM, who are typically overweight, constitute 90% of all diabetics. Obese nondiabetics require 2 to 5 times more insulin than do nonobese nondiabetics; thus, obesity may unmask latent diabetics.

Complications from diabetes are numerous. The most serious acute metabolic complication is ketoacidosis, defined as hyperglycemia in the presence of metabolic acidosis. The symptoms include nausea, vomiting, lethargy, and signs of hypovolemia due to dehydration, which is due to the osmotic effect of glucose. Causes of ketoacidosis include poor patient compliance with their insulin therapy, insulin resistance because of infection, and silent myocardial infarction. Administration of a $beta_2$ agonist to inhibit labor in the presence of IDDM has been reported to abruptly precipitate ketoacidosis, even with prior subcutaneous insulin administration. Complications of prolonged diabetes include macroangiopathies such as

75

coronary artery disease, cerebrovascular disease, and peripheral vascular disease. These complications are more common in the patient with NIDDM; sequelae such as premature myocardial infarction, angina pectoris, or peripheral vascular insufficiency often are the presenting symptoms in an undiagnosed diabetic. However, in the IDDM patient, microvascular complications and disorders of the nervous system predominate. Retinopathy, nephropathy, and autonomic and peripheral nervous system neuropathies are common. Diabetic retinopathy occurs in 80% to 90% of those with IDDM for longer than 20 years. Autonomic nervous system dysfunction may affect more than 15% of patients with diabetes. Delayed wound healing and postoperative infection are more likely in these patients. Stiff joint syndrome affects 30% to 40% of patients with IDDM and often affects all joints. Most important to anesthesia, the atlanto-occipital joint may be involved, making hyperextension of the head and subsequently, laryngoscopy, difficult.

TREATMENT

Treatment includes a diabetic diet, oral hypoglycemic drugs, and exogenous insulin. NIDDM is prevented primarily by avoidance or treatment of obesity. Transplantation of pancreatic tissue may be considered in selected patients.

ANESTHETIC CONSIDERATIONS

Anesthetic goals in the diabetic patient undergoing anesthesia/surgery are to mimic normal metabolism as closely as possible by avoiding hypoglycemia, excessive hyperglycemia, ketoacidosis, and electrolyte disturbances. Hypoglycemia is prevented by ensuring an adequate supply of exogenous glucose. Hyperglycemia and associated ketoacidosis, dehydration, and electrolyte abnormalities are prevented by the administration of insulin. The goal of blood glucose control is to maintain a level well above that considered hypoglycemic but below the level at which deleterious effects of hyperglycemia (hyperosmolarity, osmotic diuresis, electrolyte disturbances, impaired phagocyte function, impaired wound healing) become evident. Blood glucose concentration should be kept between 120 and 180 mg-dL^{-1}. Along with the careful preoperative, intraoperative, and postoperative monitoring of the blood glucose and electrolytes, thorough preoperative evaluation should determine whether other systems, such as cardiac, neurologic, and renal systems, are involved. Appropriate preoperative laboratory work and intraoperative monitoring should be directed at these complications.

B. Diabetes Insipidus

DEFINITION

Diabetes insipidus (DI) reflects the absence of antidiuretic hormone owing to the destruction of the posterior pituitary (neurogenic DI) or failure of the renal tubules to respond to antidiuretic hormone (nephrogenic DI).

ETIOLOGY

Neurogenic DI can be caused by intracranial trauma, hypophysectomy, neoplastic invasion, or sarcoidosis. Nephrogenic DI can be caused by hypokalemia, hypercalcemia, sickle cell anemia, obstructive uropathy, chronic renal insufficiency, or chronic use of lithium.

CLINICAL MANIFESTATIONS

Clinical features include polydipsia and polyuria with poorly concentrated urine despite increased plasma osmolarity. Neurogenic and nephrogenic DI are differentiated on the basis of response to desmopressin, which produces concentration of the urine in neurogenic, but not nephrogenic, DI.

TREATMENT

Treatment includes careful monitoring of urine output, plasma volume, and plasma osmolarity. Isotonic fluids may be administered until osmolarity is greater than 290; then hypotonic fluids are necessary. Neurogenic DI may be treated with desmopressin at 3 mg/kg. Nephrogenic DI may be treated with chlorpropamide, an oral hypoglycemic drug that potentiates the effect of antidiuretic hormone on renal tubules.

ANESTHETIC CONSIDERATIONS

Anesthetic management for the patient with DI should include monitoring urine output and plasma electrolyte concentrations during the perioperative period. If emergent surgery is needed, central venous pressure monitoring may aid in the evaluation of volume status.

C. Thyroid Disease

DEFINITION

Thyroid disease is the misregulation of thyroid hormone. Thyroid hormone is one of major regulators of cellular metabolic activity, altering the speed of reactions, total oxygen consumption, and heat production of the body.

ETIOLOGY

Thyroid-stimulating hormone (TSH) is released from the anterior pituitary, causing iodine to be taken up into the thyroid gland. The iodine is then incorporated into tyrosine residues, and the hormones triiodothyronine (T_3) and thyroxine (T_4) are formed and stored. Peripheral tissues convert T_4 to T_3, which is 3 times more potent than T_4 and has a shorter half-life. Both T_4 and T_3 are partially bound to the plasma protein thyroid-binding globulin (TBG), although only the unbound forms are pharmacologically active. TBG levels can increase with acute liver disease, pregnancy, acute intermittent porphyria, and medications (oral hypoglycemics, exogenous estrogens, clofibrate, opioids). They can decrease with chronic liver disease, nephrotic syndrome, anabolic steroids, and acromegaly. TBG has no direct role in cell metabolism but its concentration can alter diagnostic test results when checking for thyroid disease.

HYPERTHYROIDISM

Hyperthyroidism is an increase in thyroid function resulting from an excess supply of thyroid hormones and is associated with Graves' disease, TSH over-production, and pregnancy. In subacute thyroiditis, excess thyroid hormone leaks out of the gland owing to inflammation. Ovarian tumors or metastatic thyroid carcinoma may also produce extrathyroid gland hormone. Exogenous consumption of thyroid hormone can also lead to hyperthyroidism.

LABORATORY RESULTS

Laboratory findings in hyperthyroidism include elevated levels of T_3 and T_4. Because TBG concentration may affect the measured T_4, a resin T_3 uptake test may be performed to distinguish between protein-binding abnormalities and true metabolic changes associated with hyperthyroidism. TSH levels may be normal or decreased.

CLINICAL MANIFESTATIONS

Clinically, hyperthyroid patients present with nervousness, tachycardia, goi-ter, tremors, muscle weakness, heat intolerance, and weight loss despite high caloric intake. Exophthalmos occurs in approximately 7 of 10 cases of hyperthyroidism. Worsening of angina pectoris or unexpected onset of con-gestive heart failure or atrial fibrillation may reflect undiagnosed hyperthy-roidism, especially in elderly patients in whom the increased amount of thyroid hormones is sufficient only to aggravate underlying heart disease.

Thyroid storm (thyrotoxicosis) is an abrupt exacerbation of hyperthy-roidism caused by the sudden excessive release of thyroid gland hormones into the circulation. Hyperthermia, tachycardia, congestive heart failure, dehydration, and shock commonly occur. Thyroid storm may be precipi-tated by surgical stress but is usually seen 6 to 18 hours postoperatively. It may mimic malignant hyperthermia, sepsis, hemorrhage, or a transfu-sion/drug reaction.

TREATMENT

Treatments for hyperthyroidism include antithyroid drugs, subtotal thy-roidectomy, or radioactive iodine. Thyroid storm therapy includes active cooling, hydrating beta-adrenergic blockade, use of steroids if there is any indication of adrenal insufficiency, and institution of long-term therapy with antithyroid drugs or iodine. Six weeks are required to become euthy-roid. Only emergency surgery should be performed in thyrotoxic patients. Premedication, including β-blockers, should be given generously. Sympathetic stimulation (pain, ketamine, pancuronium) should be avoided. Eyes should be protected well, especially if exophthalmos is pres-ent. Drug metabolism and anesthetic requirements are increased. Because of muscle weakness, muscle relaxants should be titrated carefully. Hypotension should be treated with direct-acting agents, such as phenyle-phrine. Regional anesthesia may be beneficial in thyrotoxic patients because it blocks the sympathetic response. Local anesthetics with epinephrine may lead to further arrhythmias.

HYPOTHYROIDISM

Hypothyroidism can be classified as either *primary* (because of destruction of the thyroid gland, where there is an adequate level of TSH), or *secondary* (because of central nervous system dysfunction leading to decreased levels of TSH). Causes of primary hypothyroidism include chronic thyroiditis, subtotal thyroidectomy, radioactive iodine therapy, and irradiation of the neck. Thyroid hormone deficiency may occur because of antithyroid drugs, excess iodide, or a dietary iodine deficiency. Causes of secondary hypothyroidism include hypothalamic dysfunction (leading to thyrotropin-releasing hormone deficiency) and anterior pituitary dysfunction (leading to TSH deficiency).

LABORATORY RESULTS

Laboratory findings in primary hypothyroidism include decreased levels of T_3 and T_4, with an increased concentration of TSH. Secondary hypothyroidism exhibits decreased levels of T_3, T_4, and TSH. Resin T_3 uptake is decreased in both incidences.

CLINICAL MANIFESTATIONS

Onset of clinical symptoms in the adult patient is insidious and may go unrecognized. Patients experience lethargy, constipation, cold intolerance, facial edema with an enlarged tongue, a reversible cardiomyopathy, pericardial effusion, ascites, anemia, and an adynamic ileus with delayed gastric emptying. There may be adrenal atrophy with decreased cortisol production, dilutional hyponatremia, and decreased water excretion. There is a decreased cardiac output, bradycardia, hypovolemia, and diminished baroreceptor reflexes. Myxedema coma (profound hypothyroidism) may be triggered by trauma, infection, and CNS depressants, leading to respiratory depression, congestive heart failure, and depressed consciousness.

TREATMENT

Treatment for hypothyroidism involves the exogenous supplementation of thyroid hormone. T_4 requires 10 days to have an effect. T_3 begins to have an effect in 6 hours. Treatment for myxedema coma includes intravenous administration of T_3, and, if adrenal insufficiency is suspected, cortisol. Digitalis should be used sparingly to treat congestive heart failure because the drug increases myocardial contractility, and this is not well tolerated by patients with hypothyroidism. Fluid replacement is important, since these patients may be vulnerable to water intoxication and hyponatremia.

Elective surgery must be postponed in any patient who is clinically hypothyroid. In patients with hypothyroidism who must undergo emergency procedures, anesthetic considerations should include avoidance of preoperative sedation because of profound CNS and respiratory sensitivity to depressants. Cortisol supplementation should be considered, intravascular volume should be optimized, and anemia should be corrected. Anesthetic techniques must take into consideration airway problems associated with a large tongue, poor gastric emptying, and increased sensitivity to all depressant medications.

D. Cushing's Disease

DEFINITION
Cushing's disease (hyperadrenocorticism) may reflect overproduction of adrenocorticotropic hormone by the anterior pituitary (about two thirds of cases), ectopic production of adrenocorticotropic hormone by malignant tumors (especially carcinoma of the lung, kidney, or pancreas), excess production of cortisol by a benign or malignant tumor of the adrenal cortex, or exogenous (pharmacologic) administration of cortisol or related drugs.

LABORATORY RESULTS
Diagnosis is best made by measurement of plasma cortisol in the morning after a midnight dose of dexamethasone. Dexamethasone suppresses plasma cortisol concentration in normal patients but not in patients with Cushing's disease. Magnetic resonance imaging for pituitary tumors and computed tomography showing large adrenal glands are also used for diagnosis.

CLINICAL MANIFESTATIONS
Signs and symptoms include hypertension, hypokalemia, hyperglycemia, skeletal muscle weakness, osteoporosis, obesity, hirsutism, menstrual disturbances, poor wound healing, and susceptibility to infection.

TREATMENT
Transsphenoidal microadenomectomy is the preferred treatment for hyperadrenocorticism owing to excess secretion of adrenocorticotropic hormone by the anterior pituitary.

ANESTHETIC CONSIDERATIONS
Anesthetic management should account for the effects of excess cortisol secretion, especially as reflected in blood pressure, electrolyte balance, and blood glucose concentration. Osteoporosis is a consideration in positioning for the operative procedure. Plasma cortisol concentration decreases promptly after microadenomectomy or bilateral adrenalectomy. Intraoperative replacement therapy (cortisol, 100 mg IV) should be initiated.

E. Addison's Disease

DEFINITION
Primary adrenal insufficiency (Addison's disease) reflects the absence of cortisol and aldosterone owing to the destruction of the adrenal cortex. The most common cause is adrenal hemorrhage in the patient in whom coagulation is hindered, but insufficiency can also develop as a result of sepsis or accidental or surgical trauma.

Diagnosis of hypoadrenocorticism requires measurement of the plasma cortisol concentration within 1 hour of administration of adrenocorticotropic hormone.

CLINICAL MANIFESTATIONS

Symptoms of primary adrenal insufficiency include weight loss, anorexia, nausea, vomiting, skeletal muscle weakness, abdominal pain, diarrhea or constipation, and hyperpigmentation over palmar surfaces and pressure points.

LABORATORY RESULTS

Laboratory findings include hyperkalemia and hypoglycemia. Lack of catecholamines may result in hypotension, which is often indistinguishable from shock due to loss of intravascular fluid volume.

TREATMENT

Treatment for primary adrenal insufficiency entails both glucocorticoid and mineralocorticoid replacement. Acute adrenal insufficiency (Addisonian crisis) is a medical emergency, and treatment includes fluids, steroid replacement, inotropes as necessary, and electrolyte correction.

ANESTHETIC CONSIDERATIONS

Anesthetic management for patients with primary adrenal insufficiency should provide for exogenous corticosteroid supplementation. Etomidate should be avoided because it transiently inhibits synthesis of cortisol in normal patients. Doses of anesthetic drugs should be minimized since these patients may be sensitive to drug-induced myocardial depression. Invasive monitoring (arterial line and pulmonary artery catheter) is indicated. Because of skeletal muscle weakness, the initial dose of muscle relaxant should be reduced, and further doses should be governed by peripheral nerve stimulator response. Plasma concentrations of glucose and electrolytes should be measured frequently during surgery.

F. Acromegaly

DEFINITION

Acromegaly is due to excessive secretion of growth hormone in an adult, most often from an adenoma in the anterior pituitary gland. Failure of plasma growth hormone concentration to decrease 1 to 2 hours after the ingestion of 75 to 100 g of glucose is presumptive evidence of acromegaly, as is a growth hormone concentration greater than 3 mg/L.

LABORATORY RESULTS

A skull x-ray and CT scan are useful in detecting enlargement of the sella turcica, which is characteristic of an anterior pituitary adenoma.

CLINICAL MANIFESTATIONS

Clinical manifestations reflect parasellar extension of the anterior pituitary adenoma and peripheral effects produced by excess growth hormone.

An enlarged sella turcica, headaches, visual field defects, and rhinorrhea may occur with parasellar extension. Excess growth hormone is reflected by skeletal overgrowth (prognathism), soft tissue overgrowth (lips, tongue, epiglottis, vocal cords), connective tissue overgrowth (recurrent laryngeal nerve paralysis), peripheral neuropathy (carpal tunnel syndrome), visceromegaly, glucose intolerance, osteoarthritis, osteoporosis, hyperhidrosis, and skeletal muscle weakness.

TREATMENT

Treatment is trans-sphenoidal surgical excision of the pituitary adenoma. If the adenoma extends beyond the sella turcica, surgery or irradiation is no longer feasible, and medical treatment with bromocriptine may be an option.

ANESTHETIC CONSIDERATIONS

Anesthetic management must account for potentially difficult airway management and the possible need to insert a smaller-diameter tracheal tube. Awake intubation with or without a fiberoptic endoscope may be necessary. If diabetes mellitus is present, the plasma glucose concentration should be monitored. An arterial line placed in the radial artery can lead to inadequate collateral circulation at the wrist, so Allen's test should be performed or an alternative site should be selected. Muscle relaxant use should be guided by peripheral nerve stimulation, especially in patients with a history of skeletal muscle weakness.

G. Pheochromocytoma

DEFINITION

Pheochromocytoma is a catecholamine-secreting tumor that originates in the adrenal medulla or in chromaffin tissue along the paravertebral sympathetic chain, extending from the pelvis to the base of the skull.

ETIOLOGY

Pheochromocytoma typically occurs in patients 30 to 50 years of age, although one-third of reported cases are in children, principally males. Pheochromocytoma may also be part of an autosomal dominant multiglandular neoplastic syndrome, a condition called multiple endocrine neoplasia. Less than 0.1% of patients with hypertension actually have pheochromocytoma; however, nearly 50% of deaths in patients with unsuspected pheochromocytoma occur during anesthesia and surgery or parturition. Pheochromocytoma and associated hypertension and hypermetabolism may mimic other diseases, including malignant hyperthermia.

LABORATORY RESULTS

Diagnosis requires chemical confirmation of excessive catecholamine release. Measurement of "free" norepinephrine from a 24-hour urine test is thought to be a more sensitive index of pheochromocytoma than measures of catecholamine metabolites (normetanephrine, metanephrine, vanillylmandelic acid). Normotension despite increased plasma concentration of catecholamines is thought to reflect a decrease in the number of α receptors (down-regulation) in response to increased circulating concentrations of the neurotransmitter. Clonidine (0.3 mg orally) suppresses the plasma concentration of catecholamines in hypertensive patients but not in patients with pheochromocytoma, reflecting the drug's ability to suppress increases in plasma catecholamine concentration resulting from neurogenic release but not from diffusion of excess catecholamine from a pheochromocytoma into the circulation. CT scan is the initial localizing procedure in the diagnosis of pheochromocytoma.

CLINICAL MANIFESTATIONS

The classic symptom of pheochromocytoma is paroxysmal hypertension. The triad of tachycardia, diaphoresis, and headache in a hypertensive patient is highly suggestive of pheochromocytoma. Conversely, absence of this triad virtually rules out the presence of pheochromocytoma. Tremulousness, palpitations, and weight loss are common, especially in young to middle-aged patients. Symptoms may last from minutes to several hours and are often followed by fatigue. Decreased intravascular fluid volume associated with sustained hypertension may manifest as orthostatic hypotension. A hematocrit greater than 45% may reflect hypovolemia caused by this mechanism. Death resulting from pheochromocytoma is often due to congestive heart failure, myocardial infarction, or intracerebral hemorrhage.

TREATMENT

Treatment consists of surgical excision of the catecholamine-secreting tumor only after medical control is optimized. α blockade (phentolamine, prazosin) should be instituted and blood pressure normalized prior to surgery. Return to normotension facilitates an increase in intravascular fluid volume as reflected by a decrease in the hematocrit. If cardiac arrhythmias or tachycardia persist after α blockade, β blockade is indicated in the absence of congestive heart failure.

ANESTHETIC CONSIDERATIONS

Anesthetic management for the patient requiring excision of a pheochromocytoma is based on administration of drugs that do not stimulate the sympathetic nervous system. α- and β-antagonist therapy should be continued. Invasive monitoring (A-line, PA catheter) should be inserted preoperatively. The depth of anesthesia should be adequate before laryngoscopy. This may be accomplished by IV induction of anesthesia followed by establishment of a surgical level of anesthesia with a volatile agent. Halothane should be avoided because of its propensity to produce cardiac arrhythmias in the presence of increased plasma catecholamine concentrations. Administration of lidocaine (1 to 2 mg/kg IV) 1 to 2 minutes before initiation of laryngoscopy may help in attenuating the hypertensive response to intubation and decrease the likelihood of cardiac arrhythmias. Furthermore, administration of short-acting opioids (fentanyl, 100 to 200 μg IV; sufentanil, 10 to 20 μg IV) before laryngoscopy may attenuate the pressor response. Nitroprusside and phentolamine should be readily available, should persistent hypertension accompany intubation of the trachea. If surgical paralysis is required, nondepolarizing muscle relaxants devoid of circulatory effects should be selected.

Anesthesia can be maintained with an inhalation agent and nitrous oxide. If hypertension persists despite high concentration of inhalational agent, nitroprusside, esmolol, lidocaine, and phentolamine can be used as needed. A decrease in blood pressure may accompany surgical ligation of the venous drainage of pheochromocytoma, which may be treated by decreasing the concentration of volatile agent, along with rapid infusion of crystalloids, colloids, or both. Rarely, intravenous infusion of phenylephrine or norepinephrine is required until the peripheral vasculature adapts to decreased levels of endogenous catecholamine. ABGs, electrolytes, and blood glucose levels should be monitored intraoperatively. Postoperatively, invasive monitoring should be continued and pain control should be maintained.

H. Hypoaldosteronism

DEFINITION
Hypoaldosteronism is suggested by hyperkalemia in the absence of renal insufficiency. Isolated deficiency of aldosterone secretion may reflect congenital deficiency of aldosterone synthetase or hyporeninemia due to a defect in the juxtaglomerular apparatus or treatment with an angiotensin-converting enzyme inhibitor leading to loss of angiotensin stimulation.

ETIOLOGY
Hyporeninemic hypoaldosteronism typically occurs in patients older than 45 years with chronic renal disease, diabetes mellitus, or both. Indomethacin-induced prostaglandin deficiency is a reversible cause of this syndrome.

CLINICAL MANIFESTATIONS
Symptoms include heart block secondary to hyperkalemia and postural hypotension with or without hyponatremia. Hyperchloremic metabolic acidosis is common.

TREATMENT
Treatment of hypoaldosteronism includes liberal sodium intake and daily administration of hydrocortisone.

ANESTHETIC CONSIDERATIONS
Begin anesthetic management with preoperative monitoring of the serum potassium level, which should be less than 5.5 mEq/L before elective surgery. ECG monitoring for effects of hyperkalemia (tall, tentlike T waves; heart block) is recommended. Hypoventilation should be avoided to prevent an additional increase in serum potassium. Succinylcholine should be avoided when possible to prevent potassium release. Intravenous fluids should be potassium-free. If hypovolemia is suspected, fluid replacement should be initiated, possibly governed by invasive (i.e., CVP) monitoring.

I. Hyperaldosteronism

DEFINITION

Primary hyperaldosteronism (Conn's syndrome) is excess secretion of aldosterone from a functional tumor independent of a physiologic stimulus. *Secondary* hyperaldosteronism is when increased renin secretion is responsible for the excess secretion of aldosterone.

ETIOLOGY

Hyperaldosteronism should be suspected in a patient with diastolic hypertension (100 to 125 mm Hg) and a plasma potassium concentration of less than 3.5 mEq/L. Hypertension reflects aldosterone-induced sodium retention and the resultant increased extracellular fluid volume. Hypokalemic metabolic acidosis is present secondary to aldosterone-induced renal excretion of potassium. Skeletal muscle weakness is presumed to reflect hypokalemia. Hypokalemia nephropathy can result in polyuria and the inability to concentrate urine optionally.

LABORATORY RESULTS

Diagnosis of hyperaldosteronism is confirmed by increased plasma concentration of aldosterone and increased urinary potassium excretion (greater than 30 mEq/L) despite coexisting hypokalemia. Measurement of plasma renin activity permits classification of the disease as primary (low renin activity) or secondary (increased renin activity).

TREATMENT

Treatment consists of supplemental potassium and administration of competitive aldosterone antagonists, such as spironolactone. Hypertension may require treatment with antihypertensive drugs. Hypokalemia from drug-induced diuresis is decreased with a potassium-sparing diuretic such as triamterene. The definitive treatment for aldosterone-secreting tumor is surgical excision.

ANESTHETIC CONSIDERATIONS

Anesthetic management begins with preoperative correction of hypokalemia and treatment of hypertension. Unsuspected hypovolemia is evidenced by orthostatic hypotension during preoperative evaluation. Invasive monitoring (central venous pressure, pulmonary arterial catheter) may be necessary in these patients to monitor intraoperative filling pressures. Supplementation with exogenous cortisol is also a consideration.

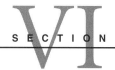

VI

Hepatic System

A. Hepatitis

DEFINITION
Hepatitis is an inflammatory disease of hepatocytes that may be either acute or chronic (lasting more than 6 months) and can progress to cell necrosis and eventual hepatic failure.

ETIOLOGY
Some of the causes of acute and chronic hepatitis include viral infections and drug-induced toxicity. The organisms responsible for viral hepatitis include hepatitis A virus, hepatitis B virus, hepatitis C virus (formerly non-A, non-B virus), Epstein-Barr virus, cytomegalovirus, and herpes simplex virus. Hepatitis A, or infectious hepatitis, is transmitted by the fecal-oral route or by ingestion of food contaminated with sewage. Hepatitis types B and C are transmitted percutaneously and by contact with body fluids. Hepatitis B, or serum hepatitis, is the most common type of viral hepatitis and may also be transmitted by nonparenteral routes (oral-to-oral and sexual). Drug-induced hepatitis may result from dose-dependent toxicity of a drug (or drug metabolite), from an idiosyncratic drug reaction, or from a combination of both. Halothane has been associated with hepatic dysfunction with repeat administration at short intervals in adults.

DIAGNOSTIC AND LABORATORY RESULTS
Laboratory evaluation should include blood urea nitrogen (BUN), serum electrolytes, serum creatinine, glucose, transaminases, bilirubin, alkaline phosphatase, albumin, prothrombin time, platelet count, and hepatitis B surface antigen. Concentrations of plasma transaminase enzymes are elevated 7 to 14 days before the onset of jaundice and begin to decline shortly after jaundice is clinically evident. Severe hepatitis is suggested by a plasma albumin concentration of less than 2.5 g/dL or a markedly prolonged prothrombin time unresponsive to vitamin K therapy. The presence of hepatitis B surface antigen in plasma indicates the potential for infectivity, and persistence for longer than 6 months in the absence of antibodies indicates that the patient is a chronic carrier and potentially infective to others.

CLINICAL MANIFESTATIONS
Symptoms of viral hepatitis include jaundice, dark urine, fatigue, anorexia, nausea, fever, and abdominal discomfort. Mild anemia and lymphocytosis also occur. Hypomagnesemia may be present in chronic alcoholics and can predispose to arrhythmias.

TREATMENT

Dehydration and electrolyte abnormalities should be corrected. Vitamin K or fresh-frozen plasma is used to correct coagulopathies. Bacterial infections should be treated and neomycin, lactulose, or both should be used to decrease plasma ammonia levels. Factors that may aggravate hepatic encephalopathy should be avoided. Orthotopic liver transplantation may be considered in selected patients.

ANESTHETIC CONSIDERATIONS

Coagulopathy should be corrected with fresh-frozen plasma. Premedication with sedatives should be avoided. Barbiturates, opioids, and some muscle relaxants may have prolonged effects due to altered hepatic metabolism. Response to succinylcholine may also be prolonged because of depression of pseudocholinesterase. Factors known to reduce hepatic blood flow, such as hypotension, excessive sympathetic activation, and high mean airway pressures during controlled ventilation, should be avoided. Hypoglycemia can be prevented by administering exogenous glucose. Blood should be administered at a controlled rate to minimize the likelihood of citrate intoxication. Alcoholic patients may develop cross-tolerance to both intravenous and volatile anesthetics.

B. Cirrhosis/Portal Hypertension

DEFINITION

Cirrhosis/portal hypertension is a chronic disease process that destroys the hepatic parenchyma and replaces it with collagen. This distorts the liver's normal architecture, leading to obstruction of portal venous flow and subsequent portal hypertension as well as impairment of physiologic functions of the liver. Other complications include variceal hemorrhage secondary to the portal hypertension, intractable fluid retention in the form of ascites and the hepatorenal syndrome, and hepatic encephalopathy or coma.

ETIOLOGY

The most common cause of cirrhosis in the United States is alcohol abuse (Laennec's cirrhosis). Other causes include chronic active hepatitis (postnecrotic cirrhosis), chronic biliary inflammation or obstruction (biliarycirrhosis), chronic right-sided congestive heart failure (cardiac cirrhosis), hemochromatosis, and Wilson's disease.

DIAGNOSTIC AND LABORATORY RESULTS

Laboratory changes in the presence of portal hypertension include a hematocrit of 30% to 35%, hyponatremia due to increased secretion of antidiuretic hormone, blood urea nitrogen greater than 20 mg/dL, and elevated plasma bilirubin, transaminases, and alkaline phosphatase concentrations.

CLINICAL MANIFESTATIONS
Gastrointestinal
Portal hypertension leads to the formation of ascites, esophageal varices, hemorrhoids, and gastrointestinal bleeding. Peptic ulcer disease is twice as common in patients with cirrhosis and may result in further hemorrhage. Patients develop anorexia and lose skeletal muscle mass. Gastric emptying is often slow, warranting premedication (cimetidine, metoclopramide) and a rapid sequence induction.

Circulatory
A hyperdynamic circulation characterized by an increased cardiac output is attributed to an increased vascular volume, decreased blood viscosity secondary to anemia, and generalized peripheral vasodilation. Cardiomyopathy can manifest as congestive heart failure. Palmar erythema and spider angiomas over the face, upper back, and arms are prominent. Hepatomegaly occurs with or without splenomegaly and ascites.

Pulmonary
Hyperventilation commonly results in primary respiratory alkalosis. Arterial hypoxemia develops because of right-to-left shunting (up to 40% of cardiac output). Elevation of the diaphragm from ascites reduces functional residual capacity, predisposing to atelectasis.

Renal
Decreased renal perfusion, enhanced proximal and distal sodium reabsorption, impaired free water clearance, hyponatremia, and hypokalemia are common. The hepatorenal syndrome may develop in these patients following gastrointestinal bleeding, aggressive diuresis, sepsis, or major surgery. This syndrome is characterized by progressive oliguria, azotemia, intractable ascites, and a high mortality rate unless liver transplantation is undertaken.

Hematologic
Anemia, thrombocytopenia, and leukopenia may be present. Coagulopathies result from decreased hepatic synthesis of coagulation factors (all except factor VIII and fibrinogen are affected) and reduced or impaired platelet function. Enhanced fibrinolysis due to decreased clearance of activators of the fibrinolytic system may also contribute to the coagulopathy.

Metabolic
Hypoalbuminemia, hyperaldosteronism, and hypoglycemia may be present.

Central Nervous System
Hepatic encephalopathy as well as coma may be manifested. Mental obtundation, asterixis (flapping motion of the hands), and fetor hepaticus (musty, sweet breath odor) are evident. Elevated intracranial pressure may require prompt treatment and continuous intraoperative monitoring.

TREATMENT

Treatment is supportive until liver transplantation can be undertaken. Variceal bleeding involves replacement of blood loss, vasopressin infusion (0.1 to 0.9 U/min IV), balloon tamponade (Sengstaken-Blakemore tube), or endoscopic sclerosis or the transjugular intrahepatic portosystemic shunt/stent (TIPS) procedure to stop the bleeding. If bleeding does not stop or recurs, emergency surgical procedures such as shunts (portocaval or splenorenal), esophageal transection, or gastric devascularization may be needed. Coagulopathies should be corrected by replacing clotting factors with fresh frozen plasma or cryoprecipitate. Platelet transfusions should be performed prior to surgery for counts less than 100,000 mm^3. Preservation of renal function involves avoiding aggressive diuresis while correcting acute intravascular fluid deficits with colloid infusions.

ANESTHETIC CONSIDERATIONS

The dosage of muscle relaxants should be reduced depending on hepatic elimination (e.g., pancuronium, vecuronium) because of reduced plasma clearance. Cisatracurium may be the relaxant of choice. The duration of action of succinylcholine may be prolonged as a result of reduced levels of pseudocholinesterase. Half-lives of opioids may be prolonged, leading to prolonged respiratory depression. The use of halothane should be avoided so as not to confuse the diagnosis if liver function test results deteriorate postoperatively. Regional anesthesia may be used in patients without thrombocytopenia or coagulopathy if hypotension is avoided (perfusion to the liver becomes highly dependent on hepatic arterial blood flow). Following removal of large amounts of ascitic fluid, colloid fluid replacement may be necessary to prevent hypotension. Whole blood may be preferable to packed red blood cells when replacing blood loss. Coagulation factors and platelet deficiencies should be corrected with fresh-frozen plasma and platelet transfusions, respectively. Citrate toxicity can occur in these patients because of impaired metabolism of the citrate anticoagulant in blood products. Intravenous calcium should be given to reverse the negative inotropic effects of a reduction in serum ionized calcium levels.

C. Hepatic Failure

DEFINITION

Hepatic failure occurs when massive necrosis of liver cells results in the development of a life-threatening loss of functional capacity that exceeds 80% to 90%. Hepatic failure can result from acute or chronic liver disease.

INCIDENCE

The major causes of hepatic failure in the United States are related to the effects of viral hepatitis or drug-related liver injury. Each year, an estimated 2000 cases of hepatic failure in the United States are related to viral hepatitis. This accounts for 1% of all deaths and 6% of all liver-related deaths.

ETIOLOGY

Following is a categorical list of the potential causes of hepatic failure.

Viral
Hepatitis A, B, C, D, E viruses
Herpes simplex virus
Cytomegalovirus
Adenovirus
Epstein-Barr virus
Varicella zoster virus
Dengue fever virus
Rift Valley fever virus
Toxic Damage
Acetaminophen
Isoniazid
Phenytoin
Halothane
Methyldopa
Tetracycline
Valproic acid
Nicotinic acid
Carbon tetrachloride
Phosphorus
Pesticides
Ethyl alcohol

Metabolic
Wilson's disease
Acute fatty liver of pregnancy
Reye's syndrome
Sickle cell disease
Galactosemia

Other
Autoimmune hepatitis
Amanita phalloides
   (mushroom) poisoning
Budd-Chiari syndrome
Veno-occlusive disease
Hyperthermia
Partial hepatectomy
Jejunoileal bypass

DIAGNOSTIC AND LABORATORY FINDINGS

Most proteins associated with the promotion or inhibition of coagulation are synthesized in the liver. When one is reviewing laboratory data, special attention should be given to coagulation studies, liver function studies, complete blood count, electrolytes, glucose, blood urea nitrogen, and creatinine.

A 12-lead ECG should be performed to rule out any possible cardiac arrhythmias related to acidemia, electrolyte abnormalities, or hypoxemia associated with hepatic failure. The patient with liver failure is at risk for the development of acid-base derangements. Respiratory alkalosis may result from hyperventilation related to an abnormality of central regulation. Respiratory acidosis may be caused by endotoxins, increased intracranial pressure (ICP), or pulmonary sequelae, which depress respiratory centers. Metabolic acidosis is also possible, related to substantial tissue damage and decreased clearance of lactic acid by the failing liver.

The hypoxemia associated with liver failure can be attributed to aspiration, atelectasis, infection, hypoventilation, or their combinations. Results of chest x-ray should be obtained to rule out evidence of pulmonary edema or adult respiratory distress syndrome (ARDS). ABGs guide respiratory management and correction of acid-base abnormalities.

Lab Study	Normal	Liver Failure
WBC	3.5 to 10.6 cells/mm^3	Decreased
Hgb	11.5 to 15.1 g/dL	Decreased
Hct	34.4% to 44.2%	Decreased
Platelet count	150 to 450 mm^3	Decreased
PT	11 to 14 s	Increased
PTT	20 to 37 s	Increased
Bilirubin	Plasma: 0.3 to 1.1 mg/dL Indirect: 0.2 to 0.7 mg/dL Direct: less than 0.5 mg/dL	Increased. Jaundice is seen with plasma bilirubin levels greater than 3 mg/dL.
SGOT (AST)	10 to 40 IU/L	Increased
SGPT (ALT*)	5 to 35 IU/L	Increased
LDH (LD-5*)	5.3% to 13.4%	Increased
ALP	87 to 250 U/L	Normal; used to differentiate biliary obstruction.
Albumin	3.3 to 4.5 g/dL	Decreased levels less than 2.5 g/dL are precarious.
NH_3	Less than 50 g/dL	Increased NH_3 is converted to urea by the normal liver.
BUN	7 to 20 mg/dL	Normal or decreased due to impaired excretion of Na and retention of H_2O; increased in hepatorenal syndrome.
Cr	0.6 to 1.3 mg/dl	Increased in hepatorenal syndrome.
Na	135 to 145 mEq/L	Usually decreased. Increased Na may result after the administration of lactulose or if replacement of free H_2O is inadequate.
K	3.6 to 5.0 mEq/L	Decreased; related to the secondary effects of hyperaldosteronism, vomiting, diuretic use, or inadequate replacement. Increased K may result from the use of blood products.
Mg	1.6 to 3.0 mEq/L	Decreased
Ca	8.8 to 10.4 mg/dL	Decreased
P	2.5 to 4.5 mg/dL	Decreased
Glucose	70 to 110 mg/dL	Decreased; related to impaired gluconeogenesis and decreased insulin clearance.

* Specific of liver damage.

CLINICAL MANIFESTATIONS

No matter the exact cause of the patient's liver failure, it inevitably affects the entire physiologic makeup. Physical examination is important for the approximation of liver and spleen size, evidence of bleeding abnormalities, identification of extravascular fluid shifts, and any other organ dysfunction.

Listed below are common clinical features of hepatic failure and their associated causes.

Clinical Feature	Cause
Anemia	Iron, B_{12}, or folate deficiency; hypersplenism; bone marrow suppression
Ascites	Portal HTN; hypoalbuminemia; Na and H_2O retention
Fetor hepaticus (pungent sour odor detected in exhaled breath)	Inability to metabolize methionine
Gynecomastia	Increased circulating estrogen
Hepatic encephalopathy (hepatic coma)	Inability to metabolize ammonia; increased cerebral sensitivity to toxins; hypoglycemia
Hepatorenal syndrome	Decreased renal blood flow, particularly to the cortex; vasoconstriction; decreased GFR; renal retention of Na
Increased bleeding tendencies, nosebleeds, gingival bleeding, menstrual bleeding, easy bruising	Anemia; thrombocytopenia; decreased production of clotting factors; decreased adherence of circulating platelets
Increased risk of infection	Endotracheal intubation with impaired cough reflex; IV catheters; central lines; urinary catheters; leukopenia; decreased neutrophil adherence; complement deficiencies
Increased skin pigmentation	Increased activity of MSH
Jaundice	Increased circulating bilirubin
Leukopenia	Hypersplenism; bone marrow suppression
Palmar erythema	Increased circulating estrogen
Pectoral and axillary alopecia	Increased circulating estrogen
Peripheral edema	Hypoalbuminemia; failure of the liver to inactivate aldosterone and ADH, with subsequent Na and H_2O retention
Spider angiomas "nevi"	Increased circulating estrogen
Testicular atrophy	Increased circulating estrogen
Thrombocytopenia	Hypersplenism; bone marrow suppression
Weight loss and muscle wasting	Nausea and vomiting; anorexia; impaired gluconeogenesis; impaired insulin functioning; hypoproteinemia

TREATMENT

Management of the patient with liver failure should include admission to the intensive care unit. The health care team should be on constant guard for complications associated with liver failure, such as sepsis, cerebral edema, hypoglycemia, and electrolyte and bleeding abnormalities. Liver failure associated with acetaminophen poisoning or mushroom poisoning should be identified immediately, because antidotes are available for both. Patients not responsive to conventional treatment should be considered for transplantation as early as possible, before they are excluded by the development of infection or encephalopathic brain damage.

General treatment modalities for the patient with liver failure include the following:

- Antibiotic prophylaxis
- Urinary catheter
- Central venous pulmonary catheter
- Histamine$_2$ antagonist or sucralfate
- Blood glucose checks every 1 to 2 hours
- Aspiration precautions
- Periodic assessment of neurologic status
     Prevent sepsis
     Monitor renal function and fluid status
     Monitor fluid volume
     Increase gastric pH and decrease risk of gastrointestinal bleeding
     Prevent hypoglycemia and guide administration of intravenous dextrose
     Prevent aspiration pneumonia and adult respiratory distress syndrome
     (Note that neurologic status may rapidly deteriorate because of increasing ammonia levels or increasing ICP)
- Early nutritional supplementation—prevent nutrition-related complications

ANESTHETIC CONSIDERATIONS

Only surgery to correct life-threatening conditions should be performed on the patient with liver failure. The patient's condition should be optimized prior to the surgical procedure. A normally "minor" procedure can become a major catastrophe when dealing with the patient with liver failure.

Premedication must be considered, taking into account the severity of the patient's disease process, the presence of altered consciousness, and the liver's diminished ability to metabolize pharmacologic agents. If the patient is thought to have a full stomach, antacids and histamine$_2$ antagonists may be administered.

Monitoring should conform to the established standards of care. The size and number of intravenous catheters should be individualized. Most cases involving liver failure require the use of an arterial line, a CVP or PA catheter, and a urinary drainage catheter to monitor the patient's fluid status.

The use of local anesthesia with sedation or regional anesthesia should be considered whenever possible. Coagulopathies must first be ruled out, and the surgical procedure itself must be considered. Patients may be considered to have a full stomach, especially in the presence of ascites. In this case a rapid-sequence induction is standard. The choice of induction agent and dosage administered should reflect the liver's diminished ability to metabolize pharmacologic agents and the patient's increased volume of distribution.

Both nondepolarizing and depolarizing muscle relaxants may be administered. Dosages may need to be individualized according to the patient's initial response. A peripheral nerve stimulator aids the practitioner in gauging the patient's response and adjusting subsequent doses. The breakdown of succinylcholine remains relatively normal despite advanced disease states. Muscle relaxants metabolized by the liver (e.g., vecuronium) should be avoided. Cisatracurium may be the muscle relaxant of choice because of its unique metabolic properties, which do not involve either the liver or the kidneys. If cisatracurium is unavailable, any other nondepolarizing muscle relaxant may be used, taking into account the patient's specific organ involvement and the drug's metabolic properties.

Isoflurane and desflurane are the inhalational agents of choice. Enflurane may also be considered, but the practitioner must consider the neurologic status of the patient. Halothane is contraindicated in patients with liver disease. Nitrous oxide may be safely instituted according to the nature of the surgery and as long as a high fraction of inspired oxygen is not required.

The use of opioids must take into account a prolonged half-life and decreased clearance. Because fentanyl does not decrease hepatic blood flow, it is often the opioid of choice for the liver failure patient.

The liver failure patient is at risk for major blood loss with any invasive procedure. Blood products should be available, and all losses should be replaced accordingly.

PROGNOSIS

In the United States, mortality rates due to liver disease have increased since the 1960s. Overall, the mortality rate from hepatic failure is 70% to 95%. Liver transplantation should be considered when conventional medical management fails; such consideration should take place early, before infection or encephalopathic brain damage renders the potential candidate ineligible. One-year patient survival rates after transplantation are 63% to 78%.

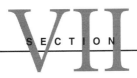

Renal System

A. Urolithiasis

DEFINITION

Urolithiasis, or "kidney stones," is the presence of calculi typically composed of calcium oxalate. These are due to hypercalciuria or hyperoxaluria. Other types of stones include magnesium ammonium phosphate, calcium phosphate, and uric acid.

ETIOLOGY

Causes of hypercalcemia and hypercalciuria are primarily hyperparathyroidism, vitamin D intoxication, malignancies, and sarcoidosis. Small bowel bypass is associated with hyperoxaluria. Alterations in urine pH or the presence of metabolic disturbances can also result in formation of renal stones, which differ in composition from the typical oxalate variety.

TREATMENT

Extracorporeal shock wave lithotripsy is a noninvasive treatment of renal stones. It transmits shock waves through water, focusing them on the stone via biplanar fluoroscopy. The shock waves are triggered by the R wave of the ECG and delivered during the heart's refractory period (approximately 20 msec after R wave) to avoid initiating any cardiac arrhythmias. Patients with artificial cardiac pacemakers risk pacemaker dysfunction with this form of therapy.

ANESTHETIC CONSIDERATIONS

General or regional anesthesia, including epidural and intercostal nerve blocks with local infiltration, may be used to provide analgesia during lithotripsy. The sitting position may be associated with peripheral pooling of blood, especially with the use of regional anesthesia and resultant vasodilatation. Immersion in water increases hydrostatic pressures on the abdomen and thorax, which can displace blood into the central circulation. This may result in acute congestive heart failure in patients with limited cardiac reserve. The hydrostatic forces on the thorax likewise result in decreases in chest wall compliance and functional residual capacity. This may produce ventilation-perfusion mismatches. Water in the immersion tub should be kept warm to avoid hypothermia. Extracorporeal shock wave lithotripsy is contraindicated in patients with abdominal aortic aneurysms, spinal cord tumors, or orthopedic implants in the lumbar region. Parturients, obese patients, and patients with coagulopathies are also not good candidates.

B. Acute Renal Failure

DEFINITION

Acute renal failure is a rapid deterioration in renal function that results in retention of nitrogenous waste products (azotemia).

ETIOLOGY

Azotemia can be divided into prerenal, renal, and postrenal types, depending on its causes. Prerenal azotemia results from an acute decrease in renal perfusion. Renal azotemia is usually due to intrinsic renal disease, renal ischemia, or nephrotoxins. Postrenal azotemia is the result of urinary tract obstruction or disruption. Up to 50% of cases are due to ischemia and nephrotoxins following major trauma or surgery. This is also called *acute tubular necrosis* (ATN). Potential toxins include aminoglycosides, x-ray contrast dyes, and (in some patients), nonsteroidal anti-inflammatory drugs. Other factors predisposing to acute renal failure include pre-existing renal impairment, advanced age, atherosclerotic vascular disease, diabetes, and dehydration.

LABORATORY RESULTS

Acute renal failure is thought of as either oliguric (urinary volume less than 400 mL/d) or anuric (urinary volume less than 100 mL/d). However, nonoliguric acute renal failure (urine volume greater than 400 mL/d) may now account for up to 50% of cases. These patients have a lower urine sodium concentration than do oliguric patients. Moreover, they appear to have a lower complication rate and require shorter hospitalization.

CLINICAL MANIFESTATIONS

Please refer to the section on chronic renal failure that follows.

TREATMENT

Standard treatment includes restriction of fluids, sodium, potassium, and protein intake. Dialysis may be employed to treat or prevent uremic complications. Peritoneal dialysis and hemodialysis can be equally effective, yet elevation and immobilization of the diaphragm associated with continuous peritoneal dialysis may predispose to respiratory complications. Standard hemodialysis may also be replaced by continuous arteriovenous hemofiltration (CAVH), which may be better tolerated in critically ill patients.

ANESTHETIC CONSIDERATIONS

Please refer to the section on chronic renal failure that follows.

PROGNOSIS

Sepsis remains the most common cause of death in patients with acute renal failure. Urinary function improves over the course of several weeks but may not return to normal for up to 1 year.

C. Chronic Renal Failure

DEFINITION
Chronic renal failure is characterized by a progressive decrease in the number of functioning nephrons, leading to an irreversible reduction in the glomerular filtration rate.

ETIOLOGY
Common diseases that lead to chronic renal failure are chronic glomerulonephritis, diabetic nephropathy, hypertensive nephrosclerosis, and polycystic renal disease.

LABORATORY RESULTS
Chest x-ray should be examined for possible fluid overload (be aware of when the patient was last dialyzed) or pulmonary edema. Electrolytes, complete blood count, and coagulation factors should be checked, because all may be affected.

CLINICAL MANIFESTATIONS
Metabolic
Hyperkalemia, hyperphosphatemia, hypocalcemia, hypermagnesemia, hyperuricemia, and hypoalbuminemia are possible. Water and sodium retention results in extracellular fluid overload and hyponatremia. Failure to excrete nonvolatile acids causes a high anion gap and metabolic acidosis.

Hematologic
Anemia is present because of decreased erythropoietin production, decreased red cell production, and decreased cell survival. Anemia and metabolic acidosis result in a rightward shift of the oxyhemoglobin dissociation curve. Both platelet and white cell function are impaired in patients with renal failure. This is clinically manifested as a prolonged bleeding time and increased susceptibility to infection. Patients who have recently undergone hemodialysis may also have residual anticoagulant effects from heparin. Observe the prothrombin time and partial thromboplastin time, especially if regional anesthesia is being considered.

Cardiovascular
Cardiac output is increased to maintain oxygen delivery. Sodium retention and abnormalities in the renin-angiotensin system result in systemic arterial hypertension. Left ventricular hypertrophy is common. Extracellular fluid overload, along with the increased demands of anemia and hypertension, predispose these patients to cardiomegaly and congestive heart failure. Arrhythmias may be due to metabolic abnormalities. Hypovolemia may develop if too much fluid is removed with dialysis.

Pulmonary
Chronic renal failure interferes with normal excretion of hydrogen ions by the kidneys, resulting in metabolic acidosis. Treatment of the acidosis may include hemodialysis or intravenous administration of sodium bicarbonate.

Pulmonary edema may result from an increase in permeability of the alveolar-capillary membrane with the appearance of "butterfly wings" on chest x-ray.

Endocrine

Diabetes mellitus is common because of peripheral resistance to insulin. Secondary hyperparathyroidism due to chronic hypocalcemia leads to osteodystrophy and vulnerability to pathologic fractures.

Gastrointestinal

Anorexia, nausea, vomiting, and ileus are associated with azotemia. Gastric fluid volume and acidity are increased. These changes, combined with delayed gastric emptying related to autonomic neuropathy, predispose these patients to pulmonary aspiration.

Neurologic

Asterixis, lethargy, confusion, seizures, and coma are manifestations of uremic encephalopathy. Autonomic and peripheral neuropathies are common. Peripheral neuropathies are typically sensory and involve the distal lower extremities. The median and common peroneal nerves are most often affected.

TREATMENT

Treatment may include intermittent hemodialysis using an arteriovenous fistula or continuous peritoneal dialysis via an implanted catheter. Renal transplantation may become necessary.

ANESTHETIC CONSIDERATIONS
Monitoring

Avoid measuring blood pressure in an arm with an arteriovenous fistula. Consider invasive monitoring, especially for procedures involving major fluid shifts. Intra-arterial monitoring is indicated for patients with poorly controlled hypertension.

Premedication

Aspiration prophylaxis with a histamine$_2$ blocker and metoclopramide may be indicated.

Induction

Rapid-sequence induction with cricoid pressure is indicated for patients with nausea, vomiting, or gastrointestinal bleeding. Reduced protein binding of drugs results in more unbound drug to act at receptor sites. Succinylcholine should be avoided in patients with a serum potassium level greater than 5 mEq/L. Atracurium, mivacurium, and cisatracurium are the muscle relaxants of choice. Expect a prolonged response to the other nondepolarizing muscle relaxants.

Maintenance

Agents that reduce cardiac output (principal compensatory mechanism for anemia) should be avoided. Isoflurane/desflurane is the preferred volatile agent because it has the least effect on cardiac output. Enflurane should be avoided because of the potential adverse effects of fluoride on the diseased kidneys. Use of meperidine may result in accumulation of the metabolite normeperidine. Morphine and its effects may be prolonged. If regional anesthesia is considered, the adequacy of coagulation should be confirmed and the presence of uremic neuropathies should be excluded. The duration of action of local anesthetics may be shortened because of elevated tissue blood flow secondary to increased cardiac output. Ventilation of the lungs should maintain normocapnia and reduce the effects of positive-pressure ventilation on cardiac output. Hypoventilation, which results in respiratory acidosis, should also be avoided. However, hyperventilation causing respiratory alkalosis shifts the oxyhemoglobin dissociation curve to the left and reduces tissue oxygen availability.

Fluid Management

The use of Lactated Ringer's injection should be avoided in hyperkalemic patients when large volumes of fluid may be required because of the potassium concentration of 4 mEq/L.

PART 1   **Common Diseases**

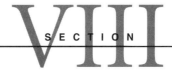

Hematologic System

A. Anemia

DEFINITION
Anemia is a deficiency of erythrocytes caused by either too-rapid loss or too-slow production of the cells. Therefore numeric concentrations of hemoglobin are reduced and the oxygen-carrying capacity of blood is decreased. This results in reduced oxygen delivery to peripheral tissues.

ETIOLOGY
Anemia may result from acute blood loss; however, iron-deficiency anemia due to persistent blood loss is the most frequent form of chronic anemia. Anemia is also associated with many chronic diseases, such as persistent infections, neoplastic processes, connective tissue disorders, and renal and hepatic disease. Other forms of anemia include aplastic anemia, which involves bone marrow depression, and megaloblastic anemias, which are related to deficiencies of vitamin B_{12} or folic acid. Lastly, various anemias can result from intravascular hemolysis of erythrocytes.

LABORATORY RESULTS
Erythrocyte production can be assessed from the reticulocyte count in peripheral blood. For instance, a low reticulocyte count in the presence of a low hematocrit suggests an erythrocyte production defect, rather than blood loss or hemolysis as a cause of anemia. A decrease in hematocrit that exceeds 1% per day is most likely related to acute blood loss or intravascular hemolysis.

CLINICAL MANIFESTATIONS
A history of reduced exercise tolerance characterized as exertional dyspnea is a frequent clinical sign of chronic anemia. A functional heart murmur and evidence of cardiomegaly may be detected on physical examination. The decreased oxygen-carrying capacity of arterial blood is compensated for by a rightward shift oxyhemoglobin dissociation curve and an increase in the cardiac output. The decreased exercise tolerance reflects the inability of cardiac output to increase to maintain tissue oxygenation when these patients become physically active.

TREATMENT
Packed erythrocytes can be transfused preoperatively to increase hemoglobin concentrations but it should be remembered that about 24 hours are necessary to restore intravascular fluid volume and blood viscosity. Compared with a similar volume of whole blood, erythrocytes produce about twice the increase in hemoglobin concentration.

ANESTHETIC CONSIDERATIONS

Minimum acceptable hemoglobin concentrations for elective surgery have changed over the years. The "old" value of 10 g/dL has been lowered to approximately 8 g/dL (depending on the patient, operation, institution, etc.). If elective surgery is performed, the anesthetic should be geared toward preventing changes that may interfere with tissue oxygen delivery. For example, myocardial depression produced by the volatile agents may reduce cardiac output and thus impair the patient's compensatory mechanisms. Likewise, leftward shifts of the oxyhemoglobin dissociation curve (as produced by hyperventilation and resulting in respiratory alkalosis) can impair release of oxygen from hemoglobin to the tissues. It is also important to maintain body temperature, since hypothermia will cause a leftward shift of the curve. Intraoperative blood loss should be promptly replaced and closely monitored. Finally, it is important to minimize shivering or increases in body temperature postoperatively, since these changes can greatly increase total body oxygen requirements.

B. Sickle Cell Disease

DEFINITION

Sickle cell disease represents an inherited group of disorders, ranging in severity from the usually benign sickle cell trait to the often fatal sickle cell anemia. All the variants of the disease have in common various quantities of hemoglobin-S. Hemoglobin-S differs from normal hemoglobin-A by the substitution of valine for glutamic acid at the sixth position on the β chain of hemoglobin molecules.

INCIDENCE AND PREVALENCE

The incidence of sickle cell trait among the black population of the United States is about 10%. Sickle cell anemia is present when patients are homozygous for hemoglobin-S and affects approximately 0.3% to 1.0% of the Afro-American population in the United States. In the homozygous state, 70% to 98% of hemoglobin is of the S-type, that may "sickle" resulting in severe hemolytic anemia.

ETIOLOGY

Sickle cell trait is the heterozygote manifestation of sickle cell disease containing the hemoglobin genotype AS. Erythrocytes of patients with the trait contain 20% to 40% hemoglobin-S; the remainder being hemoglobin-A. Affected persons are usually asymptomatic. Sickle cell anemia occurs when deoxygenated forms of hemoglobin-S result in the deformation of erythrocytes into sickle shapes instead of their usual biconcave shape. This damages the erythrocyte membranes, leading to their rupture and chronic hemolytic anemia. Formation of sickle cells is exaggerated by low oxygen partial pressures (less than 40 mm Hg). Formation tends to be greater in veins than in arteries, so maintenance of pH is important. Hypothermia also promotes formation of sickled cells due to vasoconstriction, which leads to stasis of blood flow and deoxygenation of hemoglobin.

CLINICAL MANIFESTATIONS

Most commonly, the clinical manifestations are infarctive events due to occlusion of blood vessels with sickled cells and anemia due to hemolysis. The cardiac output is generally increased to compensate for chronic anemia. The oxyhemoglobin dissociation curve for hemoglobin-S is shifted to the right (P_{50} = 31 mm Hg). Patients are susceptible to bacterial infections because splenic function is lost secondary to repeated thrombosis. Multiple organ dysfunction produced by infarctive events is the major reason that survival beyond 30 years of age is unlikely.

LABORATORY RESULTS

In steady state, hemoglobin concentrations are 5 to 10 g/dL. ABGs, electrolytes, liver function tests, and other tests should be watched depending on the patient's clinical symptoms and possible organ involvement.

TREATMENT

Treatment of a painful infarctive crisis is with hydration and mild alkalinization of blood. Partial exchange transfusions with erythrocytes containing hemoglobin-A will reduce concentrations of hemoglobin-S and decrease the incidence of further infarctive damage. The goal of exchange transfusions is to increase hemoglobin-A concentrations to at least 40%.

ANESTHETIC CONSIDERATIONS

Hypoventilation of the lungs should be avoided to prevent acidosis. Oxygenation should be maintained. To prevent circulatory stasis, improper body positioning or the use of tourniquets should be avoided. Intravascular fluid volume must be maintained in order to prevent increased blood viscosity. Normal body temperature should also be maintained. Preoperative medication should be administered judiciously to avoid depression of ventilation. Regional anesthesia may be preferred over general anesthesia, although compensatory vasoconstriction and decreased arterial oxygen partial pressures in the unblocked area may predispose patients to infarction.

C. Polycythemia Vera

DEFINITION AND ETIOLOGY

Polycythemia vera is a myeloproliferative disease that generally occurs in patients between 60 and 70 years of age. Hyperactivity of myeloid progenitor cells results in increased production of erythrocytes, leukocytes, and platelets.

LABORATORY RESULTS

Hemoglobin concentrations typically exceed 18 g/dL, and platelet counts can be greater than 400,000/mm^3.

CLINICAL MANIFESTATIONS

Clinical symptoms are due to hyperviscosity of the blood, which leads to stasis of blood flow and an increased incidence of vascular thrombosis, particularly in the cardiovascular and central nervous systems. Defective platelet function is the most likely mechanism for spontaneous hemorrhage, which may occur in these patients.

TREATMENT

Treatment entails reducing hemoglobin concentrations to near-normal levels by phlebotomy before elective surgery.

ANESTHETIC CONSIDERATIONS

Surgery in the presence of uncontrolled polycythemia vera is associated with a high incidence of perioperative hemorrhage and postoperative venous thrombosis. In emergency situations, viscosity of the blood can be reduced by intravenous infusions of cystalloid solutions or low-molecular-weight dextrans.

D. Leukemia

DEFINITION

Leukemia is the uncontrolled production of leukocytes due to cancerous mutation of lymphogenous cells or myelogenous cells. Lymphocytic leukemias begin in lymph nodes or other lymphogenous tissues and then spread to other areas of the body. Myeloid leukemias begin as cancerous production of myelogenous cells in bone marrow, with spread to extramedullary organs. Cancerous cells usually do not resemble other leukocytes and lack the usual functional characteristics of white cells.

INCIDENCE, PREVALENCE, ETIOLOGY, CLINICAL MANIFESTATIONS, AND LABORATORY RESULTS

Acute lymphoblastic leukemia accounts for approximately 15% of all leukemias in adults. CNS dysfunction is common. These patients are highly susceptible to life-threatening infections, including those produced by *Pneumocystis carinii* and cytomegalovirus.

Chronic lymphocytic leukemia accounts for approximately 25% of all leukemias and is most common in elderly males. Diagnosis is confirmed by the presence of lymphocytosis (greater than $15,000/mm^3$) and lymphocytic infiltrates in bone marrow. There may be neutropenia with an associated increased susceptibility to bacterial infections. Treatment is with cancer chemotherapeutic drugs classified as alkylating agents.

Acute myeloid leukemia can result in death in about 3 months if untreated. Patients present with fever, weakness, bleeding, and hepatosplenomegaly. Chemotherapy produces a temporary remission in about one half of patients.

Patients with chronic myeloid leukemia present with massive hepatosplenomegaly and white blood cell counts greater than 50,000/mm³. Fever and weight loss reflect hypermetabolism. Anemia may be severe. Splenectomy is routine in these patients.

TREATMENT

Cancer chemotherapy is the best available therapy for irradiation of cancerous cells anywhere in the body. Adverse clinical effects of these drugs include bone marrow suppression (susceptibility to infection, thrombocytopenia, and anemia), nausea, vomiting, diarrhea, ulceration of the gastrointestinal mucosa, and alopecia. Bone marrow transplantation is also becoming an increasingly successful treatment for leukemia.

ANESTHETIC MANAGEMENT

Management of anesthesia for the leukemia patient requires a clear understanding of the mechanisms of action, potential interactions, and likely toxicities associated with the use of cancer chemotherapeutic drugs. Patients taking doxorubicin or daunorubicin (antibiotics) may develop cardiomyopathy leading to congestive heart failure, which is often refractory to cardiac inotropic drugs. Cardiomegaly and/or pleural effusions may be found on chest x-ray. Marked LV dysfunction was found to persist for as long as 3 years after the drug was discontinued. Nonspecific and usually benign ECG changes have been observed in 10% of patients. Bleomycin is an antibiotic that can cause pulmonary toxicity, with dyspnea and nonproductive cough being the initial manifestations. PFTs demonstrate "restrictive" pulmonary disease. Inspired FiO_2 should be maintained at less than 30% during surgery because patients are susceptible to the toxic pulmonary effects of oxygen while on bleomycin therapy. Strict aseptic technique is important because of immunosuppression. Preoperatively, signs of CNS depression, autonomic nervous system dysfunction, and peripheral neuropathies should be noted. Renal or hepatic dysfunction should influence the choice of anesthesia and muscle relaxants. Volatile anesthetics may reduce myocardial contractility in patients with cardiotoxicity related to chemotherapeutic drugs. ABGs should be monitored. Replacing fluid losses with colloid rather than crystalloid solutions in patients with pulmonary fibrosis may be considered. Also, possible postoperative ventilation, depending on the length of the procedure and the degree of fibrosis, should be considered.

The use of nitrous oxide in patients donating bone marrow or undergoing bone marrow transplantation should be avoided because of the potential for drug-induced adverse effects on the bone marrow itself. Donors may be given heparin before removal of bone marrow, which influences the use of spinal or epidural anesthesia for this procedure.

E. AIDS/HIV Infection

DEFINITION

Acquired immunodeficiency syndrome (AIDS) is not a single disease but rather the appearance of various opportunistic infections due to generalized depression of the immune system. Immunodeficiency is caused by infection of helper T-lymphocytes with a retrovirus known as human immunodeficiency virus (HIV). This virus destroys T-lymphocytes, leaving the host susceptible to development of infection and neoplastic diseases.

INCIDENCE

In the United States, AIDS statistics are as follows. Over 90% of adult patients with AIDS are men, with 70% being homosexual or bisexual males. Heterosexual IV drug users account for 15% of males with AIDS and 50% of affected females. Persons with hemophilia coagulation disorders account for 1% of all AIDS cases and recipients of infected blood transfusions account for 2% of all cases.

ETIOLOGY

The virus is transmitted by sexual contact, inoculation by other body secretions, and transfusion of blood or blood products (especially factor VIII concentrates). Because HIV selectively infects lymphocytes, concentrations of the virus are probably highest in secretions containing lymphocytes, such as semen, vaginal secretions, and blood. There is no evidence of airborne transmission of AIDS.

CLINICAL MANIFESTATIONS

Patients develop severe immunosuppression due to destruction of T-lymphocytes, resulting in susceptibility to opportunistic infections. The most frequently encountered opportunistic, life-threatening infection is pneumonia due to the parasite *Pneumocystis carinii*. The most common malignant condition in AIDS patients is Kaposi's sarcoma. Of all AIDS/HIV patients, 50% develop some element of CNS dysfunction. Weight loss, fatigue, idiopathic thrombocytopenia, chronic diarrhea, and anemia are nonspecific findings. Milder manifestations of AIDS include a transient mononucleosis-like syndrome and persistent generalized lymphadenopathy.

LABORATORY RESULTS AND DIAGNOSTIC FINDINGS

Laboratory findings include lymphopenia and reduction in the ratio of helper T-lymphocytes to suppressor T-lymphocytes. Detection of HIV antibodies using an enzyme-linked immunoassay indicates that the patient has been infected with the virus. To increase reliability, a positive enzyme-linked immunoassay result is confirmed by a Western blot test. Persons infected with HIV usually develop antibody (seroconvert) against the virus within 6 to 12 weeks of being infected.

A positive antibody test result does not mean that the subject has AIDS or will develop the syndrome.

TREATMENT

Oral administration of zidovudine (formerly azidothymidine, or AZT) inhibits replication of some retroviruses, including HIV, and therefore may be useful in reducing the risk of developing opportunistic infections associated with AIDS. The drug is primarily eliminated by the kidneys following breakdown by the liver. Drugs such as probenecid, acetaminophen, aspirin, and indomethacin may competitively inhibit zidovudine's breakdown in the liver. Anemia and granulocytopenia are adverse effects of zidovudine therapy.

ANESTHETIC MANAGEMENT

Anesthetic management must assume that all patients are potentially infected with HIV or other bloodborne pathogens. Universal precautions must be followed. Disposable laryngoscope blades should be used if available and bacterial filters should be placed in the anesthesia circuit. The choice of anesthetic drugs and techniques depends on accompanying systemic manifestations of AIDS and related opportunistic infections. For example, oxygenation may be impaired in patients with *P. carinii* infection. Frequently, patients are malnourished and dehydrated. Anemia due to chronic infection may require transfusion.

PROGNOSIS

The incubation period for AIDS may be 7 years or longer. The mortality rate approaches 70% within 2 years after diagnosis.

F. Coagulopathies

HEMOPHILIA A

DEFINITION

Hemophilia A is a disorder of blood coagulation due to inadequate activity of factor VIII.

INCIDENCE AND PREVALENCE

It is estimated that hemophilia A is present in 1 of 10,000 males because the gene for factor VIII is carried on X-chromosomes.

ETIOLOGY

Plasma concentrations of factor VIII and the severity of bleeding are directly related. For example, spontaneous hemorrhage is likely when factor VIII concentrations are less than 3% of the normal values.

LABORATORY RESULTS

Classically, patients present with a prolonged partial thromboplastin time (PTT) but a normal prothrombin time and bleeding time.

CLINICAL MANIFESTATIONS

Deep tissue bleeding, hemarthrosis, and hematuria are common forms of clinical bleeding associated with hemophilia A. Central venous system bleeding is a major cause of death in these patients.

TREATMENT

Factor VIII levels should be increased to more than 50% prior to anesthesia/operation. Fresh-frozen plasma is considered to have 1 U of factor VIII activity per milliliter. Cryoprecipitate has 5 to 10 U of activity per milliliter, whereas factor VIII concentrates have 40 U of activity per milliliter. Transfusions are given twice a day following surgery because of the short half-life of factor VIII (8 to 12 hours). If cryoprecipitate or factor VIII is administered, there is an increased risk of transmission of viral diseases, such as hepatitis or acquired immunodeficiency syndrome (AIDS).

ANESTHETIC CONSIDERATIONS

All intramuscular injections should be avoided. Regional anesthesia should be avoided because of the risk of bleeding. The possibility of coexisting liver disease from hepatitis that may have occurred after blood or factor VIII transfusions should be considered. Universal precautions must always be followed.

HEMOPHILIA B

DEFINITION

Hemophilia B, also known as Christmas disease, is a disorder of blood coagulation due to the absence or decreased activity of factor IX.

INCIDENCE AND PREVALENCE

Hemophilia B is similar to hemophilia A, but much less common (1 in 100,000 males).

ETIOLOGY

Measurement of factor IX levels establishes the diagnosis. Factor IX activity should be maintained at more than 30% of normal.

LABORATORY RESULTS

The partial thromboplastin time (PTT) is prolonged in these patients.

CLINICAL MANIFESTATIONS

See under "Hemophilia A," p. 106.

TREATMENT

Fresh-frozen plasma is no longer considered adequate therapy for patients with hemophilia B. Specific pro-coagulant concentrates to raise plasma concentrations of factor IX are chosen.

VON WILLEBRAND'S DISEASE

DEFINITION AND ETIOLOGY
Von Willebrand's disease is a hematologic disease that is transmitted as an autosomal dominant characteristic affecting both sexes. It is most likely due to the deficiency of a protein (von Willebrand's factor) important for adequate activity of factor VIII and optimal function of platelets.

LABORATORY RESULTS
The classic expression is prolonged bleeding time, impaired aggregation of platelets, and decreased plasma concentrations of factor VIII.

CLINICAL MANIFESTATIONS
Epistaxis, bleeding from mucosal surfaces, and superficial bruising are common. Pregnancy produces an increase in factor VIII and von Willebrand's factor in parturients with mild to moderate forms of this disorder.

TREATMENT
Cryoprecipitate (40 units per kg) provides von Willebrand's factor as well as factor VIII. Desmopressin, the synthetic analogue of antidiuretic hormone, also effectively induces release of von Willebrand's factor.

ANESTHETIC CONSIDERATIONS
Drugs that interfere with optimal aggregation of platelets should be avoided. The patient should also be properly positioned to avoid bruising.

DISSEMINATED INTRAVASCULAR COAGULATION

DEFINITION
Disseminated intravascular coagulation (DIC) is characterized by uncontrolled activation of the coagulation system, with consumption of platelets and pro-coagulants. Thrombi develop in the microcirculation and bleeding results because of loss of coagulation factors into these thrombi.

ETIOLOGY
Normal mechanisms of controlling intravascular coagulation may be overwhelmed by extensive tissue damage in cases such as sepsis, burns, retained placenta after delivery, trauma to the central nervous system, and prolonged extracorporeal circulation. Large amounts of thromboplastic material are released into the circulation with subsequent activation of the extrinsic coagulation pathway. Consumption of platelets and pro-coagulants, including factors I, II, V, VIII, and XIII, reflects generalized activation of the entire coagulation system. Furthermore, impaired perfusion of the liver interferes with extraction of activated clotting factors.

LABORATORY RESULTS
Platelet counts are often less than $150,000/mm^3$ because of consumption. Prothrombin time (PT) and partial thromboplastin time (PTT) are pro-

longed. Decreased fibrinogen (less than 150 mg/dL) reflects consumption of this procoagulant. Levels of fibrin degradation products are elevated.

CLINICAL MANIFESTATIONS

Patients often demonstrate hemorrhage from wound sites and around sites of placement of intravascular catheters. In some cases, thromboembolic phenomena may follow.

TREATMENT

The goal is correction of the underlying disorder responsible for initiating the widespread clotting process. Platelet concentrates and fresh-frozen plasma may be administered as determined by measurement of the platelet count and of the prothrombin time and partial thromboplastin time, respectively. Heparin has been recommended as therapy, but its use is controversial.

ANESTHETIC CONSIDERATIONS

Intramuscular injections and regional anesthesia should be avoided. Coagulation factors and the DIC screen should be monitored, and be prepared to administer the necessary blood products.

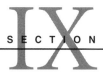

Gastrointestinal System

A. Diaphragmatic Hernia

DEFINITION

Diaphragmatic hernia is an incomplete embryologic closure of the diaphragm with herniation of abdominal contents into the thorax. Normal lung maturation is impaired because abdominal contents compress developing lung tissue. Lungs develop with varying degrees of pulmonary hypoplasia.

INCIDENCE AND PREVALENCE

Diaphragmatic hernia occurs in 1 of 4000 live births. The mortality rate is approximately 50%.

ETIOLOGY

Diaphragmatic hernia is caused by incomplete embryologic closure of the diaphragm.

LABORATORY RESULTS

Antenatal diagnosis shows that polyhydramnios is present 30% of the time. Abdominal ultrasonography is used to detect these hernias.

CLINICAL MANIFESTATIONS

Clinical manifestations depend on the degree of the hernia and interference with ventilation. They include scaphoid abdomen, reduced or absent breath sounds on the affected side, a barrel-shaped chest, arterial hypoxia, abdominal contents in the thorax (as shown on chest and/or abdominal x-ray), increased pulmonary vascular resistance, and congenital heart disease.

TREATMENT

Treatment consists of prompt decompression of the stomach and oxygenation with endotracheal intubation.

ANESTHETIC CONSIDERATIONS

The airway should be secured and anesthesia administered after awake endotracheal intubation. Invasive monitoring of blood pressure should be considered. In some patients, delaying surgery for 24 to 48 hours may be possible to allow some degree of stabilization in their condition. Anesthetic induction may then be used by raising the head of the bed and using a rapid sequence approach.

B. Hiatal Hernia/Gastric Reflux

DEFINITION

Hiatal Hernia

Hiatal hernia is bulging of the stomach and other abdominal viscera through an enlarged esophageal hiatus in the diaphragm.

Gastric Reflux

Gastric reflux relates to a reduced lower esophageal tone, which can increase the risk for regurgitation/aspiration. Reflux can occur without the presence of hiatal hernia. The lower sphincter is a physiologic sphincter with no specialized musculature. Tone is 15 to 35 mm Hg.

INCIDENCE AND PREVALENCE

Types I to IV hiatal hernias are present in 10% of the population, usually without symptoms. Only 5% of the population have reflux symptoms along with a hiatal hernia.

ETIOLOGY

In most cases the cause is unknown, whether the condition is congenital, traumatic, or iatrogenic.

LABORATORY TESTS

Chest/abdominal x-rays and "barium swallow" can be used.

CLINICAL MANIFESTATIONS

Symptoms typically involve heartburn, regurgitation, esophageal stricture, bleeding with a large hernia, sensation of food "sticking," fullness or bloating after eating, and sharp pain.

TREATMENT

No treatment is needed in the absence of symptoms. Larger hernias are treated to control reflux. Enlarging hernias require surgical intervention via a thoracoabdominal incision.

ANESTHETIC CONSIDERATIONS

Symptomatic patients require pretreatment with a nonparticulate antacid and a histamine$_2$ blocker. For induction of anesthesia, elevation of the head of the bed/stretcher and rapid sequence induction to prevent aspiration should be considered. If the hernia is large, one-lung anesthesia may be used to improve surgical access during repair. Communication with the surgical team is imperative when the thoracoabdominal approach is being considered.

PROGNOSIS

Prognosis is excellent for a Type I hiatal hernia (asymptomatic without reflux). Type II paraesophageal hernias are likely to enlarge. Prognosis is poor if a giant intrathoracic stomach is present.

C. Gallstone/Gallbladder Disease

GALLSTONES

DEFINITION

Gallstones are cholesterol-containing stones that form in the gallbladder or bile ducts. They usually form when the bile contains more cholesterol than can be held in solution.

The gallbladder, which has a capacity of approximately 40 to 50 mL, concentrates bile and delivers it to the duodenum. Surgically removing the gallbladder has little effect on the body's ability to digest fat.

INCIDENCE AND PREVALENCE

The prevalence of gallstones is high in the United States. In women, gallstones tend to form at 20 to 30 years of age; in men, they form at 30 to 60 years.

ETIOLOGY

The two most common types of gallstones are: cholesterol and mixed (containing bile pigment, calcium bilirubinate, or calcium and copper). Cholesterol stones are more likely in women.

LABORATORY RESULTS

Ultrasonography and cholangiography are used to identify stones and obstruction.

CLINICAL MANIFESTATIONS

The formation of gallstones begins with excessive cholesterol secreted into the bile. Cholesterol eventually precipitates into stones. The stones can block the cystic duct, resulting in inflammation cholelithiasis with or without jaundice.

GALLBLADDER DISEASE-CHOLANGITIS

DEFINITION

Cholangitis is an inflammation of the biliary duct that presents as Charcot's triad: epigastric, upper abdominal pain; jaundice; and fever and chills.

ETIOLOGY

Cholangitis is caused by obstruction or bacterial growth in the biliary tract.

LABORATORY RESULTS

The white blood cell count is 10,000/mm^3 and the bilirubin is 2 mg/dL. Hepatic alkaline phosphatase and blood urea nitrogen are elevated. Prerenal azotemia is due to dehydration. Ultrasonography, CT scan, and x-ray are used for diagnosis.

TREATMENT

- Cholecystectomy, common duct exploration with open or closed surgical approach
- Mechanical removal with forceps or baskets
- Disintegration (dissolve stones with chemicals)
- Gastroscope removal

ANESTHETIC CONSIDERATIONS

The patient may require preoperative pain relief if emergent surgical intervention is required. If the patient is vomiting, fluids and electrolytes should be evaluated and imbalances corrected.

PROGNOSIS

Prognosis is good. The surgical mortality rate is 1.7%, related to complications (i.e., infection and pancreatitis).

D. Pancreatitis

DEFINITION

Pancreatitis is differentiated into edematous and necrotizing types. Plasma amylase concentrations are increased in a patient experiencing intense midepigastric pain. Chronic pancreatitis is present in alcoholics and in patients with diabetes mellitus or fatty liver infiltration.

INCIDENCE AND PREVALENCE

The incidence of pancreatitis varies in different countries, depending on the incidence of causative factors such as alcoholism, gallstones, and drug use. In the United States, acute pancreatitis is more commonly associated with alcohol abuse than with gallstones. It occurs in about 0.5% of the general population.

ETIOLOGY

Biliary tract disease and alcoholism are the most common causes of pancreatitis. Other causes are obstructive pancreatic ducts, infection, primary hyperparathyroidism, uremia, renal transplantation, hyperlipidemia, pregnancy, chemical substance abuse (drugs), hypothermia, idiopathic processes, and trauma.

LABORATORY RESULTS

CT scan and ultrasonography are used. CBC reveals leukocytosis (10,000 to 20,000/mm^3). Serum amylase is normal. Serum lipase, urinary amylase, and urinary lipase are elevated. Pleural and peritoneal fluid should be analyzed. Blood sugar is elevated. Calcium less than 7.5 mg/dL is associated with necrosis. Liver function enzymes are elevated. Coagulation studies, ECG, chest x-ray, and levels of methemalbumin should be assessed.

CLINICAL MANIFESTATIONS

Clinical manifestations are based on etiologic factors that include an enlarged pancreas, pain, nausea, vomiting, diarrhea, bleeding, agitation, and fever.

Stages

- *Initiating process:* Bile reflux, duodenal reflux, lymphatic spread of inflammation
- *Initial pancreatic injury:* Edema, vascular drainage, rupture of pancreatic ducts, acinar damage
- *Activation of digestive enzymes:* Trypsin, lipase
- *Autodigestion*
- *Pancreatic necrosis:* Associated with abscesses, septicemia, pulmonary failure, acute renal failure, hyperglycemia

TREATMENT

Treatment is supportive: pain should be relieved; shock should be overcome; metabolic, fluid, and electrolyte balances should be restored; and pancreatic secretion should be suppressed (give nothing by mouth, gastrointestinal suction, antacids, histamine$_2$ blockers, calcitonin, somatostatin). Secondary infection should be prevented. Optimal respiratory care should be instituted. Renal function should be preserved and renin release should be neutralized.

ANESTHETIC CONSIDERATIONS

Laboratory results should be reviewed and the patient evaluated for shock, hemorrhage, and pain relief (meperidine is the drug of choice). Fluid and electrolyte status is of concern since the patient should receive nothing by mouth. The patient will have a nasogastric tube and histamine$_2$ blockers will be given. Also, the patient should be typed and crossmatched for possible transfusion. Plasma expanders, crystalloids, and invasive monitoring may be used.

PROGNOSIS

The mortality rate is 50% with hemorrhagic pancreatitis 3% to 10% with edematous pancreatitis. One in 90 cases progresses from acute to chronic pancreatitis.

E. Carcinoid Syndrome

DEFINITION

Carcinoid syndrome is produced by metastatic tumors that secrete excessive amounts of vasoactive substances, such as histamine, bradykinin, serotonin, and various prostaglandins.

INCIDENCE AND PREVALENCE

Carcinoid syndrome develops in about 5% of patients with a carcinoid tumor.

ETIOLOGY

Carcinoid syndrome results when carcinoid tumors in the gastrointestinal tract metastasize to the liver. The liver deactivates the hormones secreted.

LABORATORY RESULTS

Levels of those vasoactive substances mentioned are increased.

CLINICAL MANIFESTATIONS

Clinical manifestations include cutaneous flushing, hypertension, tachycardia, abdominal pain, diarrhea, bronchospasm, asthma, and rarely cardiomyopathy. The exact manifestation depends on the hormone secreted. Tricuspid regurgitation and pulmonic stenosis are possible. Other manifestations are premature atrial beats, cyanosis, venous telangiectasia, hepatomegaly, hyperglycemia, decreased plasma albumin concentration, and dehydration.

TREATMENT

Treatment consists of fluid resuscitation, histamine$_1$ and histamine$_2$ antagonists, steroids, and ketanserin (a serotonin antagonist). Bronchodilation is used. Histamine release is treated with bronchodilation and epinephrine.

ANESTHETIC CONSIDERATIONS

Volatile anesthetics will cause bronchodilation. Administering drugs associated with histamine release should be avoided. Direct-acting vasopressors should be used, and vasodilators used as needed. Drugs that block vasoactive substances (octreotide, somatostatin) are used to treat kallikrein-releasing tumors. Hypertension (which may stimulate vasoactive substance release), deep anesthesia, peripheral sympathetic nervous system block, activation of the sympathetic nervous system (since catecholamines are known to activate kallikrein) and the use of ketamine should be avoided. Muscle wasting and its effect on ventilatory function must be evaluated.

PROGNOSIS

The prognosis is related to tumor treatment.

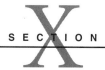

Other Conditions

A. Obesity

DEFINITION

The National Heart, Lung, and Blood Institute (NHLBI) suggests that clinicians use the Body Mass Index (BMI) to assess the degree of body fat. It is relatively simple to use and applies to both men and women. A BMI of 25 to 29.9 is considered overweight and 30 or above is considered obese. The calculation of the BMI is shown below.

$$BMI = Weight \ (kilograms) \div Height \ (meters^2)$$

INCIDENCE AND PREVALENCE

Obesity affects 25% of the U.S. population.

ETIOLOGY

Obesity is rarely a thyroid dysfunction. It is often due to a family trait, environmental factors, or psychological factors. It involves gradual accumulations of excess body weight due to a positive energy balance because of excessive caloric intake or decreased energy expenditure.

LABORATORY RESULTS

Findings include hypercholesterolemia, hypertriglyceridemia, and altered PFT results. Baseline ABGs, chest x-ray, ECG, and echocardiograms are used for diagnosis.

CLINICAL MANIFESTATIONS

Manifestations include increased cardiac output, blood volume, oxygen consumption, minute ventilation, work of breathing, and carbon dioxide production. Systemic hypertension, pulmonary hypertension, ventricular hypertrophy, decreased chest wall compliance, decreased lung volumes, arterial hypoxemia, diabetes mellitus, congestive heart failure, sleep apnea, fatty liver infiltration, and osteoarthritis are other manifestations.

TREATMENT

Medical treatment entails decreased calorie intake combined with exercise. A very-low-calorie, liquid-protein diet requires medical supervision. Surgical treatment includes gastroplasty, jejunoileal bypass, gastric stapling, and jaw wiring.

ANESTHETIC CONSIDERATIONS

Patient history must be carefully reviewed. Airway obstruction, sleep disturbance (sleep apnea), snoring, and cardiovascular disease (dyspnea, orthopnea, angina, hypertension, respiratory cyanosis) must also be evaluated. Gastrointestinal considerations are heartburn, reflux, and increased gastric volume.

Induction
Preoxygenate and denitrogenate for 3 to 5 minutes since these patients can rapidly desaturate when apneic. Rapid sequence induction and gastrointestinal prophylaxis should be considered. Awake intubation may also be considered.

Maintenance
Volatile anesthetic metabolism may be increased with fatty liver infiltration.

Emergency
If the patient is awake, intact protective reflexes should be checked. The head of the bed must be elevated. Oxygen may be needed by mask for transport to the postanesthesia care unit (PACU). Fasting patients may have electrolyte, fluid, and protein imbalances. It should also be determined if the patient is using diuretics, laxatives, amphetamines, appetite suppressants, or thyroid hormone, since anesthetics may cause adverse drug interactions.

B. Glaucoma/Open Globe

DEFINITION AND ETIOLOGY
In glaucoma/open globe, intraoccular pressure (IOP) is increased, resulting in impaired capillary flow to the optic nerve. If left untreated, loss of sight may result.

Types of Glaucoma
- *Open-angle glaucoma:* Characterized by elevated IOP with anatomically open anterior chamber. Sclerosed trabecular tissue impairs aqueous filtration and drainage. Treatment: miosis and trabecular stretching should be produced medically (eye drops, epinephrine, timolol).
- *Closed-angle glaucoma:* Peripheral iris moves in direct contact with the posterior corneal surface, mechanically obstructing aqueous flow. Caused by a narrow angle between the iris and posterior cornea. Swelling of crystalline lens.
- *Congenital glaucoma* is associated with some eye diseases (retinopathy of prematurity, aniridia, mesodermal dysgenesis syndrome). Treatment: surgical goniotomy or trabeculotomy should be performed to route aqueous flow into Schlemm's canal. Cyclocryotherapy decreases aqueous formation by destroying the ciliary body by freezing tissue with a probe.

Open Globe
This condition usually follows traumatic injury.

DIAGNOSTIC AND LABORATORY FINDINGS

Normal IOP is 10 to 25 mm Hg; abnormal IOP is greater than 25 mm Hg. Pressure becomes atmospheric when the globe is opened. Any sudden rise in IOP at this time may lead to prolapse of the iris and lens, extrusion of the vitreous humor, and loss of vision. Coagulation studies should be evaluated before instituting retrobulbar block.

CLINICAL MANIFESTATIONS

The clinical manifestations of acute glaucoma are a dilated, irregular pupil and pain in and around the eye.

TREATMENT

IOP is increased by external pressure on the eye, including venous congestion associated with coughing, vomiting, or the prone position; scleral rigidity—increased rigidity is seen in aged persons; and changes in the intraocular structure or fluids. Pilocarpine hydrochloride decreases resistance to improve drainage of aqueous humor. Acetazolamide reduces the rate at which aqueous humor is formed.

ANESTHETIC CONSIDERATIONS

Drug therapy should be continued to maintain miosis. Anticholinergic drugs are acceptable in preoperative medication. Increases of IOP, hypercarbia, and CVP should be avoided. Succinylcholine causes transient increases in IOP. Rapid sequence induction generally is acceptable for patients with open globe and a full stomach. Awake intubations are not desirable because they may contribute to increases in IOP. Techniques/drugs associated with decreasing IOP include volatile anesthetics, intravenous anesthetics, hypocarbia, hypothermia, mannitol, glycerin, nondepolarizing muscle relaxants, and timolol. General anesthesia or retrobulbar blocks are acceptable for eye surgery. General anesthesia is typically used for "open" globe repair.

Drug interactions must also be considered. Echothiophate prolongs the effect of succinylcholine. Timolol may result in bradycardia. Etomidate may induce myoclonus.

Goals of Ophthalmic Surgery

The goals of ophthalmic surgery are akinesia, profound analgesia, minimal bleeding, avoidance of the oculocardiac reflex, control of IOP, awareness of drug interactions, and smooth induction and emergence without vomiting or coughing/bucking.

PROGNOSIS

The prognosis depends on control of IOP and maintenance of capillary perfusion.

C. Hypothermia

DEFINITION

Hypothermia occurs when the body temperature falls below 37° C. It is a frequent complication of trauma.

INCIDENCE AND PREVALENCE

Patients become poikilothermic when anesthetized (i.e., subject to the temperature of their environment). When patients arrive in the PACU, 60% to 80% are hypothermic. Infants, elderly persons, and burn and trauma patients are most susceptible.

ETIOLOGY

Hypothermia is caused by trauma, burns, general anesthesia, massive resuscitation, and advanced age; it also occurs in young children, especially neonates. General anesthesia involves three phases of cooling:

Phase I   Linear decrease of 1° to 1.5° C with a decrease in muscle tone, decreased metabolism, and vasodilation with volatile anesthetics, administration of blood, and exposure to wet preparations

Phase II   A 0.5° C decrease in the first 3 to 4 hours of anesthesia, decreasing to a core temperature of 34.5° C

Phase III Vasoconstriction prevents a further decline in temperature

CLINICAL MANIFESTATIONS

Temperature is less than 37° C. Arrhythmias and respiratory depression occur as temperatures decline. Enzymatic and coagulation factor dysfunction of the humoral clotting system occurs. Bradycardia, myocardial depression, ventricular fibrillation, and shivering stops at 33° C. Coma occurs at 30° C. Relative thrombocytopenia is present.

TREATMENT

Room temperature should be increased to 21° to 25° C. Intravenous fluids should be warmed. Thermal blankets and forced hot-air heating blankets should be used, as well as a heated, humidified breathing circuit. Core rewarming must be used in severe cases, including gastric lavage, peritoneal lavage, and bladder lavage. Patients should be kept covered. Radiant heat lamps may be used.

ANESTHETIC CONSIDERATIONS

Anesthetized patients behave like poikilothermic patients. Coagulopathies may develop. Induced hypothermia is used for neurosurgery and cardiac surgery to decrease metabolism and oxygen consumption. Heat is lost through radiation, convection, conduction, and evaporation.

Cardiovascular

Decreased cardiac output (increased if the patient is shivering) and increased systemic vascular resistance occur; central redistribution of blood may cause congestive heart failure and bradycardia.

Metabolic

The metabolic rate decreases (or increases if patient is shivering). Tissue perfusion decreases and metabolic acidosis occurs. Glucose use decreases.

Pulmonary

Pulmonary vascular resistance increases, hypoxic pulmonary vasoconstriction decreases, anatomic dead space increases, and ventilation increases.

Hematologic

Blood viscosity increases, and the oxygen dissociation curve shifts to the left.

Neurologic

Cerebrovascular resistance to cerebral blood flow increases, the electroencephalogram slows to coma status, and the minimum alveolar concentration decreases.

Drug Disposition

Hepatic and renal blood decrease, and subsequently, drug metabolism and excretion. These effects can prolong drug effects, particularly muscle relaxants.

Shivering

Oxygen consumption increases by up to 500%, and CO_2 production increases.

D. Hyperthermia

DEFINITION

Hyperthermia occurs when the body temperature is above 36° C. Temperature changes with circadian rhythms, exercise, menstruation, and the environment.

INCIDENCE AND PREVALENCE

Perioperative malignant hyperthermia is rare, occurring in 1 of 250,000 patients.

ETIOLOGY

Hyperthermia is caused by sepsis, thyrotoxicosis, pheochromocytoma, anticholinergic blockade of sweating, heat stroke, and, occasionally, malignant hyperthermia syndrome.

CLINICAL MANIFESTATIONS

The temperature is elevated above 41° C because of infection or dysfunctional thermoregulation, caused by any of the following factors.
- Increased heat production due to thyrotoxicosis, pheochromocytoma, exercise, neuroleptic malignant syndrome, malignant hyperthermia

- Decreased heat dissipation due to dehydration, heat stroke, autonomic dysfunction, excessive coverings, atropine overdose
- Hypothalamic influence—stroke, tumor, trauma, infection, antipsychotic medications

TREATMENT

Treatment consists of total body cooling and treatment or removal of source.

ANESTHETIC CONSIDERATIONS

Metabolic

Metabolism changes with increased temperature. A 1° C increase raises the basal metabolic rate by 10% to 12%. Oxygen consumption increases, CO_2 production increases, fluid and electrolyte requirements increase, and the cardiovascular workload increases.

Endocrine

Antidiuretic hormone, aldosterone, growth hormone, corticosteroids, and thyroid hormones are increased.

Central Nervous System

The level of consciousness is altered and cellular edema occurs.

Hematologic

Platelets, prothrombin, fibrinogen, and factors V, VI, and VII are decreased; spontaneous fibrinolysis and consumption coagulopathies can occur.

E. Systemic Lupus Erythematosus

DEFINITION

Systemic lupus erythematosus (SLE) is a chronic inflammatory disorder of connective tissues that affects multiple organ systems with periods of remissions and exacerbations.

INCIDENCE AND PREVALENCE

Lupus occurs 8 to 15 times more often in women than in men, affecting approximately 75 people in 1,000,000 every year. It occurs most often in Asians and blacks. Exacerbations are more common in spring and summer and during stresses such as infection, pregnancy, or surgery.

ETIOLOGY

The etiology of SLE is unknown. One theory is that it is an antibody-antigen autoimmune response. Another theory deals with predisposing factors that promote susceptibility to SLE. These factors include stressors such as infection, exposure to ultraviolet light, immunizations, and pregnancy. A third theory suggests that SLE may be triggered by drugs such as procainamide, hydralazine, penicillin, anticonvulsants, oral contraceptives, and sulfa drugs.

LABORATORY RESULTS

CBC with differential may reveal anemia, a decreased WBC, and a decreased platelet count. Specific tests for SLE include antinuclear antibodies, anti-DNA, and lupus erythematosus cell tests; urine analysis may reveal both RBCs and WBCs. Chest x-ray examination may reveal pulmonary involvement, and ECG may show conduction abnormalities.

CLINICAL MANIFESTATIONS

Clinical manifestations of SLE include arthritis of the upper and lower extremities as well as avascular necrosis of the femur. Systemically, SLE affects major organ systems (heart, lungs, kidneys, liver, neuromuscular system, skin). Pericarditis, myocarditis, tachycardia, arrhythmias, and congestive heart failure may develop. Left ventricular dysfunction and endocarditis have also been associated with SLE. About 50% of SLE patients develop such cardiopulmonary abnormalities. Pneumonia, pleural effusions, cough, dyspnea, and hypoxemia are common. Glomerulonephritis and oliguric renal failure may result. Some patients develop lupoid hepatitis, which may be fatal. They may also incur intestinal ischemia. The neuromuscular system may develop myopathies. Psychological changes include schizophrenia and deterioration of the intellect. The skin may exhibit the typical lesion associated with SLE—this "butterfly rash" appears over the nose and is erythematous. Alopecia may also be seen clinically.

TREATMENT

The usual treatment of SLE includes anti-inflammatory therapy with aspirin. Corticosteroids are often used to suppress adverse renal and cardiovascular system changes. For patients who do not respond well to steroids, immunosuppressive agents may be used. Antimalarial drugs, in small doses, have been found to be effective in treating arthritis and skin lesions.

ANESTHETIC CONSIDERATIONS

Anesthesia management is based on medications being used to treat the disorder as well as the organ involvement. Care must be taken in positioning the patient to avoid hyperextension of the neck. These patients may be difficult to intubate because of their inflammatory changes, and they frequently have restrictive lung disease and therefore may be difficult to ventilate. Rapid rates with smaller tidal volumes may be helpful. Overall, a thorough preoperative evaluation should be performed in order to establish organ system involvement.

Cutaneous lesions on the nose and mouth may make mask fit difficult. Cricoarytenoid arthritis rarely occurs. Patients with advanced disease may be debilitated—chest x-ray, CBC, and electrolytes should be checked. Anemia and thrombocytopenia purpura have been identified. The partial thromboplastin time may be falsely elevated because antibodies of SLE react with phospholipids used to determine partial thromboplastin time. If renal dysfunction is advanced, renally excreted drugs should be avoided. If the patient is currently on steroids or has used them within 6 months, a steroid bolus should be used.

PROGNOSIS

Early detection and treatment improves prognosis. Prognosis, however, remains poor for those who develop cardiovascular, pulmonary, renal, or neurologic complications.

F. Immunosuppression

DEFINITION

Patients receiving medication to suppress the immune response may suffer from immunosuppression, a disease state that destroys the immune system. T_4 or T-helper cells are inhibited. Interleukin-2 production is inhibited. Blood transfusions cause nonspecific immunosuppression.

ETIOLOGY

Immunosuppression is caused by cancer, acquired immunodeficiency syndrome (AIDS), organ transplantation, and steroid use.

CLINICAL MANIFESTATIONS

Renal and liver dysfunction, as evidenced by elevated creatinine and bilirubin respectively, can occur. The normal total lymphocyte count (TLC) is 1500 to 1800 (TLC [in cubic millimeters] = white blood cells $\times$ lymphocytes).

ANESTHETIC CONSIDERATIONS

Good hand washing and protective isolation are essential. Cyclosporine may potentiate barbiturates, narcotics, and vecuronium. Transplantation patients may require more time to recover from general anesthesia.

G. Malnutrition

DEFINITION

Malnutrition, or nutritional failure, is associated with protein depletion in the presence of adequate calories or with combined protein-calorie deficiency. Protein caloric depletion is a frequent finding in surgical patients and the critically ill.

INCIDENCE AND PREVALENCE

Critically ill patients experience negative caloric intake because of the hypermetabolic state produced by their illness. Trauma, fever, sepsis, and wound healing result in a drastically increased metabolism.

ETIOLOGY

Basic energy requirements are an intake of 1500 to 2000 calories/dL. An increase in body temperature of 1° C increases daily caloric requirements by 15%. Multiple fractures increase energy needs by 25%. Major burns are the greatest manifestation, increasing energy requirements by 100%. In addition, patients with large tumors may also have their energy requirements greatly increased.

LABORATORY RESULTS

The lack of a specific test for protein-caloric malnutrition often makes diagnosis difficult. The best single index of malnutrition is evidence of weight loss from the patient's normal level of weight. Plasma albumin levels below 3 g/dL and transferrin levels below 200 mg/dL have also been used to diagnose malnutrition. Nitrogen balance, which requires the careful collection of all drainage and excretions over 24 hours, may be used to evaluate nutritional status. Nitrogen balance provides an estimate of net protein degradation or synthesis.

CLINICAL MANIFESTATIONS

Protein depletion affects the protein content of all organs. The liver and gastrointestinal tract are rapidly depleted; the brain is affected less than other organs. If protein depletion is severe, the gastrointestinal system will be unable to tolerate or digest food because protein is needed to produce digestive enzymes. Skeletal muscle is most affected and may lose as much as 70% of its protein. Patients with malnutrition are at increased risk of infections and complications in the postoperative period.

TREATMENT

The steps in planning a nutritional regimen are to first identify the need for intervention, then to determine the route of delivery, and finally to adjust the amounts of macronutrients and micronutrients the patient requires.

ANESTHETIC CONSIDERATIONS

Enteral and parenteral are the two routes of choice. At times these two routes are combined. Enteral supplements can be sipped or administered through a nasogastric feeding tube or gastrostomy tube. If the GI tract is nonfunctional, intravenous (parenteral) nutrition is instituted. Isotonic solutions can be delivered through peripheral veins. However, if the solution is hypertonic because of a greater caloric need, a central line should be used.

Patients receiving exogenous nutritional support are prone to deficits or an overabundance of certain electrolytes. Careful evaluation of laboratory values preoperatively as well as of any function tests performed is imperative. Parenteral nutrition has the greatest potential for complications. Hypoglycemia and hyperglycemia are common. Increased carbon dioxide resulting from metabolism of large amounts of glucose may hinder early extubation postoperatively. Patients with compromised cardiac function are at risk for congestive heart failure related to fluid overload. Electrolyte abnormalities include hypokalemia, hypomagnesemia, hypocalcemia, and hypophosphatemia. If parenteral nutrition is continued intraoperatively, infusions of other fluids should be minimized. Malnutrition is a clinical finding that must be partially corrected preoperatively. Therapy must be maintained postoperatively for a substantial time based on each patient's needs.

H. Geriatrics

DEFINITION
Geriatrics is the branch of medicine that deals with the physiologic effects of aging and the diagnosis and treatment of persons who are 65 years of age or older.

ETIOLOGY
Peak physiologic function is reached in the late 20s. As a person ages, physiologic function declines gradually.

CLINICAL MANIFESTATIONS
Clinical manifestations include an increased prevalence of age-related, concomitant disease (hypertension, renal disease, atherosclerosis, MI, COPD, cardiomegaly, diabetes, liver disease, CHF, angina, CVA). Basic organ function declines.

Cardiovascular Changes
There are decreases in coronary blood flow, maximum heart rate, and arterial distensibility. There are increases in peripheral vascular resistance, impediments to left-ventricular output, and increased systolic blood pressure. The cardiac index, resting heart rate, and ejection fraction undergo little or no change.

ANESTHETIC CONSIDERATIONS
The resting PaO_2 decreases, necessitating an increase in intraoperative FiO_2. A decline in the response to hypoxia and hypercapnia results in additional respiratory depression, even with small amounts of narcotics or inhalation anesthetics. The dose requirements of anesthetic agents increase because of reduced receptor sites, a decreased affinity of receptors for hormones and drugs, and decreased synthesis of CNS neurotransmitters. Circulation time decreases, and hypothermia and hyperkalemia are more likely because of decreased aldosterone levels.

In terms of general pharmacology, elimination half-lives and volumes of distribution increase, and drug clearance and protein binding decrease.

Inhalation Agents
The maximum allowable concentration decreases in relation to decreased cardiac output with a faster rate of uptake. Vasodilating effects are exaggerated and junctional arrhythmias become more prevalent.

Muscle Relaxants

The onset and elimination of muscle relaxants is slower.

Regional

The requirements of local anesthetics decrease in relation to decreased neuronal concentrations.

Epidural

Intervertebral spaces narrow; drugs may disperse; and the incidence of spinal headaches decreases.

Spinal

Hypotension from sympathetic block increases in relation to decreased cardiac reserve and decreased intravascular volume.

Positioning

Bony extremities should be well padded. Arthritis may cause airway problems—neck mobility should be assessed.

I. Scleroderma

DEFINITION

Scleroderma is characterized by widespread, symmetric lesions that cause induration of the skin and are followed by atrophy and pigmentation changes. It is a systemic disease that affects muscles, bones, heart, and lungs. Intestinal and pulmonary changes also occur. Lung volumes, vital capacity, compliance, and dead space all decrease. The respiratory rate increases and diffusion capacity is impaired. Pulmonary hypertension can occur.

ANESTHETIC CONSIDERATIONS

Tightening of the skin around the neck may limit mobility and mouth opening. Alternate methods to secure the airway (e.g., fiberoptic intubation) should be considered. Baseline PFTs and ABGs may assist in optimizing these patients preoperatively, intraoperatively, and postoperatively. Postoperative ventilatory assistance may be needed. Be alert for vasospastic phenomena following induction of anesthesia—these should be treated with a plasma expander. Regional anesthesia is acceptable. Core temperature must be maintained. Gastrointestinal pretreatment (i.e., histamine blockers, metoclopramide, etc.) may be necessary because of poor gastric emptying.

Common Procedures

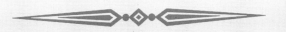

I

Gastrointestinal System

A. Cholecystectomy

1. **Introduction**
   Surgery of the upper abdomen is used in the treatment of gallstones and other diseases of the gallbladder. The mortality rate for elective cholecystectomy is less than 0.5%. In patients over the age of 70, the mortality rate rises to 2% to 3%, mostly because of preexisting cardiopulmonary disease.
2. **Preoperative assessment**
   a) *History and physical examination*
      (1) Standard
      (2) *Gastrointestinal assessment:* Pain localized in the right subcostal region. The patient may experience referred pain in the back at the shoulder level. Anorexia, nausea, and vomiting are common. Infection and fever are rare.
   b) *Diagnostic tests:* As indicated by the patient's history and medical condition.
   c) *Preoperative medication and intravenous therapy*
      (1) Use an antimicrobial to prevent bacteremia.
      (2) Narcotics must be used with caution to minimize potential spasm in the biliary tract and sphincter of Oddi.
      (3) Use a single, large-bore (18-gauge) intravenous tube with fluid replacement.
3. **Room preparation**
   a) *Monitoring equipment:* Standard
   b) *Pharmacologic agents*
      (1) Standard
      (2) Caution is advised with the use of narcotic agents due to potential changes in biliary pressure.
   c) *Position:* Supine
4. **Anesthetic technique:** General endotracheal anesthesia with muscle relaxation
5. **Perioperative management**
   a) *Induction:* Rapid sequence induction with oral endotracheal intubation if the patient is considered to have a full stomach.
   b) *Maintenance*
      (1) No specific requirements
      (2) Muscle relaxation per abdominal surgery
   c) *Emergence:* Awake extubation after airway reflexes are adequate.
6. **Postoperative implications**
   a) Retraction in the right upper quadrant during surgery can lead to atelectasis in the right lower lobe; postoperative pain and

splinting may lead to impaired ventilation.
b) Right intercostal nerve blocks improve postoperative pain management.

B. Laparoscopic Cholecystectomy

1. **Introduction**
    Surgery used in the treatment of gallstones and diseases of the gallbladder. This procedure is performed under the guidance of a laparoscope. More than 90% of cholecystectomies are performed laparoscopically today.
2. **Preoperative assessment and patient preparation**
    a) *History and physical examination:* As indicated by the patient's history and medical condition
    b) *Diagnostic tests:* As indicated by the patient's history and medical condition
    c) *Preoperative medication and intravenous therapy*
       (1) Preoperative antibiotic
       (2) Narcotics must be used with caution to minimize potential spasm in the biliary tract and sphincter of Oddi.
       (3) Use a single, large-bore (18-gauge) intravenous tube with fluid replacement.
3. **Room preparation**
    a) *Monitoring equipment:* Standard
    b) *Pharmacologic agents:* Standard
    c) *Position*
       (1) Supine
       (2) Exposure of the operative site can be optimized with the reverse Trendelenburg position and by tilting the table to the side.
4. **Anesthetic technique:** General endotracheal anesthesia with muscle relaxation
5. **Perioperative management**
    a) *Induction:* Standard or rapid sequence induction with oral endotracheal intubation
    b) *Maintenance*
       (1) Muscle relaxation with appropriate reversal
       (2) The peritoneal cavity must be insufflated for surgical exposure. Insufflation with CO_2 causes a rise in the CO_2 partial pressure unless ventilation is controlled.
       (3) Abdominal insufflation may lead to hypercarbia with inadequate ventilation. Special attention should be paid to possible adjustments in ventilator settings with insufflation.
       (4) Basal measurements should be sufficient to control CO_2 partial pressure.
       (5) Insufflation leads to increased intra-abdominal pressure.

An intra-abdominal pressure of 20 to 25 cm H_2O produces increases in cardiac output and central venous pressure secondary to changes in the volume of the venous return of blood. An IAP greater than 30 to 40 cm H_2O may lead to decreased central venous pressure and reduced cardiac output secondary to reduced right ventricular preload. Insufflation to a pressure of approximately 15 mm Hg is routine.

(6) All maintenance anesthetic drugs may be used. Some surgeons request that nitrous oxide not be used to reduce the risk of bowel expansion, which could hinder surgical exposure.

c) *Emergence:* Awake extubation after airway reflexes are adequate.

6. **Postoperative implications**

a) *Pain management:* This approach offers the benefit of reduced postoperative pain secondary to smaller abdominal incisions. Patients may experience shoulder pain from pneumoperitoneum, which is usually self-limiting.

b) *Postoperative nausea and vomiting:* Antiemetic prophylaxis

C. Liver Resection

1. **Introduction**

Patients requiring for hepatic surgery may have primary or metastatic tumors from gastrointestinal and other sources. Liver function may be entirely normal in these patients. Hepatocellular carcinoma is common in males over 50 years old and is associated with chronic, active hepatitis B and cirrhosis. Although most major resections can be performed by a transabdominal approach, some surgeons prefer a thoracoabdominal approach. The liver is transected by blunt dissection using the Cavitron Ultrasonic Suction Aspirator (CUSA) and Argon Beam Laser Coagulator (ABC).

As the principles and techniques of hepatic surgery have evolved, the overall mortality and morbidity rates have improved considerably. Because the normal liver can regenerate, it is possible to resect the right or left lobe along with segments of the contralateral lobe. In patients with cirrhoses, the regeneration process is limited; thus, uninvolved liver should be preserved.

2. **Preoperative assessment**

The following preoperative considerations are for patients *without cirrhosis:*

a) *History and physical examination:* As indicated by the patient's history and medical condition

b) *Patient preparation*

(1) *Laboratory tests:* Complete blood count, coagulation profile, liver function test, albumin, creatinine, blood urea nitro-

gen, blood sugar, bilirubin, and electrolytes. Perform other tests as indicated per history and physical examination.

(2) *Diagnostic tests:* Chest radiographs, ultrasonography, computed tomography and magnetic resonance imaging as indicated per history and physical examination.

(3) *Medications:* Standard premedication that accounts for the reduced ability of the liver to metabolize drugs. Other pre-operative medications include antiemetics.

3. **Room preparation**
   a) *Monitoring equipment*
      (1) Standard monitoring equipment
      (2) Arterial line and central venous pressure as clinically indicated
   b) *Additional equipment*
      (1) Cell saver
      (2) Consider a rapid transfusion device
   c) *Drugs*
      (1) Standard emergency drugs
      (2) Standard tabletop
      (3) *Intravenous fluids:* 14- or 16-gauge intravenous lines (2) with normal saline or lactated Ringer's solution at 10 to 20 mL/kg per hour. Warm fluids.
      (4) Two units of packed red blood cells should be available. Blood loss can be significant, and massive transfusions may be required. Appropriate blood products also include 2 units of fresh frozen plasma and 10 units of platelets.

4. **Perioperative management and anesthetic technique**
   a) *Induction*
      (1) General endotracheal anesthesia and appropriate postoperative analgesia
      (2) Restore intravascular volume prior to anesthetic induction. If patient is hemodynamically unstable, consider etomidate (0.2 to 0.4 mg/kg) or ketamine (1 to 3 mg/kg).
   b) *Maintenance*
      (1) Standard
      (2) *Combined epidural and general anesthesia:* Be prepared to treat hypotension with fluid and vasopressors. General anesthesia is administered to supplement regional anesthesia and for amnesia.
      (3) *Position:* Supine, checked and padded pressure points. Avoid stretching the brachial plexus. Limit abduction to 90 degrees.
   c) *Emergence*
      For major hepatic resections, the patient will be best cared for in an intensive care unit. Consider keeping the patient mechanically ventilated until the patient is hemodynamically stable and ventilatory status is optimized. If surgical resection was minimal, the patient can be extubated awake and after reflexes have returned.

5. **Postoperative implications**
   a) Decreased liver function—patients with normal preoperative

liver function may have significant postoperative impairment of liver function secondary to loss of liver mass or surgical trauma.

b) Pulmonary insufficiency (atelectasis, effusion, and pneumonia)—more than 90% of patients will develop some form of respiratory complication.

c) Hemorrhage

d) Disseminated intravascular coagulation

e) Electrolyte imbalance

f) Hypoglycemia

g) Hypothermia

D. Liver Transplant

1. **Introduction**

Liver transplantation is the treatment of choice for patients with acute and chronic end-stage liver disease (ESLD). The liver transplant operation can be divided into three stages: (1) hepatectomy; (2) anhepatic phase, which involves the implantation of the liver; and (3) postrevascularization, which involves hemostasis and reconstruction of the hepatic artery and common bile duct. Hepatectomy can be associated with increased blood loss. Contributing factors include severe coagulopathy, severe portal hypertension, previous surgery in the right upper quadrant, renal failure, uncontrolled sepsis, retransplantation, transfusion reaction, venous bypass induced fibrinolysis, primary graft nonfunction, and intraoperative vascular complications.

The anhepatic phase may be associated with significant hemodynamic changes. This stage consists of implantation of the liver allograft, with or without venovenous bypass. Benefits of using the venovenous bypass system include improved hemodynamics during the anhepatic phase, decreased blood loss, and possible improvement of perioperative renal function. Complications of using the system include pulmonary embolism, air embolism, brachial plexus injury, and wound seroma/infection.

Prior to revascularization, the liver must be flushed with a cold solution (i.e., albumin 5%) through the portal vein and out the infrahepatic vena cava. The reperfusion of the liver may be the most critical part of the operation. Patients may experience pulmonary hypertension, followed by right ventricular failure and profound hypotension. The hepatic artery reconstruction is performed after stabilization of the patient following revascularization. The last part involves hemostasis, removal of the gallbladder, and reconstruction of the bile duct.

2. **Preoperative assessment**

Patients requiring liver transplantation often have multiorgan system failure. Due to the emergent nature of the surgery, there may be insufficient time available for customary evaluation and correction of abnormalities.

a) *History and physical examination*
  (1) *Cardiovascular:* These patients can present with a hyperdynamic state, with increased cardiac output and decreased SVR. Many of these patients present with dysrhythmias, hypertension, pulmonary hypertension, valvular disease, cardiomyopathy (alcoholic disease, hemochromatosis, Wilson's disease), and coronary artery disease.
  (2) *Respiratory:* Patients are often hypoxic because of ascites, pleural effusions, atelectasis, V/Q mismatch, and pulmonary AV shunting. This normally results in tachypnea and respiratory alkalosis. Pulmonary infection is usually a contraindication to surgery. ARDS is usually not.
  (3) *Hepatic:* Hepatitis serology and the cause of hepatic failure should be determined. Albumin is usually low, with consequent low plasma oncotic pressure leading to edema and ascites. The magnitude and duration of drugs may be unpredictable, although these patients generally have an increased sensitivity to all drugs, and the drug actions are prolonged.
  (4) *Neurologic:* Patients are often encephalopathic and may be in hepatic coma. In fulminant hepatic failure, increased intracranial pressure is common, accounting for 40% mortality (herniation), and may require prompt treatment (mannitol, hyperventilation, etc.).
  (5) *Gastrointestinal:* Portal hypertension, esophageal varices, and coagulopathies increase the risk of GI hemorrhage. Gastric emptying is often delayed.
  (6) *Renal:* Patients are often hypervolemic, hyponatremic, and possibly hypokalemic. Calcium is usually normal. Metabolic alkalosis is often present. Preoperative dialysis should be considered.
  (7) *Endocrine:* Patients are often glucose intolerant or diabetic. Hyperaldosteronism may be present.
  (8) *Hematologic:* Patients are often anemic secondary to blood loss or malabsorption. Coagulation is impaired due to a decreased hepatic synthesis function (all factors except VIII and fibrinogen are decreased), abnormal fibrinogen production, impaired platelets, fibrinolysis, and low-grade DIC.

b) *Patient preparation*
  (1) *Laboratory tests:* See "Liver Resection," on pg. 130.
  (2) *Diagnostic tests:* Chest radiographs, pulmonary function tests, electrocardiography, echocardiogram, and cardiac catheterization
  (3) *Medication:* Standard premedication that accounts for full stomach precautions

3. **Room Preparation**
  a) *Monitoring equipment*
    (1) Standard

   (2) Arterial line, TEE, central venous pressure, or pulmonary
     artery catheter as indicated
  b) *Additional equipment*
   (1) Patient warming devices
   (2) Rapid infusion system
  c) *Drugs*
   (1) Standard tabletop
   (2) Standard emergency drugs
   (3) *Intravenous fluids:* 10 Fr × 2. Often placed in right antecu-
     bital fossa, left or right internal/external jugular. The left
     arm is avoided because the axillary vein is used for
     vasoveno bypass.
   (4) Blood loss can be significant; blood should be immediately
     available.
 4. **Anesthetic technique:** General anesthesia
  These patients are extremely complex to manage because of
  hemodynamic variability, massive blood loss, coagulopathy, and
  metabolic problems.
 5. **Perioperative management**
  a) *Induction*
   (1) Rapid sequence induction with oral endotracheal tube
   (2) May use a narcotic (fentanyl 2 to 5 mcg/kg) just prior to
     induction
  b) *Maintenance*
   (1) Standard maintenance with fentanyl 10 to 50 mcg/kg. May
     require benzodiazepine to ensure anesthesia during periods
     of hemodynamic instability and if the volatile agents are
     off.
   (2) Antibiotics and immunosuppressants are given upon
     surgeon request.
   (3) Position supine, pad pressure points. Avoid stretching the
     brachial plexus greater than 90 degrees.
   (4) Reperfusion syndrome (which occurs during the revascu-
     larization phase) is characterized by decreased heart rate,
     conduction defects, and decreased systemic vascular resist-
     ance while right ventricular pressures increase. The cause is
     unknown. Cardiac output can be maintained. An increase
     in serum potassium can lead to cardiac arrest.
 6. **Postoperative implications**
  a) *Monitor hepatic function using laboratory data:* serial liver
    function tests, prothrombin time, partial thromboplastin time,
    ammonia levels, lactate, and bile output
  b) *Possible complications:* bleeding, portal vein thrombosis, hepatic
    artery thrombosis, biliary tract leaks, primary nonfunction,
    rejection, infection, pulmonary complications, electrolyte imbal-
    ances, hypertension, alkalosis, renal failure, peptic ulceration,
    and neurologic complications

E. Pancreatectomy

1. **Introduction**

   Distal pancreatectomy is performed for tumors in the distal half of the pancreas, whereas subtotal pancreatectomy involves resection of the pancreas from the mesenteric vessels distally, leaving the head and uncinate process intact. In about 95% of patients with pancreatic cancer, the cancer is ductal adenocarcinoma, with most occurring in the head of the pancreas.

   Pancreatic cancer may appear as a localized mass or as a diffuse enlargement of the gland on computed tomography of the abdomen. Biopsy of the lesion is necessary to confirm the diagnosis. Complete surgical resection is the only effective treatment of ductal pancreatic cancer.

2. **Preoperative assessment**

   Patients requiring pancreatic surgery can be divided into three groups. (1) Those with acute pancreatitis in whom medical treatment has failed in the past. This group may be extremely ill, needing surgery during an exacerbation of pancreatitis or when the diagnosis is in doubt. (2) Patients with carcinoma of the pancreas, including hormone-secreting tumors such as insulinoma and gastrinoma (Zollinger-Ellison syndrome). (3) Patients suffering from the sequelae of chronic pancreatitis.

   a) *History and physical examination*

   (1) *Cardiovascular:* Patients with acute pancreatitis may be hypotensive and may require aggressive volume resuscitation with crystalloid and even blood prior to surgery. Patients with acute pancreatitis may show electrocardiographic change simulating myocardial ischemia. Severe electrolyte disturbances may be associated with acute pancreatitis and some hormone secreting tumors of the pancreas.

   (2) *Respiratory:* Respiratory compromise such as pleural effusions, atelectasis, and adult respiratory distress syndrome progressing to respiratory failure may occur in up to 50% of patients with acute pancreatitis.

   (3) *Gastrointestinal:* Jaundice and abdominal pain are common symptoms in this group of patients. The presence of ileus or intestinal obstruction should mandate full stomach precautions and rapid sequence induction. Electrolyte disturbances are common with acute pancreatitis and may include hypochloremic metabolic alkalosis, decreased calcium and magnesium, and increased glucose. These abnormalities should be corrected preoperatively.

   (4) *Endocrine:* Many patients with acute pancreatitis may have diabetes secondary to loss of pancreatic tissue. Hormone-secreting tumors of the pancreas are occasionally associated with multiple endocrine neoplasia syndromes. Insulinoma is the most common hormone-secreting tumor of the

PART 2 **Common Procedures**

pancreas and can result in hypoglycemia.

(5) *Renal:* Patients should be evaluated for renal insufficiency.

(6) *Hematologic:* Hematocrit may be falsely elevated because of hemoconcentration or hemorrhage. Coagulopathy may be present.

b) *Patient preparation*

(1) *Laboratory tests:* Complete blood count, prothrombin time, partial thromboplastin time, platelet count, electrolytes, blood urea nitrogen, creatinine, blood sugar, calcium, magnesium, amylase, and urinalysis. Other tests as indicated per history and physical examination.

(2) *Diagnostic tests:* Chest radiographs, pulmonary function tests, electrocardiography, and computed tomography of the abdomen. Other tests as indicated per history and physical examination.

(3) *Medication:* Standard premedication that accounts for full stomach precautions

3. **Room preparation**

a) *Standard monitoring equipment*

b) *Arterial line, central venous pressure, or pulmonary artery catheter:* As clinically indicated

c) *Additional equipment:* Patient warming devices

d) *Drugs*

(1) Standard emergency drugs

(2) Standard tabletop

(3) *Intravenous fluids:* 14- to 16-gauge intravenous lines (2) with normal saline or lactated Ringer's solution at 10 to 20 mL/kg per hour. Warm fluids.

(4) Blood loss can be significant, and blood should be immediately available.

4. **Perioperative management and anesthetic technique**

General endotracheal anesthesia is used; an epidural is used for postoperative analgesia.

a) *Induction*

(1) Standard

(2) Restore intravascular volume prior to anesthetic induction. If the patient is hemodynamically unstable, consider etomidate (0.2 to 0.4 mg/kg) or ketamine (1 to 3 mg/kg). The patient with bowel obstruction or ileus is at risk for pulmonary aspiration, and rapid sequence induction with cricoid pressure is indicated.

b) *Maintenance*

(1) *Standard maintenance:* Avoid N_2O to minimize bowel distention.

(2) *Combined epidural and general anesthesia:* Be prepared to treat hypotension with fluid vasopressors. General anesthesia is administered to supplement regional anesthesia and for amnesia. Sedatives should be minimized during this type of anesthetic since they increase the likelihood of postoperative respiratory depression. If epidural opiates are

used for postoperative analgesia, a loading dose should be
administered at least 1 hour before the conclusion of surgery.
(3)   *Position:* Supine, checked and padded pressure points. Avoid
stretching the brachial plexus. Limit abduction to 90 degrees.

c)   *Emergence*
The decision to extubate at the end of surgery depends on the
patient's underlying cardiopulmonary status and the extent of
the surgical procedure. Patients should be hemodynamically
stable, warm, alert, cooperative, and fully reversed from any
muscle relaxants prior to extubation.

5.   **Postoperative implications**
Significant third-space and evaporative losses contribute to hypovolemia. Major hemorrhage can occur during dissection of the pancreas from the mesenteric and portal vessels. Total pancreatectomy
is associated with brittle diabetes that can be difficult to control.
Subtotal resections lead to varying degrees of hyperglycemia. The
patient should recover in an intensive care unit or hospital ward
that is accustomed to treating the side effects of epidural opiates.

Tests for postoperative management include electrolytes,
calcium, glucose, complete blood count, platelets, and other tests
as indicated. Electrolyte disturbances are common with acute
pancreatitis and may include hypochloremic metabolic alkalosis,
decreased calcium and magnesium, and increased glucose. These
abnormalities should be corrected preoperatively.

F. Whipple's Resection

1.   **Introduction**
A Whipple resection consists of a pancreatoduodenectomy followed
by an anastomosis of the distal pancreatic stump into the jejunum, a
choledochojejunostomy, and a gastrojejunostomy. On entering the
peritoneal cavity, one determines the resectability of the pancreatic
lesion. Contraindications to resection include involvement of mesenteric vessels, infiltration by tumor into the root of the mesentery,
extension into the porta hepatis with involvement of hepatic artery,
and liver metastasis. If the tumor is deemed resectable, the head of
the pancreas is further mobilized. The common duct is transected
above the cystic duct entry, and the gallbladder is removed. Once the
superior mesenteric vein is freed from the pancreas, the latter is transected with care taken not to injure the splenic vein. The jejunum is
transected beyond the ligament of Treitz, and the specimen is
removed by severing the vascular connections with the mesenteric
vessels. Reconstitution is achieved by anastomosing the distal pancreatic stump, bile duct, and stomach into the jejunum. Drains are
placed adjacent to the pancreatic anastomosis. Some surgeons stent
the anastomosis until it has healed.

2. **Preoperative assessment**
   a) *History and physical examination:* See "Pancreatectomy," p. 135.
   b) *Patient preparation*
      (1) *Laboratory tests:* See "Pancreatectomy," p. 135.
      (2) *Diagnostic tests:* See "Pancreatectomy," p. 135.
      (3) *Medication:* See "Pancreatectomy," p. 135.
3. **Room preparation:** See "Pancreatectomy," p. 135.
4. **Anesthetic technique**
   General endotracheal anesthesia with an epidural for postoperative analgesia. See "Pancreatectomy," p. 135.
5. **Perioperative management:** See "Pancreatectomy," p. 135.
6. **Postoperative implications:** See "Pancreatectomy," p. 135.

G. Splenectomy

1. **Introduction**
   Typically, patients requiring a splenectomy have Hodgkin's disease or some other lymphomatous disorder. Apart from the primary disease, these patients are reasonably healthy and have not undergone irradiation or chemotherapy prior to the surgery. Patients presenting for splenectomy may be divided into two less healthy groups: trauma patients and a more complex group that includes patients with myeloproliferative disorders and other varieties of hypersplenism. Following trauma, instead of a splenectomy, a splenorrhaphy or splenic salvage is done (preservation of all or part of the spleen). This may be accomplished by using local hemostatic techniques (electrocoagulation, argon beam laser coagulator, Surgicel or Gelfoam soaked in thrombin, microfibrillar collagen, and fine sutures or mattress sutures using Teflon felt pledgets).
2. **Preoperative assessment**
   a) *History and physical examination*
      (1) *Cardiovascular:* Patients with systemic disease requiring splenectomy may be chronically ill and have decreased cardiovascular reserve. Patients who have received doxorubicin (Adriamycin) may have a dose-dependent cardiotoxicity that can be worsened by X-ray therapy. Manifestations include decreased QRS amplitude, congestive heart failure, pleural effusions, and dysrhythmia.
      (2) *Respiratory:* Patients who have splenomegaly may have a degree of left lower lobe atelectasis, which should be evaluated by physical examination. Some may have been treated with bleomycin, a chemotherapeutic drug that causes pulmonary fibrosis. Methotrexate and cytarabine may also cause pulmonary fibrosis. Toxic drug effects are potentiated by smoking, X-ray therapy, and a high fractional inspiration of oxygen.

      (3) *Neurologic:* Patients may have neurologic deficits from receiving chemotherapeutic agents. (Vinblastine and cisplatin can cause peripheral neuropathies.) Any evidence of neurologic dysfunction should be documented in the preoperative evaluation.

      (4) *Hematologic:* Patients are likely to have splenomegaly secondary to hematologic disease. Cytopenias are common.

      (5) *Hepatic:* Some chemotherapeutic agents (methotrexate) may be hepatotoxic. Evaluation of liver function tests should be considered in patients deemed at risk.

      (6) *Renal:* Some chemotherapeutic drugs (methotrexate, cisplatin) are nephrotoxic. Patients exposed to such agents may have renal insufficiency.

  b) *Patient preparation*

      (1) *Laboratory tests:* Complete blood count, prothrombin time, partial thromboplastin time, bleeding time, platelet count, electrolytes, blood urea nitrogen, creatinine, urinalysis, and other tests as indicated per history and physical examination

      (2) *Medication:* Standard premedication. A stress dose of steroids (100 mg hydrocortisone every 8 hours on the day of surgery) should be administered if the patient has received them as part of a chemotherapeutic regimen.

3. Room preparation

  a) *Monitoring equipment:* Standard and others as indicated by the patient's status

  b) *Additional equipment:* Patient warming device

  c) *Drugs*

      (1) Standard emergency drugs

      (2) Standard tabletop

      (3) *Intravenous fluids:* 16- to 18-gauge intravenous lines (2) with normal saline or lactated Ringer's solution at 10 to 15 mL/kg per hour. Warm fluids.

4. Anesthetic technique

General endotracheal anesthesia with or without an epidural for postoperative analgesia. If postoperative epidural analgesia is planned, it helps to place a catheter prior to induction to establish correct placement in the epidural space.

5. Perioperative management

  a) *Induction*

      (1) Standard

      (2) Restore intravascular volume prior to anesthetic induction. If the patient is hemodynamically unstable, consider etomidate or ketamine.

  b) *Maintenance*

      (1) Standard

      (2) Combined epidural and general anesthesia: See "Pancreatectomy," p. 135.

      (3) *Position:* Supine. Checked and padded pressure points. Avoid stretching the brachial plexus. Limit abduction to

PART 2 Common Procedures

90 degrees.

c) *Emergence:* The decision to extubate at the end of surgery depends on the patient's underlying cardiopulmonary status and the extent of the surgical procedure. Patients should be hemodynamically stable, warm, alert, cooperative, and fully reversed from any muscle relaxants prior to extubation.

6. **Postoperative implications**
   a) Bleeding
   b) Atelectasis, usually in the left lower lobe
   c) *Pain management:* Multimodal approach—epidural local anesthetics and opiates

H. Gastrectomy

1. **Introduction**
   Surgery performed for bleeding ulcers or adrenal ulcers. This procedure generally includes a gastroduodenostomy (Billroth I) or gastrojejunostomy (Billroth II). Gastric outlet obstruction from scarring or tumor is common.

2. **Preoperative assessment and patient preparation**
   a) *History and physical examination:* Gastrointestinal: Assess fluid and hydration status. The patient may be vomiting or bleeding or may have anorexia.
   b) *Diagnostic tests*
      (1) Abdominal radiography
      (2) Laboratory tests include complete blood count, electrolytes, blood urea nitrogen, glucose, Mg^{2+}, Ca^{2+}, PO_4, prothrombin time, and partial thromboplastin time. Perform other tests based on history and physical examination.
   c) *Preoperative medication and intravenous therapy*
      (1) Expect moderate fluid shift with moderate to large fluid losses. Two large bore intravenous access tubes are indicated.
      (2) Patient may be on histamine$_2$ blocker therapy. Cytochrome P450 inhibition is possible, especially with cimetidine.
      (3) Antibiotic therapy
      (4) Consider anemia from a bleeding ulcer preoperatively.
      (5) Blood transfusions

3. **Room preparation**
   a) *Monitoring equipment*
      (1) Standard
      (2) Full warming modalities
   b) *Pharmacologic agents:* Standard
   c) *Position:* Supine, with arms extended

4. **Anesthetic technique**
   a) Routine general anesthesia
   b) Epidural for intraoperative and/or postoperative management

5. **Perioperative management**
   a) *Induction:* Most patients are considered to have full stomachs; therefore rapid sequence induction is indicated.
   b) *Maintenance*
      (1) Muscle relaxation is required.
      (2) Closely monitor hydration status and blood loss.
      (3) One may avoid N_2O to minimize gastric or colonic distention.
   c) *Emergence:* Awake extubation after rapid sequence induction or placement of nasogastric tube
6. **Postoperative implications**
   a) Pain may lead to hyperventilation, reduced cough, splinting, and atelectasis.
   b) Pain control with epidural or patient-controlled analgesia.

I. Gastrostomy

1. **Introduction**
   A gastrostomy involves the placement of a semipermanent tube through the abdominal wall directly into the stomach. These tubes are used for gastric decompression or for feeding. At the time of a laparotomy, the traditional *Stamm gastrostomy* is most common. It may also be performed through a separate, small laparotomy incision in the upper midline or transverse directly over the stomach. The gastrostomy tube is introduced into the stomach and tied securely with pursestring sutures.

   The *Janeway gastrostomy* is a technical modification, also placed at the time of a laparotomy. This procedure creates a tube that rises from the main body of the stomach, which allows for permanent access to the stomach with removal of the tube between feedings. This approach is used in patients with expected long-term dependence on gastrostomy access.

   A *Percutaneous endoscopic gastrostomy* is often performed. The stomach is intubated endoscopically, and the gastric and abdominal walls punctured under endoscopic guidance. The gastrostomy tube is passed from the mouth and through the stomach and abdominal wall from the inside out.

   Temporary gastrostomies are often used after major abdominal surgery as an alternative to nasogastric suction. Feeding gastrostomy tubes are indicated in patients unable to feed by mouth but able to absorb enteral nutrition, such as patients with advanced malignancy and intestinal obstruction, inadequate oral intake, and neurologic impairment.
2. **Preoperative assessment**
   Patients undergoing gastrostomy can have neurologic impairment, which compromises their ability to handle oral secretions and

PART 2 **Common Procedures**

increases their risk for aspiration.

a) *History and physical examination*

(1) *Cardiac:* Patients are likely to be hypovolemic secondary to chronically poor oral intake and malnutrition.

(2) *Respiratory:* Patients may have difficulty swallowing and inadequate laryngeal reflexes, which places them at high risk for aspiration of gastric contents and associated pneumonitis. Hypoxemia and decreased pulmonary reserve can present with pulmonary infections.

(3) *Neurologic:* The patient is often neurologically impaired, sick, and debilitated.

(4) *Renal:* Long-term indwelling urinary catheters increase the risk of infection.

b) *Patient preparation*

(1) *Laboratory tests:* As indicated by the patient's condition

(2) *Diagnostic tests:* As indicated by the patient's condition

(3) *Medications:* Standard

3. **Room preparation**

a) *Monitoring equipment:* Standard monitoring equipment

b) *Drugs:* Standard emergency drugs

c) Standard tabletop

d) *Intravenous fluids:* One 18-gauge intravenous line with normal saline or lactated Ringer's solution at 5 to 8 mL/kg per hour.

4. **Anesthetic technique**

a) Maximum allowable concentration with local anesthesia to area of incision for gastrostomy

b) General or regional according to the site and size of the incision, the patient's physical status, and the preferences of both the patient and the surgeon

5. **Perioperative management**

a) *Induction*

(1) If general anesthesia is planned, use rapid sequence induction with cricoid pressure.

(2) Restore volume status in a hypovolemic patient before induction.

b) *Maintenance*

(1) *General anesthesia:* Standard; muscle relaxants may be necessary to facilitate closure with laparotomy incision.

(2) *Position:* Supine. Checked and padded pressure points

c) *Emergence:* Tracheal extubation after the return of protective laryngeal reflexes

6. **Postoperative implications**

Mild to moderate postoperative pain intensity may be controlled with parenteral narcotics or intercostal blocks. Postoperative complications include but are not limited to aspiration pneumonia, wound infection, and failure to function.

J. Small Bowel Resection

1. **Introduction**
   Surgery performed for abdominal trauma, abdominal structure adhesions, Meckel's diverticulum, Crohn's disease, or infection.
2. **Preoperative assessment and patient preparation**
   a) *History and physical examination: Gastrointestinal:* Assess fluid and hydration status. The patient may be vomiting or bleeding or may have third-spacing, diarrhea, or dehydration.
   b) *Diagnostic tests:* As indicated by the patient's condition
   c) *Preoperative medication and intravenous therapy*
      (1) Patients may be on steroid therapy or immunosuppressant drugs.
      (2) Expect fluid shifts requiring moderate to large fluid resuscitation. Two large bore, intravenous access tubes are indicated.
      (3) Preoperative hydration is essential.
3. **Room preparation**
   a) *Monitoring equipment:* Standard with full warming modalities
   b) *Pharmacologic agents:* Standard
   c) *Position:* Supine with arms extended
4. **Anesthetic technique**
   a) Epidural (T2 to T4 level) with "light" general anesthetic and orogastric tube
   b) General anesthesia with endotracheal tube
5. **Perioperative management**
   a) *Induction:* Most patients are considered to have full stomachs; therefore rapid sequence induction is indicated.
   b) *Maintenance*
      (1) Muscle relaxation is required.
      (2) Closely monitor hydration status and blood loss.
      (3) Avoid N_2O, which may cause bowel distention.
   c) *Emergence:* Awake extubation after rapid sequence induction or placement of nasogastric tube
6. **Postoperative implications**
   a) Pain may lead to hypoventilation, reduced cough, splinting, and atelectasis.
   b) Pain control with epidural or patient-controlled analgesia.

PART 2 Common Procedures

K. Appendectomy

1. **Introduction**
   In acute appendicitis, the long narrow tube of the appendix is obstructed, hypoxia develops, the mucosa ulcerates, and bacteria invade the wall. It is the most common surgical emergency during pregnancy.

2. **Preoperative assessment and patient preparation**
   a) *History and physical examination*
      (1) *Gastrointestinal:* Patients point to localized pain at "McBurney's point," which is midway between the iliac crest and umbilicus; rebound tenderness, muscle rigidity, and abdominal guarding are noted.
      (2) *Pregnant female:* "Alder's sign" is used to differentiate between uterine and appendical pain. The pain is localized with the patient supine. The patient then lies on her left side. If the area of pain shifts to the left, it is presumed to be uterine.
   b) *Diagnostic tests*
      (1) The white blood cell count is elevated, with a shift to the left—10,000 to 16,000 mm^3; 75% neutrophils.
      (2) Urinalysis shows a small number of erythrocytes and leukocytes.
      (3) Abdominal films demonstrate fecalith (formed, hard mass of feces in right lower quadrant or localized ileus).
      (4) Other laboratory tests include electrolytes, glucose, hemoglobin, and hematocrit. Perform tests as indicated from the history and physical examination.
   c) *Preoperative medication and intravenous therapy*
      (1) Antibiotic for enteric gram-negative bacilli, anaerobic bacteria.
      (2) Single 18-gauge intravenous tube is used because patient is dehydrated from fever, anorexia, and vomiting.
3. **Room preparation**
   a) *Monitoring equipment*
      (1) Standard
      (2) Fetal heart tone monitoring with pregnancy
   b) *Pharmacologic agents*
      (1) Standard
      (2) For fetal safety, it is essential to avoid teratogenic anesthetic during the first trimester.
   c) *Position*
      (1) Supine
      (2) Left uterine displacement with pregnancy
4. **Anesthetic technique**
   a) *Regional blockade:* Analgesia to levels T6 to T8
   b) *General anesthesia:* Endotracheal intubation is required.
5. **Perioperative management**
   a) *Induction*
      (1) Use general anesthesia with rapid sequence induction because many patients have a nasogastric tube or are considered to be on a full stomach (emergency).
      (2) In the pregnant patient, special care should be taken to prevent aspiration pneumonitis.
   b) *Maintenance*
      (1) No specific indications
      (2) Muscle relaxation is necessary.

  c) *Emergence:* Awake extubation secondary to rapid sequence induction
6. **Postoperative implications:** None

L. Colectomy

1. **Introduction**
Surgery performed for adenocarcinomas, diverticulosis, penetrating trauma, ulcerative colitis, angiodysplasia, and infarctions.
2. **Preoperative assessment and patient preparation**
 a) *History and physical examination: Gastrointestinal:* Assess hydration status, nutritional level, and electrolyte state.
 b) *Diagnostic tests:* As indicated by the patient's condition
 c) *Preoperative medication and intravenous therapy*
  (1) Patients may be on steroid therapy or immunosuppressant drugs.
  (2) Bowel preparation is usually indicated with electrolyte preparations.
  (3) Expect fluid shifts requiring moderate to large fluid resuscitation. Two large bore intravenous access tubes are indicated.
3. **Room preparation**
 a) *Monitoring equipment:* Standard with warming modalities
 b) *Pharmacologic agents:* Standard
 c) *Position:* Supine, with arms extended
4. **Anesthetic technique**
 a) Epidural (T2 to T4 level) with "light" general anesthetic
 b) General anesthesia with oral endotracheal tube (most common)
5. **Perioperative management**
 a) *Induction:* Consider possibility of full stomach; rapid sequence induction may be indicated.
 b) *Maintenance*
  (1) Muscle relaxation is required.
  (2) Closely monitor fluid and hydration status and blood loss.
  (3) Avoid N_2O, which may cause bowel distention.
 c) *Emergence:* Awake extubation after rapid sequence induction or placement of nasogastric tube
6. **Postoperative implications**
 a) Pain and splinting may lead to hypoventilation and decreased postoperative ventilation.
 b) Pain control with epidural or patient-controlled analgesia.

M. Herniorrhaphy

1. **Introduction**

   Inguinal hernias are defects in the transverse abdominal layer, where a direct hernia comes through the posterior wall of the inguinal canal, and an indirect hernia comes through the internal inguinal ring. Femoral hernia is when the hernia sac is exposed as it exits the preperitoneal space through the femoral canal. If the hernia cannot be reduced, the possibility of strangulation must be kept in mind. The peritoneal sac in most cases should be opened proximal to the femoral canal in order to gain control of the intestine before it reduces itself into the peritoneal cavity. If the bowel is ischemic, it may require resection. The repair consists of suturing the iliopubic tract to Cooper's ligament, taking care not to compromise the femoral vein.

   Incisional hernias can occur after any abdominal incision, but they are most common following midline incisions. Factors leading to herniation are wound infection, trauma, inadequate suturing, and weak tissues. Following skin incision, the skin edges and subcutaneous fat are retracted, and the dissection is carried down to the hernia defect. The redundant hernia sac is excised, and the fascia is freed up on both sides of the wound. Primary closure is preferred. In addition to primary repair, the latter may be reinforced by mesh prosthesis, or the prosthesis may be used to fill the hernia sac.

2. **Preoperative assessment**

   Predisposing factors for hernia often include increased abdominal pressure secondary to chronic cough, bladder outlet obstruction, constipation, pregnancy, vomiting, and acute or chronic muscular effort. These factors should be controlled preoperatively to avoid postoperative recurrence. The patient population may range from premature infants to the elderly with the possibility of multiple medical problems.

   a) *History and physical examination:* As indicated by the patient's condition
      (1) *Musculoskeletal:* Pain is likely in the area of the hernia; evaluate bony landmarks if regional anesthesia is planned.
      (2) *Hematologic:* If regional anesthesia is planned, check the patient's coagulation status.
      (3) *Gastrointestinal:* Hernias may become incarcerated, obstructed, or strangulated, requiring emergency surgery. Fluid and electrolyte imbalance should be assumed.

   b) *Patient preparation*
      (1) *Laboratory tests:* Complete blood count, electrolytes, and other tests as indicated per the history and physical examination
      (2) *Diagnostic tests:* As indicated per the history and physical examination
      (3) If necessary, use standard premedication.

3. **Room preparation**
   a) *Monitoring equipment:* Standard
   b) *Additional equipment:* Regular operating table
   c) *Drugs*
      (1) Standard emergency drugs
      (2) Standard tabletop
      (3) *Intravenous fluids:* One 18-gauge intravenous line with normal saline or lactated Ringer's solution at 5 to 8 mL/kg per hour.
4. **Anesthetic technique**
   General, regional, or local anesthesia with sedation are all appropriate. The choice depends on such factors as site of incision, the patient's physical status, and the preference of both the patient and surgeon. General anesthesia may be preferred for incisions made above T8. Profound muscle relaxation may be needed for exploration and repair.
5. **Perioperative management**
   a) *Standard induction:* Mask general anesthesia may be suitable for the patient with a simple chronic hernia. If there is obstruction, incarceration, or strangulation, rapid sequence induction with endotracheal intubation is indicated. General endotracheal anesthesia also may be indicated in the patient with wound dehiscence.
   b) *Maintenance*
      (1) *Standard:* muscle relaxants may be necessary to facilitate surgical repair.
      (2) *Position:* Supine. Checked and padded pressure points. Avoid stretching the brachial plexus. Limit abduction to 90 degrees.
   c) *Emergence:* Consider extubating the trachea while the patient is still anesthetized to prevent coughing and straining. Patients who are at risk for pulmonary aspiration and who require awake extubation after rapid sequence induction are not candidates for deep extubation.
6. **Postoperative implications**
   a) Wound dehiscence with coughing or straining
   b) Urinary retention. Patients with urinary retention may require intermittent catheterization until urinary function resumes.
   c) Pain management: Surgical field block or regional anesthesia should provide sufficient analgesia postoperatively.

N. Gallbladder Lithotripsy

1. **Introduction**
   a) Extracorporeal shock wave lithotripsy requires endoscopic retrograde cholangiopancreatography, sphincterotomy, and placement of a nasobiliary tube. The tube opacifies the biliary

PART 2 **Common Procedures**

> tree and helps to identify common bile duct stones.
>
> *b)* Ultrasonic shock waves are delivered to the gallbladder or common bile duct to break the stones. Gallbladder contractility is of utmost importance in removal of stone fragments and debris from the biliary system.
>
> *c)* Decreased gallbladder motility and stasis are primary causes of stone formation and may hinder expulsion of stone fragments following lithotripsy.
>
> *d)* The three basic stone types are cholesterol, pigment, and mixed.

2. **Preoperative history**

   Predisposing factors include increased age, female sex, obesity, and pregnancy.

   a) *History and physical examination*

   (1) *Cardiac:* Symptoms mimic angina and myocardial infarction.

   (2) *Respiratory:* Symptoms mimic right lower lobe pneumonia and pleurisy.

   (3) *Neurologic:* Symptoms mimic intercostal neuritis.

   (4) *Renal:* Symptoms mimic pyelonephritis and renal calculus.

   (5) *Gastrointestinal:* Symptoms mimic esophagitis, pancreatitis, intestinal obstruction, perforated ulcer, peptic ulcer, and hiatal hernia.

   b) *Patient preparation*

   (1) Laboratory tests

   (a) Complete blood count; leukocyte count is elevated.

   (b) Electrolytes—assesses effect of nausea and vomiting.

   (c) Perform tests as indicated by patient history and physical examination.

   (2) Diagnostic tests

   (a) Biliary ultrasonography

   (b) Abdominal radiographs (only 15% of stones are visible)

   (3) *Medications:* Analgesics and sedation are not necessary, although they may help the patient to lie still for the procedure.

3. **Room preparation**

   a) Procedure is completed in the radiography department (usually without anesthetic support).

   b) Standard monitors

   c) *Additional equipment:* Propofol infusion pump and airway adjuncts, nasal cannula, and oxygen cylinder

   d) *Drugs*

   (1) Fentanyl—two bolus doses of 50 to 200 mg each

   (2) Propofol—0.5 mg/kg loading dose followed by 50 mg/kg per minute infusion

   (3) *Intravenous:* 0.9% normal saline or lactated Ringer's at 2 ml/kg per hour

   (4) Tabletop standard general anesthesia setup

4. **Perioperative management and anesthetic technique**

   a) No anesthesia

b)   Monitored anesthesia care with sedation
c)   *Maintenance:* Propofol drip as necessary
5.   **Postoperative implications**
  a)   Transport to recovery room if patient has been sedated.
  b)   Transport to room if no anesthesia was given.

O. Esophagoscopy/Gastroscopy

1.   **Introduction**
Flexible, diagnostic esophagogastroduodenoscopy, a common procedure in pediatrics, is usually performed under heavy sedation in an endoscopy suite or special procedure area. Rigid esophagoscopy is usually performed for therapeutic indications, such as removal of a foreign body, dilation of an esophageal stricture, or injection of varices. The procedure is similar for each diagnosis and generally is performed with endotracheal intubation. Foreign body removal is normally a short procedure, whereas dilation and variceal injection can be prolonged and may require multiple insertions or removals of the endoscope. Compression of the trachea distal to the endotracheal tube by the rigid esophagoscope is not uncommon.

2.   **Preoperative assessment**
Esophagoscopy for foreign body removal is usually performed in healthy infants and children, although esophageal lodging of a foreign body can occur in any age group. All these patients should be treated with full stomach precautions. Esophageal dilation usually is performed in two distinct patient populations: (1) those with prior tracheoesophageal fistula repair and (2) those with prior ingestion of a caustic substance.

  a)   *History and physical examination*
    (1)   *Cardiovascular:* There may be persistent congenital cardiac anomalies in the patient with a tracheoesophageal fistula.
    (2)   *Respiratory:* Patients with prior caustic ingestion may have a history of pulmonary aspiration, with resultant chemical pneumonitis, fibrosis, or both. Prolonged intubation after tracheoesophageal fistula repair may lead to subglottic stenosis. Check any recent anesthesia records for endotracheal intubation.

  b)   *Patient preparation*
    (1)   *Laboratory tests:* Routine laboratory analyses are not required if the patient has no underlying chronic illness.
    (2)   *Diagnostic tests:* As indicated per history and physical examination
    (3)   *Medications:* For foreign body removal, intravenous access may be necessary before induction. No premedication is used if the patient is less than 1 year old.

PART 2 Common Procedures

3. **Room preparation**
   a) *Monitoring equipment:* Standard
   b) *Drugs*
       (1) Standard emergency drugs
       (2) Standard tabletop
       (3) *Intravenous fluids:* One 20- to 22-gauge intravenous line
            with normal saline or lactated Ringer's solution at 4 to
            6 ml/kg per hour.
4. **Anesthetic technique**
   Use general endotracheal anesthesia. For the pediatric patient, a pediatric circle or a nonrebreather circuit may be used. Room temperature can be maintained at 65 to 70°F as long as the patient is covered.
5. **Perioperative management**
   a) *Induction:* Rapid sequence induction is usually appropriate
       for this patient population, unless the patient is presenting
       for dilation alone and has no evidence to suggest reflux.
   b) *Maintenance*
       (1) Maintain anesthesia with a volatile agent, N_2O and O_2.
            Opiates are unnecessary because postprocedural pain is
            negligible. Maintain neuromuscular blockade. Movement
            must be avoided, particularly with rigid esophagoscopy.
       (2) *Position.* Supine. Checked and padded pressure points.
            Avoid stretching the brachial plexus. Limit abduction to
            90 degrees.
       (3) *Warming modalities for pediatric patients:* Increased room
            temperature, warming blankets, humidivent
   c) *Emergence:* Extubate when patient is fully awake. Do not attempt
       reversal of neuromuscular blockade until first twitch of train of
       four has returned.
6. **Postoperative implications**
   a) Pneumothorax—esophageal perforation is more common with
       rigid esophagoscopy and will lead to pneumothorax.
   b) Aspiration
   c) Accidental extubation
   d) Stridor secondary to subglottic edema
   e) Postoperative pain is negligible; if the patient reports marked
       substernal discomfort, suspect esophageal perforation.

P. Colonoscopy

1. **Introduction**
   Procedure used to examine the colon and rectum to diagnose
   inflammatory bowel disease, including ulcerative colitis and granulomatous colitis. Polyps can be removed through the colonoscope. The
   colonoscope is also helpful in diagnosing or locating the source of
   gastrointestinal bleeding; a biopsy of lesions suspected to be

malignant may be performed.

2. **Preoperative assessment and patient preparation**
   a) *History and physical examination:* Gastrointestinal: Assess patient's hydration status, nutritional level, and electrolyte state.
   b) *Diagnostic tests:* As indicated by the patient's condition
   c) *Preoperative medication and intravenous therapy*
      (1) Patients may be on steroid therapy or immunosuppressants.
      (2) Bowel preparation is required for visualization of the mucosa. Use colon electrolyte lavage preparations (Colyte, GoLYTELY).
      (3) One 18-gauge intravenous tube; minimal fluid replacement
      (4) Patient is lightly sedated with the use of midazolam because the procedure lasts less than 30 minutes and is an outpatient procedure.

3. **Room preparation**
   a) *Monitoring equipment:* Standard
   b) *Pharmacologic agents*
      (1) Standard
      (2) Glucagon
   c) *Position:* Left lateral decubitus; position changes are sometimes required to aid advancement of the scope at the descending sigmoid colon junction and splenic fixture.

4. **Anesthetic technique**
   a) Sedation
   b) *Intravenous sedation:* Midazolam (Versed), fentanyl, or propofol in sedative doses

5. **Perioperative management**
   a) *Induction:* Oxygenate the patient with the use of nasal cannulae or a face mask.
   b) *Maintenance:* No specific indications
   c) *Emergence:* No specific indications

6. **Postoperative implications**
   Complications of the procedure include perforation of the bowel, abdominal pain and distention, rectal bleeding, fever, and mucopurulent drainage.

Q. Esophageal Resection

1. **Introduction**
   Esophagectomy is commonly performed for malignant disease of the middle and lower thirds of the esophagus. It may also be indicated for Barrett's esophagus (peptic ulcer of the lower esophagus) and for peptic strictures that do not respond to dilation. Lesions in the lower third are usually approached via a left thoracoabdominal incision, whereas middle-third lesions are best approached via the abdomen and right side of the chest. Resections of the esophagogastric junction

for malignant disease are best performed through a left thoracoabdominal approach in which a portion of the proximal stomach is removed along with a coeliac node dissection.

Blind esophagectomy is done via the abdomen and neck by blunt dissection. This is useful primarily for benign esophageal lesions or malignant lesions of the pharynx and larynx in which the pharynx and/or upper esophagus require resection.

Total esophagectomy may be done via an abdominal and right thoracotomy approach with colonic interposition and anastomosis in the neck. Either the right or the left side of the colon can be mobilized for interposition. Both depend on the middle colic artery and the marginal artery of the colon for their vascular supply. When the proximal portion of the right colon is used, the interposed segment of bowel is isoperistaltic, but when the left colon is brought up, the segment is antiperistaltic. Although the colonic interposition is said to function primarily as a conduit for food, the isoperistaltic colonic segment functions better. In either case, the colonic segment is connected to the body of the stomach following suturing of the esophageal colonic anastomosis.

2. **Preoperative assessment**
   a) *History and physical examination*
      (1) *Cardiovascular:* The patient may be hypovolemic and malnourished from dysphagia or anorexia. Chemotherapeutic drugs (Daunorubicin, Adriamycin) may cause cardiomyopathies. Chronic alcohol abuse may also produce a toxic cardiomyopathy. Congestive heart failure, if present, may be refractory to treatment, although preoperative optimization of cardiac status is essential.
      (2) *Respiratory:* A history of gastric reflux suggests the possibility of recurrent aspiration pneumonia, decreased pulmonary reserve, and increased risk of regurgitation and aspiration during anesthetic induction. If a thoracic approach is planned, the patient should be evaluated to ensure that one lung ventilation can be tolerated.

      Determine if the patient has been exposed to Bleomycin, which may cause pulmonary toxicity; toxicity may be made worse by high concentrations of oxygen. Many patients with esophageal cancer have a long history of smoking with consequent respiratory impairment.

      Pulmonary function tests and arterial blood gases can be helpful in predicting the likelihood of perioperative pulmonary complications and whether the patient may require postoperative mechanical ventilation. Patients with baseline hypoxemia/hypercarbia on room air arterial blood gases have a higher likelihood of postoperative complications and a greater need for postoperative ventilatory support. Severe restrictive or obstructive lung disease will also increase the chance of pulmonary morbidity in the perioperative period.
      (3) *Hematologic:* Encourage preoperative autologous blood donation.

b) *Patient preparation*

   (1) *Laboratory tests:* Type and crossmatch packed red blood cells, electrolytes, glucose, blood urea nitrogen, creatinine, bilirubin, transaminase, alkaline phosphatase, albumin, complete blood count, and platelet count. Prothrombin time, partial thromboplastin time, urinalysis, arterial blood gases, and other tests as indicated per history and physical examination.

   (2) *Diagnostic tests:* Chest radiographs, electrocardiography, pulmonary function tests, and other tests as indicated per history and physical examination. If congestive heart failure or cardiomyopathy is suspected, consider cardiac or medical consultations.

   (3) *Medications:* Premedication—consider aspiration prophylaxis.

3. **Room preparation**

   a) *Monitoring equipment*

      (1) Standard monitoring equipment

      (2) Arterial line and central venous pressure or pulmonary arterial catheter as indicated

   b) *Additional equipment:* Patient warming device

   c) *Drugs*

      (1) Standard emergency drugs

      (2) Standard tabletop

      (3) *Intravenous fluids:* 14- to 16-gauge (2) normal saline or lactated Ringer's solution at 8 to 12 mL/kg per hour; fluid warmer

      (4) Blood loss can be significant, and blood should be immediately available.

4. **Anesthetic technique**

   General endotracheal anesthesia (with or without epidural anesthetic for postoperative analgesia). If postoperative epidural analgesia is planned, placement and testing of the catheter prior to anesthetic induction is helpful. If the thoracic or abdominothoracic approach is used, placement of a double lumen tube is indicated, because one lung anesthesia provides excellent surgical exposure.

5. **Perioperative management**

   a) *Induction*

      Patients with esophageal disease are often at risk for pulmonary aspiration; therefore the trachea should be intubated with the patient awake or after rapid sequence induction with cricoid pressure. Awake intubation can be done by either blind nasal or fiberoptic bronchoscopy. If the patient is clinically hypovolemic, restore intravascular volume prior to induction and titrate induction dose of sedative/hypnotic agents.

   b) *Maintenance*

      (1) Standard maintenance without N_2O. Alternatively, a combined technique with general and epidural anesthesia may be used. If epidural opiates are used for postoperative analgesia, a loading dose should be administered at least

1 hour before the conclusion of surgery.

(2) *Position:* Supine. Checked and padded pressure points. Avoid stretching the brachial plexus. Limit abduction to 90 degrees. If the lateral decubitus position is used, an axillary roll and arm holder are needed. Check pressure points, including ears, eyes, and genitals. Check radial pulses to ensure correct placement of axillary roll (a misplaced axillary roll will compromise distal pulses). Problems that can arise include brachial plexus injuries and damage to soft tissues, ears, eyes, and genitals from malpositioning.

c) *Emergence*

The decision to extubate at the end of surgery depends on the patient's underlying cardiopulmonary status and the extent of the surgical procedure. The patient should be hemodynamically stable, warm, alert, cooperative, and fully reversed from any muscle relaxants prior to extubation. With patients who require postoperative ventilation, the double lumen tube should be changed to a single lumen endotracheal tube prior to transport to the postanesthesia intensive care unit. Weaning from mechanical ventilation should begin when the patient is awake and cooperative, is able to protect the airway, and has adequate pulmonary function.

6. **Postoperative implications**

a) For atelectasis or aspiration, recover the patient in Fowler's position.

b) Hemorrhage—check coagulation times; replace factors as necessary.

c) Pneumothorax/hemothorax—decreased partial O_2 pressure, increased partial CO_2 pressure, wheezing, coughing; confirm with chest radiograph, institute chest tube drainage as necessary. In an emergency (tension pneumothorax), use needle aspiration, supportive treatment, oxygen, vasopressors, endotracheal intubation, positive pressure ventilation.

d) Hypoxemia/hypoventilation—ensure adequate analgesia and supplemental oxygen.

e) Esophageal anastomotic leak—begin surgical repair for esophageal anastomotic leak.

f) *Pain management:* Patient-controlled analgesia or epidural analgesia; patient should recover in the intensive care unit or a hospital ward that is accustomed to treating the side effects of epidural opiates (respiratory depression, breakthrough pain, nausea, and pruritus).

R. Anal Fistulotomy/Fistulectomy

1. **Introduction**

   The great majority of perianal fistulae arise as a result of infection within the anal glands located at the dentate line (cryptoglandular fistula). Fistulae may also arise as the result of trauma, Crohn's disease, inflammatory processes within the peritoneal cavity, neoplasms, or radiation therapy. The ultimate treatment is determined by the etiology and the anatomic course of the fistula. The principle behind treatment of cryptoglandular fistulae is to excise the offending gland and lay open or excise all infected tissue. Fistulae that track above the majority of the sphincter mechanism must be treated by procedures that either do not cut the overlying sphincter, cut the sphincter and repair it, or cut the sphincter gradually. A fistula may be treated at the time of drainage of a perianal abscess or as a separate elective operation. The route of a fistula tract is best determined by exploration at the time of operation. Although local anesthesia is acceptable for simple fistulae with known routes, many fistula operations require regional or general anesthesia because the ultimate route and depth of the fistula will not be known. Special consideration is given to fistulae that arise in the setting of Crohn's disease. Poor wound healing, the likelihood of recurrent or multiple fistulae, and the premium on sphincter function in patients with chronic diarrhea dictate that only the most superficial fistulae can be laid open. The primary goal is palliation, specifically to drain abscesses and prevent their recurrence. This is often accomplished by placing a Silastic seton (a ligature placed around the sphincter muscles) around the fistula tract and leaving it in place indefinitely. In the absence of active Crohn's disease in the rectum, attempts at fistula cure may be undertaken.

2. **Preoperative assessment**

   a) *History and physical examination*

      (1) *Respiratory:* A careful evaluation of respiratory status is important. If the patient has decreased respiratory reserve, the lithotomy position may be better tolerated than the prone or jackknife positions.

      (2) *Musculoskeletal:* Pain is likely at the surgical site an should be considered when positioning the patient for anesthetic induction. (If the patient has pain while sitting, perform regional anesthesia in the lateral decubitus position.)

      (3) *Hematologic:* If regional anesthesia is planned and the patient is taking acetylsalicylic acids, nonsteroidal anti-inflammatory drugs, or dipyridamole, check the platelet count and bleeding time.

   b) *Patient preparation*

      (1) *Laboratory tests:* As indicated per history and physical examination

      (2) *Diagnostic tests:* As indicated per history and physical

PART 2 Common Procedures

examination

(3) *Medication:* Standard premedication

3. **Room preparation**
   a) *Monitoring equipment:* Standard
   b) *Drugs*
      (1) Standard emergency drugs
      (2) Standard tabletop
      (3) Intravenous fluids: 18-gauge, normal saline/lactated Ringer's at 5 to 8 mL/kg per hour

4. **Anesthetic technique**
   General anesthesia; spinal or epidural techniques may be used.

5. **Perioperative management**
   a) *Induction:* Standard. Procedures done in the jackknife position may require endotracheal intubation for airway control if a regional technique is not performed.
   b) *Maintenance*
      (1) Standard
      (2) *Position:* Chest support or bolster to optimize ventilation in the jackknife position; take care in positioning the patient's extremities and genitals after turning the patient into the jackknife position. Avoid pressure on the eyes and ears after turning the patient. Avoid stretching the brachial plexus. Limit abduction to 90 degrees.
   c) *Emergence:* No special considerations. Patient is extubated awake and after return of airway reflexes.

6. **Postoperative implications**
   a) Lithotomy position can lead to damage to the peroneal nerve, which can lead to foot drop.
   b) Urinary retention
   c) Poor wound healing
   d) Atelectasis

S. Hemorrhoidectomy

1. **Introduction**
   Hemorrhoids are masses of vascular tissue found in the anal canal. Internal hemorrhoids are found above the pectinate line, arise from the superior hemorrhoidal venosus plexus, and are covered with mucosa. External hemorrhoids are found below the pectinate line, arise from the inferior hemorrhoidal venosus plexus, and are covered by anoderm and perianal skin.

2. **Preoperative assessment and patient preparation**
   a) *History and physical examination:* Rectal: Bright red blood on toilet paper or surface of the stool; iron deficiency anemia; prolapsed mass of tissue that protrudes from the anus; and thrombosis (blood clot within the hemorrhoidal vein) causing pain

b) *Diagnostic tests:* Complete blood count
c) *Preoperative medication and intravenous therapy*
    (1) A narcotic with premedication is considered if the patient experiences pain.
    (2) 18-gauge intravenous tube with minimal fluid replacement

3. Room preparation
  a) *Monitoring equipment:* Standard
  b) *Position:* Prone or lithotomy

4. Anesthetic technique
  a) Regional blockade and general anesthesia
  b) *Regional blockade:* Analgesic to S2 to S5 required
    (1) Hypobaric spinals—lithotomy position
    (2) Hypobaric spinals—flexed prone or knee chest position
  c) *General anesthesia:* Mask in lithotomy position (endotracheal intubation is necessary for the prone position).

5. Perioperative management
  a) *Induction*
    (1) *Prone:* General anesthesia induction performed on the stretcher.
    (2) Position the patient on the operating table with adequate support and padding of the extremities, head, and neck.
    (3) *Spinal:* Review principles of sympathetic blocks.
  b) *Maintenance: General anesthesia:* Deep planes of anesthesia or muscle relaxants are required to relax the anal sphincter.
  c) *Emergence:* If the prone position is used and general anesthesia is implemented, patients are usually repositioned onto the stretcher prior to emergence.

6. Postoperative implications
Bearing down to void will be painful; keep fluids to a minimum.

T. Adrenalectomy

1. Introduction
  a) A procedure in which the adrenal glands are removed by sharp or blunt dissection. The left adrenal gland is exposed by manipulating the spleen and pancreas. The right adrenal gland is exposed by retracting the liver cephalad. Adrenal veins are exposed and ligated prior to removal.
  b) *Pathophysiology:* The procedure is performed for medullary or cortical tumors, Cushing's syndrome due to adrenal calcium or hyperplasia, pituitary hypersecretion, pheochromocytoma, primary hyperaldosteronism, and adenocarcinoma.

2. Preoperative assessment
  a) *History and physical examination*
    (1) *Cardiac:* Cushing's syndrome—hypervolemia, hypertension, hypokalemia, polycythemia

    (2) *Respiratory:* Cushing's syndrome may cause truncal obesity and buffalo hump. Assess for shortness of breath. May function as a restrictive disease.

    (3) *Neurologic:* Cushing's syndrome—headache, mood changes, psychosis, muscular wasting, possibly increased response to muscle relaxants

    (4) *Renal:* Cushing's syndrome—Na^+ retention and K^+ excretion, glucose intolerance from excess steroids

    (5) *Gastrointestinal:* Cushing's syndrome—truncal obesity, muscle wasting. The patient may need rapid sequence induction and aspiration prophylaxis.

    (6) *Endocrine:* Cushing's syndrome—hypokalemia, hyperglycemia, diabetes, excess steroid production, impaired Ca^{2+} absorption

  b) *Patient preparation*

    (1) *Laboratory tests:* As indicated by the patient's condition

    (2) *Diagnostic tests:* Cushing's syndrome will cause elevated plasma and urinary cortisol levels, plasma adrenocorticotropic hormone, and 17-hydroxycorticosteroids. Hyperadrenocorticism is diagnosed when endogenous cortisol is not suppressed after exogenous dexamethasone is given. Computed tomography or magnetic resonance imaging may be useful.

    (3) *Medications:* Cushing's syndrome: Spironolactone inhibits excess aldosterone effects, mobilizes fluid, and increases K^+ level. Hydrocortisone dose: 100 mg every 8 hours.

3. Room preparation

  a) *Monitoring equipment:* Standard; central line, arterial line as indicated

  b) *Additional equipment:* Positioning devices: patient may be supine or in nephrectomy or prone jackknife position. Careful padding is needed for Cushing's syndrome patients because of their easy bruisability, thin skin, and osteopenia.

  c) *Drugs*

    (1) *Continuous infusions:* Intravenous fluids—large fluid loss is possible. Use isotonic crystalloid at 10 mL/kg per hour.

    (2) *Blood:* Estimated blood loss is 200 to 300 mL but can be significant. Type and crossmatch are needed.

    (3) Tabletop—standard. Have atropine available for unopposed parasympathetic response, lidocaine for ventricular arrhythmias (hypokalemia), and syringes of vasoactive available (ephedrine).

4. Perioperative management and anesthetic technique

  a) *Induction:* Select the appropriate induction agent based on the patient's medical condition. Use a nondepolarizer if rapid sequence induction is not used. Consider decreased muscle mass.

  b) *Maintenance:* Volatile agent, opiates, and muscle relaxant. Epidural anesthesia can improve surgical exposure by contracting the bowel.

  c) *Emergence:* The patient may be hemodynamically labile and may

have large third-space fluid accumulation. Consider postoperative ventilation.
5. **Postoperative complications**
Complications include hypoadrenocorticism after tumor resection, hypoglycemia, pneumothorax, and hypertension. Continue steroid therapy after the procedure.

U. Pheochromocytoma

1. **Introduction**
   a) Surgical procedure is 90% curative; 10% to 25% of patients have bilateral tumors. Adrenalectomy is possible, depending on tumor location.
   b) *Pathophysiology:* Pheochromocytomas are highly vascular tumors associated with adrenal medulla chromaffin tissue that secrete mostly norepinephrine but also epinephrine. Tumors usually are in the abdomen (95%) but may be found anywhere that chromaffin tissue arises. They are malignant in 10% of patients. An inherited autosomal dominant trait is involved 5% of the time. These tumors can be associated with multiple endocrine neoplasia syndrome. They are most common in early to middle adulthood. Catecholamine release does not depend on neurogenic control.
2. **Preoperative assessment**
   a) *History and physical examination*
       (1) *Cardiac:* Paroxysmal severe hypertension, dysrhythmia, myocardial infarction, orthostatic hypotension, hypovolemia, catecholamine-induced cardiomyopathy, decreased sensitivity to catecholamines
       (2) *Neurologic:* Cerebrovascular accident from hypertension, headache, tremors, sweating, hypertension retinopathy, and mydriasis
       (3) *Renal:* Impairment from hypertension
       (4) *Gastrointestinal:* None
       (5) *Endocrine:* Hyperglycemia
   b) *Patient preparation*
       (1) *Laboratory tests:* As indicated by the patient's condition
       (2) *Diagnostic tests*
           (*a*) Electrocardiogram–left-ventricular hypertrophy and nonspecific T-wave changes are common.
           (*b*) Echocardiogram for left ventricular function.
           (*c*) Chest radiography—assess cardiomegaly.
           (*d*) Magnetic resonance imaging or computed tomography to localize tumors.
           (*e*) Urinary vanilylmandelic acid, norepinephrine, and epinephrine levels usually are elevated in 24-hour collection.

PART 2 Common Procedures

(3) *Medications:* α-adrenergic blockade is recommended 10 to 14 days prior to surgery. Use phenoxybenzamine 80 to 200 mg/day or prazosin 6 to 20 mg/day. β-blockers are added only after α-blockade to help manage tachydysrhythmias that are caused from α-blockade. If β-blockers are begun prior to α-blockade, unopposed α response is possible.

3. **Room preparation**
   a) *Monitoring equipment:* Standard, arterial line, central line, and pulmonary arterial catheter as indicated
   b) *Additional equipment:* Positioning devices—may be supine, nephrectomy, or prone jackknife position, depending on whether incision is midline abdominal, bilateral subcostal, curved posterior, or dorsal flank oblique
   c) *Drugs*
      (1) Continuous infusions—nitroprusside, phentolamine, and esmolol for severe hypertension and tachycardia during tumor manipulation. Hypotension after ligation of tumor's venous supply can be treated with phenylephrine, dopamine, and fluids.
      (2) *Intravenous fluids:* Prehydrate prior to surgery because patient is usually intravascularly depleted. Large third-space loss and blood loss is possible; use isotonic fluids at 10 mL/kg per hour.
      (3) *Blood*—type and crossmatch 2 units of packed red blood cells.
      (4) *Tabletop*—have vasoactive drugs available for prompt treatment (lidocaine, nitroglycerine, nitroprusside, esmolol, phenylephrine). Syringe boluses may be used.

4. **Perioperative management and anesthetic technique**
   a) *Induction:* Slow and controlled to avoid sympathetic nervous system response to laryngoscopy. One may pretreat with esmolol. Avoid histamine-releasing drugs, ketamine, or vagolytics.
   b) *Maintenance:* Avoid halothane for increased ventricular irritability. Use isoflurane or enflurane with intravenous opiates. Desflurane may increase the heart rate. An epidural combination can also be used; however, avoid using epinephrine in test dose.
   c) *Emergence:* Pay careful attention to labile hemodynamics.

5. **Postoperative complications**
   Catecholamine levels normalize in several days. Pneumothorax, hypoglycemia, cardiac dysfunction, hypoadrenocorticism are possible.

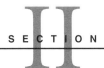

S E C T I O N

Genitourinary System

A. Transurethral Resection of the Prostate

1. **Introduction**
   Resections consists of applying a high-frequency current to a wire loop with fragments of the obstructive tissue removed under direct endoscopic vision. Hemostasis is effected by sealing vessels with the coagulating current. Continuous irrigation with fluids is required to improve visibility through the cystoscope, distend the prostatic urethra, and maintain the operative field free of blood and dissected tissue.

2. **Preoperative assessment and patient preparation**
   a) *History and physical examination: Elderly patient population:* Assess for coexisting medical diseases.
   b) *Diagnostic tests*
      (1) CBC, blood urea nitrogen, creatinine, electrolytes, coagulation profile
      (2) Postpone procedure if serum sodium is 128 mEq/L or less.
   c) *Preoperative medication and intravenous therapy*
      (1) Use an 18-gauge intravenous catheter with minimal fluid replacement.
      (2) Antibiotics

3. **Room preparation**
   a) *Monitoring equipment:* Standard
   b) *Pharmacologic agents:* Standard
   c) *Position:* Lithotomy

4. **Anesthetic technique**
   a) *Regional blockade or general anesthesia:* For regional blockade, analgesia to T10 is required. An awake patient can provide early warning of complications (hypervolemia, hyponatremia).
   b) *Technique of choice:* Spinal anesthesia

5. **Perioperative management**
   a) *Induction:* No specific indications
   b) *Maintenance*
      (1) Blood loss—difficult to assess because the irrigating fluid dilutes the blood. The average loss is about 4 mL/min of resection time.
      (2) Intravascular absorption of irrigating fluid—open venous sinuses of the prostate bed cause absorption of irrigating fluid. The primary determinants of fluid absorption are
         (a) Height of irrigation container,

PART 2 Common Procedures

161

   (*b*) Number and size of venous sinuses opened, and
   (*c*) Duration of resection.
  (3) Limit resection time to less than 1 hour (10 to 30 mL
   of fluid is absorbed per minute of resection time) and
   monitor resection time closely.
  (4) Absorption of large volumes of irrigating fluids results in
   increased intravascular volume and dilutional hyponatremia
   with early symptoms of hypertension and reflex tachycardia.
   Symptoms in an awake patient include restlessness, nausea
   and vomiting, mental confusion, and visual disturbances.
 c) *Treatment*
  (1) Terminate/complete surgical procedure.
  (2) Send blood for serum Na^+; if Na^+ level is 120 mEq/L or
   less, administer furosemide and limit fluids.
  (3) If hyponatremia is severe with neurologic symptoms,
   administer hypertonic saline (3% to 5%) at a rate no faster
   than 100 mL/hour.
   (*a*) Bladder perforation—suspect perforation of prostatic
    capsule if irrigation fluid fails to return. Initial symp-
    toms include hypertension and tachycardia followed
    by hypotension. An awake patient will experience
    suprapubic fullness and pain in the upper abdomen or
    referred from the diaphragm to the precordial region
    or shoulders.
   (*b*) Prepare for a possible open surgical procedure.
   (*c*) Glycine toxicity—a metabolite of glycine is ammonia.
    Glycine absorption can produce central nervous
    system symptoms such as mild depression, confusion,
    and transient blindness to coma.
 d) *Emergence:* No specific indications
6. **Postoperative considerations**
 Hyponatremia may not be suspected until the postoperative period.

B. Radical Prostatectomy

1. **Introduction**
 Open prostatectomy refers to removal of the prostate with or
 without the prostatic capsule. Several surgical approaches may be
 used, including suprapubic, transvesical, retropubic, perineal, and
 transcoccygeal. In suprapubic or transvesical procedures, the
 prostate is removed through the cavity of the bladder. Retropubic
 prostatectomy is performed through a low abdominal incision
 without opening the bladder. The transcoccygeal approach allows
 maximal surgical access to the posterior lobes of the prostate.
 Perineal prostatectomy is most often performed for cancer of the
 prostate when it is confined to the capsule.

2. **Preoperative assessment and patient preparation**
   a) *History and physical examination:* Individualized based on patient's condition; assess for symptoms of metastatic disease.
   b) *Diagnostic tests*
      (1) Plasma concentration of prostate-specific antigen (PSA) is increased in prostate cancer.
      (2) Blood urea nitrogen, creatinine, electrolytes, complete blood count, coagulation profile, and type and crossmatch.
      (3) Ultrasonography
   c) *Preoperative medication and intravenous therapy*
      (1) Bowel preparation will render the patient in a dehydrated state.
      (2) Minimum of two peripheral intravenous lines (18-and 16-gauge) with moderate fluid replacement.
      (3) Epidural catheter—perform test dose in preoperative area.
      (4) Antibiotics
      (5) Small incremental doses of benzodiazepines may be given to ease patient preparation.
3. **Room preparation**
   a) *Monitoring equipment*
      (1) Standard
      (2) Arterial line and central venous pressure monitoring may be necessary to tend volume status, especially if the patient is elderly with coexisting medical diseases.
      (3) Warming modalities
   b) *Pharmacologic agents*
      (1) Dopamine—may need low dose (2 to 5 mcg/kg per minute) to increase urinary output
      (2) Hetastarch (Hespan) and albumin
   c) *Position:* Supine; surgeon may request use of kidney rest and for the patient's body to be partially flexed. Expect to need to rotate the patient from side to side for optimal surgical viewing.
4. **Anesthetic technique**
   a) Regional blockade, general anesthesia, or a combination of both
   b) *Technique of choice:* General anesthesia with endotracheal intubation
   c) *Regional blockade:* Epidural catheter placement in preoperative area; analgesia to T6 to T8
   d) *General anesthesia:* Endotracheal intubation
   e) *Regional blockade with general anesthesia:* Smaller doses of each with combination technique
5. **Perioperative management**
   a) *Induction:* The patient may be dehydrated and show an exaggerated response to medications.
   b) *Maintenance*
      (1) Initiate warming modality
      (2) The Foley catheter is discontinued during the case, and volume status (blood loss) is difficult to quantify.
      (3) Muscle relaxation is necessary.
   c) *Emergence*
      (1) Initiate regional blockade through the epidural catheter for

postoperative analgesia prior to the end of the case.
   (2) Base extubation on the patient's general health, amount of
        blood loss, and overall status after the procedure.
   (3) An awake or deep extubation may be appropriate.
6. **Postoperative implications**
   a) Obtain hemoglobin and hematocrit.
   b) Continue to trend volume status.

C. Extracorporeal Shock Wave Lithotripsy (ESWL)

1. **Introduction**
   ESWL is a noninvasive technique that pulverizes renal stones with
   shock waves. Disintegrated stones are passed in the urine. The
   R wave of electrocardiogram serves as the trigger for shock waves;
   therefore the procedure length is somewhat heart rate dependent—
   usually 30 to 90 minutes.
   a) First generation lithotripters—patients are placed in a hydrauli-
         cally operated chairlift device and submerged from the clavicles
         down into a tub of water. The impact of the shock waves at the
         flank entry site is painful, requiring anesthesia.
   b) Second generation lithotripters—patients are placed on
         lithotripsy table and positioned so shock waves generated
         within an enclosed casing are directed at area of stone. Lower
         voltage shock waves are used, and pain is greatly reduced with
         this method.
2. **Preoperative assessment and patient preparation**
   a) Routine preoperative assessment with laboratory tests based on
         any abnormalities found in the history and physical examina-
         tion. Consider cardiac status; many hemodynamic changes are
         associated with this procedure.
   b) Relative contraindications include aortic aneurysm, spinal
         tumors, orthopedic implants in the lumbar region, pregnancy,
         morbid obesity, presence of a cardiac pacemaker, uncontrolled
         arrhythmias, and coagulation disorders.
   c) Urinary track obstruction distal to the stone prevents passage of
         stone fragments and is an absolute contraindication.
   d) Ureteral stent placement prior to ESWL may be used to move
         the stone upward in the ureter, where it is amenable to therapy.
   e) Adequate intravenous hydration aids in the passage of stone
         fragments.
   f) Prophylactic antibiotics may be given.
3. **Room preparation**
   a) Lithotripsy suite may be located away from the main operating
         room. All anesthetizing equipment must be available.

b)   Plan emergency and resuscitative measures in advance (immersed anesthetized patient)
c)   Gas machine and monitor connections must be long enough to extend between the patient in the tank and the anesthesia machine (immersed patient)
d)   Position the electrocardiogram electrode on the trunk and cover with transparent dressings. This results in less artifact interference with R wave triggering of shock waves.
e)   To minimize treatment times, atropine may be used to increase the heart rate.
f)   Use waterproof dressings to cover intravenous tubes and epidural catheters (immersed patient).
g)   May start an 18-gauge intravenous catheter with infusion of dimenhydrinate (Hydrate) preoperatively to ensure passage of stones.
h)   Esophageal or precordial stethoscopes are impractical because of shock discharge noise.
i)   Have vasopressors and emergency drugs available to treat hemodynamic changes.
j)   Monitor the temperature of the patient and bath. The bath should be kept at 37°C (immersed patient)

4. **Anesthetic technique**
   Use local anesthetic with sedation; general or regional anesthesia is usually required.

5. **Perioperative management**
   a)   *Monitored anesthesia care with intravenous sedation:* Usually the method of choice with newer generation lithotripters
   b)   General or regional anesthesia with older water bath lithotripters
   c)   *Regional anesthesia:* Analgesia to T4 is required.
   d)   *Epidural anesthesia:* Produces a slower onset of sympathetic block with less hypotension; can be used along with pre-ESWL cystoscopy and stent placement.
   e)   *Spinal anesthesia:* Can result in more profound circulatory changes during positioning.
   f)   *General anesthesia*
      (1)   Intubation is mandatory.
      (2)   Stones may move during ventilation of lungs. Use low tidal volume and increase the respiratory rate.
   g)   *Position*
      (1)   Patient is supported in a padded metal frame in a "lawnchair position" and lowered into the water (immersed) or positioned in supine or semilateral position based on equipment used.
      (2)   Allow shock waves to hit the kidneys and disintegrate stones but not to reach the lungs.
   h)   Considerations—Immersed Patient
      (1)   Prevent patient movement—patient may be paralyzed if general anesthesia is used; sedate with regional anesthesia.
      (2)   Hemodynamic responses to the procedure vary. Sitting

PART 2 Common Procedures

position and warm water cause vasodilation, venous pooling, and decreased cardiac output. Immersion counteracts this; hydrostatic pressure on vessels increases venous return.

(3) Slowly remove the patient from the tub or profound hypotension may occur.

(4) Pressure on the chest from immersion decreases vital capacity and functional reserve capacity and causes ventilation/perfusion mismatch.

(5) Cardiac arrhythmias may occur during immersion or emergence because of rapid changes in hemodynamics and during the procedure from the discharge of shock waves independent of the cardiac cycle.

i) Emergence: (immersed patient) Use maintenance anesthesia or sedation until the patient is removed from the tub.

6. **Postoperative implications**

a) Renal hematoma, especially in patients with preexisting hypertension

b) Cardiac dysrhythmias—bradycardia, PACs, and PVCs (primarily during the procedure)

c) Hematuria—treated with hydration and diuretics

d) Ureteral colic—evident as nausea, vomiting, or bradycardia

D. Nephrectomy

1. **Introduction**
Indications for nephrectomy include calculus, hemorrhage, hydronephrosis, hypertension, neoplasms, renal donation, trauma, and vascular disease. Partial nephrectomy is performed to preserve as much renal function as possible. Surgery of the kidney is usually accomplished through a flank incision.

2. **Preoperative assessment and patient preparation**

a) History and physical examination: Individualized for patient's condition

b) Diagnostic tests

(1) Intravenous pyelography with nephrotomography— identify renal mass.

(2) Ultrasonography—differentiates simple cysts from solid tumor.

(3) Arteriography—determines if kidney is suitable for renal transplantation.

(4) Computed tomography

(5) *Laboratory tests*

(a) Prothrombin time, partial thromboplastin time, complete blood count, electrolytes, glucose

(b) Glomerular filtration rate—blood urea nitrogen, plasma creatinine, creatinine clearance

(c) Renal tubular function—urine concentration ability,

sodium secretion, proteinuria, hematuria urine sediment, urine volume

  c) *Preoperative medications and intravenous therapy*

   (1) Identify date of last hemodialysis

   (2) Epidural catheter—perform test dose in preoperative area.

   (3) Antibiotics

   (4) Small incremental doses of benzodiazepines to facilitate axiolysis

   (5) Minimum of two peripheral intravenous tubes (16- to 18-gauge) with moderate fluid replacement

   (6) With renal failure patients, administer hypotonic solutions—5% dextrose in water or 5% dextrose and 0.45% saline.

    (*a*) Avoid normal saline—may increase sodium levels.

    (*b*) Avoid plasmolyte or lactated Ringer's solution—may increase K^+ levels.

    (*c*) Restrict fluids and consider using microdrip tubing.

3. Room preparation

  a) *Monitoring equipment*

   (1) Standard

   (2) Arterial line and central venous pressure monitoring may be necessary to trend volume status, especially if the patient is elderly with coexisting medical disease.

   (3) Noninvasive blood pressure cuff should not be placed in an arm with arteriovenous fistula.

  b) *Pharmacologic agents*

   (1) Dopamine—low dose (2 to 5 mg/kg) to increase urinary output

   (2) Furosemide (Lasix) and/or mannitol for stimulation of urinary output

   (3) Indigo carmine or methylene blue administration (intravenously to assess urinary flow)

   (4) Hetastarch (Hespan)/albumin

   (5) Heparin and protamine—with donor kidneys

  c) *Position*

   (1) Lateral decubitus position with the kidney bar raised

   (2) With low calcium levels, skin and nerve damage occur easily.

   (3) Inadequate support of the head may lead to Horner's syndrome postoperatively.

   (4) Evaluate radial pulse after placement of axillary roll.

   (5) Respiration is impaired secondary to ventilation-perfusion mismatching, decreased functional reserve capacity, decreased vital capacity, and decreased thoracic compliance.

   (6) Reassess breath sounds postmovement; an endotracheal tube may migrate into the mainstem bronchus during positioning.

4. Anesthetic technique See "Radical Prostatectomy," p. 162.

5. Perioperative management

  a) *Induction*

   (1) Opioids can be used because only a small amount of the drug is excreted unchanged by the kidneys.

  (2) Succinylcholine is contraindicated if K^+ is elevated.
  (3) Cisatracurium and atracurium do not require a functional kidney because they are degraded by Hoffman elimination and are good choices for muscle relaxation.
  (4) Vecuronium, rocuronium, and rapacuronium may be used for muscle relaxation
  (5) Regardless of blood volume status, renal patients may respond to induction of anesthesia as if they are hypovolemic.
  (6) Induction of anesthesia and intubation of the trachea can be safely accomplished with intravenous drugs plus a nondepolarizer muscle relaxant.

b) *Maintenance*
  (1) Maintain normal end-tidal CO_2 levels.
  (2) If working on a donor nephrectomy, the 11th rib may be removed—pneumothorax is a complication; therefore nitrous oxide is best avoided.
  (3) Maintain urinary output; use medications if necessary.
  (4) Volatile anesthetic is used to control intraoperative hypertension.

c) *Emergence*
  (1) If hypertension occurs on emergence, administer a vasodilator.
  (2) Renal patients are considered to have a full stomach; some practitioners require an "awake" patient prior to extubation
  (3) Initiate regional blockade through the epidural catheter for postoperative analgesia prior to the end of the case.

6. **Postoperative implications**
a) Continue to assess volume status.
b) Obtain chest film. Rule out pneumothorax or pulmonary edema, which may occur after administration of large volumes of fluid in the flank position.
c) For renal failure patients, normeperidine, the major metabolite of meperidine, may accumulate and result in prolonged depression of ventilation and seizures.

E. Kidney Transplant

1. **Introduction**
The primary indication for kidney transplantation is end-stage renal disease resulting from several causes, including chronic pyelonephritis, diabetic glomerulonephropathy, polycystic kidney disease, obstructive uropathy, lupus nephritis, hydronephrosis, hypertension, Alport's syndrome, and renal trauma. Each of these conditions can potentially lead to uremic syndrome in which the individual is unable to regulate composition and volume of body

fluids. Fluid overload, acidemia, electrolyte imbalance, and secondary dysfunction in other organ systems ultimately develop. Dialysis is used to manage volume and electrolyte status prior to transplantation. Sources for kidneys for transplants can be either cadaveric or a living donor. Ischemic time for kidneys is a least 48 hours; therefore optimization of recipient condition is possible. Timing of donor and recipient procedures is coordinated so that ischemic time for the kidney is minimized.

DONOR CONSIDERATIONS

2. **Preoperative assessment and patient preparation**
   a) *History and physical examination*
      Most are healthy adults because presence of significant systemic disease would increase the risk of general anesthesia and may increase risk of postoperative complications
      (1) *Cadaveric:* Importance of rapid procurement is based on whether circulation to the kidney is intact. If circulation fails, specimens must be removed quickly to minimize ischemic time.
      (2) *Living donors:* Usually close relatives as unrelated living donations do not produce improved results as compared to cadaveric donations.
   b) *Diagnostic tests*
      (1) Renal arteriography—used to determine if kidney is suitable for renal transplantation
      (2) IV pyelography
      (3) Computed tomography
      (4) Undergo noninvasive studies to detect coronary ischemia if donor is a male older than 45 years or a female older than 50 years.
      (5) *Laboratory tests*
         (*a*) Screened for ABO blood group compatibility and CMV titer, crossmatching of the recipient's serum with donor lymphocytes, HLA tissue typing
         (*b*) See "Nephrectomy," p. 166.
   c) *Preoperative medications and intravenous therapy*
      (1) Patient should donate several units of autologous blood 2 to 4 weeks prior to the procedure.
      (2) Starting the night before the procedure, donors are hydrated with crystalloid to promote active diuresis.
      (3) Epidural catheter—perform test dose in preoperative area.
      (4) Antibiotics
      (5) The peripheral intravenous catheter (16- to 18-gauge) is placed in a location where it will be easily accessible once patient is in lateral decubitus position; aggressive hydration since patient should be two liters positive prior to incision.

3. **Room preparation**
   a) *Monitoring equipment:* Standard and Foley catheter
   b) *Pharmacologic agents:* See "Nephrectomy," p. 166.
   c) Position
      (1) Lateral decubitus position with the kidney bar raised
      (2) With low calcium levels, skin and nerve damage occur easily.
      (3) Inadequate support of the head may lead to Horner's syndrome postoperatively.
      (4) Evaluate radial pulse after placement of axillary roll.
      (5) Respiration is impaired secondary to ventilation/perfusion mismatching, decreased functional reserve capacity, decreased vital capacity, and decreased thoracic compliance.
      (6) Reassess breath sounds postmovement; an endotracheal tube may migrate into the mainstem bronchus during positioning.
4. **Anesthetic technique** See "Radical Prostatectomy," p. 162.
5. **Perioperative management**
   a) *Induction*
      (1) Opioids can be used because only a small amount of the drug is excreted unchanged by the kidneys.
      (2) Cisatracurium and Atracurium do not require a functional kidney as they are degraded by Hoffman elimination. (Atracurium is degraded by ester hydrolysis also.) Both are good choices to use for living donors who will be losing 50% of their renal function.
      (3) Vecuronium, rocuronium, and rapacuronium may be used for muscle relaxation.
      (4) Induction of anesthesia and intubation of the trachea can be safely accomplished with intravenous drugs plus a nondepolarizing muscle relaxant.
   b) *Maintenance*
      (1) Maintain normal end-tidal CO_2 levels.
      (2) Maintain urinary output at a minimum of 1 mL/min; diuresis may need to be induced by treatment with mannitol or furosemide.
      (3) Volatile anesthetic is used to control intraoperative hypertension.
      (4) The 11th rib may be removed—pneumothorax is a complication; therefore nitrous oxide is best avoided.
      (5) Heparin is administered systemically before removal of the donor kidney to limit potential for intrarenal clotting. On removal, the kidney is flushed free of blood with cold crystalloid solution and transplanted immediately.
   c) *Emergence*
      (1) The length of the procedure, large fluid amounts, and potential for pneumothorax and pulmonary edema make an "awake" extubation an appropriate choice.
      (2) Initiate regional blockade through the epidural catheter for postoperative analgesia prior to the end of the case, since large flank incision is painful.

6. **Postoperative implications**
    a) Continue to assess volume status and urine output.
    b) Obtain chest film to rule out pneumothorax or pulmonary edema, which may occur after administration of large volumes of fluid in the flank position.

RECIPIENT CONSIDERATIONS

2. **Preoperative assessment and patient preparation**
    a) *History and physical examination:* Individualized based on patient's condition
    b) *Diagnostic tests* (based on underlying pathology)
        (1) Intravenous pyelography with nephrotomography— identify renal mass.
        (2) Ultrasonography—differentiates simple cysts from solid tumor.
        (3) Exercise stress testing and coronary angiography—assesses for potential ischemic heart disease in diabetic patients.
        (4) Computed tomography
        (5) Laboratory tests: See "Radical Prostatectomy," p. 162.
    c) *Preoperative medications and intravenous therapy*
        (1) Discuss date of last hemodialysis. Dialysis of the recipient should occur within the 24 hour period prior to scheduled transplantation to correct fluid and electrolyte derangements.
        (2) Epidural catheter (if used): Perform test dose in preoperative area.
        (3) Antibiotics
        (4) Small incremental doses of benzodiazepines to facilitate axiolysis
        (5) Minimum of two peripheral intravenous catheters (16- to 18-gauge) with moderate fluid replacement. With renal failure patients, administer hypotonic solutions— 5%—dextrose in water or 5% dextrose and 0.45% saline.
            (*a*) Avoid normal saline—may increase sodium levels.
            (*b*) Avoid plasmolyte or lactated Ringer's solution—may increase K^+ levels.
            (*c*) Restrict fluids and consider using microdrip tubing.
        (6) Noninvasive blood pressure cuff and arterial line placed on arm contralateral to arteriovenous fistula. Transplanted kidneys may not be functional immediately; therefore it is imperative to protect existing AV fistulas and other dialysis ports as post transplantation dialysis may be necessary.
        (7) Steroid replacement—full replacement doses of glucocorticoids should be considered in patients on chronic steroid therapy.
        (8) Aspiration prophylaxis—dialysis patients have delayed gastric emptying.

(9) Blood transfusion—uremic patients will have Hgb levels in the 6 to 8 g/dL range. Chronic anemia leads to compensatory changes, which promote enhanced oxygen unloading to the tissues. Therefore transfusion is not mandatory but may aid in increasing allograft survival.

3. **Room preparation**
   a) *Monitoring equipment:* See "Nephrectomy," p. 166.
   b) *Pharmacologic agents*
      (1) See "Nephrectomy," p. 166.
      (2) Indigo carmine or methylene blue administration (intravenously to assess urinary flow)
   c) *Position:* Supine

4. **Anesthetic technique**
   a) Regional blockade, general anesthesia, or a combination of both
   b) *Technique of choice:* General anesthesia with endotracheal intubation because it allows for adequate ventilation even when surgical retraction for kidney placement impinges on diaphragmatic movement.
   c) *Regional blockade:* Epidural catheter placement preoperatively; spinal impractical due to duration of transplant procedure; caution in patients with coagulopathies is warranted.
   d) *General anesthesia:* Endotracheal intubation
   e) *Regional blockade with general anesthesia:* Smaller doses of each are needed.

5. **Perioperative management**
   a) *Induction*
      (1) See "Nephrectomy," p. 166.
      (2) Succinylcholine is contraindicated if K^+ is elevated.
      (3) Select NDMR based on the patient's medical condition.
      (4) Rapid sequence induction and aspiration prophylaxis should be considered since dialysis patients have delayed gastric emptying.
      (5) Regardless of blood volume status, renal patients may respond to induction of anesthesia as if they are hypovolemic.
   b) *Maintenance*
      (1) Maintain urinary output; use medications if necessary (i.e., furosemide, mannitol).
      (2) Volatile anesthetic is used to control intraoperative hypertension.
      (3) Nitrous oxide may be omitted to avoid bowel distention, which may limit surgical exposure.
      (4) Promotion of renal perfusion after anastomoses of the kidney vessels can be achieved by maintaining high-normal blood pressures by reducing the depth of anesthesia, fluid bolus, or temporary dopamine infusion.
   c) *Emergence*
      (1) If hypertension occurs on emergence, administer a vasodilator.
      (2) Renal patients are considered at greater risk for aspiration, so an "awake" patient prior to extubation may be most

appropriate.

(3) Initiate regional blockade through the epidural catheter (if used) for postoperative analgesia prior to the end of the case or administer opioids incrementally.

6. **Postoperative implications**

   a) Continue to assess volume status since pulmonary edema can develop if urine output is slow to resume.

   b) For renal failure patients, normeperidine, the major metabolite of meperidine, may accumulate and result in prolonged depression of ventilation and seizures. Therefore meperidine should be avoided, since transplant patients are considered failure patients until adequate urine output begins.

F. Cystectomy

1. **Introduction**
   The bladder is usually removed for cancer but may also be removed for severe hemorrhagic or radiation cystitis. In a radical cystectomy for invasive cancer, the female's uterus, fallopian tubes, ovaries, and a portion of the vaginal wall are removed. In males, the ampulla of the vas deferens, prostate, and seminal vesicles are removed. There is also lymph node dissection, and a urinary diversion is created (via the intestine).

2. **Preoperative assessment**

   a) *Cardiac/respiratory/neurologic/endocrine:* Routine

   b) *Renal:* Gross hematuria may be a symptom. Check renal function tests as well as evidence of a urinary tract infection.

   c) *Gastrointestinal:* Patients are at risk for fluid and electrolyte imbalance because of bowel preparation.

3. **Patient preparation**

   a) *Laboratory tests:* Complete blood count, electrolytes, blood urea nitrogen, creatinine, glucose, prothrombin time, partial thromboplastin time, type and screen for 2 to 4 units, urinalysis

   b) *Diagnostic tests:* Electrocardiography and chest radiography for most of this patient population

   c) *Medication:* Sedation as needed

4. **Room preparation**

   a) Standard

   b) *Monitors:* Standard, arterial line, and central venous pressure. Urine output cannot be measured during this procedure. Have two large bore, reliable intravenous lines.

   c) *Additional equipment:* Epidural insertion and infusion supplies, if using, and warming devices for the patient and fluids

   d) *Position:* Supine

   e) *Drugs and fluids:* 6 to 10 mL/kg per hour of crystalloid for maintenance. Have 2 to 4 units of blood readily available.

PART 2 Common Procedures

5. **Perioperative management**
   Combined general/epidural or general anesthesia with standard
   induction. The patient may be anemic because of hematuria and
   hypovolemic because of bowel preparations. Attempt to correct these
   conditions before induction. Maintenance is routine, with special
   attention paid to fluid calculations and keeping the patient warm.
   Plan to extubate immediately postoperatively unless the patient is
   unstable during the procedure or prior respiratory complications
   prevent early extubation.
6. **Postoperative considerations**
   Epidural or patient-controlled analgesia should be planned for
   preoperative use. Watch patients for signs of hypovolemia, anemia,
   or pulmonary edema due to fluid shifts intraoperatively.

G. Cystoscopy

1. **Introduction**
   Cystoscopy is the use of instrumentation to examine the urinary
   tract. A cystoscope may be used for diagnostic or therapeutic
   procedures, such as the workup of hematuria, structure, and tumor;
   removal and manipulation of stones; placement of stents; and follow-
   up of therapy. Retrograde pyelography and other dye studies may be
   used. This procedure is usually performed on an outpatient basis.
2. **Preoperative assessment and patient preparation**
   a) *History and physical examination:* Standard
   b) *Diagnostic tests:* Standard
   c) *Preoperative medication and intravenous therapy*
      (1) Prophylactic antibiotics
      (2) 18-gauge intravenous catheter with minimal fluid
          replacement
3. **Room preparation**
   a) *Monitoring equipment:* Standard
   b) *Pharmacologic agents:* Indigo carmine, methylene blue
   c) *Position:* Lithotomy
4. **Anesthetic technique**
   Technique of choice: Regional blockade or general anesthesia
   a) *Intravenous sedation:* Versed, fentanyl, or propofol in sedation
      doses
   b) *Regional blockade:* Analgesia to T9 required
   c) *General anesthesia:* Administered by mask or oral endotracheal
      tube
5. **Preoperative management**
   a) *Induction:* No specific indications
   b) *Maintenance*
      (1) Diagnostic dyes may be administered. Use indigo carmine
          dye (α-sympathomimetic effects) cautiously with

hypertension or cardiac ischemia. Methylene blue dye may cause hypertension. Oxygen saturation readings may be altered by dye administration.

(2) Persistent erection may occur in younger males, preventing manipulation of the cystoscope. Use deeper anesthesia.

(3) Water or irrigation solution may be used to distend the bladder. See "Transurethral Resection of the Prostrate," p. 161.

(4) Quadriplegics or paraplegics may undergo repeated cystoscopies. Autonomic hyperreflexia is possible if the injury is above level T5.

   c) *Emergence:* No specific indications

6. **Postoperative considerations**
   Standard

H. Penile Procedures

1. **Introduction**
   Penile procedures are usually performed for three different indications: 1. For congenital defect–hypospadias, which is usually a pediatric procedure; 2. for penectomy/penile resection as a result of penile cancer; and 3. for implants to compensate for impotence. Organic impotence is often secondary to diabetes, hypertension and its treatment, or spinal cord trauma.

2. **Preoperative assessment**
   Individualized based on patient's condition

3. **Patient preparation**
   a) Standard preoperative laboratory testing as indicated.
   b) Preoperative medications are individualized.

4. **Room preparation**
   a) *Monitoring:* Standard
   b) *Position:* Supine
   c) *Drugs and tabletop:* Adult/pediatric setup

5. **Anesthesia and perioperative management**
   a) For pediatric patients, use an inhaled induction for general anesthetic. Intubation is desired because hypospadius repair generally takes longer than 2 hours.
   b) For penectomy or prosthetic insertion, regional or general anesthetic may be used, depending on the preferences of the patient and the anesthetist and on the medical condition. Muscle relaxation is not required, and blood loss is minimal.
   c) Some practitioners will perform a caudal block for pediatric patients just prior to awakening for postoperative pain control.

6. **Postoperative implications**
   Urinary retention is common and may be intensified with the use of a regional anesthetic.

PART 2 Common Procedures

I. Scrotal Procedures

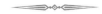

1. **Introduction**

   Scrotal procedures are considered minor operative procedures and can be performed on an outpatient basis unless there are preexisting medical conditions. In adults, most elective scrotal procedures can be performed under local anesthesia with sedation. The most common procedures include surgery for infertility, hydrocele, undescended testicle, or orchiectomy for cancer.

   The most common emergency scrotal surgery is for testicular torsion. These patients will be in acute pain and should be considered to have a full stomach.

2. **Preoperative assessment**

   a) Most patients who present for infertility concerns, hydrocele, and minor procedures are essentially healthy.

   b) Those who present for orchidectomy require careful preoperative evaluation for possible metastasis.

   c) No specific laboratory tests or medications are required except those that are suggested from the preoperative evaluation.

3. **Room preparation**

   a) *Monitoring:* Standard

   b) *Position:* Supine. Arms usually are out at the sides. Lithotomy position may be requested.

   c) *Drugs and tabletop:* Sedatives and narcotics. Tabletop should be set up for emergency general anesthetic.

4. **Anesthesia and perioperative management**

   a) The patient may receive local anesthesia with sedation, regional anesthesia, or general anesthesia depending on condition and anesthetist preference.

   b) There are no specific considerations because muscle relaxation is not required, and blood loss is minimal.

5. **Postoperative considerations**

   Pain management may be commenced intraoperatively by the use of narcotics, ketorolac, or both. Some patients, especially if being treated for malignancy, may experience nausea and vomiting.

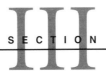

Neuroskeletal System

A. Lumbar Laminectomy/Fusion

1. **Introduction**
   Lumbar laminectomy is most commonly performed for symptomatic nerve root or cord compression. Compression may occur from protrusion of an intervertebral disk or osteophyte bone into the spinal canal. An intervertebral disk usually herniates at the L4 to L5 or L5 to S1 intervertebral spaces. A laminectomy procedure involves the complete removal of lamina. Lumbar fusion is performed when there is instability of the spine. Bone graft material can be obtained from the patient's iliac crest or from backbone.

2. **Preoperative assessment and patient preparation**
   a) *History and physical examination: Neurologic:* Assess and document neurologic deficits of the lower extremities.
   b) *Diagnostic tests:* Type and screen blood, complete blood count
   c) *Preoperative medication and intravenous therapy*
      (1) Consider a narcotic with premedication if the patient experiences pain.
      (2) Consider antisialagogue since most spinal surgery is performed in the prone position.
      (3) Use a 16- or 18-gauge intravenous catheter with minimal fluid replacement.

3. **Room preparation**
   a) *Monitoring equipment:* Standard
   b) *Pharmacologic agents:* Vasopressors, steroids, and antibiotic
   c) *Position*
      (1) Prone, lateral, knee-chest
      (2) Have foam headrest, doughnut, axillary roll, and indicated padding available.
      (3) Specially designed frames may be used to aid in positioning.

4. **Anesthetic technique**
   a) Local infiltration, regional blockade, and general anesthesia
   b) *Technique of choice:* General anesthesia
      (1) *Regional blockade:* Reduces blood loss and shrinks epidural veins, analgesia to T7 to T8 is required; regional anesthesia cannot be used if nerve function will be tested.
      (2) *Epidural:* Must be in single dose with the catheter removed.
      (3) *Spinal:* Hypotension may be accentuated with position change.

5. **Perioperative management**
   a) *Induction*

(1) If the prone or knee-chest position is used, anesthesia is induced on the stretcher.

(2) Position changes may be done in stages to avoid hemodynamic compromise. It may be necessary to lighten the anesthetic and increase fluids before the position change. A vasopressor may be needed to treat hypotension.

(3) Tape the endotracheal tube to the side of the mouth that will be positioned up. Confirm endotracheal tube placement after positioning.

b) *Maintenance*

(1) Question the surgeon regarding the use of muscle relaxants. If nerve function is to be tested, a single dose of an intermediate nondepolarizing muscle relaxant may be used for intubation.

(2) Pad all pressure points and check for pressure on face every 15 minutes during surgery.

(3) Blood loss is rarely sufficient to necessitate deliberate hypotension. The wound may be infiltrated with an epinephrine solution to decrease intraoperative blood loss.

(4) Sudden profound hypotension may indicate major intra-abdominal vessel (iliac, aorta) damage with bleeding occurring in the retroperitoneal cavity, which may not be visible to the surgeon.

(5) Infiltration of the wound with a local anesthetic will decrease postoperative pain.

c) *Emergence*
Extubation is performed when the patient is supine. The patient may need to be awake at the end of the procedure to allow the surgeon to assess for neurologic deficits.

6. **Postoperative considerations**
The patient can usually be transported in any position because stability of the back is rarely compromised.

B. Anterior Cervical Diskectomy/Fusion

1. **Introduction**
Anterior cervical fusion is most commonly performed for symptomatic nerve root or cord compression. Compression may occur from protrusion of an intervertebral disk or osteophytic bone into the spinal canal. An intervertebral disk usually herniates at the fifth or sixth cervical levels. A bone graft may be taken from the iliac crest or backbone may be used.

2. **Preoperative assessment and patient preparation**
a) Airway assessment should include thorough assessment of the range of motion of the neck. Neurologic deficits with limited neck movement may require intubation with the head in a

neutral position. Intubation can be performed using passive immobilization or in-line traction. Awake intubation with proper positioning is the safest option.

b) Neurologic deficits should be documented. Patients typically complain of neck pain radiating down one arm, which can progress to weakness and atrophy.

c) *Diagnostic tests:* Type and screen, CBC, other tests as patient condition indicates

d) *Preoperative medication and intravenous therapy:* Patients may have considerable pain preoperatively and require a narcotic with premedication. If a difficult airway is anticipated, premedication should be used sparingly. Use a 16- or 18-gauge intravenous catheter with minimal fluid replacement.

3. **Room preparation**
   a) Standard tabletop setup
   b) Supine position, arms tucked at side; a small roll may be placed under the shoulders. Pad elbows to avoid ulnar compression and use slight knee flexion since many patients have lumbar disease also. A doughnut or foam headrest may be used.
   c) Use a single, 18-gauge nonpositional intravenous catheter (arms tucked) with minimal fluid replacement.

4. **Perioperative management and anesthetic technique**
   a) *Induction*
      (1) General anesthesia with endotracheal intubation.
      (2) Tape the endotracheal tube to the side opposite of where the surgeon stands. Keep tape out of the sterile field.
   b) *Maintenance*
      (1) The trachea and esophagus are retracted laterally while the common carotid is retracted medially. The temporal artery can be palpated to monitor for carotid artery occlusion. There is the potential risk of damage to the recurrent laryngeal nerve, major arteries, veins, or esophageal perforation.
      (2) Blood loss is usually not significant, but epidural venous oozing can occur.
      (3) Patients with cord compression have an increased risk for decreased spinal cord perfusion and may not tolerate intraoperative hypotension.
      (4) Spinal cord monitoring with somatosensory-evoked potentials (SSEPs) may be performed.
      (5) The absence of muscle relaxation is required for intraoperative nerve function testing.
      (6) If a nerve stimulator is used on the face, limit twitch application to when the surgeon is not operating, as the face may move during stimulation.
   c) *Emergence*
      (1) Most patients are extubated in the operating room after the procedure.
      (2) Coughing and bucking on the endotracheal tube should be avoided, since it can dislodge the bone plug. Intravenous

PART 2 **Common Procedures**

lidocaine can be administered prior to extubation. The neck must remain in a neutral position. A neck brace may be applied.

(3) Extubate prior to application of the neck brace; a jaw lift may be required. The patient should be awake before leaving the operating room to allow the surgeon to assess neurologic function.

(4) Consider leaving the patient intubated if there is large blood loss or fluid replacement, difficult intubation, multi-level surgery, or difficult tracheal retraction that can lead to tracheal or airway edema.

(5) Assess voice for recurrent laryngeal nerve damage, which rarely causes airway obstruction and usually resolves in a few days to 6 weeks.

C. Thoracic and Lumbar Spinal Instrumentation and Fusion

1. **Introduction**
   Anterolateral, posterior, or combined anterioposterior approaches can be used to treat pathology of the thoracic and lumbar spine. Spinal instrumentation refers to implanted metal rods affixed to the spine to correct and internally splint the deformed spine. Originally designed for scoliosis, posterior spinal instrumentation is commonly performed simultaneously with spinal fusion for a variety of diagnoses, including fracture, tumor, degenerative changes, and developmental spinal deformity. The original Harrington rod is the simplest and still considered by many to be the standard. Other procedures, such as segmental spinal instrumentation, can distribute correctional forces by sublaminar wiring (Luque) or by hook or screw (Cotrel-Dubousset) procedures that apply multilevel corrective forces on the rods. Bone chips from the posterior iliac crest are placed over the site of fusion. Harrington rodding or similar extensive spinal instrumentation procedures to correct spinal column deformities put the spinal cord at risk for ischemia secondary to mechanical compression of its blood supply. This complication has been mitigated with methods to assess spinal cord function intraoperatively. These include intraoperative testing of neurologic function (wake-up test) and SSEP monitoring. Wake-up testing requires an informed cooperative patient and a practice trial of patient responses.

   The anterior approach may use the Dwyer screw and cable apparatus or Zielke rod. It offers a limited fusion area and less blood loss and can correct significant lordosis. There is a greater risk of damage to the spinal cord when compared to the Harrington rod procedure. The spinal cord can be damaged from the vertebral body screw, especially in the smaller thoracic vertebral bodies and larger number of segmental spinal arteries that require ligation. The patient is positioned laterally, and a transthoracic or retroperitoneal approach is used. The potential for respiratory compromise is significant when using the thoracoabdominal approach. Surgery above the level of T8 requires a double lumen endotracheal tube in order to collapse the lung on the operative side. The procedure may require the removal of the tenth and/or sixth rib and diaphragmatic manipulation.

An anterioposterior fusion may be required for patients with unstable spines. Usually, the anterior procedure is performed first, followed by posterior instrumentation after 1 to 2 weeks. Immediate posterior fusion is possible when the area to be fused is small, and the primary curvature is below the diaphragm. The anteroposterior approach necessitates an intraoperative position change. Anesthetic considerations are similar to those required for posterior intrumentation. Anesthetic concerns for thoracic and lumbar spine procedures are positioning, replacement of blood and fluid losses, maintaining spinal cord integrity, preventing venous air embolism, and avoiding hypothermia. The wakeup-test and SSEPs are frequently used.

2. **Preoperative assessment**
   Patients requiring spinal reconstruction usually have either idiopathic or acquired scoliosis. Scoliosis is a deformity of the spine resulting in curvature and rotation of the vertebrae, as well as an associated deformity of the rib cage. Scoliosis can be classified as idiopathic, neuromuscular, myopathic, congenital, trauma or tumor related, and mesenchymal disorders. Most cases are idiopathic with a male to female ratio of 1:4. Surgery is indicated when the curvature is severe: the Cobb is angle greater than 50 degrees or rapidly progressing. Spinal instability requiring surgery may also result from trauma, cancer, or infection. Patients with scoliosis need careful preoperative evaluation of their cardiac, pulmonary, neuromuscular, and renal systems because associated anomalies occur frequently.

   a) History and physical examination
       (1) *Cardiovascular:* High incidence of congestive heart disease, right ventricular hypertrophy, pulmonary hypertension, and cor pulmonale. Pulmonary vascular resistance is increased independent of the severity of scoliosis.
       (2) *Respiratory:* Respiratory impairment proportional to the angle of lateral curvature. Respiratory involvement is more likely when the Cobb angle is greater than 65 degrees. There may be a decreased total lung capacity and vital capacity (restrictive pattern). Ventilation perfusion mismatch and alveolar hypoventilation may result in hypoxemia. If vital capacity is less than 40% predicted, postoperative ventilation usually is required. Patients with neuromuscular disease may also have impaired protective airway mechanisms and weakness of respiratory musculature.
       (3) *Neurologic:* If an intraoperative wake-up test is planned, the

PART 2   **Common Procedures**

patient should be informed preoperatively and assured that the procedure will involve minimal pain. A practice wake-up test helps to establish a baseline assessment and teaches the patient what to expect. Careful preoperative assessment and documentation of the patient's neurologic status is essential.

(4) *Musculoskeletal:* Cardiomyopathy is a common finding in patients with muscular dystrophy. These patients are more sensitive to myocardial depression from anesthetic agents, changes in sympathetic tone, and hypercapnia. Patients with muscular dystrophy may require postoperative ventilation secondary to muscle weakness, impaired secretion removal, and atelectasis. The use of succinylcholine is contraindicated in patients with muscular dystrophy, since it may lead to hyperkalemia and cardiac arrest. These patients may be at risk for developing malignant hyperthermia. The use of nontriggering anesthetic agents and careful observation for signs of malignant hyperthermia are essential.

(5) *Hematologic:* Discontinue platelet inhibitors for 2 to 3 weeks before surgery. Autologous blood donation is recommended. Consider the use of intraoperative hemodilution (Hct 30%), controlled hypotension, and cell saver devices.

b) *Patient preparation*

(1) *Laboratory tests:* Complete blood count, prothrombin time, partial thromboplastin time, arterial blood gases, electrolytes, type and crossmatch and other tests as indicated per history and physical examination

(2) *Diagnostic tests:* Chest radiographs, pulmonary function test, spine studies, ECG, and other tests as indicated per history and physical examination

(3) *Medication:* Standard premedication, if appropriate

3. Room preparation

a) *Monitoring equipment*

(1) Standard monitoring equipment

(2) Arterial line

(3) Foley catheter

(4) Central venous pressure line (if indicated)

b) Additional equipment

(1) Patient warming devices

(2) Cell saver

(3) SSEP monitor (if indicated)

(4) Regular operating table with spinal frame or bolster

c) *Drugs*

(1) Antibiotics, vasodilators if hypotensive technique

(2) Standard emergency drugs, tabletop

(3) Intravenous fluids via one to two large bore intravenous catheters with normal saline at 8 to 10 mL/kg per hour with fluid warmer

(4) Blood loss can be significant, and blood should be immediately available.

4. Anesthetic technique

General endotracheal anesthesia. For pediatric cases, preheat room to 72° to 78° F.

5. **Perioperative management**

   a) *Induction:* Standard; for prone cases, induction is performed on the stretcher.

   b) *Maintenance*

   (1) *Standard:* If SSEPs monitored a constant state of anesthesia, stable hemodynamics and normothermia are essential. Question the SSEP technician regarding the use of N_2O. The concentration of inhalation agents should be kept below 1 MAC. A sufentanil infusion 0.25 to 1 mcg/kg/hour provides a continuous state of anesthesia and lowers the MAC of volatile agents. Muscle relaxation is acceptable and should be kept constant (1 twitch).

   (2) *Position:* Prone on spinal frame or bolster. Avoid abdominal compression, which impairs cardiac and pulmonary function as well as increases bleeding through epidural engorgement. Pressure points must be carefully padded and routinely assessed, especially during controlled hypotension. Anterior procedures are often performed in the lateral position; the dependent limb, ear, and eye should be checked frequently.

   (3) *Wakeup-test:* Performed after completion of spinal instrumentation requires 40 to 60 minutes advance notice from the surgeon. Avoid narcotic or muscle relaxant boluses, decrease inhalation agent; hand ventilate, reverse muscle relaxants and narcotics (Narcan 20 mcg increments) if necessary; monitor train of four; request hand squeeze followed by bilateral foot movement. Uncontrolled patient movement during a wake-up test can result in accidental extubation or dislodgment of the spinal instrumentation. Forceful inspiratory efforts may provoke venous air embolism. If the patient moves the hands and not the feet, the surgeon will decrease the spinal distraction. If movement still does not occur, be prepared to increase the blood pressure and transfuse to increase spinal cord perfusion. The possibility of a hematoma should also be considered. After completion of the wake-up test, the anesthetist must be prepared to rapidly anesthetize the patient (have pentothal or propofol ready).

   (4) SSEP indications of spinal cord ischemia should be treated by restoring normal blood pressure and decreasing cord traction. Discontinue volatile agents and ensure adequate oxygenation. Immediate transfusion may be necessary.

   (5) Controlled hypotension may be used to decrease blood loss. Inhalation agents, vasodilators, nitroprusside, and/or nitroglycerine are usually used to achieve a mean arterial pressure (MAP) of 65 mm Hg in normotensive patients or lowering the systolic blood pressure 20 mm Hg from baseline in hypertensive patients. A major concern with

hypotensive technique is compromising spinal cord blood supply. Blood pressure should be reduced slowly before the incision and allowed to gradually return to normal after surgery.

(6) Ischemic optic neuropathy can lead to blindness and is associated with deliberate hypotension and anemia. Consider the importance of early blood transfusion in the patient undergoing hypotensive technique.

(7) Hypotensive technique requires an arterial line and foley catheter to monitor urine output (0.5 to 1.0 cc/kg/hour).

(8) If a venous air embolism is suspected, the wound is packed, and N_2O is discontinued if in use. Attempt to aspirate air using CVP catheter; use fluids and pressors; turn patient supine; and institute CPR if necessary.

c) *Emergence*
Emergence usually occurs after the patient is positioned supine. Most patients can be extubated in the operating room if preoperative respiratory status was acceptable. Persistent narcotic or muscle relaxation may delay extubation. Assess neurologic function.

6. **Postoperative implications**

a) Pulmonary insufficiency—postoperative ventilation may be required in patients with severe respiratory impairment. A patient with a preoperative vital capacity of less than 40% usually requires postoperative mechanical ventilation. Aggressive postoperative pulmonary care should be emphasized.

b) Neurologic sequelae is the most feared complication, and it is important to assess and document the postoperative neurologic examination.

c) Postoperative pain management allows for early ambulation and compliance with the pulmonary care regimen. Opioids can be administered by the intrathecal, epidural, or parenteral route.

d) Hypothermia

e) Pneumothorax

f) Dislodgment of internal fixation

D. Spinal Cord Injuries

1. **Introduction**
Spinal cord transection is the description of damage to the spinal cord that is manifested as paralysis of the lower extremities (paraplegia) or of all extremities (quadriplegia). Spinal cord transection above the level of C2 to C4 is incompatible with survival, because innervation to the diaphragm is likely to be destroyed.

The most common cause of spinal cord transection is the trauma associated with a motor vehicle or diving accident that results in fracture dislocation of cervical vertebrae. Occasionally, rheumatoid arthritis of the spine leads to spontaneous dislocation of the C1 vertebra on the C2 vertebra, producing progressive quadriparesis. These patients can suddenly become quadriplegic. The most frequent nontraumatic cause of spinal cord transection is multiple sclerosis. In addition, infections or vascular and developmental disorders may be responsible for permanent damage to the spinal cord.

2. **Preoperative assessment**
   Spinal cord transection initially produces flaccid paralysis, with total absence of sensation below the level of injury. Temperature regulation and spinal cord reflexes are lost below the level of injury. The phase after the acute transection of the spinal cord is known as spinal shock and typically lasts 1 to 3 weeks. Several weeks after acute transection of the spinal cord, the spinal cord reflexes gradually return, and patients enter a chronic stage, characterized by overactivity of the sympathetic nervous system and involuntary skeletal muscle spasms. Mental depression and pain are pressing problems after spinal cord injury.

   a) *History and physical examination*
      (1) *Cardiovascular:* Electrocardiograph abnormalities are common during the acute phase of spinal cord transection and include ventricular premature beats and ST–T wave changes suggestive of myocardial ischemia. Decreased systemic blood pressure and bradycardia are also common secondary to a loss of sympathetic tone. Generally, this condition can be treated effectively with crystalloid and colloid infusion and atropine to increase the heart rate. Around 85% of patients with spinal cord transection above T6 exhibit autonomic hyperreflexia, a disorder that appears after the resolution of spinal shock and in association with the return of the spinal cord reflexes.

      (2) *Respiratory:* A transection between the levels of C2 and C4 may result in apnea due to denervation of the diaphragm. The ability to cough and clear secretions from the airway is often impaired because of decreased expiratory reserve volume. Vital capacity also is significantly decreased if the transection of the spinal cord is at the cervical level. Furthermore, arterial hypoxemia is a consistent early finding during the period after cervical spinal cord injury. Tracheobronchial suctioning has been associated with bradycardia and cardiac arrest in these patients, secondary to vasovagal reflex, emphasizing the importance of establishing optimal arterial oxygenation before undertaking this maneuver. Acute respiratory insufficiency and the inability to handle oropharyngeal secretions necessitate immediate tracheal intubation. Before intubation is initiated, the neck must be stabilized.

      (3) *Neurologic:* Patients with spinal cord trauma at the T1 level are paraplegic, whereas traumas above C5 may result in quadriplegia and loss of phrenic nerve function. Injuries between these two levels result in varying loss of motor and

sensory functions in the upper extremities. Careful assessment and documentation of preoperative sensory and motor deficits is important.

(4) *Musculoskeletal:* Prolonged immobility leads to osteoporosis, skeletal muscle atrophy, and the development of decubitus ulcers. Pathologic fractures can occur when these patients are moved. Pressure points should be well protected and padded to minimize the likelihood of trauma to the skin and the development of ulcers.

(5) *Renal:* Renal failure is the leading cause of death in the patient with chronic spinal cord transection. Chronic urinary tract infections and immobilization predispose to the development of renal calculi. Amyloidosis of the kidney can be manifested as proteinuria, leading to a decrease in the concentration of albumin in the plasma.

b) *Patient preparation*

(1) *Laboratory tests:* Arterial blood gases to substantiate the degree of respiratory impairment, urinalysis, complete blood count, coagulation profile, electrolytes, type and crossmatch, and other tests as indicated per history and physical examination

(2) *Diagnostic tests:* Computed tomography, magnetic resonance imaging, radiography of the injured parts, and other tests as indicated per history and physical examination

(3) *Medications:* Premedication is useful in this patient population and individualized based on patient need. Acute spinal cord injury patients often receive methylprednisolone 30 mg/kg loading dose over 15 minutes, then 5.4 mg/hour for 23 hours.

3. **Room preparation**

a) *Monitoring equipment*

(1) Standard monitoring equipment
(2) Foley catheter
(3) Arterial line
(4) Central venous pressure line as clinically indicated

b) *Additional equipment*

(1) Patient warming devices
(2) Regular operating table
(3) Cervical traction, tong traction, or pins; shoulder rolls as clinically indicated

c) *Drugs*

(1) Standard emergency drugs
(2) Standard tabletop
(3) Intravenous fluids via 16- or 18-gauge intravenous with normal saline at 4 to 6 mL/kg per hour with fluid warmer
(4) Regardless of the technique selected for anesthesia, a drug such as nitroprusside must be readily available to treat precipitous hypertension. Nitroprusside administration 1 to 2 g/kg per minute is an effective method of treating sudden hypertension.

4. **Anesthetic technique**
    Use general endotracheal anesthesia. Management of anesthesia in the patient with transection of the spinal cord is largely determined by the duration of the injury. Regardless of the duration of spinal cord transection, preoperative hydration helps prevent hypotension during the induction and maintenance of anesthesia.

5. **Perioperative management**
    a) *Induction*
        (1) All trauma patients are considered to have full stomachs, and rapid sequence induction should be performed. Succinylcholine is avoided in spinal cord injury patients after 24 to 48 hours because of the risk of hyperkalemia from potassium release from extrajunctional receptor sites. Furthermore, succinylcholine-induced fasciculations can exacerbate spinal cord injury. Rocuronium or rapacuronium have a rapid onset and can be used for rapid sequence induction. Ketamine can be used in the hemodynamically unstable patient, if head trauma is not suspected. The anesthetist should determine if the cervical spine x-ray films have been cleared prior to intubation. Avoid manipulating the head and neck, which can cause further injury. If the patient's neck is unstable, or if difficult intubation is anticipated secondary to a halo device or a body jacket, an awake fiberoptic intubation should be performed. The awake intubation has the advantage of preserving muscle tone, which may protect the unstable spine, and the patient's neurologic status can be assessed after the procedure. Blind nasal, awake fiberoptic nasal, or oral intubations are possible options depending on the patient's condition. A rigid laryngoscopy can be performed with in-line axial stabilization.
    b) *Maintenance*
        (1) Standard. A single dose of neuromuscular blocking drug (vecuronium 10 mg) may be administered to relax the neck muscles. Additional doses of relaxants are rarely necessary.
        (2) *Position:* For the anterior approach, the patient is positioned supine with a roll under the shoulders, and the head is moderately hyperextended. Check and pad pressure points. A cervical strap may be placed below the chin to apply continuous cervical traction; avoid pressure on ears and facial nerve. Accidental extubation can result if the chin strap slips off the chin. For the posterior approach, the patient is positioned either prone with horseshoe headrest or three-point stabilization, using a special frame or bolsters that allow the abdomen to hang freely to prevent venous engorgement. Occasionally, the sitting position is used, which increases the risk of venous air embolism.
        (3) *Hypotension:* The loss of sympathetic compensation response makes these patients more susceptible to hypotension from positioning, blood loss, and positive-pressure

ventilation. May need to treat with fluids and pressors. Goal is to maintain systolic blood pressure of 90 mm Hg.

(4) *Autonomic hyperreflexia:* Chronic spinal cord injury patients should be monitored for autonomic hyperreflexia. This condition is associated with injuries above the level of T6. May be precipitated by cutaneous or visceral stimuli below the spinal cord lesion. Bladder, bowel, or intestinal distention is known to produce autonomic overactivitiy. An adequate level of general or spinal anesthesia is paramount. Symptoms are hypertension, bradycardia, dysrhythmias, headache, sweating, piloerection below the lesion, vasodilation above the lesion, hyperreflexia, convulsions, cerebral hemorrhage, and pulmonary edema. Treatment consists of eliminating the stimulus, deepening the anesthetic, raising the head of the bed, and administering vasodilators, α-antagonists, or ganglionic blockers.

(5) *Hypothermia:* Warming devices are necessary, as the patient's core temperature will approach room temperature because of the interruption in sympathetic pathways to the hypothalamus.

c) *Emergence*

After a cervical fusion has been performed, the patient may have a halo device or body jacket. The patient should be fully awake and able to manage his or her airway prior to extubation. Lidocaine can be administered down the endotracheal tube or intravenously to prevent coughing and bucking. The patient should have a tidal volume of greater than 5 mL/kg, a negative inspiratory force of 20 to 25 cm H_2O, and vital capacity of greater than 15 mL/kg. Airway patency can be tested by deflating the cuff to determine if the patient can breathe around the tube prior to extubation. The patient should be assessed for airway obstruction secondary to soft tissue occlusion or superior laryngeal nerve damage after extubation.

6. **Postoperative implications**

a) Airway obstruction is usually caused by soft tissue against the posterior pharyngeal wall. The neck fusion or postoperative traction/stabilization device (halo or body jacket) may impair attempts to open the airway. An oral or nasal airway may be required.

b) Pneumonia may result postoperatively.

c) Respiratory insufficiency can result from the development of a tension pneumothorax from entrainment of air via the surgical wound, oropharyngeal laceration during tracheal intubation, or bleeding into the neck at the surgical site, with progressive compression and occlusion of the airway.

d) The patient should be assessed for the presence of neurologic deficits. Reversible causes such as a hematoma should be ruled out.

e) Deep vein thrombosis can occur from decreased blood flow and venous stasis. Heparinization and sequential compression stockings should be instituted.

f) Urinary retention may require urinary catheterization.

g) Stress ulcers and gastric ileus can be treated with a nasogastric tube, antacids, and H_2-receptor antagonists.

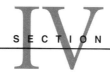

IV

Neurologic System

A. Cerebral Aneurysm

1. **Introduction**
   An intracranial aneurysm is a localized dilation most frequently located at vessel bifurcations that develop secondary to a weakness of the arterial wall. No single mechanism has been identified in the pathogenesis of an intracranial aneurysm. Possible causes are congenital structural defects in the media and elastica of the vessel wall; incomplete involution of embryonic vessels; and secondary factors such as arterial hypertension, atherosclerotic changes, hemodynamic disturbances, and polycystic disease.

   Aneurysmal rupture is prevented by maintaining a stable or low transmural pressure (TMP) within the aneurysm. TMP is defined as the difference between the mean arterial pressure (MAP) and the ICP (ICP). The relationship between the TMP and the wall stress or tension of the aneurysm is linear. Either an increase in the MAP or a fall in the ICP increases the TMP, the wall stress, and risk rupture. Cerebral perfusion pressure (CPP) is also equal to the difference between MAP and ICP; therefore when one attempts to maintain a low TMP, one should be careful not to decrease the CPP and compromise cerebral blood flow.

2. **Preoperative assessment and patient preparation**
   a) *History and physical examination* (findings depend on hemorrhage location): *Neurologic:*
      (1) Level of consciousness—brief loss of consciousness to persistent coma
      (2) Meningeal irritation—nuchal rigidity, positive Kernig's and Brudzinski's signs, fever, irritability, restlessness
      (3) Visual disturbance—blurred vision, double vision, or both; visual field defects
      (4) Cranial nerve involvement—ptosis and dilation of the pupil, inability to move the eye upward or inward, papilledema, photophobia
      (5) Autonomic function—diaphoresis, chills, heart rate and blood pressure changes, slight temperature elevation, altered respiratory rhythm
      (6) Motor function—onset and worsening of hemiparesis, aphasia, dysphagia hemiplegia, unilateral or bilateral transient paralysis of the lower extremities
      (7) Increased ICP—restlessness and lethargy, changes in level of consciousness and vital signs (Cushing's response, increased blood pressure, wide pulse pressure, decreased

pulse rate), pupillary changes (mydriasis), impaired
pupillary reflex, papilledema, vomiting, fluctuations in
temperature, seizures, and respiratory changes

   (8) Pain—sudden onset of a violent headache—usually begins
locally at frontal or temporal region, generalizing to entire
head

  b) *Diagnostic tests*

   (1) Computed tomography shows blood in the subarachnoid
space.

   (2) Magnetic resonance imaging shows blood in the
subarachnoid space.

   (3) Cerebral arteriogram identifies local or general vasospasm,
outlining of cerebral vasculature.

   (4) Skull radiographs reveal calcified walls of aneurysm and
areas of bone erosion.

   (5) Electroencephalogram reveals shifts in midline structure.

   (6) Brain scan shows local diminution of flow.

   (7) Lumbar puncture is controversial—increased opening
pressures, elevated protein count, elevated white blood
cells, cerebrospinal fluid with anthochromia (hemolyzed
red blood cells).

   (8) Regional cerebral blood flow—mean flow values for both
hemispheres and determination of cerebral vasospasm.

   (9) *Laboratory tests:* Complete blood count, electrolytes,
glucose, blood urea nitrogen, creatinine, urinalysis,
coagulation profile, type and crossmatch.

  c) *Perioperative medications and intravenous therapy*

   (1) Antihypertensives—as indicated

   (2) Antifibrinolytic agents—aminocaproic acid (Amicar); not
given with coagulopathies

   (3) Corticosteroids—dexamethasone

   (4) Analgesics/antipyretics

   (5) Pituitary hormone—vasopressin injection

   (6) Narcotic analgesics—acetaminophen with codeine

   (7) Agents to control vasospasm—calcium antagonist

   (8) Antibiotics

   (9) Premedication—should not obscure signs of neurologic
deterioration. However, some sedation may be needed to
prevent anxiety and hypertension.

  (10) Two large bore (16- to 18-gauge) intravenous tubes with
variable fluid management

3. Room preparation

  a) *Monitoring equipment*

   (1) Standard

   (2) Central venous pressure or pulmonary artery catheter
monitors cardiac function, adequacy of fluid, and blood
replacement and allows access to treat venous air embolism

   (3) Arterial line—right or left radial artery depending on
access requirement

   (4) Doppler—monitors venous air embolism

      (*a*) Place between second and third intercostal spaces just to right of sternum.

      (*b*) Use a 50 mL syringe to remove air.

    (5) Foley catheter—assess global renal function

    (6) Peripheral nerve stimulator—monitor muscle blockade

    (7) Warming modalities—minimal. Hypothermia enhances the brain's ability to tolerate ischemia and reduces the cerebral metabolic requirement.

  b) *Pharmacologic agents*

    (1) Prepare infusions of nitroglycerin, nitroprusside, phenylephrine, and dopamine.

    (2) Drugs—mannitol, furosemide, lidocaine intravenous push, β-blockers: esmolol

    (3) Volume—isotonic salt solution; glucose and water solutions are not recommended because they are rapidly and equally distributed throughout total body water.

      (*a*) Administer minimal volume prior to aneurysm clipping (2 to 3 mL/kg). The goal is to maintain hemodynamic stability, accounting for preoperative fluid and electrolyte status.

      (*b*) When the aneurysm is secured, deficits are replaced with additional volume as needed.

      (*c*) At the time of aneurysm dissection, blood must be available in case of rupture.

  c) *Position:* Sitting or supine with the head of the bed raised

    (1) Plan on the use of head-holder pins.

    (2) The airway most likely will be away from immediate reach.

4. Anesthetic technique and perioperative management

Use general anesthesia with endotracheal tube placement.

  a) *Induction:* The goal is smooth, rapid, gentle intubation and induction with control of blood pressure

    (1) During induction and laryngoscopy, avoid wide swings and variances in MAP and ICP due to noxious stimuli, thus increasing the risk of rupture.

    (2) Preoxygenate, followed by a combination of thiopental (3 to 5 mg/kg) and a nondepolarizing muscle relaxant with minimal cardiovascular effects.

    (3) To block the cardiovascular and increased ICP response to laryngoscopy, use additional thiopental, fentanyl, sufentanil, or intravenous lidocaine.

    (4) Sympathetic stimulation may be blocked with use of β-blockers; esmolol, which is ultrashort acting, may be preferred.

  b) *Maintenance*

    (1) Any spontaneous movement during surgery can be disastrous; therefore adequate depth of anesthesia and muscle paralysis is crucial.

    (2) Prepare for noxious stimuli—application of head device and scalp incision

    (3) Anesthesia can be maintained with O_2/air; a volatile

anesthetic; and intravenous supplementation with opioids, barbiturates, or both.

(4) Use caution with volatile anesthetics. Their cerebral vasodilating effects may increase CBF and thus increase ICP.

(5) Total dose of fentanyl should not exceed 10 to 12 mg/kg unless postoperative ventilation is planned.

(6) N_2O is controversial because venous air embolism is possible.

(7) Venous air embolism—associated with procedure when the operative site is above the level of the heart
   (a) *Signs and symptoms:* Decreased $EtCO_2$ and EtN_2, hypertension, mill-wheel murmur by doppler, dysrhythmias, increased right atrial and pulmonary arterial pressures
   (b) *Treatment*
      i) Alert the surgeon.
      ii) Aspirate from central venous pressure/pulmonary arterial catheter.
      iii) Use the Trendelenburg position with the left side down.
      iv) Flood the field with saline or occlude an open vein or venous sinus.
      v) Consider continuous positive airway pressure or positive end-expiratory pressure.
      vi) Compress the jugular vein.

(8) Arterial carbon dioxide pressure—maintain between 25 and 30 mm Hg; hypocarbia decreases cerebral blood flow and ICP.

(9) Controlled hypotensive technique is used to facilitate surgical exposure and control intracranial aneurysms.
   (a) Blood pressure parameters need to be individualized.
   (b) It is suggested that MAP be decreased by 30% below a patient's usual MAP.
   (c) Deepen anesthesia with volatile anesthetic.
   (d) Initiate drip—nitroprusside or nitroglycerin.
   (e) Nitroprusside may cause systemic toxicity due to production of cyanide, which is manifested by metabolic acidosis and high venous oxygen pressure.
   (f) Whichever agent is used, one should be prepared for exaggerated responses in patients made relatively hypovolemic by diuretics.
   (g) Strict attention to calibration and positioning of the arterial line transducer is necessary.
   (h) CPP decreases approximately 0.7 mm Hg for each centimeter the head is elevated above the heart.
   (i) Some suggest placing the transducer at the same level as the circle of Willis—the level of the external auditory canal.

PART 2 Common Procedures

(10) Slack brain—improves lesion exposure, reduces retractor ischemia, and decreases the chance of rupture.
  (*a*) Hyperventilate the lungs.
  (*b*) Administer thiopental.
  (*c*) Administer osmotic diuretics—mannitol (0.25 to 2 g/kg).
  (*d*) Optimize venous drainage.
(11) Aneurysm rupture—likely times of rupture include the following: dura incised and decreased ICP, excessive brain retraction and increased blood pressure, dissection of aneurysm, clip placed onto neck of aneurysm, and removal of clip holder from clip.
  (*a*) Must immediately replace blood losses.
  (*b*) Maintain MAP between 40 and 50 mm Hg—decrease the rate of bleeding.
  (*c*) Alternatively, one or both carotids may be compressed against vertebral bodies for up to 3 minutes to decrease blood in the field.
  (*d*) Intravenous thiopental (Pentothal) for cerebral protection.
(12) Post aneurysm clipping, assess hemodynamics—recommendations: Pulmonary capillary wedge pressure (PCWP) 15 to 18 mm Hg, central venous pressure taken 10 to 12 times monthly, hematocrit of 30 to 35

c) *Emergence:* The goal is to avoid coughing, straining, hypercarbia, and hypertension.
  (1) Unless the patient is to be ventilated postoperatively, deep extubation is the preferred method.
  (2) Patients require monitoring in the intensive care unit for assessment of hemodynamics and neurologic status.

5. Postoperative implications
Delayed ischemia—vasospasm; in areas of dysfunctional autoregulation, cerebral perfusion passively depends on systemic arterial pressure.

a) Therapy is directed at improving cerebral perfusion by increasing systemic arterial pressure to approximately 150 mm Hg with either dopamine or phenylephrine.

b) Increase central venous pressure approximately 10 to 12 mm Hg. Colloid is preferred to crystalloid because of the impermeability of the blood-brain barrier to low–molecular-weight proteins.

c) Use calcium channel blockers, especially nimodipine, to prevent or treat delayed ischemia.

d) Potential for rebleed—usually occurs in the first 24 hours.

B. Posterior Fossa Procedures

1. **Introduction**
   Posterior fossa craniotomies are performed for treating infratentorial tumors. The posterior fossa is a limited area that contains the medulla, pons, cerebellum, major motor and sensory pathways, lower cranial nerve nuclei, and primary respiratory and cardiovascular centers.

2. **Preoperative assessment and patient preparation**
   a) *History and physical examination*
      (1) *Neurologic:* The history and physical examination should include a thorough neurologic evaluation with documentation. Pay special attention to signs and symptoms of brain stem involvement, such as focal neurologic deficits, depressed respiration, and cranial nerve palsies. Changes in level of consciousness may be secondary to increased ICP due to obstructive hydrocephalus of the fourth ventricle.
      (2) *Cardiovascular:* Evaluate for cardiovascular disease and hypertension.
      (3) *Pulmonary:* Assess for a coexisting disease process.
      (4) *Renal:* Correct fluid and electrolyte abnormalities, if present.
      (5) *Gastrointestinal:* Infratentorial tumors may involve the glossopharyngeal and vagus nerves. This may impair the gag reflex, increasing chances of aspiration.
      (6) *Endocrine:* Steroid therapy may be in use.
   b) *Laboratory tests:* Complete blood count, electrolytes, blood urea nitrogen, creatinine, glucose, prothrombin time, partial thromboplastin time
   c) *Diagnostic tests:* Computed tomography and magnetic resonance imaging
   d) *Preoperative medications:* Anxiolytics may be given to alert and anxious patients. Patients who are lethargic or have an altered level of consciousness do not receive premedication.
   e) *Intravenous therapy:* Central line, two 16- to 18-gauge intravenous tubes; consider a pulmonary arterial catheter. Estimated blood loss is 25 to 500 mL.

3. **Room preparation**
   a) *Monitoring equipment:* Standard monitors, arterial line, central venous pressure, urinary catheter, with possible ICP monitoring, precordial Doppler, electroencephalography, electromyography, and sensory/somatosensory/brain stem auditory–evoked potential monitoring
   b) *Additional equipment:* Depending on the position of the patient, have appropriate padding available (i.e., prone pillow, doughnut, chest and axillary rolls); fluid warmer
   c) *Drugs*
      (1) Miscellaneous pharmacologic agents—vasoconstrictors, vasodilators, inotropes, adrenergic antagonists, steroids, osmotic and loop diuretics, thiopental, lidocaine, fentanyl,

PART 2 Common Procedures

nondepolarizing muscle relaxants, and antibiotics

(2)   *Intravenous fluids:* Use isotonic crystalloid solutions. Avoid glucose-or dextrose-containing solutions. Limit normal saline to less than or equal to 10 mL/kg plus replacement of urinary output. If volume is required, administer 5% albumin or hetastarch and limit to less than or equal to 20 mL/kg. Maintain hematocrit at 30 to 35. Transfuse for a hematocrit of less than 25.

(3)   Blood—type and crossmatch for 2 units packed red blood cells

(4)   Tabletop—standard

4.   **Anesthetic technique and perioperative management**

   a)   General anesthesia

   b)   *Induction:* The goal is to minimize increases in blood pressure and ICP. Once an airway has been established, induce with thiopental (4 to 6 mg/kg), an opioid (fentanyl 3 to 5 g/kg), and a nondepolarizing muscle relaxant (vecuronium 0.1 to 0.5 mg). To deepen the anesthetic, consider supplementing with fentanyl in 50-g increments to a total of 10 to 15 g/kg, midazolam and lidocaine 1.5 mg/kg 90 seconds prior to intubation.

   c)   *Maintenance:* Most commonly used maintenance anesthetics are opioid, N_2O, and volatile inhalational agents. The most common opioid is fentanyl, and the most common inhalational agent is isoflurane. High-dose narcotic technique may be also considered. Maintain arterial CO_2 pressure between 25 and 30 mm Hg. Cardiovascular instability secondary to surgical stimulation of the trigeminal, glossopharyngeal, or vagus nerves is common.

   d)   *Positioning:* Patient may be placed in the sitting, lateral, prone, park-bench, or three-quarters prone position. If the sitting position is used, (must be considered) the increased incidence of venous air embolism and cardiovascular instability.

   e)   *Emergence:* Emergence should be as smooth as possible. Avoid bucking or straining on the endotracheal tube. Consider lidocaine 1.5 mg/kg 90 seconds prior to suctioning or extubation. Antihypertensive medications are administered to control systemic hypertension.

5.   **Postoperative implications**

   Closely observe for the occurrence of seizures, hemorrhage, edema, increased ICP, neurologic deficits, and tension pneumocephalus. Impairment of cranial nerves or the respiratory center in the brain stem may require postoperative mechanical ventilation.

C. Transsphenoidal Tumor Resections

1. **Introduction**
   A transsphenoidal tumor resection is performed to access the pituitary gland. It has an advantage over a craniotomy because it results in less blood loss. It involves an incision over the maxillary gingiva or along the side of the nose.
2. **Preoperative assessment and patient preparation**
   a) *History and physical examination:* See "Craniotomy," p. 198 and "Pituitary Tumors," p. 204.
      (1) *Respiratory:* Airway changes can occur with acromegaly (the patient may require a smaller oral endotracheal tube). Problems occur with mask fit. Thoroughly evaluate the airway; check for dyspnea, stridor, and hoarseness
      (2) *Cardiac:* Common findings are hypertension, coronary artery disease, and congestive heart failure acromegaly.
      (3) *Neurologic:* A nonfunctional gland usually is discovered because of increased size, resulting in neurologic changes. A hypersecreting gland is found when small.
      (4) *Renal:* Electrolyte imbalance
      (5) *Diagnostic tests:* Complete blood count. Patients with pan-hypopituitarism require hormone replacement prior to surgery. They should be euthyroid and should be receiving corticosteroids (assess for diabetes mellitus); patients may be on intranasal vasopressin. Diabetes insipidus occurs after corticosteroid is introduced. Check electrolytes and random blood sugar as indicated by history and physical examination.
      (6) *Preoperative medications and intravenous therapy:* Replace deficits and hourly surgical loss; one large bore intravenous line
3. **Room preparation**
   a) *Monitoring equipment:* Standard if sitting position is used; central venous pressure and precordial Doppler; consider arterial line, Foley catheter. Visual-or auditory-evoked potentials may be monitored.
   b) *Additional medications and continuous infusions:* Adjunct medicines to treat hypertension and tachycardia; cocaine, epinephrine preparation
   c) *Position:* Supine, head elevated 30 degrees, table turned
4. **Anesthetic technique**
   Use general anesthesia, oral endotracheal intubation (RAE or anode tubes).
5. **Perioperative management**
   See "Craniotomy," p. 198 and "Pituitary Tumors," p. 204.
   a) *Induction:* See "Craniotomy," p. 198, if increased ICP is a concern.
   b) *Maintenance:* No further neuromuscular blocking agent is required; normocapnia is desired.

PART 2 **Common Procedures**

c) *Emergence:* One must decide whether the patient will be extubated. If so, deep extubation is the method of choice unless contraindicated by airway management at induction.
6. **Postoperative considerations**
   The patient's nose is packed, and the patient is breathing by the mouth.

D. Craniotomy

1. **Introduction**
   An opening is made into the cranium for removal of a tumor, relief of ICP, or to control bleeding. A flap is created by leaving the bone attached to the muscle so that the tissue can be turned down. The dura is then incised in the opposite direction so its base is near the midline. After the surgery is complete, closure is performed in layers: dura, muscles, fascial, galea, and scalp. Craniotomies are classified as supratentorial or subtentorial. (See, "Cerebral Aneurysm," p. 190, for in-depth explanations on the following information.)
2. **Perioperative assessment and patient preparation**
   a) *History and physical examination:*
      (1) Attempt to establish the presence or absence of intracranial hypertension.
      (2) *Neurologic focus:* Level of consciousness, meningeal irritation, visual disturbances, cranial nerve involvement, autonomic function, motor function, and pain
   b) *Diagnostic tests*
      (1) Computed tomography, magnetic resonance imaging, cerebral arteriogram, echoencephalogram, brain scan, regional cerebral blood flow
      (2) *Laboratory tests:* Complete blood count, electrolytes, glucose, blood urea nitrogen, creatinine, urinalysis, prothrombin time, partial thromboplastin time, anticonvulsant levels, type and crossmatch
   c) *Preoperative medications and intravenous therapy*
      (1) Premedication is best avoided when intracranial hypertension is suspected; hypercapnia and second-degree respiratory depression increases ICP and may be lethal.
      (2) Patients with a normal ICP may be given benzodiazepine.
      (3) Steroids and anticonvulsant therapy is continued up to the time of surgery.
      (4) Two large bore intravenous tubes
3. **Room preparation**
   a) *Monitoring equipment*
      (1) Central venous pressure for patients requiring vasoactive drugs; also allows access for treating venous air embolism.
      (2) Arterial line ensures optimal cerebral perfusion.

(3) SSEP or electroencephalogram evaluates cerebral status and prevents optic nerve damage during resections of large pituitary tumors.

(4) Doppler—monitors venous air embolism.

(5) Foley catheter—guides fluid therapy and frequent use of diuretics.

(6) Peripheral nerve stimulation—monitors on nonaffected side.

(7) ICP—usually via ventriculostomy or subdural blot.

b) *Pharmacologic agents*

(1) Prepare infusions of nitroglycerine, phenylephrine, nitroprusside, and dopamine.

(2) *Drugs:* Mannitol, furosemide, lidocaine, calcium channel blocker

(3) *Volume:* Glucose-free isotonic salt solutions

    (*a*) Hyperglycemia is common in this patient population (steroid effect) and has been implicated in increasing ischemic brain injury.

    (*b*) Colloid solutions restore intravascular volume deficits.

    (*c*) Isotonic crystalloid solutions are used for maintenance of fluid requirements.

    (*d*) Intraoperative fluid replacement should be calculated and kept at a minimum unless otherwise indicated.

c) *Position:* Supine

(1) Plan to use head-holder pins.

(2) Head elevated 15 to 30 degrees to facilitate venous and cerebrospinal fluid drainage.

(3) Head may be turned to the side to facilitate exposure; be careful not to impede jugular venous drainage, which will increase ICP.

(4) Table is usually turned 90 to 180 degrees away from anesthesia. Secure endotracheal tube and breathing circuit connections.

4. **Anesthetic technique and perioperative management**

General anesthesia with endotracheal tube placement.

a) *Induction:* Goal is to intubate the trachea in a slow, controlled fashion without compromising cerebral blood flow or increasing ICP.

(1) Induction of anesthesia and endotracheal intubation are critical periods for the patient with compromised intracranial compliance or an increased ICP. Intracranial compliance can be improved by osmotic diuresis, steroids, and removal of cerebrospinal fluid via ventriculostomy.

(2) Do not allow arterial hypertension, which increases cerebral blood volume, promotes cerebral edema, and increases ICP.

(3) Most common induction technique employs thiopental together with hyperventilation to lower ICP and blunt the noxious effects of laryngoscopy and intubation.

(4) Muscle relaxant is given to facilitate ventilation and prevent straining and coughing, which can abruptly increase ICP.

(5) An intravenous narcotic (fentanyl 5 to 10 mg/kg) just prior

to thiopental attenuates the sympathetic response.
(6) Intravenous lidocaine (1 to 1.5 mg/kg) following thiopental but prior to intubation blunts the noxious effects of laryngoscopy.
(7) Avoid succinylcholine, which may increase ICP, especially if intubation is attempted prior to establishment of deep anesthesia and hyperventilation.

b) *Maintenance*
(1) Any spontaneous movement during surgery can be detrimental; therefore adequate depth of anesthesia and muscle paralysis is crucial.
(2) Prepare for noxious stimuli—application of head device and scalp incision.
(3) Anesthesia can be maintained with oxygen/air, a volatile anesthetic, and intravenous supplementation with opioids, barbiturates, or both.
(4) Isoflurane and desflurane are the least potent cerebral vasodilators of the volatile agents.
(5) Arterial CO_2 pressure is maintained at 25 to 30 mm Hg; hypocarbia decreases cerebral blood flow and ICP; severe hypocarbia may result in ischemia.
(6) Controlled hypotensive technique is used to facilitate surgical exposure.
(7) Venous air embolism is possible at the operative site above the heart.
(8) Slack brain improves lesion exposure and reduces retraction ischemia.

c) *Emergence*
The goal is to avoid coughing, straining, hypercarbia, and hypertension.
(1) Most patients can be extubated at the end of the procedure as long as intracranial hypertension is no longer present.
(2) Patients left intubated should remain sedated, paralyzed, and hyperventilated.
(3) Patients require intensive care unit monitoring for assessment of hemodynamics and neurologic status.

5. **Postoperative implications**
Delayed ischemia, bleeding, and infection

E. Stereotactic Surgery

1. **Introduction**
Stereotactic neurosurgery is a neurosurgical technique that makes detailed use of the relationship between the three-dimensional space occupied by intracranial structures or lesions and an extracranial reference system to accurately and precisely guide instruments to such

targets. This type of technique is used when the lesion is small or is located deep within brain tissue or as a means of obtaining a biopsy of a lesion for diagnosis.

Stereotactic procedures can be frame-based or image-guided (frameless). If the frame-based procedure is used, the frame is anchored to the skull with either four pins or four screws. Application typically takes place outside the operating room using local anesthetic. In the cooperative adult, frame application takes only 5 to 10 minutes. For children, general anesthesia is used. If the image-guided procedure is used, small markers called fiducials are placed on the head with adhesive. An imaging study is then performed to provide a system of reference.

2. **Preoperative assessment**
   a) *History and physical examination: neurologic:* Neurologic symptoms vary, depending on the site and size of the lesion; they should be carefully documented. In addition to the routine test, computed tomography is performed preoperatively with the frame in place to determine stereotactic coordinates. Once the coordinates are established, the frame must not be moved on the head until the operation is complete.
   b) *Laboratory tests:* Complete blood count and other tests as indicated per the history and physical examination
   c) *Diagnostic tests:* Computed tomography of the head and other tests as indicated per the history and physical examination
   d) *Medication:* Usually not required

3. **Room preparation**
   a) *Monitoring equipment:* Standard
   b) *Additional equipment*
      (1) Stereotactic instruments
      (2) Monitoring, ventilation, and oxygenation equipment during transport
   c) *Drugs*
      (1) Standard emergency drugs
      (2) Standard tabletop
      (3) *Intravenous fluids:* 18-gauge intravenous line with standard replacement therapy

4. **Anesthetic technique**
   a) General endotracheal anesthesia or monitored anesthesia care is used.
   b) In adults, the stereotactic frame or fiducials are placed the morning of the operation, and the patient is taken to the radiologic suite for computed tomography to determine stereotactic coordinates. The patient is then brought to the operating room with the frame or fiducials still in place. If the operation is to be a biopsy, it is generally done under monitored anesthesia care.
   c) If a complete resection is planned, such as in the removal of an arteriovenous malformation, general endotracheal anesthesia is used. In children, it is usually necessary to induce general anesthesia before placing the frame, thus necessitating the maintenance of general anesthesia during the computed tomography.

The child is then moved to the operating room still anesthetized, and the operation is completed.

5. **Perioperative management**
   a) *Induction*
       (1) If monitored anesthesia care is planned, oxygen is administered by nasal prongs, and the patient is lightly sedated with combinations of droperidol to prevent nausea and vomiting, midazolam to provide amnesia, and meperidine or fentanyl to provide analgesia. The patient must be able to communicate with the surgeon as needed throughout the operation.
       (2) Stereotactic neurosurgery for movement disorders such as Parkinson's disease requires the anesthetist to limit sedation to ensure that the patient will be able to cooperate with the surgeon. If general endotracheal anesthesia is needed with frame-based stereotaxy, fiberoptic laryngoscopy is necessary before inducing anesthesia because the frame precludes intubation by direct laryngoscopy. Once endotracheal intubation is established, anesthesia may be induced with sodium thiopental or propofol, followed by a nondepolarizing-blocking drug to facilitate positioning of the patient.
   b) *Maintenance*
       (1) If general anesthesia is used, the ideal drug is one that decreases ICP and the cerebral metabolic rate of oxygen, maintains cerebral autoregulation, redistributes flow to the potentially ischemic areas, and provides protection of the brain from focal ischemia.
       (2) If children are to be transported from the site of placement of the stereotactic frame to the radiologic suite and then the operating room, it is best to use inhalational anesthesia with isoflurane and 100% oxygen with spontaneous ventilation to ensure adequate ventilation during transport and study. Opiates and neuromuscular-blocking drugs should not be administered until the child is in the operating suite.
       (3) Hyperventilation and diuresis should be avoided in image-guided stereotaxy, as this may cause the brain to shift. If a frame is used, the key to remove it from the patient's head must always be available.
   c) *Emergence*
       No special consideration. The patient is extubated awake and after the return of airway reflexes. If the surgeon suspects that the patient may have a slow recovery or a neurologic injury, or if the anesthetist believes that recovery from the anesthesia may be delayed, it is advisable to leave the endotracheal tube in place at least overnight.

6. **Postoperative implications**
   Focal bleeding may occur postoperatively, causing the onset of a neurologic deficit.

F. Cranioplasty

1. **Introduction**
   Cranioplasty can be performed for a bony tumor resulting from traumatic injury (depressed skull fracture) or, more rarely, resulting from a congenital malformation (fused suture lines). These defects may occur anywhere on the head, so the surgery may take place in varying positions such as supine, sitting, prone, or supine with the head turned. Patients range widely in age, from the newborn to the elderly.
2. **Preoperative assessment and patient preparation**
   Individualized for patient's need
3. **Patient preparation**
   Complete blood count, electrolytes, blood urea nitrogen, creatinine, glucose, prothrombin time, partial thromboplastin time (D-dimer or fibrin split products if disseminated intravascular coagulation needs to be ruled out). Type and crossmatch (for at least 2 units). Arterial blood gases if the patient is being ventilated.
4. **Room preparation**
   a) *Monitoring equipment:* Standard. Arterial line and central line if suggested by history. Use a Foley catheter if surgery is scheduled for more than 2 hours. Some patients may have an ICP monitor in place.
   b) *Additional equipment:* Determine the patient's position during surgery—if supine or supine with the head turned, a foam support aids in positioning the head. Longer ventilation tubing is needed because the table will be turned. With the sitting position, a Doppler and a central line (with a 60 mL syringe attached) are needed to assess and treat venous air embolism. With the prone position, use prone foam rest shoulder rolls and multiple pads. In all cases, a nasal endotracheal tube assists in clearing the surgical field and in stabilizing the endotracheal tube.
   c) *Drugs and tabletop:* Thiopental and etomidate are useful in cranioplasty because of their cerebral protective properties. Propofol is known to decrease ICP. Most surgeons desire antibiotics during surgery, and they should be questioned about steroids and diuretics.
   d) *Blood and fluid requirements:* Glucose-containing solutions are best avoided in neurologic surgery. It is better to err on the side of underhydration. Fluid is usually replaced with normal saline or lactated Ringer's solution at 2 to 4 mL/kg per hour. Blood loss may be substantial, and blood should be immediately available to avoid hypotension or crystalloid overload.
5. **Anesthetic technique**
   Induction is intravenous, with one of the agents known to decrease ICP. With severe trauma, one may wish to use only oxygen and to paralyze the patient. Avoid nasal intubation if there is any chance of a basilar skull fracture. For maintenance, keep the patient's mean

PART 2 Common Procedures

arterial blood pressure slightly below the baseline and maintain normocarbia to slight hypocarbia. A constant infusion of thiopental, etomidate, or propofol with or without inhalation of isoflurane will help to maintain cerebral perfusion and maximize the cerebral oxygen consumption. Muscle relaxation is not necessary if the procedure is confined to the skull, and the head is immobilized with tongs or some other type of fixator. Most practitioners leave the endotracheal tube in place until the neurologic status is certain to allow for regular respiration. Lidocaine is useful in minimizing cough.

6. **Postoperative implications**
   Assess postoperative neurologic functions. Pain is usually controlled in the altered patient with parenteral agents or a passive cutaneous anaphylaxis pump in selected patients. One must be watchful to avoid hypercarbia in neurologic patients receiving opiates.

G. Pituitary Tumors

1. **Introduction**
   Transsphenoidal resection of the pituitary gland is performed either through a nasal or a labial incision and is associated with fewer complications than a craniotomy. A tunnel to the sphenoid sinus is created, and it is entered by removing a piece of the vomer. The mucosa of the sphenoid sinus is removed, and the sella is entered by removing a portion of the sella floor. The tumor is removed with microdissectors and suctioned under fluoroscopic guidance and with the aid of the operating microscope. Fat from the abdomen or thigh may be harvested and placed in the sella to graft and seal the dura if cerebrospinal fluid is found. The floor of the sella may be reconstructed with bone salvaged from the exposure. Uncontrollable bleeding is rare but can be massive, requiring a frontal craniotomy to achieve hemostasis.

2. **Pathophysiology**
   The pituitary gland is located at the base of the skull in the sella turcica, a bony cavity within the sphenoid bone, and it is divided into the anterior (adenohypophysis) and posterior (neurohypophysis) lobes. The anterior pituitary secretes growth hormone, prolactin, gonadotropins (follicle-stimulating hormone, luteinizing hormone), adrenocorticotropic hormone, β-lipotropin, and thyroid-stimulating hormone. The posterior pituitary stores and secretes antidiuretic hormone and oxytocin.

   Nonfunctioning pituitary adenomas are the most common tumor type. Rarely, some patients have endocrine deficiencies due to hypothalamopituitary compression. Various hyperpituitary syndromes may accompany a functioning adenoma. The most frequently occurring are prolactinomas, followed by growth hormone— and adrenocorticotropic hormone—secreting adenomas.

3. **Preoperative assessment**
   a) *Cardiac:* No special considerations unless the patient has acromegaly (growth hormone–secreting adenoma), in which case they may have hypertension, ischemic heart disease, cardiomegaly, congestive heart failure, or diabetes.
   b) *Respiratory:* Mask fit and visualization of the larynx may be difficult in patients with acromegaly due to hypertrophy of facial bones, nasal turbinates, tongue, tonsils, epiglottis, and larynx. Hoarseness and dyspnea may be caused by glottic stenosis from soft tissue overgrowth; these patients may require a smaller endotracheal tube and may be predisposed to postextubation edema. Awake intubation with a fiberoptic laryngoscope is recommended for patients with glottic abnormalities and difficult airways; this obviates the need for a tracheostomy in all but the most severe cases.
   c) *Neurologic:* Secretory tumors are usually small and rarely cause ICP. Nonfunctional tumors, however, are not usually diagnosed until they extend beyond the boundaries of the sella, causing headaches, visual field defects, ICP, or cranial nerve palsies by mass effect.
   d) *Endocrine:* Adrenocorticotropic hormone–secreting adenomas can produce Cushing's disease, which has multiple systemic effects, including insulin-resistant hyperglycemia, hyperaldosteronism with hypokalemia and metabolic alkalosis, and obesity. Prolactin-secreting tumors may present with lactation and amenorrhea. Patients with growth hormone–secreting adenomas may have large hands, feet, and head.
4. **Patient preparation**
   a) *Laboratory tests:* Preoperative endocrine studies including serum and urinary levels of pituitary, thyroid, and adrenal hormones. Hematocrit and others as indicated from the history and physical examination.
   b) *Diagnostic tests:* Computed tomography or magnetic resonance imaging to delineate tumor size and site. Radiography of the neck to analyze airway conformation and lumen diameter in patients with dyspnea, hoarseness, or stridor.
   c) *Medications:* Antibiotics and appropriate replacement therapy should be established in patients with endocrine deficiencies before proceeding with surgery.
5. **Room preparation**
   a) *Monitoring equipment:* Standard monitors, arterial line, central venous pressure line, urine output, Doppler to monitor for venous air embolism in semisitting position
   b) *Additional equipment:* Anesthetic circuits and intravascular lines must be long enough to be accessible at the patient's feet. Anode or right-angle endotracheal tube may be helpful.
   c) *Tabletop:* Table turned 180 degrees; anesthetist will be at the patient's feet.
   d) *Drugs*
      (1) Continuous infusion—vasoactive infusions to maintain

mean arterial pressure and thus cerebral perfusion pressure should be readily available (phenylephrine, nitroglycerine, nitroprusside).

(2) *Intravenous fluids:* one 16- to 18-gauge tube, normal saline or lactated Ringer's solution 4 to 8 mL/kg per hour

(3) Blood—estimated blood loss is usually less than 250 mL, unless bleeding from the internal carotid artery or cavernous sinus occurs during the course of dissection and drilling into the sella.

(4) Tabletop—measures to lower ICP should be readily available (dexamethasone, mannitol, sodium thiopental).

6. **Perioperative management**

a) *Anesthetic technique:* General endotracheal anesthesia is required for this operation.

b) *Induction:* If difficult intubation is anticipated, orotracheal intubation will need to be accomplished before the induction of general anesthesia. Awake fiberoptic is the best choice. Because tumors are generally confined to the sella turcica and ICP is usually normal, standard induction techniques are appropriate. If ICP is of concern, induction should be similar to that used for patients with other kinds of brain tumors. See "Anesthetic Considerations" for "Craniotomy," p. 198. Lidocaine may be administered by topical spray or intravenously (1.5 mg/kg) to lessen cardiovascular responses to intubation.

c) *Maintenance:* Isoflurane (maximum allowable concentration is 1.15%) titrated to effect, fentanyl. Basic neuroanesthetic principles apply whether the transsphenoidal or transcranial approach is used. With the transcranial approach, measures to control ICP are instituted because brain retraction and greater blood loss are necessary. See "Anesthetic Considerations" for "Craniotomy," p. 198. Lumbar cerebrospinal fluid drainage is commonly used in transcranial procedures, and in transsphenoidal procedures subarachnoid air injection may facilitate tumor delineation. When air is injected, N_2O should be discontinued because it may increase the volume of the air-filled closed space. Neuromuscular blocking drugs are generally not necessary, because with adequate anesthesia and the head in Mayfield-Kees skeletal fixation, movement is unlikely. Ventilation is controlled with the arterial CO_2 pressure in the normal range.

d) *Position:* Supine, head elevated 30 degrees, shoulder role. Access to the patient's head is obstructed by the operating microscope, so the endotracheal tube must be firmly secured.

e) *Emergence:* When surgical conditions permit, reverse the residual muscle relaxant when at least one twitch is present in train of four ratio. Discontinue N_2O/volatile agents and administer 100% O_2.

f) *Extubation:* If the patient evidences normal emergence from anesthesia, the endotracheal tube can be removed after suctioning the oropharynx and ensuring that the throat packs placed by the surgeon have been removed. Nasal breathing will be obstructed by packs; therefore if there is any question about airway patency because of a large tongue, small mouth, or redundant soft tissue in the oropharynx, the endotracheal tube should be left in place until the patient is fully awake.

7. **Postoperative implications**
   Diabetes insipidus, evidenced by polyuria and decreased urine specific gravity, may occur after transsphenoidal hypophysectomy. Treatment with intravenous fluids or vasopressin may be necessary. Corticosteroids may be needed postoperatively for several days until testing shows an intact pituitary-adrenal axis.

H. Arteriovenous Malformation Neurosurgery

1. **Introduction**
   Arteriovenous malformations (AVMs) are congenital abnormalities that form direct communications between cerebral arteries and veins. Arterial blood flows directly into veins, causing an irregular resistance without an intervening capillary bed, leaving surrounding brain tissue ischemic (intracerebral steal). Ninety-five per cent of AVMs occur supratentorially and present as subarachnoid or intracerebral hemorrhage, focal deficits, or seizures.

2. **Preoperative assessment and patient preparation**
   a) *History and physical examination*
      (1) *Neurologic:* A documented thorough neurologic examination is essential. Altered level of consciousness, focal deficits, seizure disorders, and headaches are occasionally seen.
      (2) *Cardiovascular:* Assess for past history, usually negative. Electrocardiographic changes might reflect the degree of brain injury.
      (3) *Pulmonary:* Assess for history of smoking or other respiratory complications.
   b) *Patient preparation*
      (1) *Laboratory tests:* Complete blood count, prothrombin time, partial thromboplastin time, electrolytes, blood urea nitrogen, creatinine, bleeding time, and urinalysis
      (2) *Diagnostic tests:* Cerebral angiogram, computed tomography, magnetic resonance imaging, and lumbar puncture
      (3) *Preoperative medications:* Titrate anxiolytics to alert, anxious patients. Avoid premedicating patients with altered level of consciousness.
      (4) *Intravenous therapy:* Central line, two 16-gauge tubes, consider pulmonary arterial catheter. Estimated blood loss is 500 to 3000 mL.

PART 2 Common Procedures

3. **Room preparation**
   a) *Monitoring equipment:* Standard, Arterial line, central venous pressure, and urinary catheter
   b) *Additional equipment:* Fluid warmer, cell saver, special frame to support the head, surgical microscope
   c) *Drugs*
      (1) Miscellaneous pharmacologic agents—osmotic and loop diuretics, sodium nitroprusside, phenylephrine, ephedrine, atropine, esmolol, labetalol, lidocaine, fentanyl, nondepolarizing muscle relaxants, antibiotics and thiopental infusion
      (2) *Intravenous fluids:* Nondextrose containing crystalloids. Normal saline/lactated Ringer's solution not to exceed 10 mL/kg plus urinary output. Transfuse for a hematocrit of less than 30. If patient is hypovolemic, give 5% albumin. Avoid hetastarch.
      (3) Blood—type and crossmatch for 6 units of packed red blood cells
      (4) Tabletop—standard
4. **Perioperative management and anesthetic technique**
   Use general anesthesia.
   a) *Induction:* Thiopental, fentanyl, NDMR, and lidocaine 1.5 to 2 mg/kg. If the patient is in a stereotactic frame, endotracheal intubation via fiberoptics is done prior to induction.
   b) *Maintenance:* Isoflurane or desflurane of maximum allowable concentrations less than 1% with O_2 and fentanyl. Consider a bolus of thiopental, 3 to 5 mg/kg, followed by a continuous infusion of 3 to 5 mg/kg when the risk of cerebral ischemia is increased. Esmolol boluses can be used to prevent reflex tachycardia, rebound hypertension, or both. Techniques to reduce intraoperative bleeding, decrease cerebral blood flow, and decrease AVM wall tension include deliberate hypotension and intentional hypothermia. Deliberate hypotension may be incorporated to maintain a mean arterial pressure of 50 to 65 mm Hg. Sodium nitroprusside 0.5 to 0.8 mcg/kg per minute, increasing inhalational agent to 2% to 3% of maximum allowable concentration, or nitroglycerine 0.5 to 8.0 mcg/kg per minute may be used. Intentional hypothermia of 28° to 35° C can be achieved by using ice packs, a thermal blanket, or a cool air blower, or by lowering the operating room temperature. Resection of AVMs can be facilitated by hyperventilation (arterial CO_2 pressure of 25 to 35 mm Hg), diuretics, and erebrospinal fluid drainage.
   c) *Position:* Most common position is supine with the head turned lateral with a shoulder roll. Lateral or modified prone positions are also used.
   d) *Emergence:* Ensure full reversal from neuromuscular blockade and closely regulate blood pressure. Suppress cough, remove the endotube, or do both. The patient is placed supine with the head of the bed elevated 30 degrees, and supplemental O_2 is administered.

5. **Postoperative complications**
    Complications include neurologic deficits, cerebral edema and
    increased ICP, and intracerebral hemorrhage.

I. Electroconvulsive Therapy

1. **Introduction**
    Electroconvulsive therapy is used in the treatment of endogenous
    depression in patients in whom an adequate course of antidepressant
    drugs has failed and those who suffer from severe melancholia or are
    suicidal. It involves placement of electrodes on the scalp and applica-
    tion of a stimulus to elicit a brief grand mal seizure: a 2- to 3-second
    latent phase, followed by a tonic phase lasting 10 to 12 seconds, and
    finally by a clonic phase of 30 to 50 seconds. The clinical outcome
    from electroconvulsive therapy correlates with both duration of indi-
    vidual seizures and cumulative seizure time.
2. **Preoperative assessment and patient preparation**
    a) *History and physical examination*
        (1) *Cardiovascular:* Assess baseline status
             (*a*) Parasympathetic nervous system response to electro-
                    convulsive therapy is immediate and may cause asys-
                    tole, bradycardia, premature ventricular contractions,
                    hypotension, and ventricular escape.
             (*b*) Sympathetic nervous system discharge follows within
                    seconds manifested as increased heart rate, premature
                    ventricular contractions, bigeminy, tachycardia, and
                    severe hypertension.
             (*c*) Myocardial oxygen consumption often increases
                    significantly.
        (2) Individualized based on patient's history
    b) *Relative contraindications:* Angina pectoris, congestive heart
        failure, chronic obstructive pulmonary disease, thrombophlebitis,
        glaucoma, and retinal detachment
    c) *Absolute contraindications:* Recent myocardial infarction, recent
        stroke, intracranial mass, pheochromocytoma.
    d) *Laboratory tests:* Electrolytes, glucose
    e) *Preoperative medications and intravenous therapy*
        (1) Antipsychotic agents may compound the sedating proper-
             ties of anesthesia.
        (2) Monoamine oxidase inhibitors predispose to hemodynamic
             oxidase inhibitors, hemodynamic instability, and hyperten-
             sive crisis.
        (3) Patients receiving lithium may show delayed awakening,
             memory loss, and confusion postictally.
        (4) Anticholinergics modify parasympathetic nervous system
             response; glycopyrrolate causes tachycardia and central

PART 2 Common Procedures

nervous system confusion
(5) 18-gauge intravenous line with minimal fluid replacement
3. **Room preparation**
   a) *Monitoring equipment:* Electrocardiogram, blood pressure cuff, pulse oximeter, and tourniquet
   b) *Pharmacologic agents:* Standard
   c) *Position:* Supine, arms safely tucked to the side or secured on armboards
4. **Anesthetic technique**
   Use general anesthesia and skeletal muscle paralysis.
5. **Perioperative management**
   a) *Induction*
      (1) Methohexital (0.75 to 1.0 mg/kg intravenous)—its redistribution is more rapid than that of thiopental, thus decreasing recovery time; etomidate (0.3 to 0.4 mg/kg intravenous) may be an alternative.
      (2) Ventilate lungs with oxygen by mask.
      (3) Inflate a tourniquet on the arm opposite the intravenous catheter—permits seizure visualization because the arm is isolated from the muscle relaxant.
      (4) Administer a muscle relaxant, usually succinylcholine (1 mg/kg intravenously).
   b) *Maintenance*
      (1) Ventilation continues by mask with 100 mL oxygen.
      (2) An oral airway may be inserted to prevent tongue and tooth damage.
      (3) An electrical charge is applied to the head—avoid contact with the patient and stretcher.
      (4) Severe hypertension is expected—a short-acting intravenous agent may be needed.
   c) *Emergence:* Mask ventilation is resumed until spontaneous recovery occurs.
6. **Postoperative implications**
   None

J. Ventriculoperitoneal Shunt

1. **Introduction**
   A ventriculoperitoneal shunt is placed to relieve increasing cerebrospinal fluid pressures. The hydrocephalus may be caused by a congenital defect, cyst, tumor, trauma, infection, or cerebral blood flow absorption abnormality. Therefore patients undergoing this procedure range in age from the newborn to the elderly. Besides a conduit to the peritoneum, the ventricle can also be drained into the pleura or right atrium.
2. **Preoperative assessment**

a) Neurologic ICP monitoring is routine.

b) Assess for level of consciousness, headaches, nuchal rigidity seizures, and any presurgical neurologic defects such as stroke, spina bifida, and focal defects.

c) Review results of computed tomography of the head. Review blood pressure and heart rate trends in relation to ICP. Cushing's triad—increased ICP, increased blood pressure, and decreased heart rate.

3. **Patient preparation**

a) Complete blood count, electrolytes (especially if the patient is receiving diuretics), glucose (especially if the patient is on steroids such as dexamethasone), prothrombin time, partial thromboplastin time, type and screen.

b) Other diagnostic tests as indicated. Communicate with the neurologist if steroid and diuretic therapy are anticipated during surgery. Usually, preoperative medication is not given to patients with increased ICP.

4. **Room preparation**

a) *Monitors:* Standard and ICP monitor

b) *Position:* Supine with the head turned. A shoulder roll may be used. A foam head rest aids positioning.

c) *Additional equipment:* Table will probably be turned, requiring an adequate length of ventilation tubing. Because much of the patient will be exposed, it is helpful to have a fluid warmer and the room temperature adjusted warmer.

d) *Drugs and tabletop:* Standard. Fluids are usually run at approximately 4 mL/hour.

5. **Anesthesia and perioperative management**

a) Use general anesthesia with endotracheal intubation. Thiopental and etomidate are good choices for induction because of their cerebral protective properties. Muscle relaxation is desirable.

b) Normocarbia aids the surgeon in cannulating the ventricles. It is wise to have the thiopental or etomidate immediately available during the "tunneling," which is the most stimulating part of this procedure. Extubation is performed at the end of the procedure.

6. **Postoperative implications**

Assess neurologic status. Pain can usually be managed with oral preparations.

K. Epilepsy Surgery

1. **Introduction**

Surgery is recommended in the epileptic patient when seizure control is intractable to conventional medical treatment. The goal of epilepsy surgery is to remove a focal area of epileptogenesis without causing neurologic deficits. Epilepsy surgery consists of two types.

PART 2 Common Procedures

Intracranial electrode placement and testing may be required to localize epileptogenic foci. After localization, surgical resection may be performed. Extensive testing is required to define the focal area and its physiologic activity.

2. **Preoperative assessment and patient preparation**
   a) *History and physical examination*
      (1) *Neurologic:* Uncontrollable focal or generalized seizures. Obtain a description of seizure and prodromal symptoms. Obtain list of antiepileptic drugs. A WADA test may be performed (intracarotid injection of a barbiturate) to determine the dominance or speech function in the area of the surgery.
      (2) *Gastrointestinal:* Antiepileptic drugs may cause liver damage.
      (3) *Diagnostic Tests:* CBC. A low hematocrit can be found in patients taking phenytoin or phenobarbital. A low white blood count can be found in patients taking carbamazepine or primidone. A low platelet count can be found in patients taking carbamazepine, valporate, ethosuximide, or Primidone. Obtain laboratory levels of antiepileptic drugs as necessary (e.g., Dilantin).

3. **Room preparation**
   a) *Monitoring equipment:* Standard arterial line and CVP are used for general anesthesia. Foley catheter is used to monitor urine output.
   b) *Additional equipment:* Determine the position of the patient during surgery (supine, lateral, prone, semisitting, and/or table turned 90 or 180 degrees). A foam support aids in positioning the head. A long circuit, long intravenous tubing, and so on will be needed if the table is turned. Appropriate padding should be used according to patient position.
   c) *Drugs:* Short acting benzodiazepines, narcotics, and/or a Propofol infusion are acceptable for providing conscious sedation. If intraoperative electrocorticography is used, benzodiazepines and anticonvulsants must be avoided. It is best to avoid anesthetics that may trigger seizure activity (e.g. methohexital, ketamine). Higher drug doses (e.g., muscle relaxants and narcotics) may be needed due to enzyme induction by anticonvulsant therapy. If a semisitting position is used, the anesthetist should be prepared for VAE.

4. **Perioperative management**
   a) *Induction*
      Local anesthesia with sedation or general anesthesia with OET are the anesthetic techniques of choice. Local anesthesia with sedation is used when the seizure focus is in the dominant hemisphere or if neurologic injury may be caused by temporal lobectomy. Screening is necessary to determine patients that will be able to tolerate the procedure. Standard induction is used for general anesthesia. If a stereotactic frame is used, fiberoptic awake intubation may be necessary.
   b) *Maintenance*
      If general anesthesia is used, low-dose isoflurane, N_2O, and an

opioid infusion are generally used. Isoflurane must be turned off during intraoperative electrocorticography and can be resumed if resection follows. The anesthetist may be asked to elicit a seizure by inducing hyperventilation or administering methohexital. Muscle relaxants generally are not redosed after induction to facilitate evaluation of motor response.

c) *Emergence*
The patient should be emerged smoothly and quickly so that the patient can be assessed for any neurologic deficits.

5. **Postoperative complications**
Seizure, bleeding, and cerebral edema are postoperative complications. The patient must be monitored carefully for altered mental status. If the patient shows any signs of delayed emergence or altered mental status, a CT scan should be performed.

V

Intrathoracic and Extrathoracic

A. Mediastinoscopy

1. **Introduction**
   A mediastinoscopy is performed to diagnose and stage the spread of carcinoma of the bronchus. It permits biopsy of the subcarinal, peritracheal, and superior tracheobronchial lymph nodes under direct visualization. It may also be used to place electrodes for atrial pacing of the heart. A small transverse incision is made above the suprasternal notch. The patient's head is turned to the left, and the mediastinoscope is placed in the space between the anterior surface of the trachea and the posterior border of the suprasternal notch.
2. **Preoperative assessment and patient preparation**
   a) *History and physical examination*
      (1) *Respiratory*
          (*a*) Search for potential airway obstructions and distortions.
          (*b*) Assess smoking history.
          (*c*) May have significant airway edema in patient with SVC syndrome (edema, venous engorgement of head, neck and upper body, supine dyspnea, headache, mental status changes).
      (2) *Cardiac*
          (*a*) Assess for hypertension, angina, dysrhythmias, congestive heart failure, etc.
          (*b*) Reflex bradycardia and arrhythmias may be caused by mechanical compression on the aorta.
      (3) *Neurologic*
          (*a*) Assess for evidence of impaired cerebral circulation—stroke, carotid bruits, and transient ischemic attacks.
          (*b*) The mediastinoscope can exert pressure against the innominate artery and cause diminished blood flow to the right carotid and subclavian arteries.
   b) *Diagnostic tests*
      (1) *Chest radiography*
      (2) *Laboratory tests:* Complete blood count, electrolytes, glucose, coagulation profile, type and crossmatch, and others as indicated by patient's condition.
   c) *Preoperative medications and intravenous therapy*
      (1) Sedatives and narcotics—use with caution in patients with poor respiratory reserve.
      (2) 18-gauge peripheral intravenous line with minimal fluid replacement

3. **Room preparation**
   a) *Monitoring equipment:* Standard
      (1) Pulse oximeter on the right and a noninvasive blood pressure monitor on the left arm
      (2) Continuous assessment to identify compression of the innominate artery—repositioning of the mediastinoscope as necessary.
   b) *Pharmacologic agents*
      (1) Atropine—vagal-mediated reflexes
      (2) Cardioactive drugs
   c) *Position:* Supine; arms may need to be tucked to the side.
4. **Anesthetic technique**
   Local anesthetic with intravenous sedation and general anesthetic.
   a) *Local anesthetic with sedation:* Mediastinum has extensive autonomic nerve supply but few pain fibers. This technique allows continuous monitoring of the level of consciousness in a patient with cerebrovascular disease or an airway obstruction.
   b) *General anesthetic:* Endotracheal intubation
   c) *Technique of choice:* General anesthesia
5. **Perioperative management**
   a) *Induction:* Consider the use of reinforced/armored tubes; avoids tracheal compression from the mediastinoscope.
   b) *Maintenance*
      (1) After endotracheal intubation, either an inhalation or a balanced anesthetic may be used.
      (2) Although the procedure is not very stimulating, the patient must remain motionless.
      (3) A muscle relaxant may be used to prevent the patient from coughing because this may produce venous engagement in the chest or trauma by the mediastinoscope.
      (4) Patients with Eaton-Lambert syndrome are sensitive to succinylcholine and nondepolarizing muscle relaxants; therefore the dosage should be reduced.
      (5) Positive-pressure ventilation of the lungs minimizes the risk of venous air embolism.
   c) *Emergence*
      (1) Extubate after full return of airway reflexes.
      (2) Consider evaluation of vocal cord movement (extubate under direct vision).
6. **Postoperative implications**
   Obtain chest radiographs—pneumothorax is a complication; it is usually right sided. Signs and symptoms are tracheal shift, decreased blood pressure, cyanosis, decreased oxygen saturation (SpO_2), decreased chest movement, decreased blood sugar. Treatment—100% oxygen and prepare for chest-tube insertion.

PART 2   Common Procedures

B. Open Lung Biopsy (Wedge Resection of Lung Lesion)

1. **Introduction**
   An open lung biopsy involves the removal of a mass and 1 cm margins in a manner that does not remove an entire pulmonary segment. This procedure is appropriate for a patient with limited pulmonary reserve who cannot tolerate a lobectomy.

2. **Preoperative assessment**
   a) *Cardiovascular:* Electrocardiography (Watch for right-ventricular hypertrophy, conduction defects, and prior ischemia.)
   b) *Respiratory:* Pulmonary function tests as with an open thoracotomy. Chest radiographs if computed tomography of the chest is not available. Look for airway obstruction, which could interfere with double lumen tube (DLT) placement.
   c) *Musculoskeletal:* Patients diagnosed with lung cancer may have myasthenic (Eaton-Lambert) syndrome, causing an increased sensitivity to nondepolarizing muscle relaxants.
   d) *Hematologic:* Patients are often anemic because of their primary disease. Preoperative blood transfusions may be a consideration.
   e) *Premedication:* When epidural opioids are planned, avoid opioid or other sedative medications, which may potentiate the respiratory effects of the spinal opioids.

3. **Room preparation**
   a) Routine monitors and room setup. Consider a DLT if one-lung ventilation is needed. If so, have a fiberoptic bronchoscope available for checking tube placement. An arterial line is needed occasionally.
      The patient will be positioned in the lateral decubitus or supine position. If the patient is supine, a wedge will be placed under the back of the operative side.
   b) One large bore intravenous tube will be needed.
   c) *Fluid requirements:* Normal saline or lactated Ringer's at 2 mL/kg per hour.

4. **Perioperative management and anesthesia**
   Routine induction and maintenance. Use a balance technique of oxygen, isoflurane, and intravenous opioids (if an epidural catheter is not used). N_2O may be used with two-lung ventilation but discontinue with one-lung ventilation.
      Extubate in the operating room, transfer the patient in the head-up position to the postanesthesia care unit or intensive care unit with oxygen via mask.

5. **Postoperative management**
   Postoperative complications include atelectasis, pneumonia, and fluid overload.

C. Thoracotomy

1. **Introduction**

   A thoracotomy is usually performed in an attempt to resect malignant lung tissue but may also be performed for trauma, infections, and parenchymal abnormalities such as recurrent blebs. Because a thoracotomy involves incising the pleura, all patients require a chest tube postoperatively. Most patients are over the age of 40 years with a history of smoking. Many also have associated cardiovascular disease.

2. **Preoperative assessment**

   a) *Cardiac:* Exercise tolerance is an excellent assessment for cardiopulmonary reserve. Also question the patient about heart failure or arrhythmias. A 12-lead electrocardiogram is needed. Echocardiography and cardiac catheterization may also be useful in certain patients.

   b) *Respiratory:* Pulmonary function tests are routine for elective cases involving resections. Arterial blood gases are mandatory but cannot often predict postoperative functioning. Chest radiographs are mandatory. Most patients also have computed tomography of the chest. Question the patient about smoking history, bronchospasm, exercise tolerance, and pneumonia. Auscultate the chest carefully immediately preoperatively. Confer with the surgeon about one-lung anesthesia preferences and whether there are any foreseeable problems with tube placement (e.g., tumor in the mainstem bronchus).

   c) *Neurologic:* The incidence of Eaton-Lambert syndrome is increased in patients with lung cancer. Assess patients for any generalized weakness or any focal weaknesses that may be the result of stroke.

   d) *Gastrointestinal, renal, endocrine:* Routine

3. **Patient preparation**

   Laboratory tests include complete blood count, electrolytes, blood urea nitrogen, creatinine, glucose, prothrombin time, partial thromboplastin time, arterial blood gases; type and crossmatch for at least 2 units (depending on the type of surgery and the patient's hemoglobin.) Other tests are electrocardiography, chest radiography, pulmonary function tests, and others indicated by history. Keep preoperative medications, especially narcotics, to a minimum in patients who are CO_2 retainers. Digitalization is recommended during pneumonectomy to help prevent postoperative heart failure. It will also reduce tachyarrhythmias intraoperatively. Have bronchodilators, especially inhalants, readily available. Many practitioners administer them prophylactically. Administer an antisialagogue, such as glycopyrrolate, to ease placement and verification of the double lumen endobronchial tube.

4. **Room preparation**

    a) *Monitoring:* Standard with a reliable arterial line. Central venous pressure or pulmonary arterial catheter for patients with preexisting heart disease. Keep in mind that central venous pressure readings may be inaccurate while the chest is opened, and the pulmonary arterial catheter may interfere with a pneumonectomy.

    b) *Additional equipment:* Double lumen endobronchial tubes, at least two. (Balloon rupture on insertion is common.) Fiberoptic endoscope to check tube placement. Equipment to add continuous positive airway pressure and positive end-expiratory pressure intraoperatively. Epidural catheter insertion and infusion supplies, if used. Warming devices for the patient and fluids.

    c) *Positioning:* Lateral or supine with lateral tilt. Beanbag, arm "sled," and axillary rolls may be used. Check for lack of pressure on down arm, eye, and ear. Ensure that arms are not hyperextended.

    d) *Drugs and fluids:* It is preferable to err on the side of underhydrating because these patients are prone to pulmonary edema. Usually use no more than 4 to 5 mL/kg per hour. Have ephedrine/phenylephrine available to treat hypotension.

5. **Perioperative management and anesthetic technique**
    Use standard induction techniques, keeping in mind that the positioning and placement of a double lumen endobronchial tube requires more time than a standard tube placement. Preoxygenate these patients. Arterial blood gases are obtained after induction for baseline so that they may be compared with later results on one-lung ventilation. During one-lung ventilation, maintain tidal volume and place the patient on 100% oxygen. If hypoxemia is present (verify tube placement first), add 5 cm of continuous positive airway pressure to the "up" (surgical) lung. If hypoxemia is still present, add 5 cm of positive end-expiratory pressure to the "down" (ventilated) lung. Extubation at the end of the procedure is preferable unless the patient had a preoperative respiratory indication for remaining intubated (e.g., bronchospasm) or there were large fluid shifts. If the patient needs to remain intubated, the DLT must be replaced with a standard endotracheal tube.

6. **Postoperative considerations**
    Epidural anesthesia, patient-controlled analgesia, or another type of pain control (e.g., nerve block) should be planned preoperatively. The patient must understand and be able to perform deep-breathing exercises. Institute intensive care unit monitoring for at least 24 hours.

D. Bronchopulmonary Lavage

1. **Introduction**
    The bronchopulmonary lavage consists of irrigation of the lung and

bronchial tree. It is performed under general anesthesia with a DLT. Bronchopulmonary lavage can be used to treat alveolar proteinosis, cystic fibrosis, bronchiectasis, radioactive dust inhalation, and asthma or bronchitis.

2. **Preoperative assessment and patient preparation**
   Routine preoperative assessment, including a ventilation-perfusion scan. The lavage is performed on the most severely affected lung first. If both lungs are affected equally, the left lung is lavaged first due to better exchange on the larger right lung.

3. **Room preparation**
   A fiberoptic bronchoscope is needed to check for accurate placement of the DLT. Monitors are routine, including an arterial line. A stethoscope should be placed over the nondependent lung to check for rales, which may indicate leakage of the lavaged fluid into this lung. The patient is positioned in the left or right down position.

4. **Perioperative management and anesthetic technique**
   After intravenous induction, anesthesia is maintained with an inhalation agent. Keep the fractional inspired oxygen as high as possible. The cuff seal on the DLT should be checked and should maintain perfect separation at a pressure of 90% of the fluid cm H_2O to prevent leakage of fluid from around the cuff.

   With the patient in the head-up position, 700 to 1000 mL of warmed heparinized isotonic saline is instilled from a reservoir 30 cm above the midaxillary line into the catheter to the dependent lung. When the fluid ceases to flow, the patient is placed in the head-down position, and the fluid is allowed to drain out.

   With each lavage, inflow and outflow volumes are measured to prevent excess absorption and leakage to the ventilated side. At least 90% of the fluid should be recovered with each lavage. Two-lung ventilation is reestablished; as compliance improves, air may be added to maintain alveolar patency. Patients can be extubated in the operating room if stable.

E. Thymectomy

1. **Introduction**
   The thymus gland is a bilobate mass of lymphoid tissue located deep to the sternum in the anterior region of the mediastinum. Thymectomy involves two surgical approaches: median sternotomy or transcervical.

   The thymus gland is believed to play a role in myasthenia gravis. This is a neuromuscular disorder in which postsynaptic acetylcholine receptors are attacked, inducing rapid receptor destruction.

2. **Preoperative assessment and patient preparation**
   a) *History and physical examination*
      (1) *Respiratory* (based on the myasthenia gravis patient)

(*a*)   Weakness of pharyngeal and laryngeal muscles with a high risk of aspiration. Assess the patient's ability to cough and handle secretions.

(*b*)   "Myasthenic crisis"—an exacerbation involving respiratory muscles to the point of inadequate ventilation

(2)   *Cardiac:* potential cardiomyopathy

(3)   *Neurologic*

(*a*)   Fatigability and fluctuating motor weakness of voluntary skeletal muscles that worsens with repetitive use and improves with rest.

(*b*)   Ptosis and diplopia are initial symptoms.

(4)   *Endocrine:* Potential hypothyroidism

b)   *Diagnostic tests*

(1)   Pulmonary function studies as indicated.

(2)   Laboratory tests include electrolytes, complete blood count, type and screen, and others as indicated by the patient's medical condition.

c)   *Preoperative medications and intravenous therapy*

(1)   Cholinesterase inhibitors retard the enzymatic hydrolysis of acetylcholine at cholinergic synapses, causing acetylcholine to accumulate at the neuromuscular junction. Continue up to the morning of scheduled surgery.

(2)   Immunosuppressive drugs

(*a*)   Interfere with production of antibodies that are responsible for degradation of cholinergic receptors.

(*b*)   Patients who have been on these drugs for more than 1 month in the past 6 to 12 months need supplementary steroids.

(3)   Antisialogogues and H_2 (histamine$_2$ receptor) blockers—patients with bulbar involvement should be evaluated to determine the safety of these drugs.

(4)   Sedatives and narcotics—use with caution in patients with poor respiratory reserve.

(5)   Antibiotics

(6)   18-gauge intravenous tube with moderate fluid replacement

3.   **Room preparation**

a)   *Monitoring equipment:* Standard

(1)   *Arterial line*

(*a*)   If arterial blood gas monitoring is necessary.

(*b*)   Some suggest placing the catheter in the left radial artery for continuous monitoring in case the innominate artery is damaged.

b)   *Pharmacologic agents*

(1)   Standard

(2)   Depolarizing muscle relaxants are not to be used with myasthenia gravis patients.

(3)   Nondepolarizing muscle relaxant—myasthenia gravis patients have varying responses.

c)   *Position:* Supine

4. **Anesthetic technique**
   General anesthesia—endotracheal intubation is required.
5. **Perioperative management**
   a) *Induction*
   (1) When anesthetizing myasthenia gravis patients, avoidance of all muscle relaxants is preferred.
   (2) An inhaled anesthetic by itself should provide sufficient relaxation of skeletal muscle for intubation of the trachea.
   b) *Maintenance*
   (1) Ability to dissipate the effects of inhaled drugs at the conclusion of anesthesia is important for evaluation of muscle strength.
   (2) Prolonged effects of narcotics, especially on ventilation, detracts from the use of these drugs for maintenance.
   c) *Emergence*
   (1) Before extubating the patient, it is important to know that respiratory ability is adequate.
   (2) Minimal extubation criteria must be met.
   (3) Reversal of neuromuscular blockade is controversial—the additional anticholinesterase may increase weakness and precipitate a cholinergic crisis.
6. **Postoperative considerations**
   a) Patients may need to be observed in an intensive care unit.
   b) Anesthesia and surgery often decrease the need for anti-cholinesterase drugs in the postoperative period.

F. Bronchoscopy

1. **Introduction**
   A bronchoscopy permits direct inspection of the larynx, trachea, and bronchi. Indications include collection of secretions for cytologic or bacteriologic examination, tissue biopsy, location of bleeding and tumors, removal of a foreign body, and implantation of radioactive gold seeds for tumor treatment.
2. **Preoperative assessment**
   a) *History and physical examination*
   (1) *Respiratory:* Evaluate for chronic lung disease, wheezing, atelectasis, hemoptysis, cough, unresolved pneumonia, diffuse lung disease, and smoking history.
   (2) *Cardiac:* Question underlying dysrhythmias because they may arise with stimulation of the scope, or they could be a sign of hypoxemia during the procedure.
   (3) *Gastrointestinal:* Access drinking history and nutritional intake.

PART 2 **Common Procedures**

  b) *Diagnostic tests*
   (1) Chest radiography
   (2) Computed tomography
   (3) Pulmonary function test with lung disease
   (4) Laboratory tests include complete blood count, electrolytes, glucose, and others as indicated by patient's medical condition.
  c) *Preoperative medications and intravenous therapy*
   (1) The patient may already be on sympathomimetic bronchodilators and aminophylline.
   (*2*) Sedatives and narcotics are to be used with caution in patients with poor respiratory reserve.
   (3) Cholinergic blocking agents reduce secretions.
   (4) Intravenous lidocaine—0.5 to 1.5 mg/kg decreases airway reflexes.
   (5) Topical anesthesia—4% lidocaine using a nebulizer to anesthetize the airway by spraying the palate, pharynx, larynx, vocal cords, and trachea.
   (6) One 18-gauge peripheral intravenous with minimal fluid replacement.

3. Room preparation
  a) *Monitoring equipment:* Standard; Arterial line if thoracotomy is planned or the patient is unstable
  b) *Pharmacologic agents:* Lidocaine, and cardiac drugs
  c) *Position:* Supine—table may be turned. One must manage an upper airway that is shared with the surgeon.

4. Anesthetic technique
  a) Local infiltration or general anesthesia
  b) Technique of choice is general anesthesia. Must discuss with the surgeon if a rigid or flexible fiberoptic bronchoscopy will be performed.
  c) Nerve blocks:
   (1) Transtracheal: 2 mL of 2% plain lidocaine through the cricothyroid membrane using a 22-gauge needle attached to a small syringe.
   (2) Superior laryngeal: 25-gauge needle anterior to the superior cornu of the thyroid cartilage.
  d) If topical anesthesia is employed, consider total dosage of local anesthetic and be prepared to treat local anesthetic toxicity.

5. Perioperative management
  a) *Induction*
   (1) *Flexible bronchoscopy*
    (*a*) Endotracheal tube must be long enough (8.0 to 8.5 mm) to permit endoscope to pass easily.
    (*b*) Do not administer O_2 through the suction channel of the flexible bronchoscope to avoid gas trapping and inducing barotrauma.
   (2) *Rigid bronchoscopy*
    (*a*) Conventional ventilation
     i) Ventilation through the side port requires high

gas-flow rates and an intact glass eyepiece.
  ii) Suction, biopsy, and foreign-body manipulation require removal of the glass and loss of ventilation.
  (b) Jet ventilation
   i) Give patients high-inspired oxygen and hyper-ventilate them before apneic oxygenation.
   ii) Perform jet ventilation through the side port of a catheter alongside the bronchoscope.
   iii) Place the tracheal tube to the left side of the mouth because the surgeon will insert the scope down the right side.
   iv) The endotracheal tube must be smaller in diameter to allow surgical access.
  (3) After preoxygenation, general anesthesia is induced with the insertion of an oral endotracheal tube.
  (4) Succinylcholine may be contraindicated if the patient has severe muscle-spasm wasting or complains of myalgia.
 b) *Maintenance*
  (1) General anesthesia must provide good muscle relaxation without patient movement—coughing, laryngospasm, or bronchospasm.
  (2) Cardiac dysrhythmia may be a problem (i.e., supraventricular tachyarrhythmias, premature ventricular contraction, and atrial dysrhythmias). Plan appropriate treatment modalities.
  (3) Volatile anesthetics are useful to provide adequate suppression of upper airway reflexes and permits high-inhaled concentrations of oxygen.
  (4) Air leaks around the bronchoscope may be minimized by having an assistant externally compress the hypopharynx.
  (5) Spontaneous ventilation is preferred in cases of foreign body removal–positive airway pressures could push the foreign body deeper into the bronchial tree.
 c) *Emergence*
  (1) The patient should be awakened rapidly with complete return of airway reflexes prior to extubation.
  (2) Patient needs to have a cough to clear secretions and blood from the airway.
6. **Postoperative implications**
 a) If nerve blocks are administered, keep the patient from eating or drinking for several hours postoperatively; the blocks cause depression of airway reflexes.
 b) Subglottic edema may be treated with aerosolized racemic epinephrine and intravenous dexamethasone (0.1 mg/kg).
 c) Chest radiographs to detect atelectasis or pneumothorax

PART 2 Common Procedures

G. Lung and Heart/Lung Transplantation

1. **Introduction**
   Heart/lung transplants are performed primarily for combined heart and lung disease, e.g., Eisenmenger's syndrome due to a congenital heart defect with irreversible pulmonary hypertension and for certain types of diffuse lung disease such as primary pulmonary hypertension without significant heart failure and cystic fibrosis. A single-lung transplant is usually performed due to end-stage pulmonary disease without significant sepsis including interstitial fibrosis, lymphangioleiomyomatosis and emphysema (including α_1-antitrypsin deficiency). Pulmonary vascular diseases, such as primary pulmonary hypertension or pulmonary hypertension associated with an ASD may also be an indication for single-lung transplantation. Bilateral lung transplantation that is done as a sequential single-lung transplant is performed due to septic lung disease, e.g., chronic bronchiectasis, severe bullous emphysema, pulmonary vascular disease with or without cardiac repair, and cystic fibrosis. One-year survival rates average between 60% and 70%.

2. **Preoperative assessment and patient preparation**
   History and physical examination
   Standard preoperative evaluation supplemented with consideration for the fact that these patients are usually terminally ill, although some are still able to perform limited activity. Thorough documentation of the progression of the disease is indicated.
   a) *Respiratory*
      (1) Severe pulmonary hypertension (80/50 mm Hg) results in enlarged PAs that may cause vocal cord dysfunction (hoarseness, inability to phonate "e"- due to enlarged PA stretching the left recurrent laryngeal nerve resulting in an increased risk for pulmonary aspiration.
      (2) Assess the patient's ability to undergo one-lung ventilation (OLV). If little perfusion of nonoperative lung is present as indicated by ventilation-perfusion scan, anticipate the need for cardiopulmonary bypass. Room air PaO_2 of less than 45 mm Hg predicts need for cardiopulmonary bypass.
      (3) ABG, PFT, V/Q scan
   b) *Cardiac*
      (1) Assess for recent exacerbation of symptoms. Cardiac catheterization data reviewed and responsiveness to specific vasodilators during catheterization assessed along with severity of pulmonary hypertension.
      (2) Assess for evidence of RV dysfunction with tricuspid regurgitation.
      (3) ECG, cardiac catheterization, echocardiogram. Need for partial cardiopulmonary bypass in lung transplantation indicated by mean PAP greater than 40 mm Hg and PVR greater than 5 mm Hg/min/L.

c)   *Neurologic:* Patient with pulmonary hypertension may have right to left shunting so history of embolic episodes must be evaluated. Avoid injection of even small amounts of intravenous air.

d)   *Hematologic*
(1)   Assess for use of anticoagulants.
(2)   Hct, PTT, PT, platelet count, fibrinogen
(3)   Polycythemia due to chronic hypoxemia is common.

e)   *Laboratory tests*
(1)   Assess for renal and hepatic dysfunction.
(2)   Hematocrit, coagulation profile, others as indicated
(3)   Hypokalemia usually not treated since heart/lung transplant graft is preserved with K^+ and implantation will reverse hypokalemia.

f)   *Premedications*
(1)   No premedication is usually required by these patients since the majority of them are well motivated and psychologically prepared.
(2)   May be hypoxic and on continuous oxygen therapy.
(3)   Increased risk for pulmonary aspiration due to use of oral cyclosporine immediately preoperative, unscheduled nature of surgery, and incidence of recurrent laryngeal nerve damage.
(4)   Metoclopramide (10 mg) and ranitidine (50 mg) given intravenously prior to surgery.
(5)   Cyclosporine PO 1 to 2 hours before surgery and azathioprine intravenous 1 hour prior to surgery or before induction. Immunosuppressive regimen varies from center to center.
(6)   Continue with specific antibiotic regime. Cefazolin 1 g intravenous given for single lung transplantation. Coverage for pseudomonas in patients with cystic fibrosis.
(7)   Epidural catheter may be placed for postoperative pain management unless the patient needs cardiopulmonary bypass and full heparinization.

3.   **Intraoperative for Lung Transplantation**
a)   *Monitors and equipment*
(1)   Standard monitors
(2)   Arterial line—blood gases are sampled every 10 minutes.
(3)   PA catheter
(4)   Additional ventilator may be needed to optimally ventilate each lung.
(5)   DLT: for double-lung transplant, a left-sided tube is used, and the left-sided bronchial anastomoses is preformed distal to the tip.
(6)   FOB to verify proper tube placement. Equipment to add CPAP and PEEP intraoperative.
(7)   Agents to treat bronchospasm, right ventricular failure, and pulmonary hypertension should be available.
(8)   Two 14- or 16-gauge intravenous tubes. Crystalloids should be kept to a minimum because transplanted lung has no

lymphatics and cannot drain excess fluid.

   (9) Axillary roll and beanbag for lateral decubitis position for OLV.

b) *Anesthetic technique*

   (1) GETA—usually OLV with a DLT for single lung transplants.

   (2) Aseptic technique very important with these immunosuppressed patients.

   (3) Airway equipment is presterilized and bacterial filters are used.

   (4) Use cricoid pressure due to the risk of aspiration in these patients.

   (5) Induction agents that provide cardiovascular stability are used. Typically fentanyl, etomidate, and vecuronium for muscle relaxation are used. Midazolam (0.1 mg/kg) for amnesia.

   (6) Maintenance with narcotic/O_2/air/isoflurane (if no hypoxemia and right heart failure).

   (7) Emergence: Lungs are inflated to 35 cm H_2O prior to closure of the chest to reinflate atelectatic areas and check adequacy of bronchial closure. When surgery is done, both lumens of DLT are aspirated, and the tube replaced with a single lumen endotracheal tube.

   (8) Patient will go to intensive care unit intubated and ventilated.

c) *Lung isolation:* Achieved with DLT. (See "Thoracotomy," p. 217.)

d) *PA clamping*

   (1) PA clamped to improve V/Q mismatch and oxygenation but severe pulmonary hypertension and RV failure may develop.

   (2) Treat pulmonary hypertension and reduce RV afterload with vasodilators, but take care to avoid systemic hypotension. The patient may need inotropic support.

   (3) May need to temporarily unclamp PA to allow further pharmacologic therapy. Cardiopulmonary bypass may be needed if RV failure cannot be controlled pharmacologically.

e) *Cardiopulmonary bypass*

   (1) Performed if patient with pulmonary hypertension cannot tolerate unilateral PA clamping.

   (2) Indications: arterial O_2 saturation less than 90% following clamping of PA, CI less than 3 L/min/m^2 despite therapy with dopamine and nitroglycerin, or SBP less than 90 mm Hg.

f) *Position:* Supine to lateral decubitus for single-lung and supine with arms above head for bilateral subcostal incision for double-lung transplantation.

g) *Postoperative management*

   (1) Infusion of narcotics through an epidural catheter for postoperative analgesia.

   (2) If cardiopulmonary bypass was performed, an epidural catheter should be delayed until normal coagulation is determined.

(3) Complications include pulmonary edema due to lack of lymphatic drainage in the transplanted lung and infection.

(4) Keep the patient intubated until the transplanted lung(s) begins to function properly and there are no symptoms of pulmonary edema and acute rejection.

(5) Assess for signs of acute renal failure due to toxicity from immunosuppressive therapy.

4. **Intraoperative for Heart/Lung Transplantation**

a) *Monitors and equipment*

(1) Standard monitors

(2) Arterial line

(3) CVP/PA catheter: Invasive monitors are usually placed prior to induction, but if the patient is very dyspneic in supine position, monitors may be inserted following induction.

(4) TEE may be used to optimize selection of fluid therapy, vasodilators, chronotropic, and inotropic agents.

(5) Two 14- or 16-gauge intravenous tubes. Need to anticipate large blood loss; bleeding can be a major problem following termination of cardiopulmonary bypass.

b) *Anesthetic technique*

(1) GETA.

(2) Aseptic technique is very important with these immuno-suppressed patients.

(3) Airway equipment is presterilized, and bacterial filters are used.

(4) Anesthesia is not induced until harvesting of graft is deemed normal by direct inspection.

(5) Induction: Avoid further increases in PVR by protecting against respiratory acidosis, light anesthesia, N_2O, hypoxia, and extremes of lung volume. If hemodynamically stable, fentanyl is used to blunt pulmonary vascular response to intubation.

(6) Do not use N_2O due to exacerbation of pulmonary hypertension, reduction in the fractional inspiration of O_2(FiO_2) and expanding intravascular air bubbles.

(7) Use cricoid pressure due to risk of aspiration.

c) *Termination of cardiopulmonary bypass*

(1) When tracheal anastamosis is complete, lungs are ventilated with FiO_2 at 0. 21 at 5 breaths/min and TV of 6 mL/kg. When bladder temperature reaches 36° C, increase ventilation to 10 breaths/min and TV of 12 mL/kg.

(2) TV adjusted to eliminate atelectasis and to obtain peak inflation pressure of 25 to 30 cm H_2O with the chest open.

(3) Adjust FiO_2 in relation to pulse oximetry and arterial blood gases.

(4) PEEP may be used to enhance oxygenation.

(5) Avoid hypoxemia.

(6) A junctional rhythm is common in a denervated heart. Treat with isoproterenol to obtain a heart rate of 100 to 120. It is common to see 2 P waves with SR.

(7) Atropine and neostigmine have no affect on the heart rate in denervated heart. Hypertension will not cause reflex bradycardia.

(8) A denervated heart responds normally to norepinephrine, epinephrine and isoproterenol.

(9) Care should be taken with intravenous fluids and vasodilators since CO of denervated heart is very sensitive to preload.

(10) Use dopamine, isoproterenol, and epinephrine for inotropic support if pulmonary hypertension and RV failure are present.

(11) Methylprednisolone 500 mg is given postbypass.

(12) Exacerbation of postbypass bleeding may be due to the use of anticoagulants, trauma of CPB, and depressed synthetic liver function. Coagulation therapy may be needed such as protamine, platelets, blood components, FFP, EACA, DDAVP, and aprotinin. Severe bleeding may require cryoprecipitate or factor IX concentration.

d) *Postoperative management*

(1) PCA for postoperative pain management.

(2) Oliguria may be present; treat with mannitol and furosemide.

(3) Pulmonary edema may be present due to a lack of lymphatic drainage in the transplanted lung.

(4) May have RV failure due to pulmonary hypertension and high RV afterload.

(5) Avoid exacerbation of pulmonary hypertension by controlling for hypoxia, acidosis, and extremes of lung volume.

(6) Infection is a potential complication.

(7) There is the potential for nephrotoxicity due to cyclosporine therapy.

(8) Complications from corticosteroids include glucose intolerance, hypertension, hyperlipidemia, aseptic necrosis of the hip, bowel perforation, infection, and obesity.

(9) Complications of azathioprine include thrombocytopenia, leukopenia, hepatotoxicity, and anemia.

H. One-Lung Ventilation (OLV)

1. **Indications**
   a) *Absolute:* Control of ventilation and prevention of contamination of healthy lung.
   b) *Relative:* Surgical exposure and removal of chronic pulmonary emboli

2. **Lung Separation Methods**
   a) *Bronchial blockers*

Univent tube: single-lumen endotracheal tube with a built-in movable endobronchial blocker that is then manipulated into the right or left mainstem bronchus with the aid of a fiberoptic bronchoscope.

b) *Double lumen endobronchial tubes*
Most commonly used tubes for OLV. Two catheters are bonded together, with one lumen long enough to reach to the mainstem bronchus while the other shorter portion of the catheter remains in the trachea above the carina. Inflation of both the tracheal and bronchial cuffs results in lung separation. In a right-sided tube, the bronchial cuff is slotted to allow ventilation of the right upper lobe. Use a left-sided tube. A right-sided tube is indicated only when the left-sided double lumen tube is contraindicated (large lesion of left mainstem, tight left mainstem stenosis, and left mainstem bronchus distortion).

c) *Robershaw*
A DLT with no carinal hook. Available as a left- or right-sided tube.

3. **Insertion of a DLT (Robershaw)**
    a) Insert with distal concave curvature facing anteriorly. Once tip of tube is past the vocal cords, the tube is rotated 90 degrees toward the desired mainstem. Advance the tube until resistance is met (about 29 cm).
    b) Proper position is then checked by inflating the tracheal cuff and confirming bilateral, equal breath sounds. The bronchial cuff is then inflated, and bilateral equal breath sounds are confirmed. Then clamp each lumen individually and confirm OLV. A fiberoptic bronchoscope is then used to verify placement.

4. **Management of OLV**
    a) Maintain two-lung ventilation as long as possible. After the patient is placed in the lateral decubitus position, the position of the tube should be checked again.
    b) Verify proper placement of the tube using fiberscope if arterial hypoxemia occurs during OLV.
    c) If arterial hypoxemia persists despite proper tube placement, consider use of CPAP or PEEP.
    d) A sudden increase in airway pressure may indicate tube displacement.
    e) Reinstitute two-lung ventilation if needed.

I. Breast Biopsy

1. **Introduction**
    Breast cancer is diagnosed via excisional biopsy (by needle aspiration or open excision), followed later by a more definitive surgical procedure designed to decrease tumor bulk and thus enhance effectiveness of systemic therapy (chemotherapy, hormonal therapy, or radiation).

PART 2 Common Procedures

Carcinoma of the breast is an uncontrolled growth of anaplastic cells. Types include ductal, lobular, and nipple adenocarcinomas.

2. **Preoperative assessment and patient preparation**
   a) *History and physical examination*
      (1) The most common initial sign of carcinoma of the breast is a painless mass.
      (2) Bloody discharge is more indicative of cancer than spontaneous unilateral serous nipple discharge.
      (3) Signs of advanced breast cancer include dimpling of skin, nipple retraction, change in breast contour, edema, and erythema of the breast skin.
   b) *Diagnostic tests*
      (1) Mammography, thermography, ultrasonography
      (2) Metastases to bone are frequent; therefore a bone scan and measurement of alkaline phosphatase may be indicated.
      (3) Laboratory tests as indicated by the patient's medical condition.
   c) *Preoperative medications and intravenous therapy*
      (1) The patient may be on hormone therapy.
      (2) Use light sedation and short-acting narcotics preoperatively because the procedure lasts less than 1 hour.
      (3) Metoclopramide (Reglan)—outpatients have an increased gastric volume, and there may be insufflation of air into the stomach if one is using a mask technique.
      (4) One 18-gauge intravenous tube with minimal fluid replacement

3. **Room preparation**
   a) *Monitoring equipment*
      (1) Standard
      (2) Noninvasive blood pressure cuff on the side opposite of surgery
   b) *Pharmacologic agents:* Standard
   c) *Position:* Supine; may need to tuck the surgical arm to the side

4. **Anesthetic technique**
   a) Local infiltration and general anesthesia
   b) Technique of choice is general anesthesia with mask technique.

5. **Perioperative management**
   a) *Induction:* Consider rapid sequence induction and endotracheal intubation with a patient who is obese or on a full stomach.
   b) *Maintenance:* No indications
   c) *Emergence:* If rapid sequence induction is used, perform an awake extubation.

6. **Postoperative implications**
   None

J. Mastectomy

1. **Introduction**
   A total mastectomy (simple or complete mastectomy) removes only the breast; no axillary node dissection is involved. It is used for the treatment of duct carcinoma in situ. A radical mastectomy involves removal of the breast, underlying pectoral muscles, and axillary lymph nodes. There are two major alternatives to radical mastectomy: modified radical mastectomy and wide local excision of the tumor (partial mastectomy or lumpectomy) with axillary dissection. This treatment is followed by postoperative radiation therapy to the remaining breast.

2. **Preoperative assessment**
   Patients often have no other underlying medical problems. The anesthetic implications of metastatic spread to bone, brain, liver, lung, and other areas should be considered. Preoperative assessment should be routine, with special consideration to the following:
   a) *Cardiac:* Cardiomyopathies may result from chemotherapeutic agents (e.g., doxorubicin at doses greater than 75 mg/m^2). Patients exposed to this type of drug may experience cardiac dysfunction, and a cardiac consultation may be needed to determine ventricular function.
   b) *Respiratory:* If the patient has undergone radiation therapy, there may be some respiratory compromise. Drugs such as bleomycin (greater than 200 mg/m^2) can cause pulmonary toxicity and necessitate administration of low fractional inspiration of oxygen (0.30).
   c) *Neurologic:* Breast cancer often metastasizes to the central nervous system, and there could be signs of focal neurologic deficits, altered mental status, or increased intracranial pressure. If mental status is altered, a full medical workup should be undertaken without delay. Postpone surgery until the cause is found.
   d) *Hematologic:* The patient may be anemic secondary to chronic disease or chemotherapeutic agents.

3. **Room preparation**
   Monitors and equipment are routine. If the procedure is for a superficial biopsy, monitored anesthesia care with sedation can be used. Be sure to place the blood pressure cuff on the arm opposite the operative site. The patient is placed in the supine position during the procedure.

4. **Perioperative management and anesthesia technique**
   a) Routine induction and maintenance
   b) Pressure dressings are often applied with the patient anesthetized and "sitting up" at the conclusion of the procedure. Communicate with the surgeon if this type of dressing will be used in order to time emergence more appropriately. If there are no further considerations, the patient may be extubated in the operating room.

5. **Considerations**
    a) Deep surgical exploration may inadvertently cause a pneumothorax. The patient should be monitored for signs and symptoms of pneumothorax, which include increased peak inspiratory pressures, decreased arterial CO_2 pressure, asymmetric breath sounds, hemodynamic instability, and hyperresonance to percussion over the affected side.
    b) Diagnosis is concluded by a chest radiograph.
    c) Treatment includes placing the patient on a fractional inspired oxygen of 100% and insertion of a chest tube.

6. **Postoperative implications**
    a) If the patient is unstable hemodynamically (which may suggest a tension pneumothorax), place a 14-gauge angiocatheter in the second intercostal space while the surgeons set up for a chest tube.
    b) A postoperative chest radiograph may be needed if a pneumothorax is suspected.

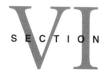

VI

Cardiac Surgery and Anesthesia Considerations

Management of anesthesia for cardiac surgery requires a thorough understanding of normal and altered cardiac physiology; knowledge of the pharmacology of anesthetic, vasoactive, and cardiac drugs; and an understanding of the physiologic alterations associated with cardio-pulmonary bypass (CPB) and the specific surgical procedures.

A. Coronary Artery Disease

The rate of coronary artery disease (CAD) has rapidly progressed to make it the predominant cause of death for patients in their 40s and 50s. More than 280,000 open-heart operations for the correction of nonvalvular heart disease take place each year, representing 80% of the total adult operations performed at most medical centers in the United States.

1. **Risk Factors**
   a) Age: Increased risk with increased age
   b) Sex: Males are at greater risk than females.
   c) Hyperlipidemia: High levels of low-density and intermediate-density lipoproteins are associated with atherosclerosis. Apoproteins are polar lipids.
   d) Hypertension: Increased risk with high blood pressure (BP), especially diastolic BP
   e) Smoking: The risk of those who smoke 1 pack per day is 70 to 200-fold that of nonsmokers.
   f) Diabetes mellitus (DM): DM increases risk for myocardial infarction (MI) by twofold.
2. **Myocardial oxygen supply and demand**
   Management of patients with CAD requires controlling the factors determining myocardial oxygen demand and optimizing oxygen delivery to the heart. When myocardial demand exceeds supply, ischemia develops.
   a) *Determinants of oxygen demand*
       (1) *Myocardial wall tension:* According to the Law of Laplace, wall tension is directly proportional to the chambers dis-tending pressure and internal radius and indirectly propor-tional to wall thickness.
           (a) *Preload:* Refers to left ventricular end-diastolic (LVED) volume, which determines the end-diastolic fiber length and in turn profoundly affects myocardial performance.

(*b*) *Afterload:* Refers to the force distributed by the ventricular wall during ejection, usually equated with the ventricular pressure during ejection and varies with time; impedance to ventricular ejection.

(*c*) *Goal:* Lowering the end-diastolic volume will decrease wall tension and therefore decrease myocardial oxygen demand. (Nitroglycerin, morphine, and Nipride all accomplish this goal.)

(2) *Contractility*

(*a*) The ability of the myocardium to develop force; not dependent on the load of the heart. In the normal heart, sympathetic stimulation and inotropes increase myocardial contractility and oxygen demand.

(*b*) *Goal:* If wall tension is constant and contractility is decreased, oxygen demand will decrease (Calcium channel blockers, β-blockers, and volatile agents decrease myocardial oxegen demand.)

(3) *Heart Rate*

(*a*) Oxygen demand increases as the number of contractions per minute increases.

(*b*) *Goal:* Avoid tachyarrythmias. (β-blockers are effective to decrease heart rate).

b) *Determinants of oxygen supply*

(1) *Coronary blood flow:* Directly related to the perfusion pressure across the coronary vascular bed and inversely related to total coronary resistance.

(*a*) *Coronary perfusion pressure:* The difference between aortic diastolic pressure and the LVED pressure.

(*b*) *Total coronary resistance:* Consists of the basal resistance during diastole and the compressive resistance during systole.

(*c*) *Goal:* A low ventricular end-diastolic pressure (LVEDP) is ideal for improving perfusion due to the higher pressure gradient.

(*d*) *Heart rate:* Coronary arteries fill during the diastolic phase of the cardiac cycle; increased heart rates decrease coronary filling time.

(*e*) *Arterial oxygen content* (CaO_2): Maintaining the blood's oxygen-carrying capacity is vital to perfusion of vital organs, including the heart. Variables affecting arterial oxygen content include the hemoglobin level and oxygen saturation.

$$CaO_2 = (SaO_2)(Hgb)(1.34) + (PaO_2)(0.003)$$

3. **Coronary Artery Bypass Grafting**

a) Methods have been devised to promote coronary blood flow since it has been determined that thrombosis causes the development of myocardial infraction. Some of these methods involve shunting collateral pericardial blood to epicardial arteries and

Improving Myocardial O$_2$ Supply-Demand Balance

---

1. **Decrease myocardial oxygen demand**
   a. Decrease wall tension by decreasing chamber size with venous and arterial vasodilators.
   b. Decrease contractility with CAE antagonists, β-blockers, or volatile agents. (Caution in patients with compromised LV function.)
   c. Slow heart rate with β-blockers and anesthetics.
2. **Increase O$_2$ Supply**
   a. Decrease heart rate to 50 to 60 bpm to maximize coronary filling time during diastole.
   b. Increase CPP by increasing aortic DP and decreasing LVEDP. (Often a combination of Neo-Synephrine and nitroglycerin will achieve these goals.)
   c. Maximize O$_2$ carrying capacity with supplemental O$_2$ and red blood cells to correct anemia.

---

      implantation of the internal mammary artery to the left ventricle without ligating side branches. Saphenous veins can also be anastomosed to the epicardial coronary arteries. The technique of coronary artery bypass involves bypass to a narrowed or occluded epicardial coronary greater than 1 mm in diameter with a small-diameter conduit distal to the narrowed segment. The proximal arterial inflow source is the ascending aorta.

b)   The surgeon approaches the heart via a median sternotomy, and the patient is supported on full coronary artery bypass. The most common strategy used is for all distal (epicardial) anastomoses to be performed during a period of aortic cross-clamping and cardiac arrest. Myocardial protection is achieved by hypothermia and occasional repercussion via anterograde or retrograde cardioplegia. Cardiac standstill and a bloodless field are mandatory when these small-diameter anastomoses are constructed with an obstruction to flow in minimal amount of time.

c)   The cross-clamp is removed, and the heart is allowed to resume beating. A partially occluding aortic cross-clamp can be applied to allow for the construction of the proximal aortic anastomoses. After an adequate period of resuscitation, the patient is weaned from cardiopulmonary bypass (CPB). Decannulation is performed, heparin is reversed, and the chest is closed.

d)   Typical target arteries requiring CPB include the distal right coronary artery (RCA) and its major terminal branch, the posterior descending artery. Typical target arteries on the left include the left anterior descending (LAD) with its diagonal and septal branches. This coronary artery courses in the posterior atrioventricular groove and is not easily accessible for bypass. Therefore this procedure is usually performed to its obtuse marginal or posterolateral branches.

e)   The choice of the vein graft depends on its availability and durability. The internal mammary artery appears to have superior long-term performance with patency rates of 90% after 10 years. On the other hand, the saphenous vein graft has a 50% patency rate at 10 years.

PART 2 Common Procedures

f) The usual preoperative diagnosis of these patients is CAD with class 3 or 4 angina. This type of angina occurs with minimal exertion or at rest.

4. **Selection of Anesthesia**
   a) *Goal:* Decrease myocardial oxygen requirements and prevent myocardial ischemia.
   b) The selection of drugs is influenced by the extent of preexisting myocardial dysfunction and the pharmacologic properties of the specific agents.
   c) Opioids lack myocardial depressant effects and are useful in patients with severe myocardial dysfunction.
      (1) In critically ill patients, fentanyl (50 to 100 mcg/kg) or sufentanil (5 to 20 mcg/kg) may be used as the sole anesthetic.
      (2) In patients with good LV function, opioids may be inadequate in suppressing sympathetic nervous system activity, requiring the addition of volatile anesthetics and sedatives/hypnotics.
   d) *Inhalation agents*
      (1) Advantages—dose dependency, easily reversible, reliable suppression of sympathetic nervous system responses to surgical stress and CPB.
      (2) Disadvantages—myocardial depression and systemic hypotension.
      (3) Combinations of opioids and volatile agents produce the advantages of each and minimize undesirable side effects.
      (4) Isoflurane is a coronary vasodilator, though effects are clinically insignificant is doses less than 1 MAC.
   e) *Sedative hypnotics:* Thiopental, propofol, ketamine, and etomidate may be useful as coinduction agents in particular situations. Of these drugs, etomidate causes the least amount of myocardial depression.
   f) *Muscle relaxants*
      (1) The best drugs are those with minimal cardiovascular effects (e.g., vecuronium, cisatracurium, rocuronium).
      (2) A "priming dose" will help to counteract chest wall rigidity that is often encountered with narcotic induction.
      (3) Succinylcholine may cause bradycardia but can be used in modified rapid sequence inductions for patients with reflux or a full stomach.
      (4) Pancuronium can be used to produce a graded increase in heart rate when desirable.

B. Valvular Heart Disease

1. **Aortic stenosis**
   Disease of the aortic valve may present as valvular stenosis, insuffi-

ciency, or a combination of both. Valvular disease is usually caused by rheumatic disease, but it may also occur secondary to calcific degeneration in the elderly. Endocarditis and congenitally bicuspid valve account for most of the remainder. It is rarely possible to repair the aortic valve; therefore most conditions require valve replacement.

a) *Pathophysiology:* Chronic obstruction to LV ejection results in concentric LV hypertrophy and myocardium that is highly susceptible to ischemia (even in the absence of CAD). Stenosis is severe when valve area is less than 0.6 cm^2 and the pressure gradient is greater than 70 torr.

b) *Hemodynamic goals:* LV filling is dependent on atrial contractions, heart rate, and normal intravascular volume. Decreases in systemic vascular resistance are dangerous due to the fixed ventricular ejection; decreased systemic vasculor resistance (SVR) results in decreased BP, coronary perfusion pressures, and resultant ischemia.

c) Dysrhythmias should be aggressively treated. Because the ventricle is stiff, atrial contraction is critical for ventricular filling and stroke volume.

d) *Anesthetic considerations*
   (1) *Induction*
      (*a*) Usually high-dose narcotic technique—fentanyl, etomidate, muscle relaxant.
      (*b*) Avoid anesthetic agents that reduce vascular tone. Vasopressors should be available for induction.
      (*c*) Maintain intravascular volume and sinus rhythm.
      (*d*) Avoid increased heart rate; avoid decreased SVR and BP
      (*e*) External cardiac massage is not effective in these patients. Ventricular tachycardia and fibrillation are usually fatal.
   (2) *Maintenance:* High-dose narcotic, low-dose volatile agent, oxygen, and air.
   (3) *Post-bypass*
      (*a*) May have higher filling pressures due to the noncompliant ventricle. Inotropic support is commonly required.
      (*b*) May be hyperdynamic or require vasodilators for hypertension.

2. **Aortic regurgitation**
   a) *Pathophysiology*
      (1) The incompetent aortic valve results in a decrease in forward LV stroke volume as part of the ejected LV volume and regurgitates back into the LV from the aorta resulting in chronic volume overload of the left ventricle and eccentric hypertrophy.
      (2) Aortic regurgitation causes a decrease in aortic diastolic pressure and decreased coronary artery perfusion pressures resulting in subendocardial ischemia and angina (even in the absence of CAD).
      (3) The magnitude of regurgitation is dependent on the

duration of flow and the pressure gradient across the valve.
Regurgitation can be reduced by increasing heart rate and
decreasing systemic vascular resistance.

(4) In chronic aortic regurgitation, as end-diastolic volume
increases, stroke volume increases so that the ejection
fraction is well maintained until LV failure occurs. When
failure occurs, cardiac output decreases, end-diastolic
volume increases, and pulmonary edema results.

(5) In acute aortic regurgitation, the sudden increase in LV
volume before ventricular hypertrophy results in sudden
cardiac failure.

b) *Anesthetic considerations*

(1) Maintenance of adequate ventricular volume in the
presence of mild vasodilation and increases in heart rate
are most likely to optimize forward left ventricular stroke
volume.

(2) Avoid increases in SVR and BP; avoid decreases in HR

3. **Mitral stenosis**

a) *Pathophysiology*

(1) Increased left atrial pressure and volume overload occur as
a result of the narrowed mitral orifice. Persistent increases
in the left atrial pressure are reflected back through the
pulmonary circulation, leading to right ventricular hypertrophy and failure, tricuspid regurgitation, and perivascular
edema in the lungs.

(2) The left atrial enlargement predisposes the patient to
formation of thrombi and systemic emboli, especially
with the development of atrial fibrillation.

b) *Anesthetic considerations*

(1) Tachycardia results in inadequate left ventricular filling
and concomitant hypotension. Continued preoperative
administration of digitalis and β-antagonists, the selection
of anesthetics with minimal propensity to increase heart
rate, and achievement of an anesthetic depth sufficient to
suppress sympathetic nervous systems responses are recommended.

(2) Administer induction agents slowly to avoid drug-induced
reductions in SVR and resultant hypotension in the presence
of a fixed LV stroke volume. Avoid ketamine due to the
increase in heart rate associated with this drug.

(3) Preoxygenation and brief laryngoscopy to reduce the
potential for hypoxia, hypercarbia, and acidosis. (These
potentiate pulmonary vasoconstriction, which will potentiate right-sided heart failure.)

(4) Avoid increases in heart rate; avoid decreases in myocardial
contractility, SVR, and BP.

4. **Mitral regurgitation**

a) *Pathophysiology*

(1) Chronic volume overload of the left atrium occurs, resulting
in a decreased left ventricular stroke volume due to part of

the stroke volume regurgitating through the incompetent valve. The increase in left atrial pressure results in elevated pulmonary pressures and right-sided heart failure. Left ventricular hypertrophy results to compensate for the decreased cardiac output.

(2) The amount of regurgitation depends on the size of the valve orifice, the heart rate, and the pressure gradient across the valve.

(3) Mild increases in heart rate improve left ventricular stroke volume. Bradycardia results in acute volume overload of the left atrium.

(4) The pressure gradient across the valve is determined by the compliance of the left ventricle and the impedance to left ventricular ejection into the aorta. Reducing systemic vascular resistance can improve forward flow.

b) *Anesthetic considerations*

(1) Select agents that promote vasodilation and increase the heart rate.

(2) Avoid myocardial depression, which will decrease cardiac output.

(3) Barbiturates, benzodiazepines, etomidate, and succinyl-choline are good choices.

(4) Maintain normocarbia and oxygen saturation to prevent increases in pulmonary hypertension associated with pulmonary vasoconstriction.

C. Cardiac Tamponade and Constrictive Pericarditis

1. **Pathophysiology**

   a) A large pericardial effusion, which can develop slowly, may cause few or no symptoms. A small and rapidly forming effusion may lead to cardiac tamponade.

   b) Right ventricular pressure waveforms are unchanged during tamponade but show a dip and a prominent Y descent in constrictive pericarditis.

   c) Severity of the condition is determined by the degree of tachycardia, hypotension, and filling pressures.

2. **Anesthetic considerations**

   a) Primary goals are to avoid decreases in myocardial contractility, peripheral vascular resistance, and heart rate.

   b) Pericardiocentesis in patients with tamponade may be advisable before induction.

   c) Induction agents include etomidate and ketamine. A dopamine infusion during induction and the preparation phase is helpful.

d) Transesophageal and transvenous pacing modalities should be readily available.

e) In severely compromised patients, an awake intubation and having the patient prepped and draped prior to induction is advisable.

D. Cardiopulmonary Bypass (CPB)

1. In order to proceed with all but the least invasive procedures involving surgery on the heart, an extracorporeal circuit (ECC) must be used. The ECC is also called the "heart-lung machine," named for the cardiovascular function it must support during open-heart surgery.

2. The primary goals of the ECC are vascular transport, oxygenation, physiologic homeostasis, hemodynamic control, thermoregulation, and organ system preservation.

3. The ECC consists of an oxygenator (membrane or bubble), venous reservoir, cardiotomy reservoir, circuit tubing, filters (arterial, prebypass, cardiotomy), tubing connectors, and cannulas (arterial, venous, and cardioplegic).

4. *Prime*

   a) Prior to bypass, the circuit is filled with fluid to eliminate air and to coat the surface of the membrane oxygenator, filters, and system tubing with the constituents of the prime solution. Establishment of an air-free circuit is essential for unimpaired fluid volume transport and prevention of air embolism.

   b) Most circuits require at least 2000 mL of a solution such as Normosol, Plasmalyte A, or Isolyte S with pH and electrolytes closely matching the composition of whole blood. Added to this base are heparin, sodium bicarbonate, mannitol, hetastarch, albumin, and possibly corticosteroids or antihyperfibrinolytic agents. The result is priming volumes in excess of 2000 mL, which when transfused to the patient at the onset of cardiopulmonary bypass, can equate to a hemodilutional bolus of 30% to 50% of the patient's circulating blood volume.

5. Safety mechanisms function to alert the operator to low venous operating reserve, high arterial pressures, disconnection from air supply, and introduction of air embolus into the arterial line.

6. A cardioplegia delivery system provides and maintains hypothermic and pharmacologic arrest of the heart during revascularization.

7. Ultrafiltration and red blood cell–sequestering devices may be incorporated into the circuit to counteract hemodilution by removing excess volume through dialysis or centrifugal separation of fluid and plasma components from the circulating blood volume.

8. Cardiac output is controlled by a pump delivery system (centrifugal or rollerhead) that maintains patient blood flow and perfusion pressure in accordance with physiologic state and requirements.

9. For control of pulmonary function, an oxygenator and blender are used to maintain appropriate oxygen saturation levels and respiratory acid-base homeostasis.
10. Core thermal regulation is maintained by a heater/cooler system that propels fluid housed separately in a compartment parallel to the blood pathway.
11. *Vascular transport*
    a) Vascular access at sites on the right side of the heart (atrial/venous) and the left side of the heart (aortic/arterial) are necessary for the shunting of deoxygenated blood away from the patient, to the heart-lung machine, and back to the aorta as propelled arterialized blood.
    b) Isolation of the heart and lungs from systemic blood flow is accomplished by right atrial or vena caval cannulation with subsequent diversion of venous blood returning to the heart into a venous reservoir situated at a level below the patient's heart to facilitate gravity exsanguination.
    c) Blood from the reservoir is propelled to the oxygenator, where it becomes arterialized. A heat exchanger mounted on the oxygenator provides for thermal control of blood temperature.
    d) Oxygenated blood passes through an arterial filter and an arterial gas monitoring device.
    e) Aortic cannula placement is distal to the sinus of Valsalva and proximal to the brachiocephalic artery.
    f) Cardiac index and mean arterial pressure are maintained according to metabolic requirements and surgical demand.
12. *Myocardial protection techniques*
    a) Rapid cardioplegia-induced cardiac arrest, decompression of the ventricles, and hypothermia are the underlying concerns for myocardial protection during cardiopulmonary bypass.
    b) The severity of preexisting ischemia determines the magnitude of injury associated with reperfusion. The duration of aortic cross-clamping time, collateral coronary blood supply, frequency of cardioplegia delivery, and composition of cardioplegia are factors influencing the extent of reperfusion injury.
    c) Intermittent doses of cold crystalloid cardioplegia help maintain cardiac arrest, hypothermia, and pH; counteract edema; wash out metabolites; and provide oxygen substrate for aerobic metabolism.
       (1) Maintenance doses are delivered in an antegrade fashion through the aortic root at intervals corresponding to completion of individual distal graft anastomosis.
       (2) Retrograde delivery of cardioplegia through the coronary sinus in the right atrium may be used in the presence of severe cardiovascular disease, emergent revascularization due to recent or ongoing MI, or high-grade stenosis, in which antegrade delivery may prove ineffective in protecting myocardium distal to the lesion.

PART 2 Common Procedures

E. Cardiac Surgery Plan of Care

1. **Patient assessment**
   a) *Cardiac evaluation*
      (1) Hypertension, heart disease (CAD, angina, MI, congestive heart failure [CHF], smoking, chronic obstructive pulmonary disease [COPD], carotid artery stenosis, transient ischemic attack/cardiovascular accident) diabetes, renal disease, age greater than 70 years, male sex
      (2) Electrocardiogram (ECG), previous history of MI, angina, causes, symptoms, treatment, number of laboratory tests performed (abnormalities always indicate increased perioperative risks)
      (3) Cardiac catheterization report:
         (*a*) Degree of vessel occlusion; presence of collaterals
         (*b*) Chamber pressures; pulmonary artery (PA) pressures
         (*c*) Ventricular function:

Good LV Function:	**Poor LV Function:**
1. History	1. History
a. Angina	a. Multiple MI
b. Hypertension/obesity	b. Symptoms of CHF
c. No sx CHF	2. Cardiac Cath
2. Cardiac Cath	a. EF < 40%
a. EF > 50%	b. LVEDP > 18 mm Hg
b. LVEDP < 12 mm Hg	c. Multiple areas of dyskinesia
c. Normal CO	d. Decreased CO

      (4) Chest radiography (heart size, pulmonary vascular flow), exercise tolerance tests, dysrhythmias, ischemic threshold, location of ischemia, ventricular dysfunction), induced ischemia, arrhythmias, and hemodynamic changes (ambulatory)
      (5) ECG (Holter 12 to 48 hours, with symptoms diary; dysrhythmias, ST depression)
      (6) Echocardiography (EF, valvular function, congenital defects, segmental wall motion)
      (7) Pharmacologic stress perfusion imaging (dipyridamole thallium scan). A vasodilator (dipyridamole) is administered to cause maximal dilation of coronary arteries. Vessels with fixed stenoses will not dilate, allowing less perfusion agent to reach the myocardium.
      (8) Dobutamine echocardiography. Abnormally contracting muscle segments seen on resting echocardiography are classified as ischemic or infarcted; good for patients on theophylline or caffeine or with COPD.
   b) *Pulmonary evaluation*
      (1) Asthma, emphysema, smoking history (to decrease

carboxyhemoglobin and nicotine tachycardia, quit at least 2 days prior)

(2) Pulmonary function tests with increased operative risk:
  (a) Forced vital capacity (FVC) less than 50% predicted.
  (b) Forced expiratory volume in 1 second (FEV_1) less than 2.0 L.
  (c) FEV_1/FVC less than 50%.
  (d) $PaCO_2$ less than 45 mm Hg on room air.

(3) Assess lung sounds; relieve bronchospasm with B_2 adrenergic agents (terbutaline sulfate, albuterol), phosphodiesterase inhibitors (aminophylline), parasympatholytics (atropine), steroids, and mast cell stabilizers (cromolyn sodium).

(4) Chest radiography

c) *Neurologic evaluation:* Carotid stenosis, TIA/CVA

d) *Renal evaluation:* Chronic end-stage renal diagnosis

e) *Laboratory tests:* Arterial blood gases, electrolytes, complete blood count, platelet count, coagulation tests, activated clotting time (ACT), type and crossmatch with blood available (2 units packed red blood cells [PRBCs] in room for redos)

f) *Medications:* Aspirin, digoxin, β-blockers

2. **Room preparation**

Monitors—5-lead ECG, arterial line/central venous pressure/PA transducers, CO setup, zero all lines

Two units of PRBCs in room and ensure availability of platelets for redos

Oxygen tank and ambu bag for transport to the surgical intensive care unit (SICU)

Transesophageal electrocardiography (TEE) in room for valves (TEE two-dimentional echo permits on-line evaluation of regional wall motion and global ventricular function)

Cordis kit and Swan-Ganz catheter with VIP port; lidocaine, 10 mg/mL; arterial line setup and 10 mL flush; intravenous materials, sterile gloves, and gown

Drips
  Nitroglycerin
  Sodium nitroprusside
  Neo-Synephrine
  Epinephrine
  Dobutamine
  Dopamine
  Levophed
  Milrinone/Amrinone

3. **Patient Preparation**

a) Assess airway, heart, and lung sounds. Review history.

b) Check laboratory values: Note K^+, RBS, H/H, blood urea nitorgen, creatinine.

c) Verify that blood is available. Keep 2 to 4 units in the operating room for redos.

d) Assess sedation needs and apply oxygen via nasal cannula.
  (1) Good LV function—heavy premedication

      (2) Poor LV function—light premedication

e) Place two large bore peripheral inravenous tubes.

f) Start arterial line. (If radial artery harvest planned, do not use that site; if LIMA planned, use right side).

g) Check allergies and give antibiotic as ordered.

h) Radial artery grafts: Cardizem and heparin are used preoperative.

      (1) Cardizem 0.1 mg/kg/hour to decrease spasm of artery with manipulation

      (2) Heparin at 1000 units/hour.

i) Redos: Aprotonin may be given preoperatively.

      (1) Test dose: 1 mL (1.4 mg); given preoperative; observe for anaphylaxis for 10 minutes.

      (2) Loading dose: 100 mL over 20 minutes. (140 mg); can't give until Swan is in.

      (3) Pump prime: 200 mL (280 mg); given by perfusionist.

      (4) Cont. infusion: 50 mL/hour (35 mg/hour); D/C at end of case.

      (5) Rationale: Used for repeat coronary bypass surgery or when transfusions are unavailable or unacceptable (Jehovah's Witnesses). During CPB, levels of plasminogen activator are markedly enhanced, and platelets are activated directly. Aprotinin is a proteinase inhibitor that inhibits the fibrinolytic activity while preserving platelet adhesion function; considered a antifibrinolytic agent; mechanism of action unknown.

      (6) Pharmacokinetics: Eliminated by the kidneys, half-life is 2 hours (reason for continuous infusion)

      (7) Adverse reactions:

         (*a*) Anaphylaxis (increased risk with repeat exposure)

         (*b*) Kidney dysfunction/failure

      (8) Drug interactions: Many (reason for central line with no other drips) ACT standard on bypass less than 400 seconds. ACT with aprotinin use less than 600 seconds.

      (9) Other considerations with Redos:

         (*a*) Have blood in the room at start of case in case of cutting through great vessels or old grafts with sternotomy.

         (*b*) Be ready for emergent on CPB (fem-fem bypass), heparin drawn up, rapid infuser and resuscitation. measures ready.

         (*c*) Will keep lungs up with sternotomy for redos.

4. Perioperative management

a) Induction

      (1) *Goal:* Minimal hemodynamic effects, reliable loss of consciousness, and sufficient depth of anesthesia to prevent vasopressor response to intubation.

      (2) Choice of drugs and speed of induction based on patients underlying LV function.

         (*a*) Poor LV function requires slow narcotic/relaxant technique.

(*b*) Good LV function permits narcotic/relaxant/pentothal induction with use of inhalation agent.

(3) 100% O_2 via mask; avoid using N_2O if possible.

(4) Muscle relaxant priming dose, 1 mL (helps decrease chest wall rigidity while the vagolytic effect of pancuronium bromide offsets the bradycardia of sufentanil citrate).

(5) Benzodiazepine: lorazepam, 2 to 4 mg; midazolam, 2 to 5 mg.

(6) Have nitroglycerin, Neo-Synephrine, and atropine ready.

(7) Lidocaine (1 to 1.5 mg/kg) to decrease SNS response to laryngoscopy.

(8) High dose narcotic technique: opioids alone are associated with minimal or no cardiac depression. Fentanyl vs. Sufentanil—conflicting data.

(*a*) Fentanyl:
Dose: 20 to 100 mcg/kg (usually 1 cc/kg)
Onset: 1 to 2 minutes.
DOA: 30 to 60 minutes.
Half-life: 3 to 4 hours
Better choice than sufentanil in very compromised patients.

(*b*) Sufentanil:
Dose: 5 to 20 mcg/kg
Onset: 1 to 3 minutes.
DOA: 20 to 45 minutes.
Half-life: 2.5 hr. (d/t smaller VD than fentanyl)
Special considerations with sufentanil: More profound analgesia than fentanyl. Suppresses catecholamine response 10 times greater than fentanyl (better for more robust person). Vagolytic effects greater than fentanyl, thus patients become bradycardic. Some sedative qualities and hypnosis (unlike fentanyl). Increased incidence of skeletal muscle rigidity.

(*c*) Sequence:
Usually give $^1/_{10}$ th MR dose before opioid administration because of chest wall rigidity r/t high dose opioid. Slowly administer opioid dose until consciousness is lost. Treat hypotension with IV fluid and then small doses of phenylephrine 25 to 50 mcg intravenously.

(*d*) Treat bradycardia with atropine 0.2 to 0.4 mg intravenously.

(*e*) If patient remains conscious after full opioid dose, give benzodiazepine (BZD).

(9) Muscle relaxant:

(*a*) Avoid those that cause release of histamine (Atracurium, DTC, Mivacron)

(*b*) Best choices: Zemuron, Norcuron, Pavulon.

(*c*) Norcuron may precipitate severe bradycardia when combined with high dose opioid.

(10) Aortic and mitral valve stenosis anesthesia goals: avoid SVR and tachycardia (keep heart rate at 60 bpm).

PART 2 Common Procedures

(11) Aortic and mitral valve regurgitation anesthesia goals: avoid SVR and bradycardia (keep heart rate at 90 bpm).

(12) While waiting for full muscle relaxation, the sapphenous veins may be drained by elevation of the legs, and the Foley catheter with thermistor may be inserted.

(13) Laryngoscopy, intubation—note patient response; confirm endotracheal tube placement.

(14) Check and pad pressure points (ulnar nerve, radial nerves, occiput, and heels).

    (*a*) Ischemia secondary to compression and compounded by decreases in temperature and perfusion pressure on CPB may cause peripheral neuropathy or damage to soft tissues.

    (*b*) Brachial plexus injury can occur if arms are hyperextended or if chest retraction is excessive.

    (*c*) Ulnar nerve injury can occur from compression of the olecranon against the metal edge of the OR table. Provide adequate padding under olecranon.

    (*d*) Radial nerve injury can occur from compression of the upper arm against the ether screen or the support post of the retractor used in internal mammary dissection. Provide adequate padding of arm.

    (*e*) Finger injury can occur secondary to pressure from members of the OR team leaning against the table. Position with hands next to body in neutral position and away from edge of table.

    (*f*) Occipital alopecia can occur 3 weeks after the operation secondary to ischemia of the scalp. Provide adequate padding of the head, reposition head frequently during procedure.

    (*g*) Heel of foot ischemia and tissue necrosis can occur. Heels should be well padded.

(15) *Postinduction:* ether screen, TEE if valve, obtain postinduction CO, draw labs (arterial blood gases, ACT, K^+, RBS, hematcrit), and give antibiotics.

5. **Prebypass**

    a) High levels of patient stimulation occur at the following times: (a) induction/intubation, (b) incision, (c) sternal split and spread (d) sympathetic nerve dissection, and (e) cardiotomy. Maintain adequate levels of anesthesia to avoid increasing catecholamine levels (treat with additional narcotic as necessary), which can precipitate hypertension, ischemia, and heart failure. Treat hypertension with nitroglycerin or sodium nitroprusside.

    b) Low levels of stimulation occur preincision and during mammary dissection and CPB cannulation. Deep levels of anesthesia may cause hypotension, bradycardia, and ischemia.

    c) Skin incision: Supplement narcotic as needed to avoid tachycardia and breakthrough hypertension.

    d) Sternotomy: Supplement narcotic as needed and keep paralyzed. Lungs must be deflated during sternal sawing by disconnecting exhalation limb and providing adequate muscle relaxation (redos need not drop lungs, decrease tidal volume, and increase respiratory rate because a different saw is used and is a slower process). Confirm equal inflation of lungs after the chest is open. This is the most common period for awareness and recall. (Redo hearts must have aminocaproic acid infusing, and 2 units PRBCs checked and ready in room because vein grafts, right atrium, right ventricle, or greater vessels may be cut or torn. The femoral vein should be identified and prepped by the team).

e) Harvesting the left internal mammary artery/right internal mammary artery and/or saphenous vein: Decrease tidal volume and increase respiratory rate while the surgeon is dissecting the mammary artery. The chest is retracted to one side, with the table up and rotated away from surgeon. Keep the BP up to prevent vasospasm, which leads to ischemia. The surgeon sprays nitroglycerin or sodium nitropnsside over the vessel to prevent vasospasm (watch for a decreasing BP and maintain normotensive state).

f) Pericardiotomy: Ensure adequate anesthetic depth. Observe wall motion and myocardial contractility. A pericardial sling is made prior to heparinization and cannulation. This provides a dam for the cardioplegia solution and iced normal saline slush. The sling can also serve to lift the heart. After the pericardium is opened, the postganglionic sympathetic nerves are dissected from the aorta to allow insertion of aortic cannula. This is a period of high-level stimulation because of sympathetic discharge with nerve manipulation. Attenuate with β-blockers and vasodilators.

g) Heparinization: Activate antithrombin III (stops blood clotting during CPB)

   (1) Onset: immediate; duration; metabolism by heparinases in liver.

   (2) Aspirate back on central line to ensure venous access.

   (3) Dose: 3 mg/kg (300 units/kg), or body surface area × 100 mg (10,000 units/kg [1 mg = 100 units]).

   (4) Give prior to aortic cannulation. Surgeon can also administer heparin directly into the heart. (Decreases viscosity; watch for decreased BP and reflex increase in heart rate.)

   (5) Check ACT 3 minutes after heparin given. Must be greater than 400 seconds prior to initiation of CPB (normal ACT, 70 to 110 seconds). Keep surgeon aware of all ACTs.

   (6) If ACT is not adequate, then one-third of original dose should be given (if necessary, up to 3 times until original dose is doubled). Check ACT every 5 minutes until greater than 400 seconds. If a double dose is given and ACT is still low, consider heparin resistance or low antithrombin III. Replace antithrombin III with fresh frozen plasma.

h) Aortic cannulation: Done first to provide access for rapid infusion if urgently required. Keep systolic BP at 100 mm Hg to avoid blood spray or aortic dissection. The cannula is placed in the ascending aorta proximal to the innominate artery and distal to the sites of saphenous vein graft, if used. Pay attention to perfusionist and surgeon communication about cannula pressure readings. Complications include entering innominate, carotid, or subclavian arteries, embolism, dysrhythmias, aortic dissection.

i) Venous cannulation: Placed in right atrium (through the appendage). Can result in hypotension due to volume depletion or mechanical compression, especially if the inferior vena cava is cannulated. Dysrhythmias, mainly atrial, can occur due to surgical manipulation. Purse string sutures are used to keep the cannulas in place and to close the incision after the cannulas are removed. Bypass can be started immediately if the patient is hemodynamically unstable.

j) Left ventricular vent: Even though venous return is bypassed from the right ventricle, 2% to 5% of the C.O. is drained into the LV from bronchial, thebesian, and pleural veins. A LV sump prevents overdistention of the LV, which may cause postpump failure.

6. **Cardiopulmonary bypass**

Cardiopulmonary bypass (CPB) sustains systemic blood flow, oxygenation, and ventilation during periods when the heart and lungs are arrested.

a) Ensure an adequate level of muscle relaxation and amnesia. The surgeon notifies the perfusionist to go on bypass (record time and maintain MAP at 50 to 70 mm Hg to maintain coronary perfusion before cross-clamping; treat with Neo-Synephrine).

b) When pulmonary blood flow ceases, stop ventilation; disconnect exhalation limb of circuit to deflate lung (increases surgeon visibility); and turn off vent, gas analyzer, and pulse oximeter. Continue O_2 flow at 2 L/min.

c) Hypotension is associated with CPB due to the 2 L of prime solution, which causes hemodilution, decreases blood viscosity, dilutes circulating catecholamines and contains no O_2; thus, hypoxic vasodilation occurs.

d) Patient assessment: 30 to 60 seconds after initiation of CPB.
    (1) Check pupils. Examine conjuctiva for chemosis and reassess pupils size and for unilateral dilation, which may indicate arterial inflow into innominate artery (unilateral carotid perfusion).
    (2) Examine face for color, symmetry, temperature, and edema.
    (3) Check carotid pulses, which should feel like trills because of nonpulsatile flow.
    (4) Examine heart for distention and contractility.
    (5) Examine pump lines for arteriovenous color differences.

e) Hypothermia

(1) Patient is cooled to 28° to 32° C, which decreases the O_2 demands of tissues and allows for lower CPB flows. Shifts autoregulation to left to 25 to 125 mm Hg. Each 1° C decrease in temperature leads to an 8% decrease in metabolic rate. A 10° C decrease in temperature leads to a decrease in metabolism by $1/2$. CO_2 and O_2 are more soluble; thus expect lower $PaCO_2$ on arterial blood gas testing.

(2) Iced saline around heart cools it to 8° to 15° C.

(3) Watch for ventricular fibrillation, which causes increased utilization of O_2 and requires immediate cardioplegia to arrest heart.

f) Cardioplegia

The goal is to obtain a motionless heart and a clean, dry, operative field.

(1) The aorta is cross-clamped. (Record time of CPB on/off and cross-clamp on/off.) Pay attention to perfusionist and surgeon communication in regard to "flow up/flow down" accompanying clamping/ unclamping. The effects of aortic cross-clamping are as follows:

   (a) Cessation of coronary perfusion—this stops the blood from the coronary sinus from flooding the operative field.

   (b) If the aortic valve is incompetent, this prevents blood from regurgitating through the valve and flooding the field.

   (c) As the heart becomes hypoxic, it relaxes and can be manipulated more easily.

   (d) If there is any question of air entering the beating heart, the clamp will prevent air from reaching the brain.

(2) *Cardioplegia* is the application of a cold solution (4° C) high in K^+ (20 to 40 mEq) that produces electromechanical quiescence. Arrests the heart in diastole and produces energy conservation. (If arrested in systole, as seen with calcium, tetany results).

   (a) This solution causes the myocardial cells to depolarize; contraction occurs, calcium goes into the cells, the myocardium relaxes, but membrane repolarization is prevented.

   (b) Four parts blood for one part of cardioplegic solution. Components of the cardioplegia solution may include K^+, Na^+, Ca^{2+}, Mg^{2+}, mannitol, and/or albumin, nitroglycerin (coronary dilator), HCO_3 (buffer), calcium channel blockers, propranolol HCl, glucose (cellular energy), hemoglobin (oxygen-carrying), and lidocaine or procaine (membrane stabilization).

PART 2 **Common Procedures**

(c) Repeat application of solution every 20 to 30 minutes, or if heart temperature is greater than 18° C to maintain hypothermia, prevent lactic acid accumulation, and deliver some minimal available O_2.

g) Keep MAP between 30 and 60 mm Hg. Patients with carotid stenosis may require higher pressures. CPP equals MAP. LVEDP = 0. PA pressures should be less than 15 mm Hg; central venous pressure less than 5 mm Hg.

h) K^+ can cause systemic hyperkalemia. Treat with 10 units of regular insulin intravenously, 50 g of glucose, hyperventilation, HCO_3, calcium, and furosemide.

i) Ventricular fibrillation usually occurs twice during CPB: during cooling and during warming. Inform the surgeon.

j) Urine output should be maintained above 1 mL/kg (notify the surgeon if it is less). Large outputs of 300 to 1000 mL/hour can be seen if mannitol is used in the priming solution. Low urine outputs can be attributed to absent pulsatile flow, hypothermia, and decreased renal blood flow; increased catecholamines cause release of ADH. Treat low urine outputs with mannitol, furosemide, adequate perfusion, and renal dose dopamine.

k) Hemodynamics during CPB

(1) Maintain MAP between 30 and 70 mm Hg with a venous saturation greater than 60%. If cerebral circulation is impaired, keep MAP at 60 mm Hg. Low MAP causes decreased peripheral perfusion. High MAP damages blood components, increases the blood in the operative field, and increases warmed the blood to the heart. Treat low SVR with Neo-Synephrine and high SVR with nitroglycerin or sodium nitroprusside.

(2) Reasons for decreased venous saturation— increased O_2 consumption with light anesthesia, low CPB flows, decreased O_2 delivery from oxygenator, or decreased O_2 carrying capacity of hemoglobin secondary to hemodilution.

l) Physiologic response to CPB

(1) Platelets—clumping and degranulation occur after contact with nonendothelial surfaces. Leads to reduction in numbers, inhibits adhesiveness and aggregation.

(2) Proteins—denaturation of oncotic and carrier proteins (albumin, lipoproteins, and γ-globulin). Leads to increased viscosity, clumping of red blood cells, and fat embolism. Amplification of "humoral system" proteins. Factor XII stimulation of coagulation and fibrinolytic cascade. Complement system activation releases kallikrein and bradykinin; generalized inflammatory response that increases capillary permeability. Altered enzymatic function.

(3) Blood—red blood cells become stiffer and less distensible, which leads to lysis and hemoglobinuria, which leads to impaired renal tubular function. Leukocyte damage and activation leads to degranulation. Complement activation causes pulmonary sequestration of neutrophils leading to inflammatory response and lung injury.

(4) Endocrine—elevated epinephrine levels during hypothermia cause peripheral vasoconstriction and impair release of insulin (hyperglycemia and release of free fatty acids). Norepinephrine levels rise early during CPB in patients, leading to postoperative hypertension. Renin and aldosterone levels are increased, promoting sodium retention and potassium excretion. Increased vasopressin produces increased sodium and water diuresis. Angiotensin elevation leads to asoconstriction.

(5) Hemodilution reduces requirements for homologous blood transfusion. Reduces blood viscosity and improves tissue perfusion. Counteracts negative effects of hypothermia on tissue perfusion (vasoconstriction and impaired O_2 release from hemoglobin). Dilutes coagulation factors and platelets, contributing to coagulopathy. May increase interstitial edema.

(6) Hypothermia reduces tissue metabolism and O_2 consumption. Improves myocardial protection. Provides end-organ (brain, kidney) protection in case of low-flow negative effects. Decreases intraoperative awareness. Increases SVR. Shifts the oxyhemoglobin curve to the left, impairing tissue O_2 release. This effect is offset by increased O_2 solubility at lower temperatures and lower metabolic demand. Contributes to decreased platelets and platelet function.

(7) Renal—renin-angiotensin-aldosterone system alterations promote increased renal vascular resistance and sodium and water retention and lead to decreased renal blood flow, glomerular filtration rate, and tubular function. Hemodilution protects kidneys by increasing cortical plasma flow. Hemaglobinuria may result from long bypass runs (greater than 4 per hour).

(8) Liver/intestines—jaundice may occur in up to 23% of patients following CPB. Mucosal ischemia may occur due to splanchnic vasoconstriction induced by elevated angiotensin, as well as to microembolism of platelets and leukocytes.

(9) Changes in cerebral autoregulation from 50 to 100 mm Hg to lower values. Embolic phenomena from fat, thrombi, platelets, foreign substances, and air embolism. Important to keep blood glucose levels between 100 and 200 mg/dL to prevent cerebral ischemic episodes.

(10) Pulmonary—lungs inactivate catecholamines under normal circumstances. This lack of degradation during CPB may contribute to increased catecholamines seen during CPB. May contribute to high PVR. The lungs have a high affinity for narcotics, especially fentanyl. May see decreased pulmonary blood flow after CPB due to embolism (ventilation-perfusion mismatch and edema), as well as localized vasoconstriction due to elevated catecholamines.

m) Potential bypass catastrophes
   (1) Aortic dissection (cannula placed within arterial wall cannulation): Cannula should always be transduced; ensure that the pulsation correlates with arterial line. Treatment is repositioning of aortic cannula by surgeon.
   (2) Carotid or innominate artery hyperperfusion; reposition catheter.
   (3) Stone heart.
   (4) Reversed cannulation: Blood is drained from the aorta, causing hypotension, and is infused into the vena cava at high pressures. Execute gas embolism protocol.
   (5) Massive gas embolism (from oxygenator reservoir vortexing or clotting, opened beating heart, or leak or kink in lines): Vigilance is the prevention. Treatment includes the following:
      a) Stop CPB and place the patient in Trendelenburg's position.
      b) Remove the aortic cannula, vent air for cannulation site, and institute retrograde SVC perfusion for 2 to 4 minutes.
      c) Perform carotid compression to allow purging of air from vertebral bodies.
      d) When no additional air can be expelled, resume anterograde CPB, maintaining hypothermia for 40 to 50 minutes. (Lower temperatures increase gas solubility and help reabsorption of gas bubbles.)
      e) Express coronary air by massaging and needle aspiration. Induce hypertension because hydrostatic pressure shrinks bubbles and "pushes" them through the vessels.
      f) Administer steroids and wean from CPB. Ventilate patient with 100% O_2 for at least 6 hours to maximize the blood-alveolar gradient for elimination of N_2. Hyperbaric chambers may accelerate reabsorption of residual bubbles.

7. **Rewarming**
   a) Rewarming is sensed as hyperthermia by the hypothalamus. Awareness is possible. Supplemental doses of pancuronium, lorazepam, and sufentanil may be required. Watch for the return of electrical activity of the heart (treat ventricular fibrillation

with lidocaine and defibrillation). Consider lidocaine drip if
ventricular fibrillation is refractory.

b)   Check TRIPLE

(1)   T = temperature (Increase operating room temperature.
Patient is rewarmed to core temperature of 37° C 20 minutes prior to termination of CPB. When temperature rises
close to 32° C, the SVR and MAP may decrease [treat with
Neo-Synephrine]. Rewarming accelerates metabolism of
drugs given.)

(2)   R = rate and rhythm (For adequate cardiac output,
patient requires sinus rhythm with a heart rate of
70 to 100 bpm. Use pacer, atropine, or cardioversion,
if needed.)

(3)   I = inhalation (FiO_2 equals 100%. Reexpand lungs with
2 to 4 breaths at 30 to 40 cm H_2O to resolve atelectasis.
Observe field to ensure that you are not affecting grafts.
Resume mechanical ventilation.)

(4)   P = pressure (Support as needed. High BP places stress on
new grafts; low BP can cause ischemia.)

(5)   L = laboratory test results (Check test results: prothrombin
time, partial thromboplastin time, ACT, fibrinogen,
Sonoclot, arterial blood gases, hematocrit, electrolytes,
glucose. If K^+ is trending less than 4.0 mEq at separation,
supplement.)

(6)   E = everything else (Level table, zero all lines.)

c)   Unclamping of aorta: Observe the heart for volume, rate, and
contractility. The perfusionist may give/take 50 to 100 mL
increments of blood. Monitor filling pressures, distention,
or hypotension as indicators that the heart cannot handle the
volume. Consider treatment with calcium chloride, epinephrine,
or dobutamine for support.

8.   **Discontinuing CPB**

a)   Flow is decreased by 50%; the heart is visually inspected for distention of chambers and wall motion abnormalities. Observe
ECG for dysrhythmias. Most patients fall into one of four
groups when coming off bypass:

b)   Ensure adequate hemodynamic parameters; use inotropes and
pressors as needed. Pulmonary capillary wedge pressure is a
poor indicator of left atrial function after CPB.

c)   Venous line is removed first.

d)   Protamine is administered, 1 mg per 1 mg of heparin.
Calcium chloride, 500 to 1000 mg, is mixed with protamine to
counteract depressed contractility, decreased pH, decreased
Ca^{2+} levels. (Extreme Caution: May lead to stone heart in
digitalized patient.)

(1)   Protamine is a base that combines with acidic heparin
to form a stable salt and inactivates the anticoagulant
effect.

(2)   Administered slowly, over 5 to 10 minutes, into a
peripheral venous site. Notify the surgeon when

	Group I Vigorous	Group II Hypo- volemic	Group III Pump Failure	Group IV Hyper- dynamic
Filling pressure	Low	Low	Normal or high	Low
Blood pressure	Normal	Low	Low or normal	Low
Cardiac Output	Normal	Low	Low	High
Systemic Vascular Resistance	Normal	High	High	Low
Treatment	None	Volume	Inotrope, afterload reduction, IABP	Vasoconstrictor

one-half is administered so that pump suckers can be turned off to prevent coagulation in the pump. Observe for hypotension and increased pulmonary artery pressure (PAP).

(3) Reactions can include histamine release, anaphylactic/ anaphylactoid reactions (IgE-mediated venodilation, decreased cardiac filling, and decreased SVR), and pulmonary vasoconstriction (increased airway pressures). Increased risk of allergic reactions in patients allergic to fish, in patients who have been treated with protamine-containing insulin, or in the presence of antiprotamine antibodies in serum of infertile or vasectomized men. Treat reaction with diphenhydramine and/or epinephrine, 0.1 to 0.3 mg.

e) Check hemoglobin, hematocrit, K^+, ACT, and arterial blood gases. Begin infusing cardiotomy blood because patient will require volume. ACT goal is to return to preoperative level. Hematocrit of 25% or less may be acceptable without transfusion. Patient will slowly hemoconcentrate.

f) Aortic line is removed, chest tubes are inserted, hemostasis is obtained, and incision is closed. Chest closure causes a transient increase in intramediastinal pressure, which may depress systemic venous return.

g) Check cardiac output when sternal wires closed and patient is stabilized.

h) Transport to SICU when hemodynamically stable. Lifepak, ambu bag with O_2 tank, Omni-Flow, and tabletop drugs. Ventilation settings: respiratory rate, 8 to 12 bpm (for $PaCO_2$ of 35 to 45 mm Hg); FiO_2, 100%; tidal volumes, 10 mL/kg; PEEP, 5 cm H_2O.

9. **Postoperative Complications**
   a) Hypokalemia
   b) MI and acute graft closure
   c) Ischemia
   d) Tamponade

  e) Hemorrhage

  f) Prosthetic valve failure

10. **"Mini" CABG procedures**

  a) Refers to those CABG procedures done off bypass with a hemisternotomy.

  b) Prepare the heart for ischemia by reducing myocardial oxygen demand with β-blockers and calcium channel blockers while increasing oxygen supply with nitroglycerin infusion.

  c) Coronary anastamosis is facilitated by inducing bradycardia with adenosine, β-blockers, and calcium channel blockers.

   (1) Usually these patients have healthier hearts and can tolerate the slow heart rate.

   (2) Adenosine will induce a sinus pause lasting 10 to 20 seconds and will decrease BP.

   (3) Pacing wires should be in place.

  d) Postanastomosis—discontinue β-blockers, continue nitroglycerin, continue calcium channel blockers to decrease vasospasm, and vigorously treat LV dysfunction and/or arrhythmias.

  e) Heparin dose requirements are half of that required for traditional CABG (150 units/kg); No Amicar is given.

  f) Less narcotic and benzodiazepine required.

  g) Left radial arterial line; right arterial system will be used for angiography.

F. Supplemental Information

1. **Hemodynamic variables: calculations and normal values**

Variable	Calculation	Normal Values
Cardiac index (CI)	CO/BSA	2.5 to 4.0 l/min/m^2
Stroke volume (SV)	CO/HR	60 to 90 mL/beat
Stroke index (SI)	SV/BSA	40 to 60 mL/beat/m^2
Mean arterial pressure (MAP)	$2(DPB) + SBP/3$	80 to 120 mm Hg
Systemic vascular resistance(SVR)	$MAP - CVP/CO \times 80$	1,200 to 1,500 dynes/cm/sec^{-5}
Pulmonary vascular resistance (PVR)	$PAP - PWP/CO \times 80$	100 to 300 dynes/cm/sec^{-5}
Ejection fraction (EF)	SV/EDV	65%
Cardiac output (CO)	$SV \times HR$	5 to 6 L/min

2. **Commonly used drugs**

Agent	Dosage	Onset	Duration	Action
Nitroprusside	0.5 to 10 mcg/kg/min	30 to 60 sec	1 to 5 min	Direct arterial and venous vascular smooth muscle relaxation
Nitroglycerin	5 to 100 mcg/min	1 min	3 to 5 min	Direct venous dilation
Esmolol	0.5 mg/kg over 1 min	1 min	12 to 20 min	Direct β_1 antagonist
Labetalol	2.5 to 20 mg	1 to 2 min	4 to 8 hr	Direct α_1, β_1, and β_2 antagonist
Propranolol	0.2 to 3 mg	1 to 2 min	4 to 8 hr	Direct β_1 antagonist
Hydralazine	2.5 to 20 mg	5 to 20 min	4 to 8 hr	Direct vascular smooth muscle relaxation
Nifedipine	10 mg	5 to 10 min	4 hr	Direct vascular smooth muscle relaxation
Epinephrine	1 to 4 mcg/min	30 to 60 sec	1 to 5 min	Direct α_1, α_2, β_1, and β_2 agonist
Ephedrine	2.5 to 10 mg	30 to 60 sec	1 to 5 min	Mixed α_1, α_2, β_1, and β_2 agonist
Aminocaproic acid	10 g loading; 1 g/hr	30 to 60 sec	3 to 5 hr	Coagulant
Protamine	1 mg per mg heparin	30 to 60 sec	2 hr	Heparin antagonist
Phenylephrine	10 to 200 mcg/min	30 to 60 sec	15 to 30 min	Pure α
Norepinephrine	2 to 20 mcg/min	30 to 60 sec	10 min	α_2, β_2

VII

Vascular Surgery

A. Abdominal Aortic Aneurysm

1. **Introduction**
   Abdominal aortic surgery may be required for atherosclerotic occlusive disease or aneurysmal dilation. These processes can involve the aorta and any of its major branches, leading to ischemia or rupture and exsanguination. Elective surgery is indicated when the aneurysm diameter is greater than 5 cm; each centimeter greater than 5 increases the chances of rupture.

   Surgical repair involves proximal and distal clamping of the aorta, opening of the aneurysm, evacuation of the thrombus, and placement of a synthetic graft. A midline transabdominal surgical approach or retroperitoneal left thoracoabdominal approach may be used.

   The aorta is the main artery from the left ventricle of the heart. It supplies oxygenated blood to all tissues and organs of the body except the alveoli of the lung. The aorta is subdivided into the ascending aorta, the aortic arch, and the descending aorta, which has thoracic and abdominal portions. The abdominal aorta is the second portion of the descending aorta. It descends through the aortic hiatus of the diaphragm, enters the abdominal pelvic cavity, and travels down the ventral surface of the vertebral column. The abdominal aorta terminates at the fourth lumbar vertebra by dividing into the right and left common iliac arteries.

2. **Preoperative assessment**
   a) *History and physical examination*
      (1) *Respiratory:* Assess for pulmonary disease—chronic obstructive pulmonary disease, chronic bronchitis, asthma, and emphysema.
      (2) *Cardiac:* Evaluate for coronary artery disease, angina, hypertension, dysrhythmias, congestive heart failure, and left ventricular dysfunction.
      (3) *Renal:* Assess baseline status because the kidneys may be affected with cross-clamping.
      (4) *Neurologic*
         (a) Spinal cord ischemia may occur with repair of the distal descending thoracic aorta.
         (b) Assess for transient ischemic attacks, strokes, and carotid bruits.
      (5) *Endocrine:* This patient population is prone to diabetes mellitus.
      (6) *Other:* Back or flank pain may indicate expanding or leaking abdominal aortic aneurysm.

   b) *Diagnostic tests*
- (1) Chest radiography
- (2) Echocardiogram with ejection fraction
- (3) 12-lead electrocardiogram
- (4) Pulmonary function test with abnormal pulmonary histories
- (5) Angiograms—estimate the difficulty of the procedure and relationship of cross-clamping to the renal arteries
- (6) *Laboratory tests:* Complete blood count, electrolytes, glucose, blood urea nitrogen, creatinine, urinalysis, coagulation profile, type and crossmatch, and others as indicated

   c) *Perioperative medications and intravenous therapy*
- (1) Antihypertensives—usually need 24 to 48 hours prior to surgery.
- (2) Antianginals—nitrates, calcium channel blockers, and β-blockers; continue until the day of the procedure.
- (3) Digoxin
  - (*a*) Assess serum level prior to procedure.
  - (*b*) Hypokalemia following intraoperative diuresis will increase the likelihood of digoxin toxicity.
- (4) Antiarrhythmics—continue until day of surgery.
- (5) Anticoagulants—warfarin should be substituted with heparin preoperatively, allowing the patient's level to normalize. Plan to hold heparin 4 hours prior to surgery.
- (6) Bronchodilators—continue until surgery.
- (7) Antibiotics
- (8) Epidural catheter (for postoperative pain management)—perform test dose on the awake patient. There is a remote risk of epidural hematoma formation from anticoagulation during surgery.
- (9) Preoperative sedatives and narcotics
  - (*a*) Use with caution in patients with poor respiratory reserve.
  - (*b*) Onset of intravenous medications may be delayed because of low cardiac outputs.
- (10) Two peripheral, large bore (16- to 18-gauge) intravenous lines with variable fluid management

3. Room preparation
   a) *Monitoring equipment*
- (1) Pulmonary artery catheter monitors cardiac function and adequacy of fluid and blood replacement.
- (2) Arterial line
  - (*a*) Right radial artery or left radial artery if the aneurysm involves the innominate artery.
  - (*b*) Maintain mean arterial pressure close to 100 mm Hg in the upper body and greater than 50 mm Hg distal to the aneurysm.
- (3) Somatosensory-evoked potential or electroencephalogram evaluates central nervous system viability during aortic cross-clamping.

(4) Transesophageal echocardiography monitors left-ventricular function during cross-clamping.

(5) Foley catheter assesses global renal function.

(6) Warming modalities.

(7) Electrocardiogram leads V_5 and II—detects myocardial ischemia.

b) *Pharmacologic agents*

(1) Prepare infusions of nitroglycerin, nitroprusside, phenylephrine, and dopamine.

(2) Drugs: mannitol, furosemide, sodium bicarbonate, heparin, protamine, and calcium

(3) Volume

(*a*) Intravascular volume is depleted by hemorrhage, third-spacing into the bowel and peritoneal cavity, and insensible losses associated with a large abdominal incision.

(*b*) Greatest blood loss occurs when aneurysm is opened and the arteries are back-bleeding.

(4) Crystalloids—use if electrolytes, glucose, and osmolarity are within normal limits.

(5) Colloids

(*a*) Albumin, hetastarch (Hespan), blood

(*b*) Maintain hematocrit in 30% range for oxygen-carrying capacity

(6) Autotransfusion—blood is obtained from the operative field.

c) *Position:* Supine

4. **Anesthetic technique**

a) Regional blockade with general anesthesia or general anesthesia

b) Technique of choice is general anesthesia with endotracheal intubation because hemodynamic changes are significant.

c) *Regional blockade:* Epidural catheter placement and test dose preoperatively; analgesia to T4 to T5

d) With general anesthesia, an endotracheal tube is needed.

5. **Perioperative management**

a) *Induction*

(1) If the patient is hypotensive with a rupturing abdominal aortic aneurysm, perform an awake intubation or rapid sequence induction with ketamine and succinylcholine.

(2) A slow, "controlled" induction is preferred with an opioid and a nondepolarizing muscle relaxant.

(3) Omit thiopental and other cardiac depressors in the patient with poor left-ventricular function.

(4) Anticipate exaggerated blood pressure changes; maintain within 20% of baseline.

(5) Minimize pressor response during intubation of trachea by limiting duration of laryngoscopy to less than 15 seconds.

b) *Maintenance*

(1) O_2/air, opioid, and volatile anesthetic

(2) Cross-clamping of the thoracic aorta at the suprarenal or supraceliac level is not necessary for surgery.

c) *Emergence*

PART 2 **Common Procedures**

(1) Recommended that these patients should remain intubated and taken to an intensive care unit because there are major fluid shifts, probably increased blood loss, and stress from surgery.

(2) Unless the patient is stable, do not reverse muscle relaxants or try to awaken the patient.

(3) Consider initiating regional blockade through the epidural catheter for postoperative analgesia.

6. **Postoperative implications**

   a) Consider ventilatory support for several hours or overnight.

   b) Potential complications include myocardial ischemia/infarction, renal failure, peripheral vascular insufficiency, stroke, intestinal ischemia/infarction, paraplegia/monoparesis, fluid shifts, electrolyte imbalance, and coagulopathies.

7. **Aortic Stent Placement**

   a) Minimally invasive procedure for repairing abdominal aortic aneurysms. Uses a stent graft (a Dacron tube inside a collapsed metal-mesh cylinder) that is threaded through the arteries, using fluoroscopy, to the site of the aneurysm.

   b) *Preoperative assessment:* Is the same as open repair of abdominal aortic aneurysm.

   c) Procedure is performed under spinal or epidural anesthesia with intravenous sedation.

   d) Central line or pulmonary artery catheter placed if patient's history/condition warrants. Radial arterial and intravenous lines are placed in the right arm, which may be tucked at the patient's side. The left arm and both groins are used for surgical access.

   e) *Intraoperative medications:* Heparin will be given, and ACTs should be checked every half hour to maintain level. Mannitol infusion will be used. Infusions of nitroglycerin, phenylephrine, and dopamine should be prepared. Protamine will be used to reverse heparin at end of case.

   f) *Additional considerations:* Keep patient warm throughout procedure. Pulmonary Artery (PA) pressure usually becomes elevated with stent placement.

B. Peripheral Vascular Procedures

1. **Introduction**

   Peripheral vascular procedures include femoral-femoral, femoral-popliteal, femoral-tibial, illeofemoral, axillofemoral, and embolectomies. Obstruction most often is in the superficial femoral artery, followed by common iliac claudication in the gastrocnemius muscle, whereas pain and ischemic ulceration gangrene occur with severe occlusion.

Clamping Stage	Goals	Drug to Prepare
Preclamping	Maintain blood pressure 20% baseline (low normal)	Volatile anesthetic • Nitroglycerin, nitroprus (Nipride) • If pulmonary capillary wedge pressure (PCWP) is increased and cardiac output is decreased, inotropic support (dopamine, epinephrine) may be needed.
	Maximize urinary output	Mannitol, furosemide (Lasix)
	Minimize fluids	Monitor crystalloid administration.
	Prevent thrombosis	Heparin-monitor activated clotting times (ACTs)
Cross-clamping	Prevent myocardial infarction	• Decrease afterload nitroglycerin and nitroprusside. • Monitor electrocardiogram for ischemia. • Monitor the cardiac output—expect a decline.
	Maintain oxygenation	• O_2/air or 100% oxygen • Monitor O_2 saturation and arterial blood gases.
	Maintain urinary output (0.5 ml/kg per hour)	• Anuria is rare. • Dopamine (1 to 5 mcg/kg)
Prerelease	Prevent myocardial infarction, declamping, hypotension	• Monitor electrocardiogram • Ask surgeon for a 10-minute warning before aortic clamp is removed. • Lighten anesthesia depth. • Discontinue vasodilating agents (nitroglycerin and nitroprusside) • Increase central venous pressure and PCWP 4 to 6 mm Hg with fluids (and blood if needed). • Have vasopressors ready.
Post-release	Maintain blood pressure and vital signs	Use vasopressors (dopamine, epinephrine, phenylephrine).
	Correct acidoses	• Mechanical ventilation • Bicarbonate administration (pH: less than 7.25) • Calcium chloride ($CaCl_2$) administration
	Correct coagulation profile	Protamine
	Maintain urine output	Volume—crystalloids and colloids, dopamine

PART 2 Common Procedures

Procedures are classified as inflow or outflow vascular reconstruction. The inflow reconstruction procedures bypass the obstruction in the aortoiliac segment (aortoiliac endarterectomy or aortofemoral bypass). These are more stressful procedures requiring cross-clamping of the aorta. Outflow procedures are performed distal to the inguinal ligament to bypass the femoropopliteal or distal obstruction.

2. **Preoperative assessment**
   a) *History and physical examination*
      (1) See "Abdominal Aortic Aneurysm," p. 257.
      (2) *Musculoskeletal:* Decreased or absent popliteal and pedal pulses, delayed capillary refill, blanching on elevation of the leg followed by dependent edema after lowering it, and pain with walking relieved by rest
   b) *Diagnostic tests*
      (1) See "Abdominal Aortic Aneurysm," p. 257.
      (2) Doppler studies
         (*a*) Determinations of systolic blood pressure at level of ankle compared with brachial.
         (*b*) Assess the severity of ischemia, urgency of revascularization, and baseline values for evaluation of operative results.
      (3) Angiography—determine the precise site of the actual lesion.
   c) *Preoperative medications and intravenous therapy*
      (1) Elderly population with coexisting medical disease requiring pharmacologic support (i.e., antihypertensives, antianginals, antiarrhythmics, digoxin). These medications may be continued up to the day of the operation.
      (2) Sedatives and narcotics.
         (*a*) Use with caution in patients with poor respiratory reserve.
         (*b*) Onset of intravenous medications may be delayed because of potentially low cardiac output.
      (3) Two peripheral large bore (16- to 18-gauge) intravenous lines with moderate fluid management
      (4) Epidural catheter—test dose on the awake patient; there is a risk of epidural hematoma from anticoagulation during surgery.

3. **Room preparation**
   a) *Monitoring equipment*
      (1) Electrocardiogram leads V_5 and II to detect myocardial ischemia and diagnose tachyarrhythmias.
      (2) Warming modalities
      (3) Foley catheter
      (4) Arterial line and central venous pressure monitoring may be necessary.
   b) *Pharmacologic agents*
      (1) Have nitroglycerin, nitroprusside drugs within quick access.
      (2) Drugs: vasopressors, heparin, β-blockers.
      (3) May be asked to administer dextran solution.
   c) *Position:* Supine

4. **Anesthetic technique**
   a) Regional blockade, general anesthesia, or a combination.
   Technique of choice is regional anesthesia—avoids airway problems and sequelae, provides greater hemodynamic stability with coexisting diseases, provides sympathetic blockade that increases circulation in the lower extremity, reduces the incidence of intravascular clotting, facilitates postoperative pain relief, suppresses the endocrine stress response, and decreases blood loss in selected cases.
   b) Regional blockade—analgesia to T10; epidural or spinal
      (1) The elderly population is more sensitive to local anesthetics; reduce dose by 50%.
      (2) Some practitioners administer ephedrine prophylactically to prevent hypotension.
      (3) Level is slightly above the skin dermatome necessary for usual incisions (T12), but sympathetic innervation of lower extremities, which contains visceral afferent fibers, is believed to occur at T10 to L2.
5. **Perioperative management**
   a) *Induction*
      (1) General anesthesia
         (*a*) Goal is smooth transition from awake state to surgical anesthesia and the maintenance of cardiovascular stability.
         (*b*) A slow "controlled" induction is preferred with an opioid and nondepolarizing muscle relaxant.
         (*c*) Muscle relaxation may be chosen on the basis of cardiovascular effect
            i) Pancuronium—if the heart rate is slowed during induction
            ii) Vecuronium—if the heart rate is in the desired range
         (*d*) Onset of drugs may be delayed with low cardiac output.
         (*e*) Omit thiopental and other cardiac depressors in patients with poor left-ventricular function.
         (*f*) Anticipate exaggerated blood-pressure changes—maintain within 20% of baseline.
         (*g*) Minimize pressor response during intubation of trachea by limiting duration of laryngoscopy to less than 15 seconds.
      (2) *Regional anesthesia*
         (*a*) Review the principles of sympathetic block.
         (*b*) Consider administering blockade with the operative side down so that the onset of sympathetic and sensory blockade is more rapid on the dependent site. Theoretically, the level will be higher on the dependent side. The total volume of anesthetic requirements may be decreased.
   b) *Maintenance*
      (1) Surgeon will ask that heparin be administered via

PART 2 **Common Procedures**

intravenous push—ensure the patency of the port prior to injection.

(2) One may perform intraoperative angiography.

(a) Allergic reactions may occur with dye.

(b) Level of surgical stimulation changes; blood pressure decreases when surgical activity stops in preparation for angiography. Blood pressure and heart rate may increase when dye is injected.

(c) Repeat injection of contrast dye during multiple attempts at angiography may cause osmotic diuresis.

(3) Hyperkalemia and acidosis due to ischemic extremities are possible, and myoglobin can be released into the circulation.

(4) Maintain the hematocrit above 30 to maximize O_2-carrying capacity; do not give too many red cells or too few crystalloids. There is an increase in blood viscosity and the possibility of graft thrombosis.

(5) Unclamping of femoral artery rarely affects hemodynamics significantly. The lower extremity receives arterial blood through collateral vessels even when the femoral artery is occluded.

(6) Regional anesthesia

(a) Attention to patient comfort is important.

(b) Sedation is aimed at reducing patient anxiety without producing respiratory depression or unresponsiveness.

c) *Emergence*

(1) Initiate regional blockade through the epidural catheter for postoperative analgesia prior to the end of the case.

(2) Base extubation on the patient's general health, amount of blood loss, and overall status after the procedure.

6. **Postoperative implications**

(a) Obtain hemoglobin and hematocrit.

(b) Assess the musculoskeletal status of the operative extremity.

C. Thoracic Aortic Aneurysm

1. **Introduction**

Aneurysms that affect the thoracic aorta include ascending and arch defects (60% to 70%) or descending lesions (30%). These dissections are sometimes classified (Crawford) into the segments and arteries that are involved (types 1 to 4). Surgery is performed to prevent rupture, repair leaking or expansion of the aneurysm, and possibly for acute or chronic dissections. Diseases of the thoracic aorta may be associated with atherosclerosis, connective tissue disorders (Marfan's syndrome), congenital abnormalities, trauma, infection (syphilis), hypertension, and inflammatory processes.

2. **Preoperative assessment and patient preparation**
   a) *History and physical examination*
      (1) *Cardiac:* Coexisting disorders may include hypertension (70% to 90% of patients), angina, coronary artery disease, congestive heart failure, myocardial ischemia, and peripheral vascular disease.
      (2) *Respiratory:* Manifestations may include hemoptysis, stridor, hoarseness, dyspnea, or pleural effusion.
      (3) *Neurologic:* Assess for any preexisting condition.
      (4) *Renal:* Kidneys may be affected secondary to coexisting diseases.
      (5) *Gastrointestinal:* Bowel ischemia has been associated with descending aneurysms.
   b) *Patient preparation*
      (1) *Laboratory tests:* Complete blood count, electrolytes, blood urea. nitrogen, creatinine, prothrombin time, partial thromboplastin time, urinalysis, and arterial blood gases
      (2) *Diagnostic tests:* Electrocardiography, echocardiography, Doppler, magnetic resonance imaging, chest and abdominal radiography
      (3) *Preoperative medications:* Anxiolytics and analgesics as indicated
      (4) *Intravenous therapy:* Central line, two 14- to 16-gauge intravenous lines; consider pulmonary arterial catheter.
3. **Room preparation**
   a) *Monitoring equipment:* standard with arterial line, pulmonary arterial catheter, and Foley catheter
   b) *Additional equipment:* fluid warmers, cardiopulmonary bypass, cell saver, and transesophageal echocardiography
   c) *Drugs*
      (1) Miscellaneous pharmacologic agents—heparin, diuretics, vasodilators/constrictors, inotropes, adrenergic antagonists, opioids, nondepolarizing muscle relaxant, and antibiotic
      (2) *Intravenous fluids:* Calculate for major blood loss. Crystalloids at 6 to 8 mL/kg per hour. Estimated blood loss is 200 to 800 mL.
      (3) Blood—Type and crossmatch for 8 to 10 units of packed red blood cells
      (4) Tabletop—standard
4. **Perioperative management and anesthetic technique**
   Anesthetic technique is general anesthesia.
   a) *Induction:* Smooth induction to maintain hemodynamic stability can be accomplished with etomidate (0.1 to 0.3 mg/kg) or thiopental (4 to 6 mg/kg), high-dose fentanyl (20 to 100 mcg/kg) or sufentanil (5 to 20 mcg/kg), pretreatment with lidocaine (1.5 mg/kg), and vecuronium (0.1 mg/kg). Consider midazolam (50 to 350 mcg/kg) and esmolol as indicated. A double lumen endotracheal tube may be required.

PART 2 **Common Procedures**

b) *Maintenance:* Maintain the mean arterial pressure at 60 to 80 mm Hg and urinary output at 0.5 to 1.0 mL/kg per hour. Inhalational agent/O_2 narcotic is used. The aorta is cross-clamped for 25 to 120 minutes, and cardiopulmonary bypass may be instituted for 30 to 150 minutes. The position is supine or lateral decubitus.

c) *Emergence:* The patient is transported to an intensive care unit intubated and remains ventilated for 24 to 48 hours.

5. **Postoperative implications**

a) Complications—cardiac, respiratory, and renal failure as immediate postoperative risks. Other complications include hemorrhage, hypertension, coagulopathy, myocardial ischemia, and arrhythmias.

b) Postoperative pain management—consider an epidural catheter.

D. Aorto-Bifemoral Bypass Grafting

1. **Introduction**
Aorto-bifemoral bypass grafting is commonly performed to correct symptomatic unilateral iliac occlusive disease, which generally occurs in males older than 55 years.

2. **Preoperative assessment and patient preparation**

a) *History and physical examination*

(1) *Cardiovascular:* 30% to 50% of patients have coexisting coronary artery disease. Other common risk factors are myocardial infarction, hypertension, angina, valvular disease, congestive heart failure, and arrhythmias.

(2) *Respiratory:* Most patients have a significant history of smoking and possibly chronic obstructive pulmonary disease.

(3) *Neurologic:* Check for coexisting cerebrovascular disease.

(4) *Renal:* Chronic renal insufficiency is common.

(5) *Endocrine:* Many patients have diabetes and its associated complications.

b) *Patient preparation*

(1) *Laboratory tests:* Complete blood count, prothrombin time, partial thromboplastin time, bleeding time, electrolytes, blood urea nitrogen, creatinine, creatinine clearance, and urinalysis

(2) *Diagnostic tests:* 12-lead electrocardiography, pulmonary function tests, arterial blood gases, chest radiography, magnetic resonance imaging, computed tomography, and arteriography

(3) *Preoperative medications:* Knowledge of daily medications is essential. Cardiac medications are continued, and anticoagulant therapy is sometimes held for 4 hours prior to surgery.

Anxiolytics, sedatives, and analgesics are used as indicated.

(4)   *Intravenous therapy:* Central line, two 14- to 16-gauge intravenous lines. Estimated blood loss is 500 mL.

3. **Room preparation**

   a)   *Monitoring equipment:* Standard with arterial line and central venous pressure catheter, pulmonary arterial catheter, or both. ST segment analysis and transesophageal echocardiography are beneficial.

   b)   *Additional equipment:* Fluid warmer; consider cell saver

   c)   *Drugs*

   (1)   Miscellaneous pharmacologic agents—osmotic and loop diuretics, local anesthetics, antibiotics, adrenergic antagonists, inotropic agents, vasodilators/constrictors, and heparin

   (2)   *Intravenous fluids:* Calculate for major blood loss. Consider rapid infusion of crystalloids, colloids, or both to treat hypovolemic states.

   (3)   Blood—type and cross–match for 4 units of packed red blood cells

   (4)   Tabletop—standard

4. **Anesthetic technique**

   General anesthesia, epidural anesthesia, or a combination of general and regional anesthesia

5. **Perioperative management**

   a)   *Induction:* Use smooth induction to preserve cerebral perfusion and to maintain hemodynamic stability. For general anesthesia, consider etomidate, fentanyl, lidocaine, and muscle relaxants to decrease episodes of tachycardia and hypotension. For regional anesthesia, consider placing an epidural catheter prior to beginning anticoagulation.

   b)   *Maintenance:* For general anesthesia, consider O_2/air, volatile agent/narcotic. For regional anesthesia, use local anesthetic/narcotic/anxiolytic. Maintain blood pressure within the high-normal range.

   c)   *Emergence:* Maintain hemodynamic stability; prevent hypertension and tachycardia. For general anesthesia, use full reversal of muscle relaxants and smooth extubation.

6. **Postoperative implications**

   Complications include hemodynamic instability, myocardial ischemia, hemorrhage, respiratory failure, renal failure, and neurologic changes.

PART 2 **Common Procedures**

E. Carotid Endarterectomy

1. **Introduction**

    Surgical excision of fibrous atherosclerotic plaque at or near the bifurcation of the common carotid artery is performed for the treatment of transient ischemic attacks. It is reserved for patients with lesions of greater than 80% blockage in the carotid artery. Cerebral angiography is used to determine the location and severity of stenosis. The operative mortality rate is 1% to 2% and is due to myocardial infarction; the operative morbidity rate is 4% to 10% and is due to stroke.

2. **Preoperative assessment and patient preparation**

    a) *History and physical examination*

        (1) *Cardiac:* Assess normal range of blood pressure and heart rate and note asymmetries in blood pressure between arms. Obtain a detailed history of cardiovascular function.

        (2) *Neurologic:* Assess and document preexisting neurologic deficits to distinguish new deficits.

        (3) *Respiratory:* Obtain preoperative blood gases if pulmonary disease is suspected. Preoperative arterial CO_2 pressure dictates this value during anesthesia.

        (4) *General:* Optimal control of hypertension, diabetes, chronic obstructive pulmonary disease, and chronic renal failure is imperative prior to surgery.

    b) *Diagnostic tests:* Electrocardiogram, complete blood count, blood urea nitrogen, blood sugar, chest radiography, creatinine, electrolytes, type and crossmatch, arterial blood gases, other cardiac tests as needed according to history

    c) *Preoperative medication and intravenous therapy*

        (1) Continue all cardiac medications until time of surgery.

        (2) Two 16- to 18-gauge intravenous lines with moderate fluid replacement

        (3) Premedication is minimal.

3. **Room preparation**

    a) *Monitoring equipment*

        (1) Standard with arterial line, electrocardiogram with lead II/V5 and ST segment monitoring

        (2) Hemodynamic monitoring

        (3) Electroencephalogram, somatosensory-evoked potential; carotid stump pressure monitoring may be used to assess cerebral ischemia.

    b) *Pharmacologic agents:* Standard tabletop setup with ephedrine, phenylephrine, esmolol, nitroglycerin, labetalol, heparin, and protamine available.

    c) *Position:* Supine; arms may be tucked at sides. A roll may be placed under the shoulder blades to extend the neck. The head may be placed on a doughnut. Determine if the table will be turned and attach monitors accordingly.

4. **Anesthetic technique**
   a) Regional blockade or general anesthesia
   b) *Regional blockade:* Cervical plexus block at the transverse process of C3 to C4 and along the inferior border of the sternocleidomastoid muscle offers advantage of an awake patient, allowing for continuous neurologic monitoring.
   c) *General anesthesia:* Allows for control of ventilation, oxygenation, and lack of patient movement. General anesthetics protect the brain by depressing the level of cerebral metabolism and the cerebral metabolic rate of oxygen.

5. **Perioperative management**
   a) *Induction*
      (1) A slow, controlled induction is preferred with an opioid and nondepolarizing muscle relaxant.
      (2) Anticipate exaggerated blood pressure changes with induction. Adequate hydration is imperative. Use of lidocaine and esmolol will attenuate the response to laryngoscopy.
   b) *Maintenance*
      (1) Maintain arterial blood pressure in the patient's normal range.
      (2) Prior to cross-clamping, increase blood pressure by 20 to 30 mm Hg. May need vasoactive agent (i.e., Neo-Synephrine).
      (3) Document the cross-clamping time.
      (4) If a shunt is used, document shunt insertion and removal.
      (5) Maintain arterial CO_2 pressure in the patient's normal range.
      (6) If the surgeon stretches the baroreceptor nerve endings, ask the surgeon to inject the area of bifurcation with 1% lidocaine 10 to 15 minutes prior to carotid artery occlusion.
   c) *Emergence*
      (1) Smooth emergence is important; use lidocaine to blunt reflexes.
      (2) The patient needs to be awake at the end of the procedure so the surgeon can assess for neurologic deficits.

6. **Postoperative considerations**
   Hypertension is common. Other complications include carotid body damage, hemorrhage with compromise of the airway, myocardial infarction, stroke, and dysfunction of cranial nerves VII, IX, X, and XII.

PART 2 **Common Procedures**

F. Portasystemic Shunts

1. **Introduction**
   Portasystemic shunt procedures are performed to prevent or cease variceal hemorrhage due to portal hypertension in patients with liver disease, cirrhosis, ascites, and hypersplenism. The redistribution of blood from the portal vein to the inferior vena cava causes variations in flow and resistance of the liver, intestine, and spleen. This hemodynamic alteration aids portal perfusion and oxygenation with net effects of increased venous return and cardiac output. Variations in procedures include portacaval, end-to-end, end-to-side, mesocaval, mesorenal, or splenorenal shunts.
2. **Preoperative assessment and patient preparation**
   a) *History and physical examination*
      (1) *Cardiac:* Associated disorders include increased heart rate, circulating blood volume, and intrathoracic pressure. Variations of cardiac output, cardiomyopathy, congestive heart failure, coronary artery disease, and decreased response to catecholamines and systemic vascular resistance may be present.
      (2) *Respiratory:* Hypoxemia may be related to ventilation-perfusion mismatch, increased closing volume, increased functional residual capacity, atelectasis, right-to-left pulmonary shunting, increased disphosphoglycerate, pulmonary infections, and impaired hypoxic pulmonary vasoconstriction.
      (3) *Neurologic:* Manifestations may include hepatic encephalopathy with associated confusion and obtundation.
      (4) *Renal:* Renal impairment and failure with electrolyte imbalance is frequently observed.
      (5) *Gastrointestinal:* Gastric or esophageal varices with gastrointestinal bleeding is common.
      (6) *Endocrine:* Abnormal glucose utilization, increased growth hormone, intolerance to carbohydrates, and irregular sex hormone metabolism may be observed.
   b) *Patient preparation*
      (1) *Laboratory tests:* Arterial blood gases, complete blood count, prothrombin time, partial thromboplastin time, bleeding time, electrolytes, blood urea nitrogen, creatinine, creatinine clearance, urinalysis, diffuse intravascular coagulation profile, albumin, bilirubin, serum glutamic-oxalo-acetic transaminase, serum glutamic-pyruvic transaminase, ammonia, alkaline phosphatase, lactate
      (2) *Diagnostic tests:* Electrocardiography, echocardiography, pulmonary function tests, chest radiography
      (3) *Preoperative medications:* Avoid intramuscular injections. Anxiolytics are administered in small doses as indicated. Consider metoclopramide (10 mg) and ranitidine (50 mg).

    (4) *Intravenous therapy:* Central line, two 14- to 16-gauge intravenous lines. Consider a pulmonary arterial catheter.

3. **Room preparation**
   a) *Monitoring equipment:* Standard with arterial line, central venous pressure catheter, and urinary catheter
   b) *Additional equipment:* Fluid warmer, cell saver, Bair Hugger, and rapid infuser
   c) *Drugs*
      (1) Miscellaneous pharmacologic agents—opioid (fentanyl), midazolam, vasodilators and vasoconstrictors, inotropes, nondepolarizing muscle relaxants, and antibiotics
      (2) *Intravenous fluids:* Calculate for major blood loss. Estimated blood loss is 1000 to 2000 mL.
      (3) Blood—type and crossmatch for 8 to 10 units of packed red blood cells, platelets, fresh frozen plasma, and cryoprecipitate.
      (4) Tabletop—standard

4. **Anesthetic technique**
   General anesthesia, epidural anesthesia, or a combination of general and regional anesthesia.

5. **Perioperative management and anesthetic technique**
   a) General anesthetic is the technique of choice.
   b) *Induction:* Rapid sequence induction with thiopental (3 to 5 mg/kg) or succinylcholine (1 to 2 mg/kg). Consider etomidate (0.2 mg/kg) or ketamine (1 mg/kg).
   c) *Maintenance:* Inhalational agent/O_2/fentanyl/midazolam and nondepolarizing muscle relaxant. Position is supine.
   d) *Emergence:* Patient generally is transported to the intensive care unit.

6. **Postoperative implications**
   a) Complications—coagulopathy, renal failure, hypothermia, encephalopathy, jaundice, and anemia
   b) Postoperative pain management—passive cutaneous anaphylaxis

VIII

SECTION

Orthopedics

A. Hip Arthroplasty

1. **Introduction**

   The replacement of joint surfaces is required primarily for inflammatory or degenerative conditions within the joint, such as those accompanying rheumatoid arthritis or osteoarthritis from degeneration of the synovium or cartilage. As one or more of the normal joint tissues deteriorate or degenerate, the bone ends are exposed, causing pain and limitation of joint movements. Joint stiffness and muscle atrophy follow further increasing pain, limiting movement, and mobility. Exposed bone surfaces will lead to bone growth that may eventually adhere to the opposing bone ends, causing bony ankylosis and loss of joint movement. Therefore replacement of the deteriorated or degenerated tissues and bones restores movement and relieves pain.

   Total joint replacement involves removal of some or all of the synovium, cartilage, and bone in both sides of the joint. One of the joint bone surfaces is then replaced with a metallic prosthesis, whereas the other surface is replaced with a ceramic or plastic, silicone-lined prosthesis. The metallic-plastic material is necessary to prevent metal-to-metal wear, friction, and possible electrolytic reactions from the interactions and intermingling of joint fluids.

2. **Preoperative assessment and patient preparation**

   a) *History and physical examination*
      (1) With this elderly population, assess for coexisting medical diseases.
      (2) Carefully assess blood volume, central venous pressure, and orthostatic hypotension because dehydration may mask hemoglobin changes due to hematoma formation.

   b) *Diagnostic tests*
      (1) *Radiographs:* Hip and chest film
      (2) *Laboratory tests:* Complete blood count, electrolytes, glucose, blood urea nitrogen, creatinine, urinalysis, prothrombin time, partial thromboplastin time, bleeding time of the patient on aspirin, and type and crossmatch

   c) *Preoperative medications and intravenous therapy*
      (1) Anticoagulants—heparin
      (2) Antirheumatic or anti-inflammatory medications
      (3) Antibiotics
      (4) Sedatives and narcotics—use with caution in the elderly population.
      (5) Two peripheral, large bore (16- to 18-gauge) intravenous tubes with moderate fluid replacement

(6) Epidural catheter placement—perform test dose on awake patient.

3. **Room preparation**
   a) *Monitoring equipment*
      (1) Standard
      (2) Indwelling urinary catheter—controversial
          (a) Absence of bladder drainage can cause overdistention, affecting bladder function.
          (b) Insertion may cause urinary tract infection.
      (3) Central venous pressure—trend volume status.
      (4) Warming modalities
      (5) Electrocardiography leads V_5 and II detect myocardial ischemia and diagnose tachyarrythmias in the elderly population.
      (6) Transesophageal echocardiography—assess fat and bone deposits when acetabulum is reamed and curetted.
      (7) X-ray shields for self-protection
      (8) Arterial line monitoring if hypotensive techniques
   b) *Pharmacologic agents:* Vasopressors
   c) *Position:* Lateral; Special orthopedic table may be used.

4. **Anesthetic technique**
   a) *Considerations:* Regional blockade, general anesthesia, or a combination of both
   b) Technique of choice
      (1) Regional anesthesia
      (2) Reduced blood loss and postoperative deep venous thrombosis/pulmonary embolism
   c) *Regional blockade*
      (1) Epidural catheter placement and preoperative test dose OR
      (2) One-time spinal for analgesia to T10
   d) *General anesthesia*
      (1) Endotracheal tube must be inserted.
      (2) Combination with regional anesthetic allows reduced dosages of agents and control of airway.
   e) *Induction*
      (1) *General anesthesia*
          (a) Thorough airway assessment with arthritic population
          (b) Induction performed on stretcher
          (c) Succinylcholine may be contraindicated with crush injuries if large amounts of muscle tissue are devitalized.
      (2) *Regional anesthesia:* spinal/epidural—review principles of sympathetic blocks.
   f) *Maintenance*
      (1) Laminar flow is used to minimize infections and can increase evaporative fluid and heat losses from the operative site.
      (2) Controlled hypotensive techniques facilitate surgical exposure and decrease blood loss.
          (a) Blood pressure parameters need to be individualized.
          (b) Maintain mean blood pressure of 50 to 70 mm Hg.
          (c) Deepen anesthesia with volatile anesthetic.

(*d*)   Initiate vasoactive (nitroprusside) drip.
(3)   Methylmethacrylate cement is used to distribute the forces of the femoral and acetabular prosthetic components.
   (*a*)   Mixing the cement causes the monomer portion to polymerize—exothermic reaction.
   (*b*)   Problems with methylmethacrylate relate to cementing the femoral prosthesis—unpolymerized monomer can be absorbed into the circulation.
      i)   Causes direct vasodilation, usually within the first minute; can last as long as 10 minutes.
      ii)   Venous embolism can occur when the femoral prosthesis is inserted into the femoral canal.
      iii)   Hypotension, hypoxia, and cardiovascular collapse following prosthesis insertion have been reported.
   (*c*)   High-risk arteriosclerotic patients (who compensate poorly for sudden cardiovascular dynamic changes) and those whose fluid and blood replacement was inadequate.
   (*d*)   Prevent complications—communicate with the surgeon regarding application
   (*e*)   Use 100% O_2, decrease vasodilating agent, maximize fluid status, and have vasopressor support available.
   (*f*)   Use of methylmethacrylate during total knee or total shoulder surgery is of less concern with decreased risk of complications due to the use of a tourniquet and much smaller exposure to cement.
g)   *Emergence*
   (1)   If general anesthetic is implemented, patients are usually repositioned onto the stretcher prior to emergence.
   (2)   Base extubation on the patient's status.
   (3)   Initiate regional blockade through the epidural catheter for postoperative analysis prior to the end of the case.
5.   **Postoperative implications**
   a)   Obtain laboratory results—hemoglobin and hematocrit; watch for hidden bleeding
   b)   Fat embolism typically appears 12 to 48 hours after a long bone fracture.
      (1)   *Signs and symptoms*
         (*a*)   Arterial hypoxemia
         (*b*)   Adult respiratory distress syndrome
         (*c*)   Central nervous system dysfunction (confusion, coma, seizures)
         (*d*)   Petechial (neck, shoulders, and chest)
         (*e*)   Coagulopathy
         (*f*)   Fever
      (2)   *Treatment*
         (*a*)   Supportive
         (*b*)   Oxygenation
         (*c*)   Corticosteroids

(*d*)   Immobilization of long bone fractures

c)   Other potential complications include deep venous thrombosis and pulmonary embolism

B. Knee (Total Knee Replacement) Arthroplasty

1. **Introduction**

   Arthroplasty of the knee joint is performed when metallic and plastic components are used for the replacement of knee joint surfaces. The femur, patella, and tibia are exposed, and cartilage and a small amount of bone are removed with a saw. The new components may or may not be cemented.

2. **Preoperative assessment**

   Routine, including history and physical examination. These patients have been diagnosed with arthritis of the knee.

   a)   *Respiratory:* These patients may have rheumatoid arthritis and associated pulmonary conditions. Pulmonary effusions may be present. Rheumatoid arthritis involving the cricoarytenoid joints may exhibit itself by hoarseness. A narrow glottic opening may lead to a difficult intubation. Arthritic involvement of the cervical spine and temporomandibular joint may also complicate airway management.

   b)   *Cardiovascular:* Depending on the severity of the arthritis, the patient may have a lowered exercise tolerance. Rheumatoid arthritis is associated with pericardial effusion. Cardiac valve fibrosis and cardiac conduction abnormalities can occur with possible aortic regurgitation. Test electrocardiogram and, if possible, echocardiogram and dipyridamole thallium imaging.

   c)   *Neurologic:* A thorough preoperative neurologic examination may yield evidence of cervical nerve root compression. If indicated, obtain lateral neck films for the determination of stability of the atlanto-occipital joint.

   d)   *Musculoskeletal:* Positioning may be difficult because of pain and the decreased mobility of the joint

   e)   *Hematologic/laboratory:* Hemoglobin and hematocrit, other tests related to the history and physical examination

   f)   *Premedication:* Individualized based on patient need.

3. **Room preparation**

   a)   Standard monitoring equipment. A tourniquet may or may not be used.

   b)   The patient should have one large bore intravenous tube.

   c)   Fluid requirements include normal saline or lactated Ringer's at 6 mL/kg/hour.

   d)   Standard drugs for general or regional anesthesia

PART 2 Common Procedures

4. **Anesthetic technique**
   a) This procedure can be done under general or regional anesthesia.
   b) Regional anesthesia could be with a subarachnoid block or placement of an epidural catheter.
5. **Perioperative management**
   a) *Induction:* Standard induction with routine medications. Muscle relaxation will be needed for the placement of the prosthesis.
   b) *Emergence:* These patients are usually extubated in the operating room unless there was preoperative respiratory compromise.
6. **Postoperative implications**
   Watch for posterior tibial artery trauma, peroneal nerve palsy (foot drop), hemorrhage from the posterior tibial artery, and tourniquet nerve injury, if indicated.

C. Shoulder (Total Shoulder) Arthroplasty

1. **Introduction**
   Total shoulder arthroplasty is usually done for end-stage arthritis or following trauma. Rheumatoid arthritis and psoriatic arthritis are inflammatory conditions that may require shoulder replacement for correction of pain relief. These conditions are often associated with massive rotator cuff tears.
2. **Preoperative assessment**
   a) *Respiratory*
      (1) Rheumatoid arthritic patients may show signs of pleural effusion or pulmonary fibrosis. Hoarseness may be due to cricoarytenoid joint involvement. This patient may be difficult to intubate.
      (2) Tests: Chest radiography, pulmonary function tests (if indicated; arterial blood gases in compromised patients
   b) *Cardiovascular:* Patients with rheumatoid arthritis may suffer from chronic pericardial tamponade, valvular disease, and cardiac condition defects.
   c) *Neurologic*
      (1) Arthritic patients may have cervical or lumbar radiculopathies. Preoperative documentation of these conditions is essential. Head flexion may cause cervical cord compression.
      (2) Tests: Cervical spine films to rule out subluxations in rheumatoid patients with neck or upper-extremity radiculopathy
   d) *Musculoskeletal:* With the possibility of limited neck and jaw mobility, special intubation may be indicated. Special attention must be paid to positioning in patients with bony deformities or contractures.

e) *Hematologic:* Almost all nontrauma patients will be on some type of nonsteroidal anti-inflammatory drug, which should be stopped approximately 5 days before the procedure.

f) *Endocrine:* Rheumatoid patients will most likely be on some type of corticosteroid and therefore should have a supplemental dose of steroids to treat adrenal suppression (e.g., intravenus hydrocortisone 100 mg).

g) *Laboratory tests:* Hemoglobin and hematocrit from healthy patients, other tests as indicated from the history and physical examination

h) *Premedication:* If a regional block is done, moderate to heavy premedication is indicated.

3. **Room preparation**
    a) Standard monitoring equipment
    b) The patient will be in a semisitting position. A precordial Doppler device may be used to detect venous air embolism.
    c) One large bore intravenous tube will be needed on the nonoperative side.
    d) If the patient is more hemodynamically compromised, hemodynamic monitoring may be indicated.
    e) Fluid replacement—normal saline or lactated Ringer's at 6 mL/kg/hour

4. **Anesthetic technique**
    This procedure can be performed under a general or a regional anesthetic technique. The interscalene approach to the brachial plexus alone or combined with a general anesthetic could be used for this procedure.

5. **Perioperative management**
    a) *Induction:* Standard. If the patient has limited range of motion, awake fiberoptic intubation may be indicated.
    b) *Maintenance:* Standard maintenance with muscle relaxation; consider a continuous opioid infusion because of the length of the procedure.
    c) *Position:* Semisitting or lawn chair position or lateral decubitus position
    d) *Considerations:* If using N_2O during placement of the humeral component, discontinue it because of the increased risk of a venous air embolism with moderate muscle relaxation at that time.
    e) *Emergence:* The patient can be extubated in the operating room. Reverse muscle relaxant after positioning the patient back to a supine position.

6. **Postoperative implications**
    Consider a patient-controlled anesthesia pump or regional block technique for postoperative pain.

PART 2 Common Procedures

D. External Fixator Placement and Open Reduction and Internal Fixation of Extremities

1. **Introduction**
   Tibial fractures are fixed with percutaneous pins that are clamped to an external frame. Pins made of stainless steel are drilled into the proximal and distal fragments of the fracture through stab wounds through the skin and subcutaneous tissue.

   Open reduction and internal fixation is performed under direct vision. The fractures are fixed and stabilized with pins, plates, or a combination thereof. Radiographs are taken intraoperatively to confirm placement of hardware. After the incisions are closed, a splint or cast is applied.

2. **Preoperative assessment**
   a) *History and physical examination*
      (1) *Respiratory:* 10% to 15% of patients with bone fractures will develop fat emboli. Symptoms include hypoxemia, tachycardia, tachypnea, respiratory alkalosis, mental status changes, and conjunctival petechiae. Urinalysis shows fat in the urine. These patients should be adequately hydrated and mechanically ventilated, and the hypoxemia should be corrected.
      (2) *Cardiovascular:* If blunt chest trauma occurs during the injury, cardiac contusion or tamponade are possible. Tachycardia, hypotension, or orthostasis should be managed with crystalloids (10 to 40 mL/kg/hour) or blood accordingly. Electrocardiography, creatinine, cardiac enzymes, and echocardiography help to determine the presence of cardiac injury.
      (3) *Neurologic:* A thorough evaluation including mental status and peripheral sensory examination is indicated.
      (4) *Musculoskeletal:* Consider a cervical spine injury if the mechanism of injury included rapid deceleration or trauma to the head or neck
   b) *Laboratory tests:* Routine and indicated tests should be performed, including hemoglobin and hematocrit.
   c) *Premedication:* For trauma patients, minimal or no premedication is given. If the patient has severe pain on movement, opiates can be titrated for pain relief.

3. **Room preparation**
   a) Standard monitoring equipment
   b) Lead apron for protection during radiography
   c) One large bore intravenous tube. If the patient is hemodynamically compromised, consider an arterial line and central venous pressure monitoring.
   d) Fluid replacement—normal saline or lactated Ringer's at 4 to

8 mL/kg/hour
   e)   If blood loss has been significant, type and crossmatch for
        appropriate blood replacement.
4. **Perioperative management and anesthetic technique**
   a)   Same as for knee or shoulder replacement
   b)   This procedure may be performed under general or regional
        anethesia. If the patient has suffered trauma, use general
        anesthesia with rapid sequence induction and cricoid pressure.
   c)   *Maintenance:* Routine maintenance for general or regional
        anesthetic
   d)   *Position:* Supine
   e)   *Emergence:* If the procedure is performed under a general anes-
        thetic, the patient should be extubated in the operating room.
5. **Postoperative implications**
   a)   Complications of hypoxemia may develop secondary to a fat
        embolism.
   b)   Pain management can be controlled under a continuous
        epidural infusion.

E. Pelvic Reconstruction

1. **Introduction**
   A pelvic reconstruction is a surgical procedure that involves the open
   reduction of pelvic fractures, which are then maintained by the
   application of plates and screws. Bone grafting may be used to repair
   any defects. The surgical time for the procedure is 3 to 6 hours.
   These fractures may be caused by minor trauma, especially in elderly
   persons, but most result from high-impact trauma (i.e., motor vehicle trauma). Evaluation of the patient for potential coexisting trauma
   should include a thorough neurologic, thoracic, and abdominal
   assessment. The extremities may also be involved.
2. **Preoperative assessment**
   a)   *History and physical examination:* Obtain a verbal history from
        the patient or family member. Note any preexisting disease
        processes, social history, current medications, past surgical his-
        tory, and allergies.
        (1)   *Cardiac:* Assess for cardiac contusion or aortic tear. Tests:
              12-lead electrocardiography, creatinine, isoenzymes, chest
              radiography (wide mediastinal silhouette suggests aortic
              tear). Transesophageal echocardiography or angiography
              if aortic tear is suspected. Consult with a cardiologist if
              indicated.
        (2)   *Respiratory:* Assess for possible hemothorax, pneumotho-
              rax, pulmonary contusion, fat embolism, or aspiration. The
              patient may require supplemental O_2 or mechanical venti-
              lation to correct hypoxemia. Coexisting trauma to the head

or cervical spine may require fiberoptic intubation. Tests: chest radiography, arterial blood gases.

(3) *Neurologic:* A thorough neurologic evaluation including mental status and peripheral sensory examination. Note any preexisting deficits. Consult with a neurologist if necessary. Tests: Computed tomography of the head is indicated for patients who experience a loss of consciousness prior to anesthesia.

(4) *Renal:* Renal injury is possible with high-impact trauma. Rule out urethral tear before the Foley catheter is placed. A suprapubic catheter may be necessary. Intraoperative monitoring of urine output is mandatory to assess adequate renal perfusion. Consult an urologist if necessary. Tests: urinalysis, blood urea nitrogen, serum creatinine, hematuria, and myoglobinuria.

(5) *Musculoskeletal:* Cervical spine clearance may be required prior to neck manipulation (i.e., laryngoscopy). Consider evaluating thoracic and lumbar radiographs to rule out any deformity or instability prior to anesthesia. Tests: cervical spine radiography, others as indicated from the history and physical examination.

(6) *Hematologic:* Large blood loss associated with traumatic injury may occur. The patient's hematocrit should be restored to greater than 25% prior to induction of anesthesia. Type and crossmatch for 6 units of packed red blood cells. Consider the use of cell saver intraoperatively.

(7) *Gastrointestinal:* Patients should be assessed for abdominal injury associated with trauma. Test: diagnostic peritoneal lavage.

b) *Patient preparation*

(1) *Laboratory tests:* Hemoglobin, hematocrit, electrolytes, prothrombin time, partial thromboplastin time, others as indicated from the history and physical examination

(2) *Medications:* Anxiolytics, narcotics, antibiotics, and others as indicated from the history and physical examination. The patient may also be on anticoagulant therapy for the prevention of deep venous thrombosis. A broad-spectrum antibiotic should be administered preoperatively.

3. **Room preparation**

a) *Monitoring equipment:* Standard, arterial line, central venous pressure, pulmonary arterial catheter if indicated, two large peripheral intravenous tubes

b) *Additional equipment*

(1) Positioning devices and operating table—the patient may be placed in the supine, lateral, or prone position. A fracture table may be used. Meticulously pad the chest, axilla, pelvis, and extremities to prevent potential nerve injury and ischemia. Prevent pressure to down ear and eye if the patient is in the lateral position. Maintain the neck in neutral alignment.

(2) Because of the length of the procedure and surgical exposure, warming devices should be implemented (i.e., fluid warmer, warming blanket).

(3) A nasogastric tube should be used to decompress the stomach if rapid sequence induction is performed.

c) *Drugs*

(1) *Continuous infusions:* Consider the use of an intravenous narcotic infusion. If an epidural catheter is placed for postoperative pain control, consider an intraoperative continuous infusion to decrease anesthetic requirements.

(2) *Intravenous fluids and blood:* Estimated blood loss is greater than 1000 mL. Type and crossmatch the patient for 6 units of packed red blood cells. Blood loss is replaced 1:1 with blood products of colloid solutions or 3:1 if crystalloid solutions are used. Consider the intraoperative use of a cellsaver. Maintain urine output at 0.5 mL/kg/hour. Consider the use of deliberate hypotension to control blood loss in those patients without cardiovascular disease or carotid stenosis. Isoflurane, esmolol, sodium nitroprusside, or a combination thereof, titrated to decrease mean arterial pressure by 30% (but not less than 60 mm Hg), is commonly used. Any fluid deficits must be replaced prior to the institution of deliberate hypotension.

(3) Tabletop—standard

4. **Perioperative management and anesthetic technique**

a) *Induction and maintenance*

(1) Rapid sequence induction must be used for trauma patients to decrease the risk of aspiration.

(2) A standard induction may be used if the procedure is performed electively.

(3) Because of the painful nature of the injury, induction is best performed on the patient's bed or stretcher before moving to the operating table.

(4) Drugs for induction and maintenance should reflect the patient's history and physical examination, accounting for any significant medical history, current physiologic states, and drug allergies.

(5) Consider the use of a nondepolarizing muscle relaxant during induction if there are no airway concerns.

(6) Anesthetic gases should be warmed and humidified. Continued muscle relaxation is optional and left to the discretion of the anesthetist or the request of the surgeon.

b) *Emergence*

(1) An epidural catheter may be placed for supplemental use intraoperatively and for postoperative pain control.

(2) Trauma patients undergoing rapid sequence induction should be fully awake and reflexive prior to extubation.

(3) Patients who suffer pulmonary complications related to trauma or the surgical procedure (i.e., fat embolism, pulmonary contusion, or aspiration) should not be extubated.

c)   *Fat embolization*
   (1)   Thirty to 90% of patients with fractures are reported to
      experience fat embolization. Most patients remain asymp-
      tomatic. The incidence of fat embolization is higher in
      patients with long bone or pelvic fractures.
   (2)   Signs and symptoms include hypoxemia; tachycardia;
      tachypnea; respiratory alkalosis; mental status changes;
      petechiae on the chest, upper extremities, axilla, and
      conjunctiva; fat bodies in the urine; and diffuse pulmonary
      infiltrates.
   (3)   Treatment is supportive and prophylactic—O_2 therapy and
      continuous positive air pressure via mask or endotracheal
      tube, judicious fluid management to help decrease the
      severity of pulmonary capillary leaks, heparin, or high-dose
      corticosteroids may all be considered.
5.   **Postoperative implications**
   a)   Consider the use of continuous epidural infusion or patient-
      controlled anesthesia for postoperative pain control.
   b)   The L4 to S5 nerve roots may be damaged from the primary
      traumatic event or the operation. The result is hemiplegia with
      bladder and bowel dysfunction. Intraoperative pressure on the
      ilioinguinal ligament may cause neuropathy of the femoral
      genitofemoral or femoral cutaneous nerve.
   c)   A marked postoperative decrease in blood pressure may be
      related to retroperitoneal hematoma formation.
   d)   Deep venous thrombosis prophylaxis should be instituted
      postoperatively (i.e., support hose and deep vein thrombosis
      prophylaxis).

F. Hip Pinning (Open Reduction and Internal Fixation)

1.   **Introduction**
   Hip pinning involves the open reduction of a hip fracture that is
   maintained by the application of plates and screws. Bone grafting
   may be used to repair any defects. Hip fractures may result from
   high-impact trauma, but most result from minor trauma in elderly
   persons. If the fracture is related to high-impact trauma, a coexisting
   trauma should be thoroughly evaluated.
2.   **Preoperative assessment and patient preparation**
   History and physical examination: Obtain a verbal history from the
   patient or family member. Note any preexisting disease processes,
   social history, current medications, past surgical history, and allergies.
3.   **Patient preparation**
   a)   *Laboratory tests:* Hemoglobin, hematocrit, complete blood

count, prothrombin time, partial thromboplastin time, others as indicated by the history and physical examination

b) *Diagnostic tests:* 12-lead electrocardiography, chest radiography, others as indicated by the history and physical examination

c) *Preoperative medications:* Individualized

4. **Room preparation**
   a) *Monitoring equipment:* Standard, arterial line, central venous pressure catheter, pulmonary arterial catheter as indicated.
   b) *Additional equipment*
      (1) Positioning devices and operating table—the patient is usually placed in a lateral position. Aging skin atrophies and is prone to trauma from adhesive tape, electrocautery pads, and electrocardiographic electrodes. Arthritic joints may interfere with positioning; when possible, the elderly patient should be positioned for comfort. Meticulous padding of the axilla and all bony prominences decreases the risk of nerve injury and ischemia. Prevent pressure to the ears and eyes. Maintain the neck in neutral alignment.
      (2) Because of the length of the procedure, the patient's usual age, and surgical exposure, warming modalities should be implemented (fluid warmer, warming blankets).
   c) *Drugs*
      (1) *Continuous infusion:* Consider the use of a continuous epidural infusion intraoperatively or for postoperative pain control.
      (2) *Intravenous fluids:* Estimated blood loss is greater than 1000 mL. Type and crossmatch for units of packed red blood cells. Blood loss is replaced 1:1 with blood products or colloid solutions or 3:1 if crystalloid solutions are used. Maintain urine output at 0.5 mL/kg/hour. Keep in mind any preexisting disease processes that may easily place the elderly patient in a state of fluid overload. Consider the use of a cell saver intraoperatively.
      (3) Tabletop—standard. All equipment needed to implement the anesthetic plan should be available.

5. **Perioperative management and anesthetic technique**
   a) Regional and general anesthesia are both options for the elderly patient.
   b) Hip pinning may be performed using subarachnoid block or continuous epidural infusion extending to the T8 sensory level. Keep in mind the expected length of the procedure, the patient's history and physical examination findings, and the patient's level of cooperation and ability to lie still. One major advantage of regional anesthesia is a decreased incidence of postoperative thromboembolism. This is thought to be due to peripheral vasodilation and maintenance of venous blood flow in the lower extremities. Local anesthetics also inhibit platelet aggregation and stabilize endothelial cells. Difficult patient positioning and altered landmarks related to degenerative changes of the spine may increase the technical difficulty of performing a regional

block. Postpuncture headaches are not as prevalent in the elderly population.

c) If a general anesthetic is the best choice for the patient, drugs for induction and maintenance should reflect findings from the patient's history and physical examination. One advantage of general anesthesia is that the anesthetic can be induced with the patient on the bed or stretcher before moving to the operating table, thus avoiding painful positioning. A disadvantage of general anesthesia is that the elderly patient cannot be positioned for maximal comfort. Consider the use of nondepolarizing muscle relaxants during induction if there are no airway concerns. Continued muscle relaxation is optional and left to the discretion of the anesthetist or the request of the surgeon. The effects of nondepolarizing muscle relaxants that are renally excreted may be slightly prolonged in elderly persons because of reduced drug clearance.

d) *Emergence:* An epidural catheter may be placed for supplemental use with general anesthesia or for postoperative pain control.

e) *Fat embolization:* See "Pelvic Reconstruction," p. 279.

6. **Postoperative implications**
   a) Consider the use of a continuous epidural infusion of patient-controlled anesthesia for postoperative pain control.
   b) A marked decrease in blood pressure postoperatively may be related to hematoma formation.
   c) Deep venous thrombosis prophylaxis should be instituted postoperatively (support hose and deep vein thrombosis prophylaxis).

G. Open Reduction and Internal Fixation of Extremities

1. **Introduction**
   A surgical procedure involving a longitudinal incision is made over the fractured bone so that it may be reduced and realigned under direct visualization; the bone is then stabilized and fixed using pins, plates, screws, and a prosthesis when applicable. Intraoperative radiography is used to confirm reduction and placement of hardware. Bone grafting may be utilized for bone defects needing repair.

   Trauma and falls in the elderly are common indications for these procedures. Severely injured trauma patients require aggressive fluid therapy, large bore intravenous tubes, and invasive monitors (arterial line and central venous pressure). Elderly patients may present with different concurrent disease processes.

2. **Preoperative assessment**
   a) Individualized based on patient history and previous medical condition.

b) *Patient preparation:* Laboratory and diagnostic tests as indicated.
c) *Premedication:* Individualized based on patient's history and medical condition.

3. **Room preparation**

a) *Monitoring:* Standard monitors, central venous pressure, arterial line, pulmonary artery pressure monitoring as indicated.

b) *Additional equipment:* Tourniquets are used for lower-extremity fractures. The fracture table is needed for repairs of the pelvis and hips.

c) *Drugs:* The patient's history helps determine the availability of adjunct drips.

d) *Fluid and blood replacement:* Follow the standard replacement guidelines. Replenish fluids secondary to NPO time in the first 2 hours of surgery, 1 mL blood loss = 3 mL crystalloid replacement, to 2 to 15 mL/kg maintenance depending on fracture site, blood loss, and history and physical examination results. Trauma patients should be hemodynamically stable prior to the induction of anesthesia, if possible.

4. **Anesthetic technique**

a) General anesthesia is indicated with hip and pelvis surgery because of the duration and varied positions necessary to accomplish pelvic fixation.

b) Regional anesthesia permits evaluation of mental status, provides intact airway reflexes, and decreases blood loss in trauma patients.

c) With combative patients, those requiring multiple concurrent surgical procedures, or procedures lasting more than 2 hours, general anesthesia may be preferred.

d) Regional anesthesia also has the advantage of decreased blood loss, decreased deep venous thrombosis, minimal respiratory impairment, and effective postoperative analgesia. Anesthesia extending from S2 to T8 (if tourniquets are used) is adequate for lower-extremity surgery. Subarachnoid block and epidural blocks are useful.

5. **Perioperative management**

a) *Induction*

(1) Trauma patients who are to receive general anesthesia should undergo rapid sequence induction with cricoid pressure to prevent aspiration.

(2) Otherwise, anesthesia may be initiated with any induction agent, volatile anesthetic, or muscle relaxant unless contraindicated by history and physical examination.

b) *Maintenance*

(1) With regional anesthesia, a propofol infusion may be indicated.

(2) With general anesthesia, N_2O, volatile anesthetics, O_2, and narcotics may be used.

(3) Muscle relaxation is needed in procedures requiring prosthesis insertion so that a full range of motion (passive) may be performed. Pad all pressure points. Unless the fracture is

pelvic, the patient will be supine. Pelvic fractures may be treated with the patient in the lateral decubitus, supine, or prone position.

    c) *Emergence*

        (1) Trauma patients must be extubated fully awake and after airway reflexes have returned.

        (2) Do not extubate patients with evolving pulmonary injuries (fat embolism, aspiration, or contusion).

        (3) When a tourniquet is used, controlled ventilation should be continued for 3 to 5 minutes after deflation of the tourniquet to help facilitate the metabolism of the lactic acid that has developed in the leg. This is especially imperative in patients with moderate to severe lung disease who may be unable to increase ventilation to buffer this acid load.

6. Postoperative implications

    a) Pain management is the most prominent postoperative concern

    b) Patient-controlled analgesia and epidural infusion are two modes of therapy used for pain relief.

    c) Nerve damage related to positioning or tourniquet placement is a potential problem. Post-tourniquet syndrome is a self-limiting condition in which the affected limb is edematous, pale, and weak.

H. Arthroscopy

1. Introduction

Arthroscopic surgery may be performed for diagnostic or therapeutic indications most often involving the ankle, knee, shoulder, or wrist. Advances in arthroscopy permit many procedures to be performed primarily or adjunctively through the arthroscope, replacing a number of procedures that previously were performed through open techniques. The majority of these procedures are done in young, healthy patients. The advantages include minimal incisions, decreased postoperative morbidity, and potentially faster rehabilitation.

2. Preoperative assessment and patient preparation

    a) *History and physical examination:* Individualized

    b) *Diagnostic tests*

        (1) Radiographs of affected extremity

        (2) CXR, ECG, laboratory tests as indicated

    c) *Preoperative medicines and intravenous therapy*

        (1) Anti-inflammatory meds—stop 5 to 7 days before surgery

        (2) Antibiotics—cefazolin 1 gm IV

        (3) Sedatives and narcotics

        (4) One peripheral large bore intravenous line

        (5) Epidural catheter placement—perform test dose on awake patient.

    d) *Choice of anesthetic method:* Local, general, and regional anesthesia have all been used successfully.

3. Room preparation
    a) Standard monitoring equipment
    b) Standard drugs for general or regional anesthesia
    c) Special orthopedic tables

4. Perioperative management
    a) *Induction:* Standard induction with routine medications
    b) *Positioning:* Usually supine
        (1) Shoulder procedures can be semisitting (40 degrees to 70 degrees)
        (2) Knee procedures—foot of table 90 degrees; thigh holder
    c) *Tourniquet use:* Often employed in surgery of the extremities to decrease bleeding and to provide a bloodless field.
        (1) Nerve injury and damage to blood vessels and skeletal muscle have been reported with tourniquets—most often a function of tourniquet pressure and the duration of inflation .
        (2) Tourniquet cuffs are usually inflated to 100 mm Hg above patient's systolic blood pressure for the leg and 50 mm Hg above for the arm.
        (3) The duration of safe tourniquet inflation is generally believed to be less than 2 hours; it may be extended longer with 5 minutes of intermittent perfusion.
        (4) Transient systemic metabolic acidosis and increased $PaCO_2$ (1 to 8 mm Hg) may follow tourniquet deflation.
        (5) Tourniquet pain is a potential complication—frequently described as a dull ache, the intensity of which increases until it becomes unbearable.
            (*a*) The induction of general anesthesia is often necessary, especially if it occurs early in the procedure.
            (*b*) The only efficacious treatment of tourniquet pain is releasing the pressure of the cuff.
    d) *Emergence:* Usually extubated in the operating room, unless there was preoperative respiratory compromise.

5. Postoperative Concerns
    a) Pain is usually minimal to moderate, unless reconstruction was performed.
        (1) Intra-articular injections of local anesthetics and/or opioids are now widely used in an attempt to provide postoperative analgesia.
        (2) Inadequate pain control can lead to decreased mobility and increase incidence of postoperative complications
    b) Swelling/edema—assess capillary refill in the affected extremity and avoid over hydration intraoperatively.
    c) Nerve damage—assess neurologic function after surgery

PART 2 Common Procedures

IX

Head and Neck

A. Thyroidectomy

1. **Introduction**
   Hyperthyroidism results from excess secretion of T_3 and T_4 by the thyroid gland. Subtotal thyroidectomy may be used in the treatment of hyperthyroidism as an alternative to prolonged medical therapy. Extensive but incomplete removal of the thyroid gland induces remission in most patients.

2. **Preoperative assessment and patient preparation**
   a) *History and physical examination: Individualized*
      (1) *Respiratory:* Palpate the thyroid gland to determine its size and relationship to the trachea.
      (2) *Cardiac:* Assess the heart rate, blood pressure, and electrocardiogram.
   b) *Diagnostic tests*
      (1) Complete blood count, electrolytes, glucose, blood urea nitrogen, creatinine, Ca^{2+}, electrocardiography, chest radiography
      (2) Radiographs may be needed to visualize the trachea and thyroid gland.
      (3) Tests specific to the thyroid gland—T_3, T_4, and thyroid stimulating hormone levels
   c) *Preoperative medication and intravenous therapy*
      (1) Maintain euthyroid state and control hyperkinetic circulation. Propylthiouracil, methimazole, potassium iodide, and β-adrenergic antagonists may be used.
      (2) Continue all antithyroid medications.
      (3) Normal thyroid function tests and a resting heart rate of less than 85 bpm are recommended prior to surgery. If the systolic blood pressure is above 140 mm Hg and the heart rate is above 100 bpm, surgery may be canceled and more antithyroid medication given. With tachycardia associated with cardiac irregularities, surgery may be postponed.
      (4) Give adequate premedication to prevent an increase in sympathetic activity.
      (5) Consider two large bore 16- to 18-gauge intravenous lines. The proximity of surgery to vessels of the neck could necessitate aggressive fluid resuscitation if one is accidentally incised.

3. **Room preparation**
   a) *Monitoring equipment:* Standard
   b) *Pharmacologic agents:* β-adrenergic blockers

   c) *Position:* Supine with the arms tucked at the side; a small pad may be placed between the shoulder blades to hyperextend the neck.

4. Anesthetic technique

   a) *General anesthesia:* Endotracheal intubation is required.

   b) *Goal of anesthetic management:* To achieve a depth of anesthesia that prevents an exaggerated sympathetic response to surgical stimulation and to avoid the administration of medications that stimulate the sympathetic nervous system.

5. Perioperative management

   a) *Induction*

     (1) Awake fiberoptic intubation may be indicated if the gland impinges on the airway.

     (2) An anode tube may be used to decrease the risk of kinking and airway obstruction.

     (3) Lidocaine and narcotics may be used prior to laryngoscopy to blunt the sympathetic nervous system response to intubation. An inhalational agent may be used to increase the depth of anesthesia prior to intubation.

     (4) Induction agent of choice is thiopental due to its antithyroid properties. Avoid ketamine due to its tendency to elicit sympathetic nervous system stimulation.

     (5) Administer muscle relaxants that lack effect on the cardiovascular system.

   b) *Maintenance*

     (1) Inhalational agents or opioids combined with N_2O are recommended to blunt the sympathetic nervous system response to surgical stimulation.

     (2) If the patient is not euthyroid, maintenance of β-blockade is highly desirable.

     (3) The incidence of myasthenia gravis is increased in hyperthyroid patients.

     (4) Treat hypertension with direct acting agents.

     (5) Patients with exophthalmus are susceptible to corneal ulceration and drying. Care must be taken to ensure protection of the eyes.

     (6) Monitor temperature, which may indicate thyroid storm or a hypermetabolic state.

   c) *Emergence*

     (1) Reverse muscle relaxation completely. Use glycopyrrolate (Robinul) rather than atropine (less chronotropic effect) in combination with neostigmine.

     (2) Extubate the patient wide awake with protective reflexes intact. Assess the vocal cords by direct visualization for bilateral or unilateral paralysis from recurrent laryngeal nerve damage.

6. Postoperative considerations

   a) Complications include recurrent laryngeal nerve damage, tracheal compression, hematoma formation, hypoparathyroidism.

   b) Thyroid storm may occur intraoperatively but is more likely in the first 6 to 18 hours after surgery.

PART 2 Common Procedures

(1)   The signs and symptoms include tachycardia, hyperthermia, congestive heart failure, dehydration, shock, full bounding pulse, hypertension, atrial fibrillation, sweating, tremors, vomiting, and diarrhea.

(2)   Treatment must be instituted immediately due to the high mortality associated with thyroid storm and should be aimed at both the symptoms and precipitating cause.

(3)   β-blockers (e.g., propranolol or esmolol) are given to control heart rate and blood pressure,

(4)   Sodium iodide or ipodate helps in reducing the size and activity of the thyroid gland.

(5)   Antithyroid drugs (e.g., propylthiouracil or methimazole) should be given several hours prior to the iodides to prevent accumulation in the thyroid gland.

(6)   Steroids may also be given.

(7)   Other supportive measures should be aimed at maintaining optimal oxygen levels, cooling the patient, and keeping the patient relaxed.

(8)   Aspirin should be avoided for temperature control because of its tendency to remove T_4 from its carrier protein.

B. Parathyroidectomy

1.   **Introduction**
Primary hyperparathyroidism results from excessive secretion of Parathyroid hormone due to benign parathyroid adenomas (89% of cases), hyperplasia (9%), or parathyroid carcinoma (2%). Symptoms result from accompanying hypercalcemia. Definitive treatment requires surgical removal of the adenoma or malignant gland. Hyperplasia of all four glands is treated by excision of all parathyroid tissue except half of one gland. Parathyroidectomy may be indicated in some cases of secondary hyperparathyroidism.

2.   **Preoperative assessment and patient preparation**

a)   Assess for clinical manifestations of hypercalcemia. Renal, cardiac, and central nervous system abnormalities are associated with chronic hypercalcemia.

b)   Laboratory tests should include a current C^{2+} level. Consider hemoglobin and hematocrit, electrolytes, magnesium, phosphate, blood urea nitrogen, creatinine, electrocardiography, and radiography.

c)   Correct volume status and electrolyte irregularities. Hypercalcemia can cause nausea and vomiting; subsequently, these patients may be markedly dehydrated and anorexic. Hypercalcemia can cause nephrogenic diabetes insipidus, thus inhibiting urine concentration by the kidneys. The resultant polyuria can compound the problem of dehydration.

    d) Elevated Ca^{2+} levels may be lowered initially with intravenous normal saline and furosemide. Emergency treatment is necessary with levels greater than 15 mg/dL. Treatment includes intravenous phosphates, mithramycin, calcitonin, glucocorticoids, and dialysis.

3. Room preparation
    a) Standard tabletop setup
    b) Supine position with arms tucked at the side; a small pad may be placed between the shoulder blades to hyperextend the neck. The operating table may be tilted to elevate the head and decrease bleeding.
    c) Consider two large (16-gauge) intravenous lines. The proximity of surgery to vessels of the neck could necessitate aggressive fluid resuscitation if one is accidentally incised. Vigorous fluid therapy is indicated to correct hypervolemia and dilute the hypercalcemia. Volume frequently is contracted.

4. Perioperative management and anesthetic technique
General anesthesia is the usual choice. Rarely is this surgery performed using local anesthetic with sedation.

5. Considerations
    a) Avoid hypoventilation as acidosis increases ionized Ca^{2+}.
    b) Renal dysfunction coexists; adjust anesthetic techniques accordingly.
    c) Somnolence before induction may decrease anesthetic requirements.
    d) The response to muscle relaxants may be altered. A nerve stimulator is important. The patient may be sensitive to succinylcholine and resistant to a nondepolarizer. Use caution with long-acting muscle relaxants if the surgeon wants to test nerve function.
    e) Osteoporosis predisposes patients to vertebral compression during laryngoscopy and to bone fractures during transport. Position the patient gently to avoid pathologic fractures.
    f) Monitor the electrocardiogram for short QT interval and prolonged PR interval.

6. Postoperative considerations
    a) Complications include recurrent laryngeal nerve damage, bleeding, and transit or complete hypoparathyroidism.
    b) Patients with significant preoperative bone disease may develop decreased calcium (hungry bone syndrome); therefore, monitor serum Ca^{2+}, magnesium, and phosphorous levels closely.

C. Tracheotomy

1. Introduction
A tracheotomy is an incision into the trachea to form a temporary or permanent opening, the latter of which is called a tracheostomy. The

incision is made through the second, third, or fourth tracheal ring, and a tube is inserted through the opening to allow passage of air and the removal of tracheobronchial secretions. Except in cases of head, neck, and face trauma, a tracheotomy is rarely performed as an emergency procedure.

2. **Preoperative assessment and patient preparation**
    a) *History and physical examination:* These patients may or may not be already intubated. If not intubated, the patient's airway should be carefully assessed. Information regarding any abnormal pathology that may make intubation difficult should be sought from the surgeon or reports from specific tests such as triple endoscopy. If intubated, the patient's respiratory status and the following should be assessed: vent settings, peak airway pressures, respiratory rate, amount and color of tracheal secretions, need for and frequency of suctioning, lung sounds, arterial blood gases, chest radiography, and presence of pulmonary infections.
    b) *Diagnostic tests*
        (1) Electrocardiography, chest radiography
        (2) Laboratory tests: as indicated by the patient's medical condition
    c) *Preoperative medication and intravenous therapy*
        (1) Preoperative medication as tolerated by patient.
        (2) One 16- or 18-gauge intravenous line. with minimal fluid replacement

3. **Room preparation**
    a) *Monitoring*
        (1) Routine, central venous pressure or pulmonary arterial catheter, as well as an arterial line as indicated by patient's history.
        (2) If peak airway pressures are greater than 60 mm Hg, may need a vent from the intensive care unit.
        (3) A sterile 6-inch connector to attach endotracheal tube to vent or sterile circuit.
        (4) Consider a bronchial adapter. Patients frequently have a bronchoscopy adapter after tracheotomy placement.
        (5) Warming modalities
    b) *Pharmacologic agents:* No special considerations

4. **Anesthetic technique**
    Use general anesthesia and skeletal muscle paralysis or local anesthesia.

5. **Perioperative management**
    a) *Induction:* If a difficult airway is anticipated, awake fiberoptic intubation should be performed. The surgeon should be on standby for an emergency tracheotomy in the event that intubation attempts are unsuccessful. If the patient is already intubated, titrate anesthetic agents to the patient's need.
    b) *Maintenance*
        (1) Adjust the O_2/air mixture to maintain saturation at greater than 95%.
        (2) If the patient is stable, N_2O, an inhalation agent, and a

narcotic may be introduced.
(3) Avoid 100% O_2 as this increases the chance of airway fires.
(4) If an airway fire occurs:
   (*a*) Pour saline into the pharynx to absorb the heat.
   (*b*) Temporarily discontinue the O_2 source.
   (*c*) Extubate and reintubate with a new endotracheal tube.
   (*d*) Follow up with chest radiography, bronchoscopy, steroids, and blood gases.
(5) Maintain constant communication with the surgeon! Use a team approach. Use hand ventilation with 100% O_2 during insertion of the tracheotomy tube. The surgeon will ask the anesthesia provider to gently pull back the OET prior to insertion of the tracheostomy tube.
c) *Emergence*
   (1) The patient may be transferred to the intensive care unit after the procedure. The nondepolarizing muscle relaxant may not have to be reversed if prolonged ventilation is planned.
   (2) 100% O_2 via ambu bag, monitoring devices functioning, returned to unit
6. **Postoperative implications**
   a) Assess patients for any symptoms suggesting pneumothorax, pneumomediastinum, cardiac tamponade, hemorrhage, and subcutaneous emphysema.
   b) Suction the airway as often as necessary to maintain airway and remove secretions.

D. Laryngectomy

1. **Introduction**
Most cancers of the upper respiratory tract are squamous cell carcinomas. When the laryngeal musculature or cartilage is invaded, a total laryngectomy is performed. Intractable aspiration, with resultant pneumonia that has been unresponsive to other treatments, is another indication for laryngectomy.

A total laryngectomy involves removal of the vallecula and includes the posterior third of the tongue if necessary. Surgical exposure is from the hyoid bone to the clavicle. A tracheostomy is performed, and an anode tube is placed. The larynx is usually transected just above the hyoid bone. The trachea is brought out to the skin as a tracheostomy without the need for an endotracheal tube or tracheostomy tube as the pharynx is closed.

A supraglottic laryngectomy leaves the true cords by resection of the larynx from the ventricle to the base of the tongue. Surgical exposure is similar to that for a total laryngectomy. The specimen includes the epiglottis, the false vocal cords, the supraglottic lesions, and a portion of the base of the tongue. The thyroid perichondrium is approximated to the base of the tongue along with the strap muscles for closure. A temporary tracheostomy is required.

A hemilaryngectomy or vertical partial laryngectomy retains the epiglottis but involves removal of a unilateral true and false cord. Surgical exposure is similar to that of supraglottic laryngectomy, and a tracheostomy is required.

A near total laryngectomy involves removal of the entire larynx. One arytenoid is used to construct a phonatory shunt for speaking. A permanent or temporary tracheostomy is created, and the procedure may be combined with neck dissection and pharyngectomy with flap reconstruction.

2. **Preoperative assessment**

Most patients will be older and have a long history of tobacco and alcohol abuse. Associated medical problems may include chronic obstructive pulmonary disease, hypertension, coronary artery disease, and alcohol withdrawal.

a) *History and physical examination:* Individualized

   (1) *Respiratory:* Smoking (more than 40 packs/year) is associated with bronchitis, pulmonary emphysema, and chronic obstructive pulmonary disease, which impair respiratory function. Arterial blood gases may reveal CO_2 retention and hypoxemia. Pulmonary function tests demonstrate decreased forced expiratory volume, forced vital capacity, and the ratio of forced expiratory volume to forced vital capacity. Preoperative airway assessment is imperative because edema may distort airway anatomy, and tumor and edema may cause airway compromise. Tracheal deviation must be considered. Fibrosis, edema, and scarring from prior radiation therapy may distort the airway as well.

   (2) Assess for signs of alcohol withdrawal (altered mental status, tremulousness, and increased sympathetic activity).

   (3) *Gastrointestinal:* Weight loss, malnutrition, dehydration, and electrolyte imbalance can be significant.

   (4) *Hematologic:* Anemias or coagulopathies may be present.

b) *Patient preparation*

   (1) *Laboratory tests:* Baseline arterial blood gases, electrolytes, hemoglobin, hematocrit, prothrombin time, partial thromboplastin time, and, if indicated from the history and physical examination, hepatic function tests

   (2) *Diagnostic tests:* Chest radiography, electrocardiography, pulmonary function test, echocardiography, and stress tests as indicated from the history and physical examination. Indirect and direct laryngoscopies preoperatively and review of computed tomography may help in planning intubation.

   (3) *Medications:* Treatment with a long-acting hypnotic, such as chlordiazepoxide or diazepam, as a precaution for delirium tremens can be considered, unless sedation would be

contraindicated because of concerns of airway compromise. An intravenous antisialagogue (glycopyrrolate 0.2 mg) facilitates endoscopy by the surgeon.

3. **Room preparation**
   a) *Monitoring equipment*
      (1) Standard monitoring equipment
      (2) Foley catheter
      (3) Arterial line—useful for serial laboratory and arterial blood gas studies
      (4) Central venous pressure—if indicated by coexisting disease (prefer basilic/cephalic vein)
   b) *Additional equipment*
      (1) Regular operating table—may be turned 180 degrees
      (2) Extension tubes
      (3) Fluid warmer and humidifier
      (4) Fiberoptic laryngoscope with anticipated difficult airway or potential for airway obstruction
      (5) Tracheostomy under local anesthesia occasionally is necessary for severe airway management.
   c) *Drugs*
      (1) Standard emergency drugs
      (2) Standard tabletop
      (3) Intravenous fluids
      (4) Two 16-to 18-gauge or larger intravenous lines with normal saline/lactated Ringer's solution at 3 to 5 mL/kg/hour
      (5) Sudden large blood losses do not occur; transfusion usually is not necessary.

4. **Perioperative management and anesthetic technique**
   a) General endotracheal anesthesia
   b) *Induction:* Standard intravenous induction is appropriate with a normal airway. The choice of an induction drug should be based on the patient's medical condition. If airway difficulty is possible, direct laryngoscopy can be performed while the patient is breathing spontaneously, and a muscle relaxant may be administered once the glottis is visualized. In more difficult cases, awake intubation or fiberoptic laryngoscopy may be required.
   c) *Maintenance:* Supine position, head elevated 30 degrees; standard maintenance, considering the patient's preexisting medical problems. An inhalation agent and supplemental narcotics will benefit patients with reactive airway disease. Use of nondepolarizing muscle relaxants should be discussed with the surgeon because nerve stimulation for facial nerve localization may be performed.
   d) *Emergence:* Many patients undergo tracheostomy. If no tracheostomy is performed, the amount of airway edema and distortion needs to be discussed with the surgeon prior to determining extubation. A gradual emergence with stable hemodynamic parameters is an important consideration in the patient with coronary artery disease.

5. **Postoperative implications**

a) Injury to the facial nerve can cause facial droop. Recurrent laryngeal nerve injury can result in vocal cord dysfunction; diaphragmatic paralysis may result from phrenic nerve injury.

b) Pneumothorax may occur with low-neck dissection.

c) Airway impingement is due to restrictive neck dressings or hematoma development.

d) Communication difficulties following laryngectomy

E. Radical Neck Dissection

1. **Introduction**
   Neck dissection is often performed when there is local tumor extension. A radical neck dissection involves a complete cervical lymphadenectomy with resection of the sternocleidomastoid muscle, internal jugular vein, and select cranial nerves. A functional neck dissection is a complete cervical lymphadenectomy, preserving the sternocleidomastoid muscle, internal jugular vein, and select cranial nerves. A modified neck dissection is a variation between a radical neck dissection and a functional neck dissection. Neck dissections are usually combined with resection of the primary lesions, such as those of the tongue, pharynx, and larynx. In a composite resection, a radical neck dissection, normally done first, is followed by a partial mandibulectomy and possibly a partial glossectomy. A tracheostomy is almost always performed with these resections.

   Usually, one or two neck incisions, occasionally extending vertically to expose the neck from the mandible to the clavicle, are performed. The accessory nerve (XI), hypoglossal nerve (XII), and lingual nerves are identified and preserved. The sternocleidomastoid muscle, internal jugular vein, and submental triangle may or may not be resected. Drains are placed posteriorly, and the wound is closed in layers.

2. **Preoperative assessment**
   Most patients will be older and have a long history of tobacco and alcohol abuse. Associated medical problems may include chronic obstructive pulmonary disease, hypertension, coronary artery disease, malnourishment, and alcohol withdrawal.

   a) History and physical examination: See "Laryngectomy," p. 293.

   b) Patient preparation: See "Laryngectomy," p. 293.

3. **Room preparation**

   a) Monitoring equipment

   (1) Standard monitoring equipment

   (2) Foley catheter

   (3) Arterial line—useful for serial laboratory and arterial blood gas studies

   (4) Central venous pressure line—if indicated by coexisting disease (prefer basilic/cephalic vein)

  b) *Additional equipment*
    (1) Regular operating table turned 180 degrees
    (2) Extension tubes
    (3) Fluid warmer and humidifier
    (4) Fiberoptic laryngoscope with anticipated difficult airway or potential for airway obstruction
    (5) Tracheostomy under local anesthesia occasionally is necessary for severe airway management.
  c) *Drugs*
    (1) Standard emergency drugs
    (2) Standard tabletop
    (3) *Intravenous fluids:* two 16- to 18-gauge or larger intravenous lines with normal saline or lactated Ringer's solution at 3 to 5 mL/kg/hour. Uncontrolled bleeding of the internal jugular vein at the skull base is rare but can result in sudden significant blood losses.
4. **Perioperative management and anesthetic technique**
  a) General endotracheal anesthesia
  b) *Induction:* Standard intravenous induction is appropriate with a normal airway. The choice of an induction drug should be based on the patient's medical condition. If airway difficulty is possible, direct laryngoscopy can be performed while the patient is breathing spontaneously, and a muscle relaxant may be administered once the glottis is visualized. In more difficult cases, awake intubation or fiberoptic laryngoscopy may be required.
  c) *Maintenance:* Supine position, head turned to the opposite side; pillow below the shoulders; standard maintenance, considering the patient's preexisting medical problems. An inhalation agent and supplemental narcotics benefit patients with reactive airway disease. Use of nondepolarizing muscle relaxants should be discussed with the surgeon, because nerve stimulation for cranial nerve (XI) localization may be done. With right radical neck dissection, a prolonged QT interval on the electrocardiogram can progress to ventricular dysrhythmia and even cardiac arrest. These changes are due to interruption of cervical sympathetic outflow to the heart via the right stellate ganglion. The left cardiac sympathetic fibers most likely have different effects on cardiac excitability because prolongation of the QT interval does not occur after left radical neck dissection. Manipulation of the carotid sinus during dissection can result in hypotension and cardiac dysrhythmia. Treatment includes cessation of manipulation and, if necessary, infiltration of surrounding tissues with a local anesthetic or administration of intravenous atropine. Unexplained hypotension or dysrhythmia may indicate venous air embolism via large open neck veins. *Treatment:* Give 100% O_2, notify the surgeon, flood the field with normal saline, place the head down, aspirate air through the central venous pressure line, increase venous pressure via positive-pressure ventilation, and administer circulatory support as required.
  d) *Emergence:* Many patients undergo tracheostomy. If no

tracheostomy is performed, the amount of airway edema and distortion needs to be discussed with the surgeon prior to determining extubation. A gradual emergence with stable hemodynamic parameters is an important consideration in the patient with coronary artery disease.

5. **Postoperative implications**
   a) Injury to the facial nerve can cause facial droop. Recurrent laryngeal nerve injury can result in vocal cord dysfunction, and diaphragmatic paralysis may result from phrenic nerve injury.
   b) Painful shoulder syndrome
   c) Pneumothorax may occur with low-neck dissection.
   d) Airway impingement is due to restrictive neck dressings or hematoma development.
   e) Communication difficulties after laryngectomy

F. Maxillofacial Trauma

1. **Introduction**
   Two common etiologies for facial fractures are fights and gunshot wounds. Because of the forces required to cause facial fractures, other traumas (e.g., subdural hematoma, pneumothorax, cervical spine injury, and intra-abdominal bleeding) often occur with these fractures. These patients are at increased risk for aspiration and should be considered as having full stomachs. Therefore securing of the airway is of utmost importance. Rapid sequence intubation should be done on these patients, provided the nature of their injuries will allow for this. Airway management can be difficult because of soft tissue injury to the tongue or airway. A tracheostomy under local or awake intubation should be strongly considered if any doubt exists about securing the airway. Nasal intubation is usually indicated for mandible or maxillary fractures, because at the end of the procedure intermaxillary fixation is performed. The surgeon may require monitoring of the facial nerve; if so, muscle relaxants are contraindicated. The surgical approach depends on the type and complexity of the fracture. Approach can vary from reduction for nasal fractures to the Caldwell Luc approach for extensive maxillary bone fractures. Intermaxillary fixation may be required for zygomatic and maxillary fractures. Mandibular fractures are usually reduced and fixed with wires or plates.

2. **Preoperative assessment**
   a) *Respiratory/airway management:* The extent of fractures is evaluated to determine appropriate airway management. Fractures of the middle face are not usually nasally intubated. Access to the oropharynx may be difficult with mandibular fractures. An urgent tracheostomy is indicated for massive facial trauma.
   b) *Neurologic:* Thorough documentation of any neurologic deficits

and review CT scan if head injury is suspected. Potential for meningitis is possible postoperatively.

c) *Musculoskeletal:* Careful positioning is imperative, with special consideration for other trauma-related injuries. C-spine and CT scans should be reviewed to rule out cervical fracture if suspected.

d) *Laboratory tests:* Hematocrit and others as indicated from the history and physical examination

e) Standard premedication for neurologically intact patients

3. **Room preparation**

a) *Monitoring equipment:* Standard; invasive monitoring may be needed for intracranial or other trauma.

b) *Additional equipment:* Regular operating table; some surgeons like the table turned 90 or 180 degrees or to have extension tubings available for the circuit.

c) *Drugs*
   (1) Standard emergency drugs
   (2) Standard tabletop
   (3) *Intravenous fluids:* one 16- to 18-gauge intravenous tube (the patient may have significant blood loss with maxillary repairs); normal saline/lactated ringer's solution at 6 to 8 mL/kg/hour for trauma-related injuries or 2 to 4 mL/kg/hour if surgery is elective. If the fracture is trauma-related and intracranial injury is suspected, solutions containing dextrose should be avoided, as this can increase cerebral edema.

4. **Perioperative management and anesthetic technique**

a) General endotracheal anesthesia

b) *Induction:* Awake fiberoptic laryngoscopy should be performed if any doubt exists concerning the ease of intubation. For patients with LeFort (mandibular or maxillary) fractures, nasal intubation is preferred. Patients with nasal, orbital, or zygomatic fractures are usually orally intubated. Standard induction is appropriate for patients having elective surgery who have normal airways and whose NPO status can be determined. Trauma patients should be considered with full stomachs, and induction should be performed using a rapid sequence technique. Nasal or oral rae endotracheal tubes are used to optimize the surgical field. If these patients arrive at the operating room already intubated, proper endotracheal tube placement should be confirmed.

c) *Maintenance:* Muscle relaxation is usually required. An antiemetic is helpful for patients who will have their jaws banded or wired together.
   (1) Standard maintenance
   (2) *Position:* Supine; check and pad all pressure points; abduct arms less than 90 degrees to avoid overstretching of brachial plexus.

d) *Emergence:* Suction oropharynx carefully to avoid aspiration. Verify that any packs are removed prior to emergence. Patients with difficult airways or wired jaws should be fully awake and

PART 2   Common Procedures

have protective reflexes before extubation. Wire cutters should be at the bedside at all times. Depending on the amount of trauma and soft tissue swelling, the patient may require extended intubation and ventilation postoperatively.

5. **Postoperative implications**
   a) Due to the possibility of airway obstruction, wire cutters should be available at all times for airway management. A throat pack may be obstructing the airway.
   b) Aggressive treatment of nausea and vomiting is imperative.
   c) Pain management includes intravenous narcotics and antiemetics as needed.

G. Tonsillectomy and Adenoidectomy

1. **Introduction**
   Tonsil and adenoid surgery are among the most common surgical procedures performed in the United States. Such surgery is indicated for the treatment of hypertrophic tonsil and adenoids and recurrent or chronic upper respiratory tract and ear infection.

2. **Preoperative patient assessment and patient preparation**
   a) *History and physical examination*
      (1) *Upper airway:* Externally inspect tonsilar and adenoid hypertrophy. Adenoid hypertrophy can be determined by having the patient breathe with the mouth closed and evaluate the degree of nasal airway obstruction.
      (2) *Oral:* Because most of these procedures are performed in children, careful inspection for loose or missing teeth is necessary.
   b) *Diagnostic tests:* Routine laboratory tests
   c) *Preoperative medication and intravenous therapy*
      (1) Light sedation with benzodiazepine
      (2) Administration of an antisialogogue may assist in improving the surgical view.
      (3) Minimal blood loss is expected, but massive hemorrhage can occur. One large bore intravenous catheter is suitable.

3. **Room preparation**
   a) *Monitoring equipment:* Standard
   b) Pharmacologic agents
      (1) Standard
      (2) Short-acting muscle relaxants may or may not be used for maintenance.
   c) *Position:* Supine, arms tucked to the sides; table turned 90 degrees

4. **Anesthetic technique**
   General anesthesia with endotracheal intubation. The major goals of anesthesia are to provide an adequate depth of anesthesia such that protective reflexes are blunted, rapid return of these reflexes after the

procedure, and adequate postoperative analgesia.

5. **Perioperative management**

   a) *Induction:* Nonspecific intubation with an oral rae endotracheal tube is beneficial but not necessary. Confirm the surgeon's preference in type of tube and placement after intubation.

   b) *Maintenance:* Nonspecific; the use of short-acting agents is suggested. Muscle relaxants may or may not be used. If used, they must be completely reversed prior to extubation. Close monitoring of breath sounds is essential. The tube can easily be dislodged during placement of a mouth gag or during manipulation of the patient's head.

   c) *Emergence*

   (1) Prior to the end of surgery, the surgeon may release the mouth gag to ensure hemostasis. At this time, an orogastric tube should be inserted gently by the surgeon or anesthesia provider, and the stomach decompressed. Extubate awake after careful suction of oral pharynx with tonsil suction. Never suction the nasopharynx after adenoidectomy. Gently suction the oropharynx. The airway should be free from blood and secretions before extubation is performed.

   (2) Maintain the patient in a head down Sim's position (also referred to as the "tonsil position") to facilitate drainage of secretions.

6. **Postoperative implications**

   Postoperative bleeding is the most significant complication. This usually happens 4 to 9 hours or 5 to 10 days postoperatively (the latter time frame is usually due to infection). These patients should be rehydrated and transfused if necessary. The extent of bleeding is often hidden because of swallowing of blood. Rapid sequence induction should be performed due to the presence of swallowed blood, as these patients should always be considered as having full stomachs.

H. Nasal Surgery

1. **Introduction**

   Nasal surgery is performed for cosmetic reasons, to restore the caliber of the nasal airway, or sometimes for both reasons. Whether for rhinoplasty, septoplasty, or septorhinoplasty, the nasal cavity can be anesthetized by placing 4% cocaine-soaked pledgets up each nostril for 5 to 10 minutes. To ensure vasoconstriction and minimize bleeding, the site is infiltrated with 1.0% lidocaine and 1:100,000 epinephrine.

   An incision is made in the septum down to the cartilage, and a submucoperichondral flap is elevated. This may be repeated on the contralateral side. Bone and cartilaginous deformities are resected or weakened either on the face, or they are removed first, shaped, then replaced. Once the surgeon is satisfied with the resection, the incision is closed with an absorbable suture. In rhinoplasty, depending on the area needing work, the nasal contours can be remodeled by tip remodeling, humps can be reduced, bone osteotomies can be

PART 2 Common Procedures

performed to shape the contour of the nose, or combinations thereof. After surgery, both nasal cavities are packed, and external splints may be used.

2. **Preoperative assessment and patient preparation**

   Generally, these procedures are elective and can be performed on an outpatient basis. It is important to identify patients with obstructive apnea. These patients often have chronic airway obstruction, redundant pharyngeal tissues, or both. Such patients, as well as asthmatic patients, should undergo arterial blood gas and pulmonary function testing. Ketorolac and acetylsalicylic acid should be avoided in patients who also have nasal polyps, because they often are hypersensitive to acetylsalicylic acid, a condition that can precipitate bronchospasm.

   a) *History and physical examination:* Carefully evaluate cardiovascular status because the use of local vasoconstrictors may cause dysrhythmia, coronary artery spasm, hypertension, and seizures.

   b) Patient preparation

   (1) *Laboratory tests:* As indicated by the history and physical examination

   (2) *Diagnostic tests:* As indicated by the history and physical examination

   (3) Standard premedication

3. **Room preparation**

   a) *Monitoring equipment:* Standard

   b) *Additional equipment:* Regular operating table; the table is turned 90 to 180 degrees. Have an anesthesia circuit extension available.

   c) *Drugs*

   (1) Standard emergency

   (2) Standard tabletop

   d) *Intravenous fluids:* Two 18-gauge lines with normal saline/lactated Ringer's solution at 4 to 6 mL/kg/hour

4. **Perioperative management and anesthetic technique**

   Use general endotracheal or local anesthesia with sedation; the choice depends on the preferences of the surgeon and the patient, as well as on the acetylsalicylic acid status of the patient.

   a) *Induction:* Routine. Use of an oral rae endotracheal tube is convenient for the surgeon but is not necessary. If sedation technique is chosen, short-acting agents are best because these procedures are usually minor, and patients are usually sent home.

   b) *Maintenance:* Routine

   c) *Emergence:* Counsel patients that nose will be packed with bandaging and possibly splinted, so mouth breathing will be necessary on awakening.

5. **Postoperative implications**

   Elevate head of bed. Nasal packing and swallowed blood may contribute to postoperative nausea and vomiting. Mild analgesics after discharge are usually sufficient.

I. LeFort Procedures

1. **Introduction**
   a) The usual preoperative diagnosis for patients with maxillary fractures is facial trauma. LeFort fractures are frequently associated with other skull fractures, zygoma fractures, and possible intracranial fractures and thus with cerebrospinal fluid rhinorrhea.
   b) Maxillary fractures are grouped by the LeFort system:
      (1) *Type 1*—horizontal fracture separating the teeth and maxillary components from the upper facial structures
      (2) *Type 2* (*pyramidal*)—triangular fracture across the ethmoid and the nose through the intraorbital rims and extending to the entire maxillary structure
      (3) *Type 3* (*craniofacial dysfunction*)—essentially, the cranium and face are dissociated. Common coexisting injuries include cerebral contusions, intracranial hemorrhage, and cervical spine trauma.

2. **Preoperative assessment and patient preparation**
   The airway is a priority. If the airway cannot be managed, emergency intubation becomes necessary. Avoid blind nasal intubation in patients with cerebrospinal fluid rhinorrhea, periorbital edema, "raccoon's eyes" bruising, or other evidence of nasopharyngeal trauma.
   a) *Neurologic:* Document any neurologic deficit; intracranial trauma may require invasive monitoring.
   b) *Laboratory tests:* Hematocrit and any other tests as indicated by the history and physical examination

3. **Room preparation**
   a) *Monitoring equipment:* Standard
   b) *Additional equipment:* Fiberoptic cart
   c) *Drugs*
      (1) Standard emergency
      (2) Standard tabletop
   d) *Intravenous fluids:* one 18-gauge line with normal saline/lactated Ringer's solution at 6 to 8 mL/kg/hour

4. **Perioperative management and anesthetic technique**
   a) General endotracheal anesthesia
   b) *Induction:* Fiberoptic laryngoscopy should be performed if there is any doubt about the ease of intubation. Patients with mandibular and maxillary (LeFort I and II) fractures should undergo intubation. Patients with nasal orbital or zygomatic fractures usually are intubated orally. Consider using anode or rae endotracheal tubes. A LeFort type II or III fracture is a relative contraindication for nasal intubation or nasogastric tube placement.
   c) *Maintenance:* Muscle relaxation is usually required. Consider the prophylactic use of antiemetics for patients with wired jaws.
   d) *Position:* Supine; check and pad pressure points. Avoid stretching

the brachial plexus, and limit abduction to 90 degrees. Protect eyes with ophthalmic ointment.

e) *Emergence:* Extubation should be performed when the patient is fully awake in the case of difficult airway or wired jaws. A wire cutter should be available at all times. Verify that throat packing has been removed before extubating. Patients with facial or airway swelling and those involved in multiple trauma may need continued postoperative intubation and ventilation.

5. **Postoperative implications**
   a) For airway obstruction, wire cutters must be available.
   b) Aggressive treatment of nausea and vomiting is important.
   c) Pain management narcotics—antiemetics as needed
   d) Cerebrospinal fluid leak

J. Uvulopalatopharyngoplasty (UPPP)

1. **Introduction**
   Uvulopalatopharyngoplasty is performed primarily for the treatment of obstructive sleep apnea. A tonsillectomy is often performed concurrently. Nasopharyngeal airway obstruction is relieved by removing redundant and obstructing tissues of the posterior pharynx.

   Inspiratory muscle tone is lost during rapid eye movement sleep, resulting in relaxation of the pharyngeal muscles, thus creating airway obstruction. Adults with obstructive sleep apnea are often obese.

2. **Preoperative assessment**
   a) *History and physical examination*
   (1) *Cardiac:* Hypoxia and hypercapnia may lead to pulmonary hypertension, cor pulmonale, cardiac arrhythmias, and failure of the left side of the heart.
   (2) *Respiratory:* Frequent nocturnal arousals (up to 50 times per hour) are common. Periods of apnea may last up to 2 to 3 minutes. These patients often have a long history of snoring.
   (3) *Neurologic:* Loss of rapid eye movement sleep results in excess daytime somnolence, fatigue, and impaired judgment.
   b) *Patient preparation:* Medical management includes weight reduction in obese patients, decreasing alcohol consumption, and nasal continuous positive airway pressure.
   (1) *Laboratory tests:* As indicated by the history and physical examination
   (2) *Diagnostic tests:* As indicated by the history and physical examination
   (3) *Medications:* Use minimal preoperative narcotics or sedatives because these patients have heightened sensitivity to them. Anticholinergics are helpful to decrease secretions.

3. **Room preparation**

    a) Standard monitoring equipment
    b) *Additional equipment:* airway adjuncts, difficult airway cart
    c) Positioning devices
    d) Operating room table—ensure appropriate weight limit
    e) *Drugs*
        (1) *Intravenous fluids:* 0.9% normal saline or lactated Ringer's solution, 4 mL/km/hour via an 18-gauge intravenous line.
        (2) Blood—type and screen
        (3) Tabletop—rapid sequence induction setup

4. Perioperative management and anesthetic technique
    a) *Induction*
        (1) Awake fiberoptic laryngoscopy and intubation may be indicated.
        (2) Inhalation with maintenance of spontaneous respiration and succinylcholine only after visualization of the larynx.
        (3) Intravenous rapid sequence induction after 3 to 4 minutes of preoxygenation, cricoid pressure, and elevation of the head of the bed.
    b) *Maintenance*
        (1) Inhalation agent: isoflurane or desflurane
        (2) 50% O_2 (may require high fractional inspired oxygen)
        (3) Rose position: Supine, shoulder roll, head extension
        (4) Operating table turned 90 to 180 degrees
    c) *Emergence*
        (1) Lidocaine 1 to 1.5 mg/kg before extubation
        (2) As with tonsillectomy, the surgeon may release the mouth gag to see if there is any uncontrolled bleeding. At this time, patients should have an orogastric tube placed, and the stomach should be suctioned. The nasal and oropharynx should also be gently suctioned and care taken not to dislodge any clots that may precipitate bleeding and incur laryngospasm
        (3) *Extubation criteria*
            (a) Patient is awake, alert, and following verbal commands
            (b) Adequate muscle relaxant reversal
            (c) Acceptable respiratory mechanics

5. Postoperative implications
    a) Head of the bed is elevated
    b) Humidified oxygen
    c) Hemoglobin and hematocrit if blood loss was excessive
    d) Careful titration of narcotics

6. Postoperative complications
    Airway obstruction due to swelling is the most common postoperative complication from a Uvulopalatopharyngoplasty. Typically, a patient will receive a dose of steroids intraoperatively to aid in reducing this swelling. Patients who have this procedure usually will be admitted to the hospital where their respiratory and airway status may be monitored carefully. If the tonsils have been removed, the possibility of rebleeding must also be considered.

K. Ocular Procedures

OPEN EYE

1. **Introduction**
   Intraocular pressure (IOP) is determined by the balance between production and drainage of aqueous humor and by changes in choroidal blood volume. Resistance to outflow of aqueous humor in the trabecular tissue maintains IOP within physiologic range. Normal IOP is 12 to 16 mm Hg in the upright posture and increases by 2 to 3 mm Hg in the supine position.
   When the globe is open, the IOP is equal to ambient pressure. If the volume of choroid and vitreous should increase while the eye is opened, the vitreous may be lost. Any deformation of the eye by external pressure on the globe will cause an apparent increase in intraocular volume.

2. **Preoperative assessment and patient preparation**
   a) *History and physical examination:* Standard; the patient may come in as an emergency with full stomach; ensure no other injuries.
   b) *Diagnostic and laboratory tests:* As indicated by the history and physical examination
   c) *Preoperative medication and intravenous therapy*
      (1) Aspiration prophylaxis
      (2) Atropine or glycopyrrolate reduces oral secretions and may inhibit the oculocardiac reflex.
      (3) Avoid narcotics—may cause nausea and vomiting.
      (4) Sedatives in preoperative hold area, titrated to effect
      (5) One 18-gauge intravenous tube with minimal fluid replacement

3. **Room preparation**
   a) *Monitoring equipment:* Standard
   b) *Pharmacologic agents:* Standard, lidocaine and atropine
   c) *Position:* Supine; table may be turned for the surgeon's access

4. **Anesthetic technique**
   General anesthesia with endotracheal intubation because a retrobulbar block causes a transient rise in IOP, which may cause intraocular contents to be expelled.

5. **Perioperative management**
   a) *Induction (general)*
      (1) The goal is to avoid increasing IOP.
      (2) When preoxygenating, avoid pressing face mask onto the eyeball.
      (3) Awake intubation is contraindicated because it may cause coughing and bucking.
      (4) Intravenous lidocaine, 1 mg/kg, may alternate coughing and bucking.
      (5) The use of succinylcholine in open eye-globe injuries is controversial. Many practitioners believe that when suc-

cinylcholine has been preceded by pretreatment with a nondepolarizing muscle relaxant and a barbiturate for induction, it is a safe combination for rapid sequence induction in the open eye, full stomach situation.

(6) Induction may be with thiopental plus a large dose of a nondepolarizing muscle relaxant.

(7) Use of ketamine is contraindicated—causes moderate increase in IOP and nystagmus or blepharospasm.

b) *Maintenance*

(1) Inhalation agents cause dose-related decreases in IOP; the degree of IOP reduction is proportional to the depth of anesthesia.

(2) Oculocardiac reflex

(*a*) Caused by traction on the extraocular muscles (medial rectus), ocular manipulation, or manual pressure on the globe.

(*b*) Signs and symptoms are bradycardia and cardiac dysrhythmias.

(*c*) Treatment is to stop surgical stimulus, ensure dysrhythmia is not due to lack of oxygen (via SpO_2 confirmation) or ventilation, and administer atropine if needed.

c) *Emergence*

(1) The goal is smoothness.

(2) Empty the stomach with a nasogastric tube and suction the pharynx while the patient is still paralyzed or deeply anesthetized.

(3) Administer an antiemetic prior to the end of surgery.

(4) Administer lidocaine, 1 mg/kg, to prevent coughing during emergence.

(5) The trachea should be extubated before there is a tendency to cough.

6. **Postoperative implications**

a) Transport the patient to the recovery room with the head up 10 to 20 degrees to facilitate venous drainage from the eye.

b) The patient can be placed on the side with the operative side up.

c) Shivering and pain can increase IOP and should be prevented.

STRABISMUS REPAIR

1. **Introduction**

Strabismus repairs are performed to correct ocular malalignment. This malalignment may be esotropia (eyes deviate inward) or exotropia (eyes deviate outward). This procedure straightens the eyes cosmetically and allows the patient binocular vision by the lengthening or shortening of individual muscles or pairs of muscles. The specific muscles involved are the horizontal rectus and the oblique muscles.

A forced duction test is performed by the surgeon after induction and intubation by manipulating the sclera of the operative eye in order to aid the surgical plan. An incision is made through the conjuctiva in the area of the muscle to be manipulated. The muscle is then isolated and sewn back farther on the globe if the muscle tension is to be increased. If the muscle tension needs to be decreased, a segment of the muscle is removed.

2. **Preoperative assessment**
   Strabismus repair is the most common ophthalmic surgical procedure performed on children. These children are usually otherwise healthy. There is, however, a higher incidence of strabismus in children with cerebral palsy and myelomeningocele with hydrocephalus. Malignant hyperthermia also is more common with children undergoing strabismus repair.
   a) *History and physical examination*
      (1) A careful family history should be obtained preoperatively, including any history of family problems with anesthesia.
      (2) *Respiratory:* For patients with signs and symptoms of an acute respiratory infection, surgery should be postponed because these children are at greater risk for laryngospasm and bronchospasm.
   b) *Patient preparation*
      (1) *Laboratory tests:* As indicated by the history and physical examination. Caffeine and halothane contracture tests may be indicated if the patient is believed to be susceptible to malignant hyperthermia.
      (2) *Diagnostic tests:* As indicated by the history and physical examination
      (3) *Medications:* Midazolam 0.5 to 0.7 mg/kg orally as a premedication

3. **Room preparation**
   a) *Monitoring equipment:* standard monitors
   b) *Additional equipment*
      (1) Standard emergency drugs (including lidocaine and atropine)
      (2) Pediatric standard tabletop
      (3) *Intravenous fluids:* 20- or 22-gauge intravenous tube with normal saline or lactated Ringer's solution at 5 to 10 mL/kg/hour

4. **Perioperative management and anesthetic technique**
   a) *Induction:* General endotracheal anesthesia is the technique of choice. Nondepolarizing muscle relaxants may be used after the forced duction test is performed by the surgeon. Bradycardia is common owing to the oculocardiac reflex, so atropine is commonly used.
   b) *Maintenance:* Routine. Watch for signs and symptoms of malignant hyperthermia.
   c) *Emergence:* Nausea and vomiting are very common.

5. **Postoperative implications**
   Aggressive prophylaxis and treatment of postoperative nausea and vomiting is required. Minimal analgesia is necessary.

INTRAOCULAR PROCEDURES

1. **Introduction**
   Intraocular procedures may refer to vitrectomy, glaucoma drainage, corneal transplant, and open-eye injury. These procedures involve entry into the vitreous humor. It is crucial to avoid increases in IOP with all intraocular procedures.

   The most common of these procedures, a vitrectomy, is performed by making three openings into the vitreous cavity. One of these openings is used to instill balanced salt solution; another is made for insertion of a fiberoptic light. The third opening is made for the insertion of various instruments used to remove abnormal tissue from the vitreous cavity. Frequently, a gas bubble is introduced during vitrectomy to tamponade retinal tears.

2. **Preoperative assessment**
   a) *History and physical examination:* Individualized based on patient's history and medical condition
   b) *Patient preparation*
      (1) *Laboratory and diagnostic tests:* As indicated from the history and physical examination
      (2) *Medications:* Midazolam (1 to 2 mg) may be given intravenously in divided doses as a premedication. The anesthesia provider must be aware that ocular drugs applied topically can have systemic effects. These include hypertension, arrhythmias, nausea and vomiting, agitation, excitement, disorientation, seizures, hypotension, and metabolic acidosis.

3. **Room preparation**
   a) *Monitoring equipment:* Standard
   b) *Additional equipment:* Standard emergency drugs, long breathing circuit (table will be turned), rae endotracheal tubes
   c) *Intravenous fluids:* 18-gauge intravenous line with normal saline or lactated Ringer's solution at 5 to 10 mL/kg/hour.
   d) A hudson hood may be used to provide O_2 to the patient if a regional block with sedation is to be used. Care must be taken if there is any electrocautery, as this will create an O_2-rich environment under the drape.

4. **Perioperative management and anesthetic technique**
   a) These procedures can be done under general anesthesia or under a regional block (retro or peribulbar block) with sedation.
   b) General anesthesia with endotracheal intubation is indicated for infants; young children; patients with severe claustrophobia; patients unable to cooperate, communicate, or lie flat for long periods of time; or patients with a history of acute anxiety attacks.
   c) Most adult patients will do well with a regional block with sedation, which is the preferred anesthetic technique. If this method of anesthesia is used, it is important to determine the patient's response to sedatives/narcotics prior to administration of the block. Once the table is turned and the patient draped, it can be difficult to maintain an airway if necessary. Care must be taken to avoid oversedation. If oversedated, patients tend to be startled

when they arouse and may be confused and move about. A short-acting hypnotic (propofol) may be useful immediately prior to administration of the block. The surgeon does need to have the patient's cooperation during the block, because the surgeon may ask the patient to look from side to side.

d) General endotracheal tube anesthesia is also appropriate.

(1) *Induction:* Standard intravenous induction. Ketamine is not a drug of choice because increased IOP is to be avoided. Care must be taken to avoid pressure on the eyes with the mask. Nondepolarizing muscle relaxants are used for intubation and continued throughout the procedure, titrated to patient response. It is imperative the patient does not move during the procedure. All connections in the breathing circuit should be secured.

(2) *Maintenance:* Continuous intravenous anesthesia is an option. Another option is the use of inhalational agents. N_2O may or may not be used. If used, however, and the surgeon performs a gas-fluid exchange, the N_2O should be discontinued 5 to 10 minutes prior to this exchange. Consider an antiemetic because of the high incidence of postoperative nausea and vomiting.

e) *Emergence:* Smooth emergence and extubation is important. Coughing, bucking, and straining should be avoided to prevent increasing the IOP. Consider deep extubation, although care must be taken not to place pressure on the operative eye with the facemask.

5. **Postoperative implications**
Again, coughing, straining, and bucking should be avoided. The patient may be positioned prone or to one side (as ordered by the surgeon) for correct positioning of the gas bubble. The patient's respiratory status should be ensured before turning the patient postoperatively.

L. Orbital Fractures

1. **Introduction**
Surgical access to the orbit may be needed to repair orbital fractures. The orbit may be divided into several compartments, including the peripheral surgical space, subperiosteal space, central surgical space, and subtenon's space. The approach for orbital wall fractures depends on the location and the pathology involved. The common approach to these fractures is the transperiosteal or extraperiosteal approach. A skin incision is made in the desired quadrant just outside the orbital rim. The periosteum is identified and incised and then resected from the wall and orbital margin.

2. **Preoperative assessment and patient preparation**

    a) *History and physical examination:* Patients are usually healthy aside from the underlying trauma. Evaluation should focus on any coexisting disease and systemic manifestations of the trauma.

    b) *Laboratory tests:* As indicated by the history and physical examination

    c) *Diagnostic tests:* As indicated by the history and physical examination

    d) *Premedication:* Standard

3. **Room preparation**
   a) *Monitoring equipment:* Standard
   b) *Additional equipment:* Regular operating table, which will be turned 90 to 180 degrees; an anesthesia circuit extension must be available.
   c) *Drugs:* Standard emergency and standard tabletop
   d) *Intravenous fluids:* One 18-gauge intravenous line with normal saline/lactated Ringer's solution at 4 to 6 mL/kg/hour

4. **Perioperative management and anesthetic technique**
   a) Use general endotracheal anesthesia.
   b) *Induction:* Standard; an oral rae endotracheal tube may be preferred.
   c) *Maintenance:* Standard; muscle relaxation is not required.
   d) *Position:* Supine; check and pad pressure points. Table is turned 90 degrees; have extension tubes or long tubes for anesthesia circuit. Check the eyes and tape or use ointment (or do both).
   e) *Potential complication:*
       (1) Oculocardiac reflex is triggered by pain, direct pressure on the eye, and pulling on the extrinsic muscle of the eye. It has both trigeminal afferent and vagal efferent pathways. Bradycardia is usual with oculocardiac reflex, although junctional rhythm, atrioventricular block, ventricular premature contractions, ventricular tachycardia, and asystole also occur.
       (2) To treat, tell the surgeon to stop the stimulus, ensure adequate oxygenation and ventilation and administer atropine as needed. Lidocaine infiltration near the eye muscles may help to attenuate the reflex, which is self-limiting (i.e., it will tire itself with repeated manipulations).

5. **Postoperative implications**
   a) For nausea and vomiting, begin prophylactic treatment prior to the end of the surgical procedure.
   b) *Pain management*—parenteral opiates

PART 2 **Common Procedures**

M. Rhytidectomy/Facelift

1. **Introduction**

   Rhytidectomy is a reconstructive plastic procedure in which the skin of the face is tightened, wrinkles (rhytid-) are removed, and the skin is made to appear firm and smooth. In the preoperative area, the surgeon marks where the planned incisions will be made; prior to incision, the surgeon will localize the area. Typically, lidocaine 1% with 1:100,000 epinephrine is infiltrated along the incision lines and lidocaine 0.5% with 1:400,000 epinephrine is infiltrated into the anticipated dissection line.

   The facelift incision begins in the temporal scalp area about 5 cm above the ear and 5 cm behind the hairline, curves down parallel to the hairline toward the superior root and continues caudally in the natural preauricular skin crease. The dissection will begin in the temporal hair-bearing area; dissection continues through temporoparietal fascia, down to the loose areolar layer. The facial nerve branches the facial muscles on their deep surface; dissection during this procedure must be done carefully. The only large sensory nerve that is important is the great auricular nerve. This nerve crosses the surface of the sternocleidomastoid muscle below the caudal edge of the auditory canal and is found posterior to the external jugular.

2. **Preoperative assessment and patient preparation**

   a) *History and physical examination*
      (1) The majority of patients are older and have some effects of aging, but the age range may be anywhere from 40 to 70. Therefore cardiovascular status should be evaluated due to the use of epinephrine in the local anesthetic.
      (2) Due to the inaccessibility of the face to the anesthesia provider and the need for sedation, careful airway evaluation and a history of sleep apnea should be identified.

   b) *Patient preparation*
      (1) *Laboratory tests:* As indicated by the history and physical examination.
      (2) *Diagnostic tests:* ECG if indicated by the history and physical examination.
      (3) *Premedication:* Standard

3. **Room preparation**

   a) *Monitoring equipment:* Standard including $EtCO_2$ nasal cannula or using a second nasal cannula attached to the capnograph.
   b) *Additional equipment:* An extra long anesthesia circuit should be available due to the turning of the table 90 to 180 degrees and an oral rae endotracheal tube if general anesthetic is to be used.
   c) *Drugs:* Standard emergency and standard tabletop
   d) *Intravenous fluids:* Due to use of vasoconstrictors in local anesthesia, blood loss should be minimal.
   e) One 18-gauge intravenous line with normal saline or lactated

Ringer's at 2 mL/kg/hour or KVO, with replacement of NPO deficit.

4. **Perioperative management and anesthetic technique**
   a) The majority of facelifts are done with deep sedation. The surgeon will need the patient to remain asleep throughout the procedure.
   b) The choice will depend on the patient and surgeon's preference.
   c) If a general technique is chosen, an oral rae endotracheal tube may be used to facilitate exposure of the surgical field.
   d) If local anesthetic with intravenous sedation is the technique chosen, a nasal airway may be placed if the patient easily obstructs.
   e) *Induction:* Routine. If local anesthetic with sedation is chosen, a short-acting agent (i.e., propofol) should be used because the majority of these surgeries are done on an outpatient basis, with the patient going home the same day.
   f) Prior to administration of localization, the patient must be motionless and deeply sedated.
   g) *Maintenance:* Routine. Deep sedation can be maintained with an infusion. Hypertension should be controlled as this may result in hematoma. Vital signs should be maintained within normal limits. Depending on the patients' anatomy and the skill and experience of the surgeon, this procedure could last up to 6 hours.
   h) *Emergence:* No special considerations

5. **Postoperative Complications**
   a) Hematoma is the most common complication of this procedure, with most occurring at the end of the procedure; but it may also present within the first 10 to 12 hours.
      (1) The cause of this is usually intraoperative hypertension.
      (2) This complication most commonly presents itself with the patient appearing restless and having unilateral pain to the face or neck.
      (3) The patient should be relatively pain free.
      (4) However, if these symptoms are noticed, the surgeon should be notified, as treatment must be surgical.
      (5) If left untreated, this could compromise the patient's respiratory status.
      (6) A general anesthetic technique or intravenous sedation technique may be done for evacuation of the hematoma. If the hematoma is large, a general technique may be performed if the patient is restless and anxious.
   b) This procedure disrupts branches of the sensory nerves to the face. Numbness may last several months postoperatively, usually 2 to 6 months. This numbness is usually limited to the area of the lower two-thirds of the ear, preauricular area, and the cheeks.

PART 2 **Common Procedures**

N. Dacryocystorhinostomy

1. **Introduction**

   Dacryocystorhinostomy (DCR) is for patients who have chronic tearing or obstruction at the level of the nasolacrimal duct. This procedure restores drainage into the nose from the lacrimal sac. The surgeon will inject lidocaine 1% with 1:100,000 epinephrine, Marcaine 0.75%, and Wydase in the operative site along the lacrimal crest. An additional injection may be given along the medial orbital wall, anesthetizing the ethmoidal nerve. This will help anesthetize the nasal mucosa by blocking the ethmoidal nerve. This block may cause a temporary dilated pupil or medial rectus muscle paralysis.

   A small incision is made near the medial canthus to allow a subperiosteal dissection to the lacrimal sac. The bone between the lacrimal fossa and middle fossa is broken and cut, making a small caniculi. The mucosa of the lacrimal sac is anastomosed to the mucosa of the nose. To prevent closure of the newly formed path by scarring, a silicone tube may be placed inside the duct. Muscles and tissues in the area are then closed. The patient is then asked to open their eyelids, and when proper height is obtained, the incision is closed.

2. **Preoperative assessment and patient preparation**

   a) *History and physical examination:* This procedure may be done in patients with varying age. The patient's cardiac history should be determined, since epinephrine is to be used for vasoconstriction. Infections in the surgical area should be treated with antibiotics several days prior to surgery. Due to the inaccessibility of the anesthesia provider to the head, patients with obstructive sleep apnea should also be identified and anesthesia planned accordingly.

   b) *Patient preparation*

      (1) *Laboratory tests:* As indicated by the history and physical examination

      (2) *Diagnostic tests:* ECG is indicated by the history and physical examination

      (3) *Premedication:* Standard

3. **Room preparation**

   a) *Monitoring equipment:* Standard

   b) *Additional equipment:* $EtCO_2$ sensing nasal cannula may be used to give additional information about ventilation.

   c) An extra long circuit should be available due to turning of the table 90 to 180 degrees.

   d) *Drugs:* Standard emergency and standard tabletop

   e) *Intravenous fluids:* Age appropriate intravenous line and fluid for pediatrics. One 18-gauge intravenous line for adults with normal saline/lactated Ringer's at 2 cc/kg/hour (blood loss should be minimal due to use of epinephrine).

4. **Perioperative management and anesthetic technique**

a) The majority of these procedures can be done with local anesthesia with sedation; very rarely is general anesthesia used.

b) The choice depends on the preferences of the surgeon and the patient.

c) *Induction:* Routine for general surgery.

d) For local with sedation, short-acting agents are best because these procedures are usually done on an outpatient basis.

e) *Maintenance:* Routine

f) *Emergence:* For general anesthetic, the patient should be emerged awake, unless their condition dictates (i.e., reactive airway disease).

5. **Postoperative implications**

As stated earlier, there may be some temporary dilation of the pupil or medial rectus paralysis.

O. Ptosis Surgery

1. **Introduction**

If ptosis is severe, the function of the levator palpebrae is poor. Most frequently, this procedure involves shortening or reattaching the muscle at its site of insertion on the superior tarsus. The upper eyelid is marked at the desired height so it matches the opposite eyelid. Local anesthetic is injected by the surgeon. The skin is incised along the upper eyelid crease, and dissection proceeds until the orbicularis oculi is reached. At the medial and lateral ends of the tarsus, scissors incisions are made, and a clamp is placed between the two incisions. The levator muscle is resected as desired, and the eyelid height is evaluated. The skin incision is then closed, with any excess being excised.

2. **Preoperative assessment and patient preparation**

a) This type of procedure in adults is preferably performed under local anesthesia so that the patient can keep their eyes open and the lid position can be adjusted.

b) *History and physical examination:* Routine

c) *Patient preparation*

(1) *Laboratory tests:* As indicated by history and physical examination

(2) *Diagnostic tests:* As indicated by history and physical examination

(3) *Premedication:* Light sedation as needed

(4) *Intravenous fluids:* One 18- or 20-gauge needle with normal saline/lactated Ringer's at KVO; blood loss should be minimal.

3. **Perioperative management and anesthetic technique**

a) Patients are kept awake such that they are able to open their eyes in order to facilitate adjustment of the lids.

b) Deep sedation is only required for localization, then the patient is kept awake.

4. **Postoperative implications**
   a) Antibiotic steroid ophthalmic ointment is applied to the suture line.
   b) Sometimes, an eye pad is applied or the patient receives iced saline pads in the postanesthesia care unit.

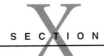

SECTION X

Obstetrics and Gynecology

A. Cesarean Section

1. **Introduction**
   A cesarean section (C-section) is the surgical removal of a fetus via an abdominal/uterine incision. A low transverse incision is the most common; in an emergency, a rapid vertical midline incision may be used. Indications for a C-section are failure of labor to progress, previous C-section, fetal distress, malpresentation of the fetus or cord, placenta previa, and genital herpes or other local infections.

2. **Perioperative assessment**
   In emergency cases, the time for assessment will be brief. Special attention should be paid to airway assessment because failed intubation is a major cause of maternal morbidity and mortality.

   a) *Cardiac*

   (1) Full-term pregnancy causes an increase in cardiac output of 30%. Twenty percent of the cardiac output goes to the uterus; with each contraction, blood flow to the uterus increases 15% to 20%.

   (2) Immediately postpartum is the largest increase in cardiac output, an up to 80% increase.

   (3) Cardiac output returns to normal 2 weeks postpartum.

   (4) By 24 to 34 weeks, blood volume increases 35% to 40% (1000 to 1500 cc). Blood volumes return to normal 1 to 2 weeks after delivery.

   (5) Blood loss for a normal delivery is 500 cc or less; for a twin vaginal delivery or C-section, it is 1000 cc or less.

   (6) There is also, normally, a mild decrease in blood pressure and systemic vascular resistance.

   (7) Evaluate for pregnancy-induced hypertension.

   (8) There is dilutional anemia due to an increase in plasma volume and increased total body water content; hemoglobin is usually greater than 11 g/dL. Postdelivery there is diuresis, and the hemoglobin returns to normal 2 to 4 weeks postpartum.

   (9) Parturients greater than 28 weeks gestation should not be placed supine without left uterine displacement. Supine hypotension syndrome occurs after the 28th week when patients lie in the supine position, causing decreased venous return that leads to decreased cardiac output and decreased blood pressure. Symptoms include pallor, nausea and vomiting, sweating, and dizziness. Aortic compression

PART 2 Common Procedures

occurs when patients lie in the supine position, causing decreased blood flow to the lower extremities and uteroplacental insufficiency. The arm blood pressure reading does not reflect such changes. Most patients are asymptomatic or feel tingling in the legs with fetal asphyxia. Aortocaval compression occurs as early as 20 weeks; with regional and increased vasodilation, there is a decrease in venous return. Systemic hypotension, increased uterine venous pressure, and uterine arterial hypoperfusion can compromise uterine and placental blood flow. When combined with anesthesia, fetal asphyxia may result

b) *Respiratory*
   (1) Oxygen consumption increases 20% at term, minute ventilation increases 50%, tidal volume increases 40%, respiratory rate increases 20%, and alveolar ventilation is increased, all leading to respiratory alkalosis with $PaCO_2$ decreased to 32 torr.
   (2) During labor, the minute ventilation increases 300%, causing hypocarbia and hypoventilation between contractions.
   (3) The oxyhemoglobin dissociation curve is shifted to the left, resulting in less oxygen available to the fetus.
   (4) Functional residual capacity decreases by 20%, causing a rapid desaturation with apnea; must preoxygenate before induction. Maximum allowable concentration (MAC) is decreased by 25 to 40%.
   (5) There is decreased airway resistance due to progesterone-induced relaxation.
   (6) Capillary engorgement of the respiratory mucosa predisposes to upper airway trauma.
   (7) Decreased glottic opening, edematous false cords, and arytenoids and nasal congestion. Never place a nasal airway; use a smaller endotracheal tube (6.0 to 6.5).

c) *Gastrointestinal:* All pregnant patients past 16 weeks of gestation are considered to be on a full stomach and require pretreatment with 30 cc of a nonparticulate antacid and rapid sequence induction.

d) The enlarged uterus obstructs the inferior vena cava, causing a decrease in the CSF volume, a decrease in the potential volume of the epidural space, and an increase in the epidural space pressure due to epidural vein engorgement. Decrease dose of epidural and spinals by $1/2$ to $1/3$. Don't push drugs during contractions, as the pressure in the epidural space increases 6 to 12 times normal.

e) *Other:* Evaluate for a history of gestational diabetes, HELLP syndrome (hemolysis, elevated liver enzymes, low platelet count), placenta previa, seizures, preterm labor, multiple gestation, drug abuse, pregnancy-induced hypertension and nonpregnancy-related illnesses and surgeries.

3. **Patient preparation**
   a) A nonparticulate antacid (such as sodium citrate, 30 mL) is

routinely administered at most institutions, regardless of the anesthetic technique chosen. Sedation is best avoided. Benzodiazapines have been implicated as possible teratogens, and it is best to avoid maternal amnesia during childbirth.

  b) Laboratory tests should include a type and screen, complete blood count, electrolytes, blood urea nitrogen, creatinine, glucose, prothrombin time, and partial thromboplastin time. In emergency C-sections, there may not be time to complete these tests.

4. **Room preparation**
  a) *Monitoring:*
    (1) Standard.
    (2) If there is a history of pregnancy-induced hypertension, an arterial line is recommended.
    (3) If there is severe preeclampsia, a central line is also recommended, with a pulmonary catheter in cases of hemodynamic instability.
  b) *Positioning:* Supine with left lateral uterine displacement. This is accomplished by placing a wedge under the right hip. Failure to use left lateral uterine displacement can result in aortocaval compression.
  c) *Drugs and tabletop:*
    (1) Tabletop should be set up for a general anesthetic.
    (2) Set out a smaller endotracheal tube (6.0 to 6.5) as well (because of airway edema).
    (3) Have ephedrine and oxytocin drawn up.
    (4) Have difficult airway equipment available.
    (5) Unless there is maternal hypoglycemia, avoid giving intravenous solutions with glucose because they may lead to neonatal hypoglycemia.

5. **Perioperative management and anesthetic techniques**
  a) Always be ready for general anesthesia. Rapid sequence induction should be done after the patient is prepped and draped; notify the surgeon immediately after the endotracheal tube is through the cords. Thiopental (4 mg/kg)/succinylcholine (1.5 mg/kg) is the most common combination for induction. Ketamine (1 mg/kg) is a useful adjunct in cases of instability or bleeding.
  b) An oral-gastric tube should be inserted after induction, and the gastric contents should be aspirated.
  c) Volatile agents can be used and then substituted with narcotics after the fetus is delivered. Begin at a 0.5 MAC because requirements for obstetrics are typically 30% to 50% reduced. The maximum end-tidal for isoflurane should not exceed 0.50%.
  d) Avoid hypotension because uterine flow is pressure dependent.
  e) Extubation is always performed with the patient awake because the danger of aspiration will be high.
  f) Regional anesthesia is the most common technique used on C-section patients. For spinal anesthesia, 0.75% bupivicaine, 11 to 12 mg, is usually enough to provide a dense block to T4. Volume loading should be accomplished before performing a

PART 2 Common Procedures

spinal block with 1 to 2 L of crystalloid. Ephedrine is also commonly needed in addition to volume loading.

g) An epidural is also an attractive regional anesthetic, especially if the parturient has a catheter in place for laboring. "Topping up" the epidural with 10 to 20 cc of 2% lidocaine or 3% Nesacaine along with narcotic and perhaps ketamine just prior to delivery are two techniques.

h) If the patient is in danger of losing consciousness or reflexes, the airway must be protected and general anesthesia induced.

6. **Postoperative considerations**

a) For pain relief, narcotics may be administered parenterally, with patient-controlled analgesia, orally when tolerated, or intrathecally/epidurally if a catheter is in place.

b) Nausea and vomiting are common in the immediate postpartum period and may be treated with an antiemetic.

7. **Obstetrical Pharmacology**

a) Placental transfer is dependent on the concentration gradient, molecular weight, lipid solubility and drug ionization state.

b) Drugs that are nonionized, lipid soluble and weigh less than 500 d cross the placenta easily.

c) Uterine stimulating agents are used for the induction and augmentation of labor, the induction of uterine contraction after a C-section or uterine surgery, the induction of a therapeutic abortion, and control of postpartum atony. The uterine vascular bed is not autoregulated. α-receptors elicit hypertonus when stimulated, and β-receptors elicit a reduction in uterine tone and contractility when stimulated.

(1) Oxytocin increases intracellular calcium, resulting in a sustained decrease in the uterine resting membrane potential. The frequency and force of contractions increases. The dose for the induction of labor is 1 to 2 milliunits/min, and is increased milliunits by 1 to 2 milliunits/min every 15 to 30 min until optimum response. The average dose is 8 to 10 milliunits/min. For control of postpartum bleeding, 10 to 40 milliunits added intravenously may be given after delivery of the placenta.

(2) Methergine causes an increase in the strength of the contractions, leading to a firm tetanic contraction followed by a series of clonic contractions. α-agonist effects result in vasoconstriction; coronary artery spasm and myocardial ischemia can occur. Side effects include severe hypertension and bradycardia. The dose is 0.2 mg intramuscularly every 2 to 4 hours.

(3) Prostaglandins act on specific receptors to stimulate synthesis of cyclic adenosine monophosphate (AMP) by the activation of adenylate cyclase. This stimulates the smooth muscle of the uterus and results in the induction of strong uterine contractions. Bronchiole smooth muscle contracts in response to prostaglandins and may result in severe bronchoconstriction. The dose is 200 to 500 mcg intramuscularly or intramyometrially.

d) Muscle relaxants are all polar quaternary ammonium compounds that do not cross the placenta in any significant amounts. They are 100% watersoluble and have a small volume of distribution. Plasma cholinesterase activity declines with pregnancy and is due to the patient's expanded blood volume. A modified succinylcholine dose is usually not needed. None of the muscle relaxants relax the uterine muscle.

e) Inhalational agents are lipid soluble, nonionized, and have a low molecular weight. Levels rise quickly in the fetal brain. The degree of neonatal depression is proportional to the depth and duration of the maternal anesthesia. Nitrous oxide has been implicated as a teratogen to the fetus; there is generally little harm at delivery if less than 50% is used.

f) Narcotics cause varying degrees of respiratory depression in the neonate and can prolong the progress of labor. Generally avoid if delivery is thought to occur within the next 30 to 45 minutes. The peak effect of meperidine occurs 40 to 50 minutes after intramuscular administration, 5 to 10 minutes after intravenous administration. The greatest incidence of respiratory depression occurs 3 to 4 hours after administration. At this time, meperidine is metabolized to the more respiratory-depressing metabolite normeperidine.

g) Benzodiazepines should not be given during the first trimester due to the risk of cleft palate. Avoid in labor and delivery due to amnesic properties.

h) Ephedrine is the drug of choice to treat hypotension due to the mixed α and β effects that maintain maternal cardiac output and uterine perfusion. It can increase the fetal heart rate.

i) Tocolytics are β-adrenergic agonists that are most commonly used to treat preterm labor. All have β-1 and β-2 effects. β-1 stimulation can result in an increased heart rate and cardiac output; β-2 stimulation can result in hyperglycemia and hypotension. Ritodrine and terbutaline are more specific β-2 agonists that are Food and Drug Adminnstration (FDA) approved for the treatment of preterm labor. The intravenous infusion rates are 0.05 to 0.1 mg/min ritodrine and 0.01mg/min terbutaline. These can cause profound tachycardia, and it is recommended that induction be delayed 10 minutes after an infusion is stopped to allow the heart rate to decrease.

j) Magnesium sulfate is a central nervous system depressant that decreases the quantity of acetylcholine released by the motor nerve impulses which blocks neuromuscular transmission, causing smooth muscle relaxation and decreased blood pressure. It is used for preeclampsia, eclampsia, and preterm labor. The dose is 3 to 4 g intravenously over 20 minutes followed by an infusion of 1 to 1.5 mg/hour; titrate by 0.5 mg/hour until contractions cease. The therapeutic range is 4.0 to 8.0 g/dL. Side effects include sweating, nausea, rag doll syndrome, confusion, and pulmonary edema. As it crosses the placenta, there will be a transient decrease in fetal heart rate, low apgar sores, hypotonia,

PART 2 Common Procedures

and respiratory depression. Magnesium increases the sensitivity
to depolarizing and nondepolarizing muscle relaxants. Avoid
long-lasting muscle relaxants and decrease the dose of all others
by $^1/_2$ to $^1/_3$.

B. Anesthesia for Vaginal Delivery

1. **Preoperative assessment**
   See "Cesarean Section," p. 317.
2. **Patient preparation**
   a) All patients should have an intravenous catheter placed and
      should receive 500 to 1000 mL bolus prior to an epidural
      placement.
   b) Lumbar epidural anesthesia provides segmental levels of
      analgesia that block pain impulses from the uterus but maintain
      sensation in the perineum and avoid motor blockade.
      (1) Generally only administered when labor is well established,
          the cervix is dilated 5 to 6 cm in primiparas and 3 to 4 cm
          in multiparas with regular contractions.
      (2) Bupivacaine is frequently used because it has little effect on
          the fetus and a longer duration of action. Solutions com-
          monly used are $^1/_8$% or $^1/_{16}$% with fentanyl 1 to 2 mcg/cc,
          with an infusion at 8 to 12 cc/hour and a bolus of 5 to 10 cc.
      (3) Monitor blood pressure frequently for the first $^1/_2$ hour and
          treat any blood pressure less than 100 mm Hg with
          ephedrine, fluids, and left uterine displacement.
      (4) Epidural topoffs may be used for forceps delivery or an
          extensive episiotomy repair with 5 to 10 cc of the infusion
          or 3% nesicaine.
   c) Saddle block may be used for forceps delivery to block the per-
      ineum and inner thigh; 7.5 to 10 mg of lidocaine may be given
      in the sitting position.
   d) Pudendal nerve block—blocks the pudendal nerves of S2 to S4
      during the second stage of labor; results in low forceps delivery
      and episiotomy. It is administered transvaginally, with the local
      anesthetic injected posterior to the ischial spines beneath the
      sacrospinus ligaments. There is risk of puncture of the fetal scalp.
   e) Paracervical block—injected into the fornix of the vagina lateral
      to the cervix. Nerve fibers from the uterus, cervix, and upper
      vagina are anesthetized; fibers from the perineum are not
      blocked. There is a high frequency of fetal bradycardia, so it is
      generally avoided.

C. Gynecologic Laparoscopy

1. **Introduction**
   Laparoscopy is a common endoscopic technique in gynecologic procedures. It is frequently used to diagnose or treat pelvic etiologies that may include sterilization, adhesions, pain, endometriosis, ectopic pregnancies, ovarian cysts and tumors, infertility, and vaginal hysterectomy. A pneumoperitoneum is achieved by insertion of a trocar and insufflation of CO_2.
2. **Preoperative assessment and patient preparation**
   a) *History and physical Examination:* As indicated by the patient history and medical condition
   b) *Patient preparation*
      (1) *Laboratory tests:* Complete blood count and other tests as indicated
      (2) *Diagnostic tests:* Pregnancy testing and as indicated
      (3) *Preoperative medications:* As indicated.
      (4) *Intravenous therapy:* One or two 16- to 18-gauge intravenous catheters
3. **Room preparation**
   a) *Monitoring equipment:* Standard.
   b) Consider others if indicated.
   c) *Additional equipment:* Fluid warmer and Bair-Hugger
   d) *Drugs*
      (1) Anesthetic and adjunct agents, antibiotics
      (2) *Intravenous fluid:* Depends on the procedure performed; calculate as indicated. Estimated blood loss is less than 50 to 100 mL.
      (3) Blood—type and screen
      (4) Tabletop—standard
4. **Perioperative management and anesthetic technique**
   a) General anesthesia is preferred.
   b) *Induction:* Standard, as indicated
   c) *Maintenance:* Inhalational agent/O_2/opioid and nondepolarizing agent as indicated. Consider antiemetics.
   d) *Position:* Lithotomy; Trendelenburg to improve pelvic exposure
   e) *Emergence:* Standard
5. **Postoperative implications**
   Complications include nausea, vomiting, and anemia.

PART 2 Common Procedures

D. Hysterectomy—Vaginal or Total Abdominal

1. **Introduction**
   A hysterectomy is commonly performed to treat uncontrolled uterine bleeding, dysmenorrhea, uterine myoma, gynecologic cancer, adhesions, endometriosis, and pelvic relaxation syndrome. Frequently, laparoscopy is used; for ovarian cancer prophylaxis, a bilateral salpingo-oophorectomy may be performed as well.

2. **Preoperative assessment**
   a) *History and physical examination:* As indicated by the patient's history and medical condition
   b) *Patient preparation*
      (1) *Laboratory tests:* As indicated by the patient's history and medical condition
      (2) *Diagnostic tests:* As indicated by the patient's history and medical condition
      (3) *Preoperative medications:* Anxiolytics as indicated. Consider prophylaxis for PONV.
      (4) *Intravenous therapy:* Two 16- to 18-gauge intravenous lines; consider central line and/or arterial line if radical procedure.
      (5) An epidural catheter may be placed for intraoperative or postoperative pain relief.

3. **Room preparation**
   a) *Monitoring equipment:* Standard
   b) Consider an arterial line and central venous pressure catheter if large blood loss is expected.
   c) *Additional equipment:* Fluid warmer and Bair-Hugger
   d) *Drugs*
      (1) Anesthetic and adjunct agents, antibiotics
      (2) *Intravenous fluids:* Vaginal—calculate for moderate blood loss; crystalloids at 4 to 6 mL/kg/hour. Estimated blood loss is 750 to 1000 mL. Abdominal—calculate for a moderate to large blood loss; crystalloids at 6 to 10 mL/kg/hour. Estimated blood loss is 1000 to 1500 mL.
      (3) Blood—type and crossmatch for 2 to 4 units of packed red blood cells
      (4) Tabletop—standard

4. **Perioperative management and anesthetic technique**
   a) General or regional anesthesia; subarachnoid block or epidural with a sensory level of anesthesia of T6 to T8
   b) *Induction:* Standard. Choice as indicated.
   c) *Maintenance*
      (1) *General anesthesia:* Inhalational agent/O_2/opioid/anxiolytic and nondepolarizing muscle relaxant.
      (2) *Regional:* Local anesthetic of choice; supplemental anxiolytic and sedation.

(3) *Position:* Abdominal—supine. Vaginal—lithotomy.
(4) *Emergence:* Standard
5. **Postoperative implications**
    a) *Complications:* Nausea, vomiting, anemia
    b) *Pain management:* Patient-controlled anesthesia; epidural
        opiates or an epidural local anesthetic such as 0.125% or 0.25%
        Marcaine with fentanyl 1 mcg/cc at an infusion of 8 to 10 cc/hour.

E. Loop Electrosurgical Excision Procedure

1. **Introduction**
    The loop electrosurgical excision procedure (LEEP) is performed for
    the diagnosis and treatment of cervical intraepithelial neoplasia. This
    form of electrosurgery uses a loop electrode for excision and fulgura-
    tion to prevent cervical bleeding. Other types of therapy that may be
    used to ablate cervical lesions are cryosurgery and CO_2 laser surgery.
2. **Preoperative assessment and patient preparation**
    a) *History and physical examination:* As indicated by the patient's
        history and medical condition
    b) *Patient preparation*
        (1) *Laboratory tests:* Pregnancy test, hemoglobin and hemat-
            ocrit, urinalysis
        (2) *Preoperative medications:* Anxiolytics may be used if
            the patient is not pregnant, such as midazolam (0.01 to
            0.02 mg/kg)
        (3) *Intravenous therapy:* One 18-gauge intravenous catheter
3. **Room preparation**
    a) *Monitoring equipment:* Standard. If a pregnancy is over
        16 weeks, fetal monitoring may be used.
    b) *Drugs:* Standard tabletop
    c) *Intravenous fluids:* Calculate for minimal blood loss, 2 to
        4 mL/kg/hour. Estimated blood loss is 50 to 200 mL.
4. **Perioperative management and anesthetic technique**
    a) Local, monitored anesthesia care, or regional or general
        anesthesia.
    b) *Induction:* Standard induction is indicated.
    c) In pregnant patients, rapid sequence induction is used.
    d) In nonpregnant patients, mask ventilation may be appropriate.
    e) *Maintenance:* Standard, inhalational agent/O_2/opioid. Muscle
        relaxation is not required.
    f) *Position:* Lithotomy.
    g) *Emergence:* Standard
5. **Postoperative implications**
    a) *Complications:* Peroneal nerve injury due to the lithotomy

position, nausea and vomiting, bleeding, postdural headache, and premature labor

b) *Pain management:* Oral analgesics if the patient is not pregnant

F. In Vitro Fertilization

1. **Introduction**
   Laparoscopic in vitro fertilization and embryo transfer are frequently performed for the treatment of infertility. This outpatient procedure is indicated for the treatment of tubal disease, endometriosis, and idiopathic infertility.
2. **Preoperative assessment and patient preparation**
   a) *History and physical examination:* As indicated by the patient's history and medical condition
   b) *Patient preparation*
      (1) *Laboratory tests:* Hemoglobin and hematocrit; other tests as indicated
      (2) *Intravenous therapy:* One 18-gauge intravenous catheter
3. **Room preparation**
   a) *Monitoring equipment:* Standard
   b) *Additional equipment:* No special considerations
   c) *Drugs*
      (1) Miscellaneous pharmacologic agents—opioid, short-acting nondepolarizing muscle relaxant, anesthetic agent
      (2) *Intravenous fluids:* Calculate for minimal blood loss; crystalloids at 2 mL/kg/hour. Estimated blood loss is less than 50 mL.
      (3) Blood—No special considerations
      (4) Tabletop—Standard
4. **Perioperative management and anesthetic technique**
   a) General anesthesia is most common and preferred.
   b) Local, regional, subarachnoid block, or epidural techniques can be used.
   c) *Induction:* Standard, as indicated. Outpatient procedure is a consideration.
   d) *Maintenance:* Standard inhalation agent/O_2/opioid.
   e) Consider complications of pneumoperitoneum (i.e., hypercapnia, hypoxia, pneumothorax, ventilation-perfusion mismatch, increased inspiratory pressures, dysrhythmias, altered cardiac output, and hemorrhage).
   f) *Position:* Supine with Trendelenburg.
   g) *Emergence:* Standard
5. **Postoperative implications**
   Complications include abdominal pain and referred shoulder discomfort.

G. Pelvic Exenteration

1. **Introduction**

   A pelvic exenteration is performed for the treatment of advanced, recurrent, radioresistant cervical carcinoma. It is considered a radical surgical approach because all pelvic tissues, including the cervix, bladder, lymph nodes, rectum, uterus, and vagina, are resected. Vaginal reconstruction and appropriate colon and urinary diversions are also performed.

2. **Preoperative assessment and patient preparation**

   a) *History and physical examination:* As indicated by the patient's history and medical condition

   b) *Patient preparation*

      (1) *Laboratory tests:* Complete blood count, electrolytes, blood urea nitrogen, creatinine, calcium, magnesium, phosphate, prothrombin time, partial thromboplastin time, urinalysis, and renal function tests

      (2) *Diagnostic tests:* As indicated by the patient's history and physical examination

      (3) *Premedication:* Anxiolytics as indicated

      (4) *Intravenous therapy:* Two 14- to 16-gauge intravenous tubes

      (5) Central and arterial line; consider a pulmonary arterial catheter if the patient has a significant cardiac history

      (6) An epidural catheter may be placed for postoperative pain relief.

3. **Room preparation**

   a) *Monitoring equipment:* Standard; consider arterial line and central venous pressure and pulmonary arterial catheters

   b) *Additional equipment:* Fluid warmer and Bair Hugger

   c) *Drugs:* standard

      (1) Miscellaneous pharmacologic agents—opioid, anxiolytic, nondepolarizing muscle relaxant, local anesthetic, and antibiotics

      (2) *Intravenous fluids:* Calculate for major blood loss, 10 to 15 mg/kg/hour. Estimated blood loss is 1000 to 4000 mL.

4. **Perioperative management and anesthetic technique**

   a) General anesthesia with epidural

   b) *Induction:* Standard, as indicated

   c) *Maintenance:* Inhalational agent/O_2/opioid

   d) Consider local anesthetic via an epidural catheter.

   e) Use long-acting nondepolarizing muscle relaxants.

   f) Maintain normocarbia, mean arterial pressure of 60 to 88 mm Hg, and urinary output at 0.5 to 1 mL/kg/hour, transfuse as indicated.

   g) *Position:* Both lithotomy and supine positions are used throughout the procedure.

   h) *Emergence:* The patient generally is transported to the intensive care unit for 2 to 3 days; postoperative ventilation may be

PART 2 Common Procedures

necessary. If the patient is hemodynamically stable, extubation may be considered.

5. **Postoperative implications**
   a) *Complications:* Bleeding, fluid maintenance due to large fluid shifts and mobilizations, and peroneal nerve damage due to the lithotomy position
   b) *Pain management:* Epidural, opiates, or both

H. Dilatation and Curettage (D & C)

1. **Introduction**
   A D & C involves dilation of the cervix and scraping of the endometerial lining of the uterus. The procedure is done to diagnose and treat uterine bleeding, cervical lesions or stenosis. D & Cs are also used to complete an incomplete or missed abortion and are then boarded as suction D & Cs with the gestational week.

2. **Preoperative assessment and patient preparation**
   a) *History and physical examination:* Assess for any cardiac, respiratory, neurologic, or renal abnormalities. Assess for a history of hiatal hernia or reflux; if a suction D & C, assess gestational week; if greater than 16 weeks, consider the patient to be on full stomach.
   b) *Patient preparation*
      (1) *Laboratory tests:* HCG, UA, CBC
      (2) *Medications:* Evaluate any medications patient is taking
      (3) *Intravenous therapy:* One 18-gauge peripheral intravenous line

3. **Room preparation**
   a) *Monitoring equipment:* Standard
   b) *Additional equipment:* Bair Hugger

4. **Perianesthetic management**
   a) *Drugs:* Anxiolytic (versed 0.01 to 0.02 mg/kg), narcotic (fentanyl 1 to 2 mcg/kg), Pitocin for suction D & Cs, induction agent (propofol 2.5 mg/kg or Pentothal 4 mg/kg).
   b) This procedure can be done either with a short-acting spinal or saddle block with lidocaine 7.5 to 10 mg as a general anesthetic by mask, laryngeal mask airway, or with an endotracheal tube with inhalation agent/N_2O or with heavy sedation (Versed, fentanyl, and propofol).
   c) Postoperatively assess for bleeding, nausea, and cramping. Treat with narcotics, nonsteroidal anti-inflammatory drugs (NSAIDs), and antiemetics.

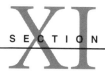

SECTION

XI

Pediatrics

A. Anatomy and Physiology

1. **Cardiovascular physiology**
   a) During fetal development, oxygenation and CO_2 elimination are accomplished through the placenta. Oxygenated blood to the fetus travels from the placenta via the umbilical vein through the ductus venosus near the liver, to the inferior vena cava. The foramen ovale, the opening between the right and left atria, allows the oxygenated blood direct access to the left circulation. From the left atrium the blood is transferred to the left ventricle then to the body. The blood returns to the placenta via the umbilical arteries. Deoxygenated blood from the superior vena cava is deposited into the right atrium. It is then ejected into the pulmonary artery. Due to high pulmonary vasculature pressure, the blood bypasses the lungs and is instead transferred through the ductus arteriosus to the aorta. The blood travels to the placenta via the umbilical arteries.
   b) Clamping of the umbilical cord increases systemic vascular resistance, increasing aortic and left-sided pressures, allowing the foramen ovale to close and the lungs to assume their role in oxygenation. Pulmonary vascular resistance decreases, and the ductus arteriosus closes as PaO_2 levels increase.
   c) Hypoxia, hypercarbia, and acidosis lead to persistent pulmonary hypertension and maintenance of fetal circulation. Diagnosis made when right radial (preductal) and umbilical line (postductal) samples reveal a difference of 20 mm Hg. Shunting continues across a patent ductus arteriosus, resulting in increased hypoxemia and acidosis.
   d) Treatment of persistent pulmonary circulation includes hyperventilation, maintenance of adequate oxygenation, and alkalosis.
   e) Neonatal cardiac output is heart rate dependent due to a noncompliant left ventricle and fixed stroke volume.
   f) The pediatric basal heart rate is higher than that of adults, although parasympathetic stimulation, hypoxia, or deep anesthesia can cause profound bradycardia and decreased cardiac output.
   g) Sympathetic nervous system and baroreceptor reflexes are immature. Infants have low catecholamine stores and decreased responsiveness to exogenous catecholamines. Infants cannot respond to hypovolemia with vasoconstriction. Therefore hypovolemia is suspected when there is hypotension in the absence of an increased heart rate.

PART 2 **Common Procedures**

329

h) *Normal parameters*

Age	Respiratory Rate	Heart Rate	Systolic Blood Pressure	Diastolic Blood Pressure
Neonate	40	140	65	40
1 year	30	120	95	65
3 years	25	100	100	70
12 years	20	80	110	60

i) Physiologic anemia of the newborn—hematocrit at birth is 50%, 80% of which is fetal hemoglobin. Fetal hemoglobin binds more strongly to oxygen than adult hemoglobin. This facilitates O_2 uptake in utero. After birth, the presence of fetal hemoglobin causes a shift in the oxyhemoglobin curve to the left, and a decrease in O_2 delivery to the tissues. At age 1 to 3 months, hemoglobin levels decrease, and levels of 2,3 DPG increase, causing a shift of the oxyhemoglobin curve to the right and increased O_2 delivery to tissues.

2. **Respiratory physiology**
   a) Increased metabolic rate, CO_2 production, and O_2 consumption.
   b) Decreased functional residual capacity and O_2 reserves.
   c) Infants have a paradoxical response to hypoxia—initial hyperpnea followed by respiratory depression and depressed response to hypercarbia.
   d) The larynx is at C2 to C4 in children, at C3 to C6 in the adult. This results in increased difficulty in alignment of the pharyngeal and laryngeal axes. A straight blade is useful for laryngoscopy in children.
   e) Children have a stiff, omega-shaped epiglottis. The vocal cords slant up and back.
   f) The narrowest part of the pediatric airway is the cricoid cartilage, as opposed to the adult glottis. The cricoid cartilage can form a seal around the endotracheal tube, eliminating the need for a cuffed tube. The cartilage is funnel shaped. Do not force fit the endotracheal tube. Properly fitted tubes allow a leak at 15 to 25 cm H_2O.
   g) Children have large occiputs that flex the head onto the chest, large tongues, and small chins. Tonsils and adenoids grow rapidly from ages 4 to 7 and may obstruct breathing.
   h) Infants are "obligatory nasal breathers". The position of the epiglottis in relation to the soft palate allows simultaneous breathing and sucking/drinking.
   i) The neonatal trachea is 4 cm. Flexion of the head onto the chest forces the endotracheal tube to extend deeper into the right mainstem. Extension of the head may dislodge the tube.
   j) The number of alveoli increase until age 6 years. Mature levels of surfactant are reached at 35 weeks gestation. Decreased amounts of alveoli and surfactant in the neonatal period increases the risk of infant respiratory distress syndrome.
   k) Increased work of breathing in the infant is due to a decreased

amount of Type I muscle fibers in the diaphragm; predisposition to fatigue. Poor chest wall mechanics, lack of rib cage rigidity, horizontal orientation of the ribs, weak intercostal muscles, and increased fatigue result in paradoxical chest movements in the newborn.

3. **Nervous system**
   a) Cranial sutures are not fused in the infant; the cranium is pliable. Fluid status is indicated by fullness of the fontanelles.
   b) Myelination of the nervous system continues until age 3. The spinal cord ends at L1 in adults, at L3 in pediatric patients. This is important to consider when using regional anesthesia techniques in the pediatric population.
   c) Preterm and low-birth-weight infants are at risk for intracranial hemorrhage due to fragile cerebral vessels. Intracranial bleeding may result from hypoxia, hypercarbia, hyperglycemia or hypoglycemia, hypernatremia, or wide variations in blood pressure.

4. **Renal system**
   a) The total body water in proportion to body weight is higher in neonates than adults. Kidneys function in utero to eliminate urine into the amniotic fluid, while the placenta eliminates waste.
   b) Neonates have the complete number of nephrons at birth. Nephrons are immature in function until age 6 to 12 months.
   c) The glomerular filtration rate (GFR) is decreased due to renal vasoconstriction, low plasma flow in the renal system, and low blood pressure. GFR increases until age 1 year.
   d) Infants are "obligate sodium excretors" because of their inability to conserve sodium. Renal tubules are not responsive to the renin-angiotensin-aldosterone system. The infant kidney cannot concentrate urine, leading to an increased risk of dehydration. The ability to reabsorb glucose is also impaired. If excessive glucose is given intravenously, the result is an osmotic diuresis.
   e) Pediatric patients have a tendency toward acidosis, as the metabolic rate and CO_2 production is double that of the adult. There is a decreased ability to conserve bicarbonate and excrete acids.

5. **Hepatic system**
   a) Near birth, the fetal liver increases glycogen stores. Preterm infants are at increased risk for hypoglycemia due to a lack of glycogen stores.
   b) Hepatic metabolism of drugs is decreased in the early weeks of life. The liver functions at the adult level by age 2.

6. **Impaired thermogenesis**
   a) Infants are at risk for hypothermia due to
      (1) increased surface area to body weight ratio,
      (2) ineffective shivering mechanism, and
      (3) decreased amounts of subcutaneous fat present in preterm infants.
   b) Heat loss is due to
      (1) radiation—the transfer of heat between two objects of different temperatures not in direct contact. Reduce radiant

loss by decreasing the temperature gradient (raise the room temperature closer to patient temperature).

(2) convection—transfer of heat to moving molecules such as air or liquid. Cover exposed skin.

(3) evaporation—occurs through the skin and respiratory systems, including sweat, insensible water loss via skin, wounds, respiratory tract, and evaporation of liquids applied to the skin.

(4) conduction—transfer of heat from warm infant to cool object in direct contact.

c) Patients assume room temperature under anesthesia—"poikilothermia."

d) Nonshivering thermogenesis—infants have impaired shivering capabilities. Autonomic nervous system activation during periods of cold results in metabolism of brown fat stores. Brown fat is located around the neck, kidneys, axilla, and adrenals, in addition to spaces between shoulders, under the sternum, and along the spine. Fatty acids in the brown fat stores are oxidated in an exothermic reaction to produce heat. Nonshivering thermogenesis is used until age 1 to 2.

e) Hypothermia in the neonate results in the release of norepinephrine, peripheral and pulmonary vasoconstriction, increasing acidosis, increased pulmonary pressures and right to left shunting, and eventually hypoxia, further perpetuating the cycle.

f) Avoid hypothermia by instituting the following: Increase room temperature, cover the head and exposed extremities, and use overhead warming light. Beware of burns. Use recommended distances for safe use. Heat and humidify delivered gases.

B. Pharmacology

1. **Introduction**

a) Neonates have less adipose tissue and muscle in proportion to body weight and have increased total body water. These differences result in higher plasma levels and decreased uptake into inactive tissues.

b) Infants have decreased renal and hepatic function. Therefore the half-life of drugs is increased in the neonate.

c) Neonates have decreased protein binding and a more permeable blood brain barrier. Therefore morphine and barbiturates have longer lasting effects.

2. **Inhalation agents**

Pediatric patients have an increased cardiac output, low systemic arterial blood pressure, and a greater blood flow per unit to vessel-rich organs. The neonate also has an increased minute ventilation and decreased functional residual capacity. These changes result in a more rapid uptake of inhalation agents and emergence from anesthesia. Maximum allowable concentration (MAC) requirements increase the greatest at ages 1 to 6 months, decreasing thereafter until puberty. All inhalation agents cause dose-related decreases in myocardial function and ventilation. Halothane and sevoflurane are preferred for mask inductions; may switch to less expensive Isoflurane after induction. N_2O provides second gas effect for increased agent delivery. N_2O may increase pulmonary vascular resistance and distend open spaces (bowel, middle ear).

3. **Intravenous agents**
    a) Barbiturates
        (1) Thiopental, 4 to 6 mg/kg intravenously
        (2) Methohexital, 7.7 mg/kg intramuscularly (add 14.5 cc 0.9 NS to vial of 500 mg to yield 3.5% solution to give 0.1 cc/lb or 7.7 mg/kg)
    b) Diprivan
        (1) Dose—2 to 2.5 mg/kg
        (2) Bradycardia may accompany use; pretreat with atropine or Robinul.
    c) Ketamine
        (1) Dose—1 to 3 mg/kg intravenously; 3 to 6 mg/kg intramuscularly. Provides cataleptic, dissociative state with analgesia.
        (2) Pretreat with benzodiazepine to prevent hallucinations. Increases heart rate, blood pressure, and O_2 consumption. May maintain respiratory drive or cause apnea; increases oral secretions.
    d) Narcotics
        (1) Morphine, 0.1 mg/kg
        (2) Demerol, 1 mg/kg
        (3) Fentanyl, 1 to 2 mcg/kg
        (4) Demerol causes less respiratory depression than morphine in neonates.
        (5) Narcan, 0.01 mg/kg
    e) Benzodiazepines—Versed, 0.08 to 0.5 mg/kg intramuscularly; 0.5 to 0.75 mg/kg orally; 0.2 to 0.5 mg/kg nasal
    f) Muscle relaxant reversal
        (1) Neostigmine, 0.03 to 0.07 mg/kg
        (2) Regonal, 0.2 mg/kg
        (3) Edrophonium, 0.7 to 1.4 mg/kg
        (4) Atropine, 0.01 to 0.02 mg/kg
        (5) Robinul, 0.01 mg/kg
    g) Miscellaneous
        (1) Epinephrine, 0.01 mg/kg
        (2) Lidocaine, 1 to 1.5 mg/kg
        (3) $NaHCO_3$, 1 to 2 mEq/kg
        (4) $CaCl_2$, 20 mg/kg

Overall, pediatric patients require increased anesthetic doses due to increased metabolic rate, greater cerebral blood flow, greater O_2 consumption, higher extracellular water content, and larger volumes of distribution.

PART 2   Common Procedures

4. **Neuromuscular blockers**
    Pediatric patients are resistant to depolarizing muscle relaxants
    due to increased extracellular water and volume of distribution.
    Administer succinylcholine, 1 to 2 mg/kg intravenously or 2 to
    4 mg/kg intramuscularly. Nondepolarizers are given in mg/kg doses
    recommended in adults. Theoretically, infants have increased sensi-
    tivity to nondepolarizers due to limited myelination and immaturity
    of the neuromuscular junction. This may be offset by the increased
    extracellular water levels, allowing standard doses to be adequate.

C. Fluids

1. **NPO (nothing by mouth) times**
    a)   2 to 3 hours after clear liquids
    b)   4 hours after breast milk
    c)   6 to 8 hours after formula or solid food
    Less irritability, less hypoglycemia, and less hypotension on
    induction are benefits of adjusted NPO times.
2. **4-2-1 rule for calculating fluids**
    a)   *Maintenance*
        (1)   < 10 kg   4 cc/kg/hour
        (2)   10 to 20 kg   40 cc/hour + 2 cc/kg >10 kg up to 20 kg
        (3)   > 20 kg   60 cc/hour + 1 cc/kg > 20 kg
    b)   *NPO*—Maintenance calculation times number of hours NPO
    c)   *Insensible loss/translocation*
        (1)   Mild (bone marrow transplantation [BMT], EUA),
              0 mL/kg/hour
        (2)   Moderate (inguinal hernia repair), 2 mL/kg/hour
        (3)   Severe (intra-abdominal cases), 4 to 6 mL/kg/hour
        (4)   Massive (spinal fusion, craniofacial), 15 to 20 mL/kg/hour
3. **Estimated blood volumes**
    a)   Preterm infants, 90 to 100 cc/kg
    b)   Newborn, 80 to 90 cc/kg
    c)   Age 3 months to 1 year, 75 to 80 cc/kg
    d)   Age 3 to 6 years, 70 to 75 cc/kg
    e)   Greater than 6 years, 65 to 70 cc/kg
4. **Lowest allowable hematocrit**

Age	Normal Hematocrit	Lowest Allowable Hematocrit
a) Preterm	40% to 45%	36%
b) Newborn	45% to 65%	30% to 35%
c) 3 months	30% to 42%	27%
d) 1 year	34% to 42%	24%
e) 6 years	35% to 43%	24%

5. **Maximum allowable blood loss**

$$EBV \times \frac{\text{Patient hematocrit} - \text{Lowest allowable hematocrit (in decimal)}}{\text{Patient hematocrit (decimal)}}$$

4. **Blood replacement**

Blood Volume Lost	Replacement
10% to 20%	Crystalloid 3 cc: 1 cc loss
25% to 33%	Colloid 1 cc: 1 cc
50%	Packed red blood cells (PRBCs) 1 cc: 1 cc Bolus 10 cc/kg IVP first, then remainder of calculated replacement
50% to 66%	PRBCs along with FFP (10 to 15 cc/kg calculated) FFP has high citrate content; check for decreased calcium levels post-transfusion
greater than 66%	PRBCs, FFP, and platelets (0.1 to 0.3 units/kg or 1 unit/10 kg weight)

D. Equipment

1. **Circuits**
   a) Pediatric circuits are designed to
      (1) eliminate valves within the circuit to decrease the resistance to breathing,
      (2) decrease the amount of deadspace within the circuit, and
      (3) minimize heat loss (Bain circuit).
   b) Commonly used circuits in pediatrics—Mapelson D, Bain, Modified T piece, Pediatric circle
   c) Disadvantages
      (1) Require high, fresh gas flows to prevent rebreathing.
      (2) Heat and moisture loss in all circuits except Bain.
      (3) Pediatric circle does contain valves and CO_2 absorber, which can increase resistance.
2. **Calculation of fresh gas flow**
   a) FGF = 2.5 times minute ventilation
   b) Minute ventilation = Respiratory rate × Tidal volume (6 mL/kg)
3. **O_2 delivery systems**
   a) Spontaneously breathing patient—nasal cannula, simple mask, oxygen hood
   b) Patient requiring ventilatory assistance—positive-pressure delivery system attached to mask or endotracheal tube
4. **Airways**
   Oral airway sizes:

Age	Size	Centimeters
a) Preterm	000 or 00	3.5 or 4.5
b) Neonate to 3 months	0	5.5
c) 3 to 12 months	1	6
d) 1 to 5 years	2	7
e) over 5 years	3	8

PART 2 **Common Procedures**

5. **Laryngoscope blades**

Age	Blade
a) Preterm/newborn	Miller 0
b) Neonate to 2 years	Miller 1
c) 3 years+	Miller 2
d) 2 to 5 years	WisHippel 1.5
e) 3 to 6 years	Macintosh 2

6. **Endotracheal tubes**

Age	Tube Size
a) Preterm under 2 kg	2.5
b) over 2 kg	3.0
c) Neonate	3.0 to 3.5
d) 0 to 6 months	3.5
e) 6 to 12 months	4.0
f) 12 to 18 months	4.0 to 4.5
g) 2 years	4.5
h) 2 to 3 years	4.5 to 5.0
i) over 4 years	Age (yr) + 16/4 or Age/4 + 1

E. Myringotomy

1. **Introduction**

   Myringotomy is a common outpatient procedure in children. Myringotomy is usually associated with the insertion of ventilation tubes into the tympanic membrane as a treatment for recurrent otitis media. Typically, a small incision is made with the use of a microscope in the tympanic membrane, and fluid is suctioned via a transcanal approach.

2. **Preoperative assessment**

   Other than a history of frequent and recurrent otitis media, this patient population is generally healthy.

   a) History and physical examination

   (1) A careful family history should be obtained preoperatively, including any history of family problems with anesthesia.

   (2) *Respiratory:* Many pediatric patients presenting for myringotomy have a history of frequent upper respiratory tract infections. If currently exhibiting signs and symptoms of upper respiratory tract infections, these children are at greater risk for laryngospasm intraoperatively and postoperatively. Because this procedure is elective, it is commonly recommended to postpone the procedure until the signs and symptoms of upper respiratory tract infection have subsided.

   (3) *Dental:* Inspection of the airway and questioning of the parents should identify any loose teeth.

   b) Patient preparation

(1) *Laboratory tests:* As indicated from the history and physical examination
(2) *Diagnostic tests:* As indicated from the history and physical examination
(3) *Medications:* Midazolam (0.2 to 0.5 mg/kg) orally may be given with 20 to 30 mL of apple juice as a premedication. Also available as an elixir.

3. **Room preparation**
   a) *Monitoring equipment:* Standard
   b) *Additional equipment:* None
   c) Standard emergency drugs (including atropine, lidocaine, and succinylcholine)
   d) Pediatric standard tabletop
   e) *Intravenous fluids:* Depending on the age of the patient, expected length of procedure, and history and physical findings, an intravenous catheter may be available for emergency use but is not started routinely. If necessary, use a 20- or 22-gauge peripheral tube, normal saline, or lactated Ringer's solution at 2 to 4 mL/kg/hour.

4. **Perioperative management and anesthetic technique**
   a) Mask general anesthesia is usually adequate for uncomplicated myringotomy of otherwise healthy patients.
   b) *Induction:* Mask inhalation induction with halothane or sevoflurane, N_2O, and O_2. If an existing intravenous catheter is present, routine intravenous induction is appropriate. Routine intravenous induction is preferred with older children and adults.
   c) *Maintenance:* standard maintenance with halothane, sevoflurane, or Forane, N_2O, and O_2. No need for muscle relaxation, and opiates are not routinely used. If the patient is an adult, isoflurane or desflurane are preferred to halothane due to increased risk of halothane hepatitis in adults.
   d) *Emergence:* Airway is maintained until the patient is fully awake. In older children and adults, antiemetics should be considered.

5. **Postoperative complications**
   Nausea and vomiting can be treated with
   a) Metoclopramide, 0.15 mg/kg/dose intravenously; maximum is 10 mg
   b) Droperidol, 30 to 75 mcg/kg/dose
   c) Ondansetron, 0.15 mg/kg/dose intravenously; maximum is 4 mg
   Note that these patients are often sensitive to sounds in the immediate postoperative period.

F. Tonsillectomy and Adenoidectomy

1. **Introduction**
   Children may present for tonsillectomy or adenoidectomy with a history of recurrent infections (chronic tonsillitis) or a history of obstruction and sleep apnea.
2. **Preoperative assessment and patient preparation**
   a) *History and physical examination*
      (1) *Cardiac:* Echocardiography may be useful to determine the presence of right-sided heart failure from chronic obstruction. These patients are at increased risk for negative pressure pulmonary edema and volume overload.
      (2) *Respiratory*: Evaluate for potentially difficult airway management. If child exhibits signs and symptoms of upper respiratory tract infection, there is an increased risk of laryngospasm intraoperatively and postoperatively. It is best to postpone this elective procedure until the upper respiratory tract infection resolves.
   b) *Patient preparation*
      (1) Judicious use of preoperative medication in children with obstructive apnea.
      (2) Midazolam (0.5 mg/kg) orally in children without obstruction
      (3) *Laboratory tests:* As indicated by the history and physical examination. Usually none in the healthy child.
      (4) *Diagnostic tests:* as indicated by the history and physical examination. Usually none indicated in the healthy child.
3. **Room preparation**
   a) *Monitoring equipment:* Standard
   b) *Additional equipment:* None
   c) Standard emergency drugs—Atropine, 0.01 to 0.02 mg/kg; lidocaine, 1 to 1.5 mg/kg; epinephrine, 0.01 mg/kg; and succinylcholine, 1 to 2 mg/kg
   d) Standard pediatric tabletop—endotracheal tubes, laryngoscope blade and handle, oral airways, lubricant, gauze, and emergency drugs
   e) *Intravenous fluids:* Depending on age and size of patient, a 22- or 24-gauge catheter should be sufficient. Infuse normal saline or lactated Ringer's solution at 2 to 4 mL/kg/hour.
4. **Perioperative management and anesthetic technique**
   a) Mask induction with O_2, N_2O, sevoflurane/halothane.
   b) Obtain intravenous access, administer narcotic, atropine as indicated, and muscle relaxant if desired (not necessary).
   c) Intubate with appropriate size endotracheal tube. Assure correct placement via auscultation of breath sounds, movement of chest, noted end-tidal CO_2 wave.
   d) *Maintenance:* Standard with sevoflurane, halothane, or isoflurane, O_2 and N_2O. Muscle relaxation not required. Opiates given at induction.

e)   At end of case, reverse remaining muscle relaxant if used. Carefully suction stomach and oropharynx. Extubate when the patient is fully awake due to increased risk of laryngospasm with presence of blood in the airway. Alternative method is true deep extubation after patient initiates first breath. Transfer patient to recovery unit in lateral position so secretions do not pool in back of airway, thus increasing risk of laryngospasm.

5. **Postoperative complications**
   a)   Nausea and vomiting can be treated with
      (1)   Metoclopramide, 0.15 mg/kg/dose; maximum is 10 mg
      (2)   Droperidol, 30 to 75 mcg/kg/dose
      (3)   Ondansetron, 0.15 mg/kg/dose; maximum is 4 mg
   b)   Pain
      (1)   Severity of pain depends on history of chronic infections and surgical technique.
      (2)   Site may be infiltrated with local anesthetic.
      (3)   Opioids may increase nausea and vomiting.
      (4)   Nonsteroidal anti-inflammatory agents are not recommended due to increased risk of bleeding.
      (5)   Pain usually resolves in 7 to 10 days with sloughing of tissue.
      (6)   Admission to hospital may be required if pain prevents adequate oral intake.
   c)   Bleeding
      (1)   Occurs in first 8 hours postoperatively or 7 to 10 days postoperatively when the eschar sheds.
      (2)   Bleeding tonsil forcing returning to OR has several implications:
         (a)   Patient is hypovolemic—establish intravenous access and infuse balanced salt solution or lactated Ringer's solution.
         (b)   Airway may be compromised due to presence of blood and edema. Have alternative plan for establishing a protected airway. Recommend use of endotracheal tube 0.5 mm smaller than original tube due to presence of edema.
         (c)   Plan rapid sequence induction. Patient is considered to be on a full stomach due to the presence of blood.

G. Pediatric Intra-abdominal Procedures

1. **Introduction**
   Abdominal procedures may be indicated for a variety of reasons: pyloric stenosis, necrotizing enterocolitis, omphalocele, gastroschisis, megacolon, biliary atresia, intestinal atresia, incarcerated hernia,

PART 2 Common Procedures

malrotation and volvulus, imperforate anus, and exstrophy of the cloaca or bladder.

2. **Preoperative assessment and patient preparation**
   a) *History and physical examination*
      (1) *Cardiac:* Other anomalies (patent ductus arteriosis, ventricular septal defect) may lead to congestive heart failure or murmur. The patient may have a labile blood pressure and hypovolemia from dehydration.
      (2) *Respiratory:* Premature infants may have immature respiratory centers and apneic/bradycardic episodes from hypoxemia. Respiratory compromise is possible with a large abdominal mass.
      (3) *Neurologic:* Premature infants may be prone to seizure disorders, myelomeningocele, hydrocephalus. Hypoxemia may predispose to intracranial hemorrhage.
      (4) *Renal:* Wilms' tumor may lead to hematuria and other genitourinary anomalies.
      (5) *Gastrointestinal:* The patient may have esophageal/gastric reflux, jaundice, anemia from hepatic disease, diarrhea with malabsorption states, a colostomy, bowel preparation, or intestinal compression.
      (6) *Endocrine:* Hypochloremia and hypokalemia; metabolic alkalosis from vomiting. Neuroblastomas are associated with increased catecholamine production.
   b) *Patient preparation*
      (1) *Laboratory tests:* Vary with pathology, procedure, and the history and physical examination—hemoglobin and hematocrit, type and crossmatch, electrolytes, glucose, liver function tests, prothrombin time, partial thromboplastin time.
      (2) *Premedication:* Midazolam (0.2 to 0.5 mg/kg) orally if at least 1 year old, 30 min prior to procedure.

3. **Room preparation**
   a) *Monitoring equipment:* Standard; depending on the procedure and health status, consider an arterial line, central venous pressure catheter, pulmonary arterial catheter, Foley catheter, and peripheral nerve stimulation.
   b) *Additional equipment:* Heated humidified circuit, heating pad, hot lamps, fluid warmers.
   c) *Position:* Supine
   d) *Fluids:* Therapy to address fluid deficit, maintenance, third-space loss, and blood loss. Insensible losses may be elevated because of phototherapy light or radiant heaters.
      (1) Deficit volume is calculated by multiplying the number of hours since the last fluid intake by hourly maintenance
      (2) Maintenance is calculated by 4 mL/kg/hour for 0 to 10 kg; 40 mL/kg/hour plus 2 mL/kg/hour for every kilogram above 10 for those weighing 10 to 20 kg; 60 mL/kg/hour plus 1 mL/kg/hour for every kilogram over 20 for those weighing more than 20 kg.
      (3) Third-space loss depends on the site and extent of surgery.

Replace with isotonic solutions. For peripheral/superficial, 1 to 3 mL/kg/hour; for abdominal/chest/hip, 3 to 4 mL/kg/hour; for extensive intra-abdominal, 6 to 10 mL/kg/hour.

(4) Replace blood when hematocrit is less than 30% and hemoglobin is less than 10 g/dL.

4. **Perioperative management and anesthetic technique**
   a) General anesthesia
   b) *Induction:* Decompress the stomach prior to induction. Preoxygenate for 2 to 3 minutes. Administer atropine (0.02 mg/kg) prior to laryngoscopy. Use rapid sequence or awake intubation. Upper extremity intravenous catheter is preferred. A leak should be present at 15 to 25 cm H_2O if the endotracheal tube is an appropriate size.
   c) *Maintenance:* Volatile inhalation agents. N_2O is avoided due to its tendency to distend the bowel. Decreases in central venous pressure of 4 mm H_2O or more are associated with vena cava compression. Use long- or intermediate-acting muscle relaxants. Vecuronium (0.05 mg/kg) or pancuronium (0.05 mg/kg). Use narcotic generously (fentanyl, 1.0 to 2.0 mcg/kg/dose). Consider intraoperative infusion, especially if postoperative ventilation is planned. Keep the oxygen saturation (SpO_2) at 95% to 97%. Avoid hypovolemia. The surgeon may infiltrate the site with local anesthetic prior to closure. Note peak inspiratory pressure (PIP) prior to abdominal closure.
   d) *Emergence:* Neostigmine (0.05 to 0.07 mg/kg) and glycopyrrolate (0.01 mg/kg) if postoperative ventilation is not desired. Suction the stomach prior to extubation. Extubate awake.

5. **Postoperative complications**
   a) Postoperative ventilation may be needed.
   b) Residual anesthesia can contribute to postoperative apnea.
   c) Peristalsis is usually delayed; may need total parenteral nutrition.
   d) Sepsis
   e) Abdominal third-space loss can continue immediately postoperatively; additional fluid resuscitation may be required.

H. Repair of Congenital Diaphragmatic Hernia

1. **Introduction**

A congenital diaphragmatic hernia results from abdominal viscera herniating into the chest through a defect in the diaphragm. The left side is affected more frequently. It occurs in 1 of 2000 to 3000 neonates; half are stillborn or die immediately after birth. Stillborn babies have a 95% incidence of other anomalies. Live births have a 20% incidence of other anomalies (patent ductus arteriosis is common). Herniated abdominal contents occupy the thoracic cavity and compromise lung development, leading to hypoplasia and mediastinal shift. The contralateral lung also has decreased amounts of alveoli. Symptoms usually are present after birth (dyspnea, cyanosis, dextrocardia, bowel sounds in the chest, bulging chest, decreased breath sounds). Infants may have to be intubated after delivery and placed in the neonatal intensive care unit.

2. **Preoperative assessment and patient preparation**
   a) *History and physical examination*
      (1) *Cardiac:* Check for other anomalies (patent ductus arteriosis). Mediastinal shift may compress the great vessels.
      (2) *Respiratory:* Check for pulmonary shunting and right-to-left shunting. A pneumothorax of the contralateral lung may occur from high positive inspiratory pressure (PIP). Check serial arterial blood gases, EtCO$_2$, oxygen saturation (SpO$_2$), chest radiographs, and ventilator setting. Adequate ventilation may correct acidosis.
      (3) *Neurologic:* Infants may be paralyzed while intubated in the neonatal intensive care unit. Severe hypoxia can lead to neurologic damage.
      (4) *Renal:* Peripheral perfusion may be increased by dopamine at 1 to 5 mcg/kg/min.
      (5) *Gastrointestinal:* A nasogastric tube should be placed for intermittent suction to prevent further distention and pulmonary compression.
   b) *Patient preparation*
      (1) *Laboratory tests:* Arterial blood gases, complete blood count, electrolytes
      (2) *Diagnostic tests:* Chest radiography with bowel gas pattern and mediastinal shift

3. **Room preparation**
   a) *Monitoring equipment:* Standard. The internal jugular vein can be used for central venous pressure monitoring. The contralateral side precordial is used to monitor for pneumothorax. Venous access in the lower extremities is not recommended because of possible vena cava compression.
   b) *Additional equipment:* All warming devices to prevent hypothermia, which increases O$_2$ consumption and desaturation.
   c) *Position:* Supine. Abdominal incision is usual, but the transthoracic or thoracoabdominal approach may be used.

4. **Perioperative management and anesthetic technique**
   a) General anesthesia
   b) *Induction:* Rapid sequence or awake intubation
   c) *Maintenance:* Need a high O$_2$ concentration. Avoid N$_2$O because it can diffuse across the viscera and increase lung compression. High-dose narcotics with low concentrations of volatile anesthetics may be used to maintain cardiovascular stability. High ventilation rates are used for adequate oxygenation. High pressure may increase the incidence of pneumothorax. Perform frequent arterial blood gases, and keep the arterial CO$_2$ pressure at 25 to

30 mm Hg. With sudden hemodynamic compromise, suspect a contralateral pneumothorax. Increase FiO$_2$ to 100% and obtain a chest x-ray. A small pneumothorax may spontaneously resolve; larger ones may compromise respiratory and hemodynamic stability, necessitating chest tube placement.

d) *Emergence:* Infants usually remain intubated, paralyzed, and ventilated in the neonatal intensive care unit.

5. **Postoperative complications**

a) Depend on the severity of pulmonary hypertension and hypoplasia. Some infants show a "honeymoon" period followed by deterioration with right-to-left shunting, hypoxia, hypercapnia, acidosis, pulmonary hypertension, and death.

b) High-frequency oscillation ventilators may be used to reduce pulmonary arterial pressure.

c) Patent ductus arteriosis may be ligated.

d) The infant may need extracorporeal membrane oxygenation (ECMO) to decrease pulmonary workload. The internal jugular vein may be cannulated with one venovenous cannula, or the internal jugular and common carotid may be cannulated with two venoarterial cannulas. The infant is kept paralyzed.

e) Prostaglandins may be used to decrease pulmonary vascular resistance.

f) Tolazoline (Priscoline) relaxes vascular smooth muscle with α-adrenergic blockade. Drip 100 mg/100 cc for a concentration of 0.1mg/cc. Infuse at 1 to 10 mg/kg/hour (usually 1 mg/kg/hour).

g) Intravenous medication can be used for hemodynamic support.
   (1) Dobutamine—vasopressor, increases heart rate and contractility
       200 mg/250 cc D5W (0.8 mg/cc = 800 mcg/cc)
       Infuse at 2.5 to 15 mcg/kg/min (MAX 40 mcg/kg/min)
   (2) Dopamine—vasopressor, increases heart rate and contractility
       200 mg/250 cc D5W (0.8 mg/cc = 800 mcg/cc)
       Infuse at 1 to 20 mcg/kg/min
   (3) Epinephrine—inotrope, increases heart rate
       1 mg/100 cc D5W (0.01 mg/cc = 10 mcg/cc)
       0.1 to 1 mcg/kg/min
   (4) Norepinephrine—inotrope
       Bolus 0.01 mcg/kg
       Drip 1 mg/100 cc D5W (10 mcg/cc)
   (5) Phenylephrine—α-agonist
       Drip 10 mg/250 cc D5W (40 mcg/cc)
       Bolus 5 to 20 mcg/kg/dose every 15 minutes
   (6) Nitroglycerine—vasodilator, reduces preload
       Drip 100 mg/250 cc D5W (0.04 mg/cc = 400 mcg/cc)
       1 to 5 mcg/kg/min

PART 2 Common Procedures

I. Pediatric Hernia Repair

1. **Introduction**

   Inguinal hernia repair is the most common procedure performed in children. Premature infants are more likely to have incarcerations, mostly due to failure of the processus vaginalis to obliterate. The procedure is performed through an inguinal crease incision. Complications of hernia repairs are rare. Umbilical hernias are more common in blacks and may close spontaneously (95% to 98% by age 5). Repair is performed through a transverse infraumbilical incision. Intraperitoneal exploration is rarely done.

2. **Preoperative assessment**

   a) *History and physical examination*
      (1) *Cardiac:* Routine
      (2) *Respiratory:* Prolonged ventilation and immature lungs are more susceptible to tracheomalacia, subglottic stenosis, and bronchopulmonary dysplasia.
      (3) *Neurologic:* Premature infants may display transient apneic and bradycardic episodes in response to hypoxemia. Premature infants are more prone to seizure disorders. Complications from general anesthesia may occur from effects on the immature central nervous system.
      (4) *Renal:* Routine
      (5) *Gastrointestinal:* The patient may have abdominal compression if the umbilical hernia is large. Consider rapid sequence induction for incarcerated hernia and bowel obstructions.
      (6) *Endocrine:* Premature infants are more prone to hypoglycemia. Check the blood glucose level.
   b) *Patient preparation*
      (1) *Laboratory tests:* As indicated from the history and physical examination
      (2) *Diagnostic tests:* None
      (3) *Medications:* Midazolam 0.2 to 0.5 mg/kg orally 30 minutes before surgery for children over 1 year of age

3. **Room preparation**

   a) *Monitoring equipment:* Standard
   b) *Additional equipment:* Use pediatric circle or bain circuit. Warm and humidify gases. Warming pad may be used on the table.
   c) *Position:* Supine
   d) *Fluids:* 0.9 normal saline or lactated Ringer's solution at 4 mL/kg/hour for 1 to 10 kg of weight. Add 2 mL/kg/hour for 11 to 20 kg. Dextrose solutions may be used for infants less than 1 month old.
   e) *Blood:* Negligible loss

4. **Perioperative management and anesthetic technique**

   a) General anesthesia, mask, or endotracheal tube. Caudal block may be performed after induction for postoperative pain.

b) *Induction:* Mask with halothane or sevoflurane/O_2/N_2O. Obtain intravenous line after induction. Administer atropine intravenously (0.02 mg/kg) prior to laryngoscopy. Vecuronium (0.1 mg/kg) or cisatracurium (0.1 to 0.2 mg/kg). If the child is healthy and more than 1 year old, the mask may be used. If applicable, caudal block with bupivacaine (0.25%) with epinephrine (1:200,000), 1 mL/kg after induction (onset of 15 minutes).

c) *Maintenance:* Caudal block will decrease the amount of volatile agent. Increase the MAC prior to incision to avoid laryngospasm.

d) *Emergence:* Extubate fully awake. Intravenous reversal, neostigmine (0.07 mg/kg) and glycopyrrolate (0.01 mg/kg).

5. **Postoperative complications**
Postoperative apnea can occur in infants at 50 to 60 weeks of gestational age, especially if premature. These patients should be admitted for postoperative observation.

J. Genitourinary Procedures

1. **Introduction**
    a) A cystoscopy is usually a brief procedure, allowing for administration of general anesthesia via a mask. A laryngeal mask airway may also be used.
    b) Hypospadias repair, chordee release, or repair of undescended testicles are usually performed under general anesthesia with an endotracheal tube. If the testicle cannot be located directly, an intra-abdominal approach with muscle relaxation may be required.

2. **Preoperative assessment and patient preparation**
    a) *History and physical examination*
        (1) Review systems to determine presence of comorbidities.
        (2) *Laboratory tests:* As indicated by the history and physical examination
        (3) *Diagnostic tests:* As indicated by the history and physical examination
    b) *Patient preparation:* Administer midazolam (0.5 mg/kg) orally 20 to 30 minutes prior to procedure if desired

3. **Room preparation**
    a) *Monitoring equipment:* Standard
    b) *Additional equipment:* Warming devices for prolonged procedures
    c) *Position:* Supine for orchipexy, chordee release, and hypospadias repair. Lithotomy position for cystoscopy. Pad all pressure points; maintain proper body alignment to prevent nerve and soft tissue injuries.
    d) *Standard pediatric tabletop*
    e) *Intravenous fluids:* Depending on patient age and size, a 22- or 24-gauge catheter should be sufficient. Infuse normal saline or

lactated Ringer's solution at a rate of 2 to 4 mL/kg/hour plus NPO and blood loss replacements.

4. **Perioperative management and anesthetic technique**
   a) Mask induction with O_2, N_2O, and sevoflurane/halothane. If patient has preexisting intravenous line established, administer propofol (2 mg/kg) or Pentothal (4 to 6 mg/kg). Muscle relaxation if desired for intubation purposes. Muscle relaxation is not required for procedure.
   b) Obtain protected airway with appropriately sized endotracheal tube. Assure proper placement and secure with tape.
   c) *Maintenance:* O_2, N_2O, and sevoflurane/halothane/isoflurane. Intravenous fluid rate as calculated. Maintain normothermia. Manipulation of the testicles or peritoneum may produce a profound vagal response. Pretreat with atropine or glycopyrrolate prior to occurrence. Caudal anesthesia prevents the response. If bradycardia occurs and is refractory to atropine, treat with fluid bolus (10 to 20 mL) or epinephrine (10 to 20 mcg) intravenously.
   d) *Emergence:* Extubate patient awake.

5. **Postoperative complications**
   a) Pain
   b) Opioids may increase incidence of nausea and vomiting.
   c) Caudal anesthesia is appropriate in children under age 7 and may be performed after induction to decrease volatile agent requirements or prior to emergence. Bupivacaine (0.25%) for a total of 0.5 to 1 mL/kg will provide approximately 6 to 12 hours of pain relief postoperatively.

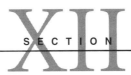

SECTION XII

Anesthesia for Therapeutic/ Diagnostic Procedures

A. Overall Anesthetic Care Plan

1. **Introduction**
   a) There are a number of diagnostic and therapeutic procedures performed outside the operating room environment that require anesthesia services. These services include providing anesthetic care adhering to the AANA/ASA standards and institutional accreditation guidelines.
   b) Examples of areas that use off-site anesthesia services are as follows:
      (1) Computer tomograghy (CT) scan
      (2) Magnetic resonance imaging (MRI)
      (3) Nuclear medicine
      (4) Interventional radiology
      (5) Radiation oncology
      (6) Cardiac catheterization laboratory
      (7) Endoscopy
2. **Monitoring**
   Follow AANA/ASA/institutional requirements.
3. **Check room for essential equipment**
   a) Oxygen and suction
   b) Anesthesia machine and ancillary supplies (i.e., endotracheal tube, laryngoscope/blades, oral and nasal airways, oxygen mask, and nasal cannulas)
   c) Adequate monitoring equipment to allow adherence to standards of practice (i.e., ECG, NIBP, pulse oximeter, capnograph, and thermometer)
   d) Intravenous supplies and fluid
   e) Sufficient electrical outlets to satisfy anesthesia machine and monitoring equipment requirements
   f) Adequate illumination of the patient, anesthesia machine, and monitoring equipment
   g) Emergency cart with defibrillator, emergency drugs, and other resuscucitative equipment equivalent to that in the operating room
4. **Disadvantages of off-site procedures**
   a) *Physical setup*
      (1) Unfamiliar and isolated location limits anesthesia department backup (i.e., emergencies, labs, staffing, transportation, and availability of drugs).

      (2) O_2 source—wall outlet inaccessibility or piped in gases

      (3) Available scavenging system

      (4) Availability of wall suction

      (5) Availability of electrical outlets

      (6) Dim lighting conditions

      (7) Recovery staff availability

  b) *Limited patient access*

      (1) Crowded spaces

      (2) Shields

      (3) Fluoroscopy and imaging tables moving and turning

  c) *Potential contact with hazardous materials*

      (1) Radiation exposure or exposure to magnetic field

      (2) Inhalation agents due to lack of adequate scavenging system

5. Potential hazards of off-site procedures

  a) *Temperature control*

      (1) Problems include cold rooms and tables and vasodilation under anesthesia

      (2) Temperature monitors are inaccessible.

      (3) Turn the internal fans of the MRI unit off during scanning.

      (4) Cover the infant's head with a cap.

      (5) In MRI, compatible, disposable, crushed warming devices may be used on neonates.

      (6) Place patient under warmer after procedure.

  b) *Monitor access and interference from machinery.*

      (1) All monitors must be placed and functioning well prior to the beginning of procedure.

      (2) Monitors should be placed at the point of least distortion.

      (3) Equipment should have good artifact suppression characteristics; however, most artifact cannot be eliminated.

      (4) Use only MRI–compatible monitors to avoid burns from coiling from an amplified antenna effect.

  c) *Fluid management*

      (1) Intravenous access is limited. It is recommended that all pediatric patients under the age of 1 year be placed on a medfusion pump for fluid volume control. Children between ages 1 and 3 years should have intravenous fluids controlled by a medfusion pump or buritrol chamber in line to avoid fluid overload. Microinfusion extension tubing has 2 mL volume per 5 ft, and this volume should be considered in fluid calculations.

      (2) Intravenous line should be taped securely to avoid loss of access.

      (3) Run fluids judiciously according to needs (i.e., bowel prep or contrast infusion, prolonged fasting, and NPO [nothing by mouth] times).

  d) *Airway management*

      (1) There is limited access of patient, so vigilance and observation is key.

      (2) Respiratory pattern may be difficult to observe; monitor $EtCO_2$ and pulse oximeter closely.

6. **Selection of anesthetic agents and techniques**
   a) *Goals*
      (1) Ventilation and perfusion of tissues should not be compromised.
      (2) Airway should remain patent with spontaneous respirations and protective reflexes intact if using sedation technique. Protect airway.
      (3) Induction of anesthetic should be rapid, painless, and 100% effective.
      (4) The patient should remain motionless for the duration of the procedure.
      (5) Recovery should be rapid, and there should be no nausea or dysphoria.
   b) *Considerations*
      (1) The patient's condition, age, and underlying medical problems must be evaluated. Many children scheduled for these procedures are chronically ill and may have multiple anomalies and disorders.
      (2) The location of the procedure may influence airway and access to patient and intravenous lines.
      (3) Requirements of procedure, such as duration, position, and the possibility of pain
7. **Preoperative considerations**
   a) *Patient preparation*
      (1) All patients should undergo a full preanesthetic assessment to determine their fitness and the type of anesthetic required for the procedure. This should consist of a full history and examination with the appropriate laboratory work.
      (2) The parent/guardian must be present for underage children. Adults should have a companion for discharge.
      (3) Strict NPO guidelines are adhered to—children under 12 months of age should have no solids after midnight on the day of surgery, formula and breast milk are allowed up to 6 hours prior to surgery, and clear liquids up to 4 hours prior to surgery. Children 1 to 3 years old should have no solids after midnight; clear liquids may be given up to 6 hours before the time of surgery. Adults should be NPO after midnight.
      (4) Appropriate premedication is given for specific procedures; assess patient medical condition and level of maturity and anxiety.
   b) Premedication has many purposes—relief of anxiety, sedation with rapid recovery, analgesia, amnesia, reduction of salivary and gastric secretions, elevation of gastric pH, and decreased cardiac vagal activity.
      (1) Versed—nasal or oral administration (0.5 to 0.75 mg/kg); 0.05 mg/kg intravenously
      (2) Methohexital—rectal 20 to 25 mg/kg (diluted to 100 mg/mL; 7 mg/kg intramuscularly of 3.5% concentration

(3) Ketamine—3 mg/kg intramuscularly or 6 mg/kg orally in conjunction with an antisialagogue glycopyrrolate

(4) Consider atropine (0.01 to 0.02 mg/kg) to provide protection against a cholinergic response.

8. **Anesthetic techniques for maintenance**

a) Safe choices may include monitored sedation, dissociative, and general anesthesia.

b) Monitored sedation is appropriate for nonpainful, simple diagnostic examinations that require patient cooperation.

c) TIVA—in children undergoing noninvasive procedures, nonintubated intravenous general anesthesia techniques are commonly used. Light levels of general anesthesia allow for prompt recovery. When a deep level of sedation is obtained, reflex activity is minimized; response to painful stimuli is attenuated; and obstruction, laryngospasm, and apnea are increased.

d) Dissociative anesthesia (ketamine) spontaneous respirations are usually maintained, with anesthesia intramuscularly prior to intravenous placement. Heart rate and blood pressure are usually increased. Disadvantages include increased airway irritability; painful injection; prolonged; unpredictable; or delirious emergence; nausea; and increased intracranial pressure.

e) General anesthesia is indicated when the airway cannot be assured because of positioning, procedure is lengthy and painful, or airway must be protected (i.e., upper endoscopy). Patient must remain motionless for long periods or neuromuscular blockade is needed (percutaneous ASD [atrial septal defect] closure).

9. **Postanesthesia care**

a) Infants and children generally recover more quickly from anesthesia and are less disturbed by minor complications than adults.

b) Transport to recovery should include appropriate monitoring, oxygen, and emergency airway equipment and medications.

c) Ability to deal with adverse reactions in a timely fashion (i.e., contrast dye anaphylaxis, laryngospasm, bronchospasm, cardiovascular collapse).

B. Anesthesia for CT Scan and MRI

1. **Introduction**

a) To obtain successful CT scan and MRI, the patient must lie absolutely still throughout the entire procedure.

b) Anesthesia may be needed for cooperative patients with movement disorders and for patients who are confused or uncooperative, such as for patients with closed head injuries or pediatric patients.

2. **Potential problems associated with anesthesia**
   a) Patient inaccessibility
   b) Airway management
   c) Effects of the MRI magnetism on the monitoring equipment
3. **Considerations on the use of radiopaque dye**
   a) Ionic contrast media (sodium meglumin, salts of iodinated acids, or combinations) can be used for imaging studies.
   b) The hyperosmolarity of ionic compounds can cause a typical (nonallergic) reaction characterized by flushing, tachycardia, and nausea, probably caused by endothelial disruption and the subsequent nonimmunologic release of vasoactive substances from mast cells.
   c) Some patients will exhibit a true allergy to iodine. Patients at risk are allergic to shellfish or have iodine, asthma, or drug allergies.
   d) Pretreatment for patients at risk for an allergic reaction include methylprednisone (0.5 mg/kg orally) and diphenhydramine (0.5 to 1.0 mg/kg orally or intravenously).
   e) Treat anaphylaxis with epinephrine (10 mcg/kg).
4. **Positioning problems**
   a) Examination of the posterior fossa with CT requires extreme flexion of the head, which may obstruct the airway or kink the endotracheal tube.
   b) Patients are secluded in a room away from the anesthesia personnel's reach.
   c) Pressure points should be padded to avoid positioning injuries.
5. **Recommended anesthesia management**
   a) *Preprocedure:* Versed (0.5 to 0.75 mg) orally 20 minutes before the scan if the patient is uncooperative.
   b) Start with mask induction with O_2, N_2O and halothane or sevoflurane.
   c) *Maintenance*
      (1) Patients should be spontaneously breathing. O_2 with nasal cannula or mask can be used. For children less than 3 months, patients with difficult airways, or patients exhibiting sleep apnea, the airway may be secured with LMA or an endotracheal tube.
      (2) Propofol—initial bolus 1 mg/kg. Atropine may be needed in children to offset cardiac depressive effects.
      (3) Propofol infusion—5 mg/kg/hour up to a maximum of 10 mg/kg/hour.
      (4) Deepening anesthesia during infusion—bolus propofol (0.3 to 0.5 mg/kg) and Versed (0.02 mg/kg).

PART 2 Common Procedures

C. Nuclear Medicine

1. **Terminology**
   a) Positron emission tomography (PET), is an advanced imaging system that provides a three-dimensional view of human organs to help diagnose disease and other abnormalities. The system is made up of three parts: a cyclotron, a PET scanner, and a computer.
   b) Radionuclides—energy-charged atoms of carbon, nitrogen, oxygen, and fluorine
   c) Half-life is the period of time that it takes for one-half of the radioactive material to lose its radioactivity.
2. **Principles**
   a) A PET image is obtained by using a cyclotron-produced radionuclide to make short-lived radiopharmaceutical compounds with half-lives of 2 to 110 minutes. These short half-lives allow lower radiation exposure.
   b) Moments after the radioactive compound is prepared, it is quickly transported to the scanner room through an underground pneumatic tube system. After injection or inhalation by the patient, the compound travels through the patient's bloodstream to the organ being scanned, where it decays and emits positively charged electrons called positrons.
   c) In the body, positrons interact with negatively charged electrons to produce gamma rays that light up at the area being examined. The PET scanner's circular array of detectors is positioned around the patient's body to detect gamma ray activity. The activity is translated by the computer into an image on the computer monitor. The image captures a cross-sectional (tomographic) slice of the organ to show its circulation of metabolism. The glucose base of many compounds used for brain scans will have an uptake quality related to the patient's cerebral metabolic rate. Maintaining the metabolic rate normality is essential to the scanning outcome.
   d) The PET scan image distinguishes parts of the organ to pinpoint where cells are dead or alive, and it helps to determine the best form of treatment for the patient.
3. **Anesthetic Considerations**
   a) The PET scan is pain free; however, the patient must be absolutely still during the scanning. The patient lies flat on a table placed in the center of the scanner and his or her arms may be strapped to the sides to prevent movement. During a brain scan, the patient wears a custom-fitted plastic face mask, and the sides of the mask are hooked onto the PET scanner table to prevent head movements during an exam. This positioning is very hard for anyone who cannot fully cooperate (pediatric, claustrophobic, and neuromuscular disease patients). Anesthesia service will often be requested for head/brain scans.

b) *Cerebral metabolism:* The outcome of the scan can be effected by depression of cerebral metabolic rates related to anesthesia. The suggested doses of propofol (1 to 2 mg/kg) initial bolus followed by a 5 to 10 mg/kg/hour maintenance infusion have provided excellent scan results, while higher doses and other synergistic sedation combinations have resulted in poor cerebral glucose metabolism and the lack of radioactive compound uptake required for scanning.

c) *Radiation:* The equipment is not the source of radiation. The patient is the source of radiation only after the intravenous injection of the radioactive material. The care provider needs to remain as far from the patient as possible and limit access time of any close or hands-on patient care.

d) *Occupational exposure:* If an anesthesia provider used complete disregard for radiation safety principles in minimizing exposure, the provider could receive a maximum 4.5 mrem/patient in a 3-hour exposure, which is 0.009% of the legal limit for occupationally exposed individuals and 4.5% of the annual limit to the general public. (Each anesthesia staff member could perform 22 such cases and not exceed the exposure limit to the general public.) In spite of legal concerns, protect staff from any unnecessary radiation exposure.

e) *Limit patient access:* Assure depth of sedation and ventilatory status; a certified registered nurse anesthetist (CRNA) should be positioned for adequate patient/monitor observation prior to the patient receiving a radioactive injection.

4. **PET Scan Room Setup**
   a) The CRNA is positioned outside the scanner room and can view the infusion pump, anesthesia monitors, and the patient (assisted by a camera focused on the patient's head) through an observation area. The room may be entered at any time without interfering with the scanning series.
   b) The CRNA can be positioned inside the scanner room, but it is highly recommended that the majority of the observation time be at distances as far from the patient as the room will allow.

5. **Nuclear Scan Setup**
   a) The CRNA must be positioned inside the scanner room.
   b) Obtain anesthesia gas machine with long ventilatory circuit, full monitoring capabilities, anesthesia sedation drugs (i.e., propofol, Versed), portable oxygen, and oximeter with ambu or Jackson-Reese for transport.
   c) Intravenous maintenance is the preferred method for the scanning period. Avoid oral medications since they will have prolonged cerebral metabolic depression and adversely effect the glucose medial/injectate uptake, resulting in poor scan quality. A brief period of halothane or sevoflurane and N_2O for intravenous start has not effected test outcome, if the expired gas sample is allowed to return to zero prior to the initial EEG. Propofol initial bolus of 1 to 2 mg/kg and 5 to 10 mg/kg/hour for continuous infusion maintenance.

D. Brachytherapy

1. **Introduction**
   Palladium-103 prostate implants are being used as an optional treatment for prostate cancer. The sources are permanently implanted directly into the tissue. The seeds are encased in a lead-lined cartridge, that attaches to lead-lined placement needles. The seeds are placed by the radiation oncologist via these needles into the prostate through the perineum. Placement is guided by ultrasound.
2. **Preoperative assessment and patient preparation**
   a) The treatment is performed in the radiation oncology department.
   b) Each patient will be prescreened and admitted as an outpatient through the short stay unit.
   c) The procedure will last a maximum of 2 hours.
   d) Patients may undergo a bowel prep at home prior to the procedure.
   e) An 18-gauge intravenous tube with a 2-inch angiocath will be placed prior to procedure.
   f) Each patient will require intravenous antibiotics prior to the procedure. One gram of Ancef is required. If the patient has an allergy to penicillin, then Cleocin (600 mg) is given.
3. **Room preparation**
   Required monitoring equipment, anesthesia, and airway supplies
4. **Anesthetic management**
   a) Anesthesia is usually maintained via spinal anesthesia. A minimal T8 level is desired. If the patient is required to have consecutive treatments, an epidural may be placed.
   b) Sedation is given as needed.
   c) The patient is placed in a lithotomy position for the procedure. A foley is inserted with hypaque in the balloon. An ultrasound probe and perineum template are placed prior to needle placement.
   d) The time of treatment is the time of radiation. Everyone must leave the room. Visual contact is always present via monitors. Treatment time is usually 5 to 15 minutes.
5. **Radiation precautions**
   a) Occasionally, seeds can become dislodged from the implanted tissue. Therefore dressings and linens must not be removed from the room until they have been checked and cleared by the oncology physicist.
   b) If a seed is discovered, ***do not*** touch it with your hands. Use long forceps to place it in a lead storage container.
   c) Some seeds may pass in the urine for the first few days. Therefore urine must be strained before being discarded.
   d) Pregnant personnel are not to attend these patients.
   e) All personnel remaining in the room during the procedure should be properly badged. No person or material should leave the room without being surveyed with a Geiger counter.

E. Cardioversion

1. **Introduction**
   Synchronized cardioversion is the electrical conversion of a tachyrhythmia, such as atrial fibrillation, atrial flutter, or supraventricular tachycardia, unresponsive to intravenous drugs, to a normal sinus rhythm. A synchronized electrical shock is released through the chest wall, depolarizing the myocardium and simultaneously making it refractory, thereby enabling the sinoatrial node to resume its function as a primary pacemaker.
2. **Preoperative assessment and patient preparation**
   a) *History and physical examination:* Standard
   b) *Diagnostic tests:* 12-lead electrocardiography
   c) *Preoperative medication and intravenous therapy*
      (1) One may desire to hold the daily dose of digoxin.
      (2) One 18-gauge intravenous tube with minimal fluid replacement
3. **Room preparation**
   a) *Monitoring equipment*
      (1) Standard
      (2) Artificial cardiac pacing
   b) *Pharmacologic agents:* Atropine, lidocaine
   c) *Position:* Supine
4. **Anesthetic technique**
   a) Sedation
   b) Intravenous sedation—midazolam, methohexital (Brevital), or propofol in sedative doses until the patient's lid reflex is gone.
5. **Perioperative management**
   a) *Induction:* Preoxygenate the patient with the use of nasal cannula or face mask.
   b) *Maintenance:* As soon as consciousness is lost, the synchronized charge should be delivered with the R-wave on the electrocardiogram to avoid causing ventricular fibrillation.
   c) *Emergence:* Support the airway and maintain ventilation until consciousness is regained.
6. **Postoperative implications**
   Monitor the electrocardiogram; complex ventricular arrhythmias may appear, especially if the patient was taking digoxin.

PART 2 **Common Procedures**

F. Automatic Implantable Cardioverter Defibrillator (AICD)

1. **Introduction**
   Indications for AICDs include sustained ventricular tachycardia (VT) and syncope due to VT and ventricular fibrillation (VF). Electrical countershock is the only reliable treatment for VF. AICDs resemble large pacemakers and contain a power generator that is implanted over the pectoral muscle under local anesthesia and sedation. AICDs contain a single intracardiac countershocking electrode; this electrode also serves as a ventricular pacing lead. This device senses electrical activity and will emit an electrical countershock if a tachydysrhythmia is sensed.

2. **Preoperative assessment**
   a) Most patients who present for an AICD have severe coronary artery disease, which may include a recent infarct, cardiomyopathy, and coronary artery bypass graft (CABG).
   b) *History and physical examination*
   (1) Document indications for AICD and preexisting medical conditions.
   (2) Evaluate left ventricular function and echocardiogram results.
   (3) Obtain recent ECG and cardiac catheterization results if available.
   (4) Assess chest X ray for left ventricular hypertrophy.
   c) *Patient preparation*
   (1) Obtain electrolytes, prothrombin time, and partial thromboplastin time if patient is taking anticoagulants.
   (2) Explain to patient that the procedure is performed locally with sedation.

3. **Room preparation**
   a) Fluoroscopy is used during the entire procedure, and lead shields should be worn.
   b) Full monitoring and standard tabletop needs to be available.
   c) Invasive monitoring during the procedure is usually not necessary, unless the patient has preexisting lines.
   d) Know where the crash cart, wall suction, and oxygen source is located.
   e) Alternative means of providing emergency pacing should be available.

4. **Perioperative management and anesthetic technique**
   a) Verification of AICD placement involves the induction of VT or VF and tests the device's capability to convert the tachyarrhythmia to a normal sinus rhythm.
   b) While the device is being tested, the patient should be ventilated with a 100% O_2 with administration of Versed for amnesia.

5. **Postoperative implications**
    a) Patients with AICDs should not enter a room with an MRI machine, since the MRI magnetic field will deactivate the AICD.
    b) AICDs should be deactivated prior to lithotripsy.
    c) Be aware of potential pacemaker and AICD interaction with other tachyarrhymthias such as sinus tachycardia or atrial fibrillation.
    d) Patients should be instructed of the need to have the AICD turned off and deactivated prior to any subsequent surgeries, as electrocautery can cause the AICD to discharge inappropriately during surgery.

G. Cardiac Radiofrequency Ablation

1. **Introduction**
    a) Cardiac ablation procedures can be performed either surgically or through a transvenous catheter.
    b) Transvenous catheter ablation involves the use of radiofrequency energy to deliver direct high-energy current shocks to the heart so as to ablate atrial and ventricular tachycardia and associated accessory pathways.
    c) Indications for ablation include SVT and recurrent accessory pathway disorders such as Wolff-Parkison-White Syndrome or Lown-Ganong Levine.
2. **Preoperative assessment**
    a) Patients are usually young with normal ventricular function.
    b) A thorough history and physical examination should be obtained.
    c) Drugs used to treat dysrhythmia are usually discontinued prior to surgery to make the dysrhythmia more inducible.
    d) External defibrillator-cardioverter pads are placed before the procedure.
    e) Sedation should be given for femoral and IJ catheter placement by the cardiologist.
3. **Room Preparation**
    Standard monitors and tabletop with fluoroscopy are used.
4. **Perioperative management and anesthetic technique**
    a) Radiofrequency ablation is not considered extremely painful because muscles and nerves are not stimulated. Most patients do experience a burning sensation when ablation is applied, and sedation is necessary at this time.
    b) Mapping of the target foci and accessory pathways requires inducing a reentry tachycardia, using a stimulator to initiate premature atrial and ventricular beats.
    c) Usual procedure time is 4 to 6 hours with intermittent stimulation used.
5. **Postoperative implications**
    The patient should be monitored overnight for any arrhythmias.

H. Endoscopy

1. **Equipment**
   As with any procedure, wall O_2 and suction, ECG, pulse oximeter, NIBP, and crash cart should be available.
2. **Anesthesia considerations**
   a) Conscious or deep intravenous sedation is used with the majority of these patients.
   b) Sedation medications can include propofol, Versed, and fentanyl.
   c) Antibiotics are not required for endoscopy patients.

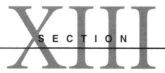

Other Procedures

A. Burns

1. **Introduction**
   Patients who sustain full-thickness burns are seen in the operating room, probably repeatedly, for debridement and grafting. The initial assessment of the emergency burn patient is begun as for any trauma patient and begins with airway intubation. Keep in mind that airway edema happens rapidly in a burn patient, and intubation after the edema occurs is difficult. Burn patients must be aggressively fluid resuscitated in the first 48 hours.

2. **Preoperative assessment**
   a) *Cardiac:* Assess for any preexisting cardiac problems. In the acutely burned patient, there is a large increase in circulating catecholamines, which will manifest as tachycardia and possibly as increased blood pressure.

   b) *Respiratory:* Intubate the patient if there are any signs of upper airway burn. This could include oral burns, cough productive of soot, and stridor. Assess arterial blood gases with a carboxy-hemoglobin level. Intubate with controlled ventilation. Burn patients are also prone to adult respiratory distress syndrome. They may need higher minute ventilation and increasing amounts of positive end-expiratory pressure. Assess edema, chest wall compliance, and neck mobility; there may be sufficient edema or scar formation to cause an unexpected difficult intubation.

   c) *Neurologic:* Assess and document preoperative neurologic function as accurately as possible.

   d) *Renal:* Relative hypovolemia from increased permeability causes renal hypoperfusion. Also, acute tubular necrosis due to myoglobinuria and cellular debris can cause acute renal failure.

   e) *Gastrointestinal:* All emergency burn patients are considered to have a full stomach. Many will develop a paralytic ileus. They are also predisposed to develop a "stress ulcer."

   f) *Endocrine:* There is an increased level of stress hormones, leading to hyperglycemia and insulin resistance. There is also a substantial increase in basal metabolic rates due to increasing catecholamines causing increased O_2 consumption and CO_2 production.

   g) *Hematologic:* Coagulopathies have been associated with both the burn process and the relative clotting factor dilution that occurs with volume resuscitation. Decreased plasma proteins, such as albumin, will increase plasma protein bound drugs (benzodiazepines). Blood loss can be extensive, especially with debridements. Estimate blood loss at 4 cc/cm^2 for surface that is excised/harvested. Start infusing blood prior to beginning the procedure. Since visual estimates are inaccurate, monitor hemoglobin, hematocrit, and urine output. Patients are susceptible to hypothermia due to hypermetabolism, evaporation of fluid loss, exposure, and multiple blood transfusions.

3. **Patient preparation**
   Complete blood count, electrolytes, blood urea nitrogen, creatinine, glucose, urinalysis, prothrombin time, partial thromboplastin time (dimer or fibrin split products if disseminated intravascular coagulation is suspected), type and crossmatch (number of units depends on the area to be debrided/grafted), chest radiography, arterial blood gases (with carboxyhemoglobin if indicated). Other tests as suggested by the history and physical examination.

   Begin volume replacement with crystalloid or blood or both preoperatively. If patient condition permits, an anxiolytic (such as benzodiazepine) and narcotic may be useful preoperatively.

4. **Room preparation**
   a) *Monitors:* Standard. Needle electrodes may be needed for electrocardiography. Blood pressure can be measured on the lower extremities; an arterial line or a cuff can be placed over the burned area with a sterile lubricated dressing after consultation with the burn specialist. Most patients with burns of more than 40% to 50% require an arterial line, a central line, and a pulmonary arterial catheter if hemodynamically unstable. Use caution in placement and avoid burned areas.

   b) *Additional equipment:* Blood and fluid warmers. A heated circuit and warming blanket are used. Room temperature is increased. Burn patients are poikilothermic.

   c) *Positioning:* Various positions may be required intraoperatively depending on the area being worked on. Assess limb contractures and stabilize fractures.

   d) *Drugs and tabletop:* Succinylcholine can cause life-threatening hyperkalemia (especially 4 to 70 days after the burn occurs) due to massive potassium release from muscle cells, thus it is contraindicated in the burn patient. These patients also have an increased need for nondepolarizing relaxants because of up regulation of ACH receptors. The plasma of burn victims has an anticurare effect. Most surgeons request that antibiotics be given intraoperatively.

5. **Perioperative management and anesthetic technique**
   Unless the burn covers a small body surface area percentage, general anesthesia is usually used. Review previous anesthesia records if the patient is receiving repeat procedures, such as debridements. The choice of induction agent depends on the patient's condition. Thiopental or propofol is appropriate in the hemodynamically stable patient. If the patient is already intubated, a narcotic/inhaled induction may be indicated. In the hemodynamically unstable patient, ketamine or O$_2$/paralysis may be used.

Several concerns intraoperatively are for fluid and blood replacement and maintenance of body temperature and respiratory parameters. Fluid should be replaced at 4 cc/kg of balanced salt solution every hour of body surface area burned or according to hemodynamics and urine output (0.5 to 1.0 cc/kg/hour). Room temperature should be increased, intravenous fluids warmed, and a humidivent added to the breathing circuit. Also use low gas flows and warming blankets. An epinephrine solution is often applied for hemostasis.

Whenever significant airway or head and neck injury occurs, the patient remains intubated and is ventilated postoperatively. Burn patients may require a large amount of narcotic titrated for their pain. Continuous infusions of narcotics manage pain better than bolus injections.

6. **Postoperative implications**
   Pain management, prevention of respiratory complications, and fluid management are the top priorities.

B. Trauma

1. **Introduction**
   Trauma is the fourth leading cause of death in the developed world. Mortality is related to the age and prior condition of the patient, type and severity of the trauma, and rapidity and quality of the emergency treatment received.

2. **Preoperative assessment**
   The time allowed for preoperative assessment is limited and based on the severity of the trauma. A rapid assessment and review of pertinent patient data available are essential. The availability of blood therapy and the initiation of adequate intravenous lines are to be prioritized.

   a) *Cardiac:* Assess for symptoms of shock. Assess the chest wall for obvious contusion and stability of vital signs.

   b) *Respiratory:* Assess breath sounds and patterns of respiration.

   c) *Neurologic:* Assess patient using the Glasgow Coma Scale; assume a cervical spine injury until it is definitely ruled out by x-ray examination. Assess the level of consciousness and pupillary response.

   d) *Renal:* Assess the color and amount of urine.

   e) *Gastrointestinal:* All trauma patients are considered to have a full stomach. Gastric emptying slows or stops at the time of the trauma. The presence of a nasogastric tube also provides a "wick" that allows gastric fluid to be aspirated.

   f) *Endocrine:* The release of stress hormones transiently elevates blood sugar levels.

   g) *Hematologic:* Severe physical stress can lead to coagulopathies, as can dilution of clotting factors during massive volume resuscitation.

PART 2 **Common Procedures**

    h) *Patient preparation*
        (1) Baseline laboratory tests as available; hemoglobin, hematocrit, and others as indicated by history and physical examination.
        (2) Type and crossmatch for at least 4 units.
        (3) Other diagnostic tests as indicated by history and physical examination.
        (4) Premedication is usually avoided but is individualized in the trauma patient.

3. **Room preparation**
    a) Standard
    b) Arterial line, arterial blood gas measurement, pulmonary artery catheters, blood warmers, and patient warming equipment
    c) The full range of standard and emergency resuscitative drugs must be immediately available.
    d) Position is usually supine unless otherwise indicated.

4. **Anesthetic technique**
General anesthesia with minimal depressant drugs is used until the patient's status and extent of injury can be determined. Immediate establishment of the airway is the priority. Anesthetics are introduced depending on the stability of the patient.

5. **Perioperative management**
    a) *Induction*
        (1) Individualized based on the patient's condition and the severity of trauma.
        (2) Rapid sequence induction and immediate establishment of the airway are necessary.
        (3) Ketamine, propofol, and Pentothal may be administered depending on hemodynamic status.
        (4) If facial or head and neck trauma is evident, then awake intubation, fiberoptic technique, or tracheostomy may be required. Oral intubation is preferable to nasal intubation. If a Philadelphia cervical collar is present, keep the neck in well-maintained axial stabilization of the head.
        (5) If central nervous system trauma is suspected, take precautions to prevent increased intracranial pressure.
    b) *Maintenance*
        (1) Oxygen and muscle relaxants are required in the critically injured patient.
        (2) After assessment and stabilization, anesthetics are administered as appropriate.
        (3) Aggressive management of fluid (blood 1 cc/1 cc, crystalloid 3 cc/1 cc) electrolyte, blood gas parameters, blood loss, and coagulation status may be required.
    c) *Emergence:* Continued ventilation and management of all major systems are required in the immediate postanesthesia period.

6. **Postoperative implications**
Continued ventilation and observation of cardiac, respiratory, renal, and coagulation status are required for at least the first 24 hours in severely injured patients. These patients are transferred to the critical

care unit for long-term management of multiple sequelae. Pain control may include narcotics, patient-controlled analgesia, or regional blockade.

C. Laser Procedures Involving the Airways

1. **Introduction**
   Laser is an acronym for "light amplification by stimulated emission of radiation." Laser procedures of the airway usually involve the CO_2 laser because such lasers can excise lesions precisely and cause minimal edema. Tumor debunking of lesions found in the lower trachea and bronchi may require the Nd:YAG laser, which produces its effects at greater depth. There are many hazards of lasers to both the patient and members of the healthcare team. Damage can be caused to the lips and skin. Fire and explosion are possible with the use of lasers and volatile anesthetics. Toxins produced by the use of the laser on tissues may be mutagenic. They may also cause infection, acute bronchial inflammation, and altered gas exchange. Because the airway will be shared by the surgeon and the anesthesia provider, much communication and cooperation is necessary.

2. **Preoperative assessment**
   a) *History and physical examination*
      (1) A careful history should be obtained, with a great deal of emphasis on airway and respiratory concerns. A thorough airway assessment is necessary. This should include thyromental distance, airway classification, cervical range of motion, dentition, phonation, hoarseness, shortness of breath, pain on swallowing, and edema. The need for awake fiberoptic intubation should be considered. Often, these patients have long smoking histories and may have chronic obstructive pulmonary disease. Such findings should be noted on the history and physical examination. Focus on any history of asthma, emphysema, and respiratory patterns. A complete respiratory assessment should be performed and documented.
      (2) Nutritional status should be evaluated because this patient population may have undergone chemotherapy or radiation therapy for the treatment of airway lesions.
      (3) Complete systems review
   b) *Patient preparation*
      (1) *Laboratory tests:* Based on the history and physical examination
      (2) *Diagnostic tests:* Based on the history and physical examination

PART 2 Common Procedures

(3) *Medications:* Preoperative sedation is minimal in patients with severe airway obstruction. Additional sedation could cause complete airway obstruction. An antisialagogue should be given to enhance visualization and to decrease secretions. Avoid ketamine because it will increase airway reflexes. Consider Decadron to decrease airway inflammation in the postoperative period.

3. **Room preparation**
   a) *Monitoring equipment:* Standard, arterial line set up and available.
   b) *Additional equipment*
      (1) Standard emergency drugs
      (2) Eyes must be protected. The patient's eyes should be taped closed and covered with wet gauze. Do not use oil-based eye lubricants because they are flammable. Others in the room should wear goggles (clear for CO_2, green for argon, and amber for Nd:YAG lasers).
      (3) Emergency airway cart and instruments for an emergency cricothyroidotomy and tracheostomy should be available and in the room during induction. A surgeon experienced in tracheostomy should be present during induction for the patient with a compromised airway.
      (4) Jet ventilator—a copper tube is attached to the jet ventilator prior to laryngoscopy; the brass ball tip should be 2 to 3 cm distal to vocal cords. Ventilate at 30 to 35 psi, 10 to 12 breaths/minute lasting 1 to 2 seconds. Assure full expiration to avoid pneumothorax. Contraindications are full stomach, obesity, hiatal hernia, and severe lung or heart disease.
      (5) Appropriate endotracheal tubes and a variety of blades and airways should be available to decrease the risk of airway fire, including metal tubes, red rubber, polyvinyl chloride (PVC), or silicone tubes. Regardless of the endotracheal tube chosen, one should use the lowest FiO_2 possible so as to decrease the risk of airway fire. Have a 50 cc syringe of normal saline on tabletop.
      (6) If an airway fire should occur, ventilation should be stopped, and the O_2 source should be discontinued. Flood the area with water. Remove the burned endotracheal tube. Mask ventilate with 100% O_2, maintain anesthetic, and reintubate the patient. Bronchoscopy, laryngoscopy, chest radiography, and arterial blood gas measurements should be performed to determine injury and to provide therapy. The patient should be monitored for at least 24 hours. Short-term steroids may be administered, as should antibiotics and ventilatory support as needed. Also monitor arterial blood gases and chest x-ray films.
      (7) Long breathing circuits may be needed if the operating table is to be turned.
      (8) *Intravenous fluids:* 18-gauge or larger tube, normal saline or lactated Ringer's solution at 2 to 4 mL/kg/hour

4. **Perioperative management and anesthetic technique**
   a) General anesthesia with endotracheal intubation is appropriate. Some surgeons advocate local anesthesia with heavy sedation for certain minor base procedures of the upper airway. However, the patient must not move; remember that sedation may lead to complete airway obstruction.
   b) *Induction:* Standard intravenous induction if the patient has airway obstruction. With airway obstruction or an awake patient, fiberoptic bronchoscopy may be performed, and the airway may be secured prior to induction. Muscle relaxants should be avoided until the airway is secured.
   c) *Maintenance:* Isoflurane, desflurane, air, and O_2 are standard. Avoid N_2O because it is combustible. Avoid FiO_2 above 0.40 to decrease the risk of airway fire.
   d) *Emergence:* Use awake extubation because there may be some airway edema. Avoid coughing, bucking, and straining on the endotracheal tube to prevent further edema. Consider lidocaine intravenously (1 mg/kg).
5. **Postoperative implications**
   Airway complications and PONV

PART 2   Common Procedures

PART THREE

3

Drugs

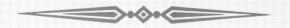

Name

Adenosine (Adenocard)

Classification

Antiarrhythmic

Indications

Supraventricular tachycardia

Dose

6-mg bolus given over 1 to 2 sec followed by normal saline line flush; may increase to 12-mg bolus if arrhythmia persists past 2 min. May repeat 12-mg bolus once. How supplied: 3 mg/mL 2-mL and 5-mL vials.

Onset and Duration

Onset: 10 to 20 sec; duration = 1 min.

Adverse Effects

Flushing, dyspnea, chest pain, headache, nausea, cough, malaise

Precautions and Contraindications

Adenosine should not be used in patients receiving methyl xanthine therapy, i.e., aminophylline, theophylline. Dipyridamole (Persantine) inhibits cellular uptake of adenosine. Use with caution in asthmatics. Contraindicated in patients with second- or third-degree heart block.

Anesthetic Considerations

An excellent agent for use under anesthesia in lieu of or preceding administration of calcium channel blockers for long-term suppression.

Name

Albuterol sulfate (Proventil, Ventolin)

Classification

β_2-adrenergic agonist, sympathomimetic, bronchodilator

Indications

Treatment of asthma and other forms of bronchospasm

Dose

Inhaler (metered dose): 2 deep inhalations 1 to 5 min apart; may be repeated every 4 to 6 hr. (Daily dose should not exceed 16 to 20 inhalations. Each metered aerosol actuation delivers approximately 90 μg per puff.) P.O.: 2 to 4 mg t.i.d. to q.i.d. (total dose not to exceed 16 mg). Syrup: 2 mg/5 mL is available.

Onset and Duration

Onset: Inhalation: 5 to 15 min; P.O.: 15 to 30 min. Peak effect: Inhalation: 0.5 to 2 hr; P.O.: 2 to 3 hr. Duration: Inhalation: 3 to 6 hr; P.O.: 4 to 8 hr.

Adverse Effects

Tachycardia, arrhythmias, hypertension, tremors, anxiety, headache, nausea, vomiting, hypokalemia

Precations and Contraindications

Safe use not established during pregnancy. Cautious use in patients with cardiovascular disease, hypertension, and hyperthyroidism. Monitor glucose and electrolyte levels.

Anesthetic Considerations

Tolerance/tachyphylaxis can develop with chronic use. Additive effects with epinephrine and other sympathomimetics. Antagonized by betareceptor antagonists.

Name

Alfentanil HCl (Alfenta)

Classification

Opioid agonist; produces analgesia and anesthesia

Indications

Perioperative analgesia

Dose

Induction: I.V.: 50 to 150 µg/kg; Infusion: 0.1 to 3 µg/kg per min.

Onset and Duration

Onset: I.V.: 1 to 2 min; I.M.: < 5 min; epidural: 5 to 15 min. Duration: I.V.: 1 to 15 min; I.M.: 10 to 60 min; epidural: 30 min.

Adverse Effects

Bradycardia, hypotension, arrhythmias, respiratory depression; euphoria, dysphoria, convulsions, nausea and vomiting, biliary tract spasm, delayed gastric emptying, muscle rigidity, pruritus

Precautions and Contraindications

Reduce dose in elderly, hypovolemic, high-risk surgical patients, and with concomitant use of sedatives and other narcotics. Crosses the placental barrier, and usage in labor may produce depression of respiration in the neonate. Resuscitation may be required; have naloxone available.

Anesthetic Considerations

Circulatory and ventilatory depressant effects potentiated by narcotics, sedatives, volatile anesthetics, nitrous oxide; ventilatory depressant effects potentiated by amphetamines, monamine oxidase, phenothiazine, tricyclic antidepressants; analgesia enhanced by α_2-agonists; reduced clearance and prolonged respiratory depression with concomitant use of erythromycin; muscle rigidity in higher dose range can be sufficient to interfere with ventilation.

Name

Alprostadil, PGE 1 (Prostin VR_R)

Classification

Prostaglandin E

Indications

Neonates: to maintain temporary patency of the ductus arteriosus until corrective or palliative surgery can be performed

Dose

Children: Continuous infusion into large vein 0.05 to 0.1 µg/kg/min initially; when a therapeutic response occurs, decrease to lowest possible dose to maintain response (maximum dose: 0.4 µg/kg/min). Dosage forms: 500 µg/mL 1-mL ampules (refrigerate at 2 to 8° C. Must be diluted in D_5W or normal saline for continuous infusion to final concentration of 5 to 20 µg/mL.

Onset and Duration

Onset: 30 min. Elimination $t_{1/2}$: 5 to 10 min. Duration: 30 min to 2 hr.

Adverse Effects

Apnea (10% to 12%), fever (14%), flushing (10%), bradycardia and seizures (4%), thrombocytopenia (less than 1%), disseminated intravascular coagulation (1%), anemia, tachycardia, hypotension (4%), diarrhea (2%), gastric outlet obstruction secondary to antral hyperplasia (related to cumulative dose)

Precautions and Contraindications

Apnea is most frequent in infants under 2 kg within the first hour of administration; ventilatory assistance may be required. Contraindicated in neonates with respiratory distress syndrome. Use with caution in patients with bleeding tendencies due to alprostadil's ability to inhibit platelet aggregation. In all neonates, monitor arterial pressure; should arterial pressure fall significantly, decrease the rate of infusion.

Name

Aminocaproic acid (Amicar)

Classification

Hemostatic agent; prevents the conversion of plasminogen to plasmin

Indications

Control of clinical bleeding where hyperfibrinolysis is a contributing factor. Hyperfibrinolysis should be confirmed by laboratory values such as prolonged thrombin time, prolonged prothrombin time, hypofibrinogenemia, or decreased plasminogen levels. Also: open-heart surgery; postoperative hematuria following transurethral prostatic resection, suprapubic prostatectomy, and nephrectomy;

hematologic disorders such as aplastic anemia, abruptio placentae, cirrhosis, neoplastic diseases, and prophylaxis in hemophiliacs pre-tooth and post-tooth extraction and other bleeding in the mouth and nasopharynx. Reduction of blood loss in trauma and shock; possible prevention of ocular hemorrhaging and bleeding in subarachnoid hemorrhage.

Dose

Acute bleeding: 5 g infused during the first hour, followed by a continuous infusion of 1 g/hr for 8 hr or until bleeding is controlled.

Chronic bleeding: 5 g preoperatively intravenous piggyback (IVPB) over 1 hr, then 5 g IVPB every 6 hr. Do not exceed 30 g in 24 hr. Decrease dose by 15% to 25% in patients with renal disease.

Children: 100 mg/kg IVPB over 1 hr, then 30 mg/kg/hr until bleeding is controlled. (Maximum dose: 18 g/m^2 in 24 hr.)

Dosage forms: 250 mg/mL 20 mL parenteral vial (5 g).

Administration: Dilute each dose in a proper volume of D$_5$W normal saline or lactated Ringer's solution.

Onset and Duration

Onset: 1 to 72 hr; t$_{1/2}$ 1 to 2 hr in patients with normal renal function. No single concentration fits all. It must be diluted. Consult package insert, I.V. reference, or pharmacy. Duration: 8 to 12 hr.

Adverse Effects

Convulsions, myopathy, rarely muscle necrosis, nausea, vomiting. Rapid infusion is associated with hypotension, bradycardia, arrhythmias.

Precautions and Containdictions

A definitive diagnosis of hyperfibrinolysis must be made before administration. Caution when using in cardiac, renal, or hepatic disease. Administration in presence of renal or ureteral bleeding is not recommended because of ureteral clot formation and possible risk of obstruction. Owing to the substantial risk of serious or fatal thrombus formation, aminocaproic acid is contraindicated in patients with disseminated intravascular coagulation unless heparin is given concurrently.

Anesthetic Considerations

Do not administer without a definite diagnosis of laboratory findings indicative of hyperfiberinolysis.

Name

Aminophylline

Classification

Bronchodilator

Indications

Chronic therapy for bronchial asthma; reversal of bronchospasm associated with chronic obstructive pulmonary disease.

Dose

Loading dose: For patients not already receiving a theophylline preparation, I.V.: 5 to 6 mg/kg (given over 20 to 30 min) or P.O./Rectal: 6 mg/kg. Maintenance: I.V.: 0.5 mg/kg/hr; P.O.: 2 to 4 mg/kg every 6 to 12 hr. Therapeutic range: 10 to 20 μg/mL.

Dosage forms: Injection: 25 mg/mL; Tablets: 100 mg, 200 mg; Tablets (sustained release): 225 mg; Oral solution: 105 mg/5 mL; Rectal solution: 60 mg/mL (rectal solution not marketed in U.S.); Rectal suppositories: 250 mg, 500 mg. Dilution for infusion loading dose: dilute 500 mg in 500 mL D_5W or normal saline (1 mg/mL). Children 9 to 16 years: 1 mg/kg per hour for 12 hr, then 0.8 mg/kg/hr. Children 6 months to 9 years: 1.2 mg/kg/hr for 12 hr, then 1 mg/kg/hr.

Onset and Duration

Onset: I.V.: within a few min; P.O.: within 30 min. Duration: P.O.: 4 to 8 hr.

Adverse Effects

Palpitations, sinus tachycardia, supraventricular and ventricular tachycardia, flushing, tachypnea, seizures, headache, irritability, nausea, vomiting, hyperglycemia.

Elevated serum levels in patients receiving cimetidine, quinolone antibiotics, macrolide antibiotics, and in patients with cardiac failure or liver insufficiency. Decreased serum levels with phenobarbital, phenytoin, rifampin, and smokers. Toxicity occurs with plasma levels greater than 20 mg/mL. Avoid rapid infusions, which may cause hypotension, arrhythmias, and possibly death.

Anesthetic Considerations

Potentiates pressor effects of sympathomimetics and may produce seizures, cardiac arrhythmias, cardiorespiratory arrest, ventricular arrhythmias with excessive plasma levels or in patients receiving volatile anesthetics. Use isoflurane or enflurane in patients who must be given aminophylline or other exogenous sympathomimetic drugs before or during surgery. Use of halothane may potentiate cardiac dysrhythmia.

Name

Amiodarone (Cordarone)

Classification

Class III antiarrhythmic

Indications

Treatment of life-threatening ventricular arrhythmias that do not respond to other antiarrhythmics (i.e., recurrent ventricular fibrillation and hemodynamically unstable ventricular tachycardia). Selective treatment of supraventricular arrhythmias.

Dose

Loading: P.O.: 800 to 1600 mg/day for 1 to 3 wk. Maintenance: P.O.: 200 to 600 mg/day. Therapeutic level: 1.0 to 2.5 µg/mL. Dosage form: Tablets: 200 mg. I.V.: 100 to 300 mg.

Onset and Duration

Onset: 2 to 4 days; $t_{1/2}$ between 2 weeks and months. Duration: 45 days.

Adverse Effects

Arrhythmias, pulmonary fibrosis or inflammation, hepatitis or cirrhosis, corneal deposits, hyperthyroidism, hypothyroidism, peripheral neuropathy, cutaneous photosensitivity

Precations and Contraindications

Amiodarone increases serum levels of digoxin, warfarin, quinidine, procainamide, phenytoin, and diltiazem. The likelihood of bradycardia, sinus arrest, and atrioventricular block increases with concurrent beta-adrenergic antagonist and calcium channel-blocker therapy.

Anesthetic Considerations

Antiadrenergic effects are enhanced in the presence of general anesthetics, manifesting as sinus arrest, atrioventricular block, low cardiac output, or hypotension. Drugs that inhibit the automaticity of the sinus node such as halothane and lidocaine could accentuate effects of amiodarone and increase the likelihood of sinus arrest. The potential need for a temporary artificial cardiac (ventricular) pacemaker and administration of sympathomimetics such as isoproterenol should be considered in patients receiving this drug.

Name

Amrinone lactate (Inocor)

Classification

Positive inotrope (phosphodiesterase inhibitor)

Indications

Short-term management of congestive heart failure

Dose

Loading dose: 0.75 mg/kg over 2 to 3 min. A second bolus may follow after 30 min. Maintenance is by continuous infusion of 5 to 10 mg/kg/min (maximum 24-hour dose: 10 µg/kg). Dosage forms: Injection: 5 mg/mL. Dilution for infusion: 500 mg in 500 mL normal saline solution.

Onset and Duration

Onset: within 5 min. Duration: 30 min to 2 hr.

PART 3 Drugs

Adverse Effects

Hypotension, arrhythmia, thrombocytopenia, abdominal pain, hepatic dysfunction

Precautions and Contraindications

Use with caution in hypotensive patients. Avoid exposure of ampule to light. Do not mix in solutions containing dextrose or furosemide. Use with caution in patients with allergies to bisulfites. Fluid balance, electrolyte concentrations, and renal function should be monitored carefully during treatment. Monitor platelet counts chronically. Amrinone contains sodium metabisulfite, a sulfite that may cause allergic-type reactions including anaphylactic symptoms and life-threatening or less severe asthamatic episodes in certain susceptible people. Sulfite sensitivity is seen more frequently in asthmatic than in nonasthamatic people.

Anesthetic Considerations

An alternative to conventional inotropes. Useful when both inotropic and vasodilating properties are desired and/or to lower pulmonary vascular resistance.

Name

Atracurium (Tracrium)

Classification

Nondepolarizing skeletal muscle relaxant

Indications

Relaxation of skeletal muscles during surgery; adjunct to general anesthesia or mechanical ventilation; facilitation of endotracheal intubation.

Dose

Initially for paralyzing: I.V.: 0.3 to 0.5 mg/kg. Maintenance: I.V.: 0.08 to 0.1 mg/kg. Dosage form: Injection: 10 mg/mL.

Onset and Duration

Onset: less than 3 min. Duration: 20 to 35 min. Elimination: plasma (half-man elimination, ester hydrolysis), hepatic, renal. The primary metabolite is laudanosine, a cerebral stimulant, excreted primarily in the urine.

Adverse Effects

Vasodilation, hypotension, sinus tachycardia, sinus bradycardia, hypoventilation, apnea, bronchospasm, laryngospasm, dyspnea, inadequate block, prolonged block, rash, urticaria

Precautions and Contraindications

Use with caution in patients with conditions in which histamine release may prove hazardous, in patients with myasthenia gravis, bradycardia, or electrolyte disturbances, and in pregnant or nursing women.

Anesthetic Considerations

Monitor response with peripheral nerve stimulator. Reverse effects with anticholinesterase. Pretreatment doses may induce sufficient neuromuscular blockade to cause hypotension in some patients.

Name

Atropine sulfate

Classification

Competitive acetylcholine antagonist at muscarinic receptor

Indications

Symptomatic bradycardia, asystole, cardiopulmonary resuscitation (CPR); antisialogogue; for vagolytic effects to block bradycardia during surgery from stimulation of the carotid sinus, traction on abdominal viscera, or extraocular muscles; blockade of muscarinic effects of anticholinesterases; adjunctive therapy in the treatment of bronchospasm, peptic ulcer disease

Dose

Adults: sinus bradycardia, CPR: I.V., I.M., SQ, via endotracheal tube (diluted in 10 mL sterile water or normal saline: 0.5 to 1.0 mg every 3 to 5 min as indicated (maximum dose: 40 µg/kg). Preoperative: 0.4 mg I.M., SQ, or P.O. 30 to 60 min preinduction.

Blockade of muscarinic effects of anticholinesterases: 7 to 10 µg/kg with edrophonium, 15 to 30 µg/kg with neostigmine, 15 to 20 µg/kg with pyridostigmine.

Bronchodilation: Inhalation: 0.025 mg/kg every 4 to 6 hr. Dilute to 2 to 3 mL normal saline and deliver by compressed air nebulizer (maximum dose 2.5 mg/dose). Pediatric bronchodilatory dose: 0.05 mg/kg diluted in normal saline 3 or 4 times daily.

Children: sinus bradycardia, CPR: I.V., I.M., SQ, or via endotracheal tube: 0.02 mg/kg every 5 min up to a maximum of 1 mg in children and 2 mg in adolescents (minimum dose: 0.1 mg).

Preoperative: P.O., I.M., SQ: 0.02 mg/kg for neonates, 0.1 mg for children weighing 3 kg, 0.2 mg for those weighing 7 to 9 kg, and 0.3 mg for those weighing 12 to 16 kg.

Dosage forms: Injection: 0.05, 0.1, 0.3, 0.4, 0.5, 0.8, and 1 mg/mL. Inhalation solution: 0.2%, 0.5%.

Tablets: 0.4, 0.6 mg.

Onset and Duration

Inhibition of salivation occurs within 30 min to 1 hr and peaks in 1 to 2 hr following P.O. or I.M. administration. Increase in heart rate occurs within 5 to 40 min after I.V. or I.M. administration. Duration: 15 to 30 min after I.V. administration and 2 to 4 hr following I.M. administration.

Plasma $t_{1/2}$ is 2 to 3 hr.

Adverse Effects

Transient bradycardia due to a weak peripheral muscarinic cholinergic agonist effect in small doses (less than 0.5 mg in adults), tachycardia (high doses), urinary hesitancy, retention, mydriasis, blurred vision, increased intraocular pressure, decreased sweating, excitement, agitation, drowsiness, confusion, hallucinations, dry nose and mouth, allergic reactions, constipation. Children and the elderly are more susceptible to adverse effects.

Precautions and Contraindications

Avoid where tachycardia would be harmful, i.e., thyrotoxicosis, pheochromocytoma, coronary artery disease. Avoid in hyperpyrexial states because it inhibits sweating. Contraindicated in acute-angle glaucoma, obstructive disease of the gastrointestinal tract, obstructive uropathy, paralytic ileus or intestinal atony, and acute hemorrhage where cardiovascular status is unstable. Use with caution in patients with tachyarrhythmias, hepatic or renal disease, congestive heart failure, chronic pulmonary disease (since a reduction in bronchial secretions may lead to formation of bronchial plugs), autonomic neuropathy, hiatal hernia, gastroesophageal reflux, gastric ulcers, gastrointestinal infections, and ulcerative colitis.

Anesthetic Considerations

Additive anticholinergic effects may occur when atropine is given concomitantly with meperidine, some antihistamines, phenothiazines, tricyclic antidepressants, and antiarrhythmic drugs that possess anticholinergic activity (e.g., quinidine, disopyramide, procainamide).

Name

Bretylium (Bretylol)

Classification

Class III antiarrhythmic

Indications

Ventricular fibrillation and other ventricular arrhythmias resistant to initial lidocaine or procainamide treatment

Dose

I.V. loading I.M. ventricular tachycardia: 5 to 10 mg/kg over 1 min or may be repeated in 1 to 2 hr. IV loading ventricular fibrillation: 5 to 10 mg/kg over 1 min (every 15 to 30 min to maximum 30 mg/kg). Infusion: 1 to 2 mg/min. Therapeutic level: 0.5 to 1.0 µg/mL. Dosage form: 50 mg/mL.

Onset and Duration

Onset antifibrillatory: few minutes; I.V./I.M. suppression of ventricular arrhythmia: 20 min to 2 hr. Duration: I.V./I.M.: 6 to 24 hr.

Adverse Effects

Hypotension, transitory hypertension and arrhythmias, anginal attacks, shortness of breath, dizziness, syncope, nausea, vomiting, diarrhea, rash, hiccups

Precautions and Contraindications

Use with caution on patients with pheochromocytoma, aortic stenosis, and pulmonary hypertension.

Anesthetic Considerations

Tricyclic antidepressants may prevent uptake of bretylium by adrenergic nerve terminals. Treat severe hypotension with appropriate fluid therapy and vasopressor agents such as dopamine or norepinephrine.

Name

Bumetanide (Bumex)

Classification

Loop diuretic

Indications

Treatment of edema of cardiac, hepatic, or renal origin. Hypertension, pulmonary edema. Usually reserved for patients who do not respond to thiazide diuretics or in whom a rapid onset of diuresis is desired.

Dose

Initial dose: 0.5 to 1 mg I.V. over 1 to 2 min. If response is not adequate following the initial dose, a second or third dose may be administered at intervals of up to 2 to 3 hr, up to a maximum of 10 mg/day. Children: Dosage forms: 0.5-, 1-, 2-mg tablets; 0.25 mg/mL solution for injection in 2-mL, 4-mL, and 10-mL vials.

Onset and Duration

Onset I.V.: few minutes; Peak effect: 15 to 30 min. Duration: 4 hr with normal doses of 1 to 2 mg and up to 6 hr with higher doses. Elimination $t_{1/2}$: 1 to 1.5 hr.

Adverse Effects

Transient leukopenia, granulocytopenia, thrombocytopenia, hypotension, chest pain, dizziness. Electrolyte abnormalities such as hyperuricemia, hypomagnesemia, hypokalemia, hypochloremia, azotemia, hyponatremia, metabolic alkalosis. Hyperglycemia, diarrhea, pancreatitis, nephrotoxicity, muscle cramps, arthritic pain, ototoxicity (less frequent than with furosemide).

Precautions and Contraindications

Anuria, hypersensitivity to bumetanide, severe fluid and electrolyte imbalance, hepatic coma, if increase in blood urea nitrogen or creatinine occurs. Patients allergic to sufonamides may have hypersensitivity to bumetanide.

Anesthetic Considerations

Loop diuretics may increase the neuromuscular blocking effect of tubocurarine, probably because of their potassium depleting effects.

Name

Bupivacaine HCl (Marcaine, Sensorcaine)

Classification

Amide-type local anesthetic

Indications

Regional anesthesia

Dose

Infiltration/peripheral nerve block: less than 150 mg (0.25% to 0.5% solution). Epidural: 50 to 100 mg (0.25% to 0.75% solution), children: 1.5 to 2.5 mg/kg (0.25% to 0.5% solution). Caudal: 37.5 to 150 mg (15 to 30 mL of 0.25% or 0.5% solution), children: 0.4 to 0.7 mL/kg. Spinal bolus/infusion: 7 to 17 mg (0.75% solution), children: 0.5 mg/kg, with minimum of 1 mg. Do not exceed 400 mg in 24 hours. Maximum single dose is 175 mg.

Onset and Duration

Onset: Infiltration: 2 to 10 min; epidural: 4 to 7 min; spinal: less than 1 min. Peak effect: Infiltration and epidural: 30 to 45 min. spinal: 15 min. Duration: Infiltration/spinal/epidural: 200 to 400 min (prolonged with epinephrine).

Adverse Effects

Hypotension, arrhythmias, cardiac arrest, respiratory impairment, arrest, seizures, tinnitus, blurred vision, urticaria, anaphylactoid symptoms. High spinal: urinary retention, lower-extremity weakness and paralysis, loss of sphincter control, backache, palsies, slowing of labor.

Precautions and Contraindications

Use with caution in patients with hypovolemia, severe congestive heart failure, shock, and all forms of heart block. Not recommended for obstetrical paracervical block or in concentrations above 0.5% due to incidence of intractable cardiac arrest. Contraindicated in patients with hypersensitivity to amide-type local anesthetics.

Anesthetic Considerations

Prior use of chloroprocaine may interfere with action. I.V. access is essential during major regional block. Toxic plasma levels of bupivacaine may cause cardiopulmonary collapse and seizures.

Name

Chloroprocaine HCl (Nesacaine)

Classification

Ester-type local anesthetic

Indications

Regional anesthesia. Local anesthesia including infiltration, epidural (including caudal), peripheral nerve block, sympathetic nerve block.

Dose

Infiltration and peripheral nerve block: less than 40 mL (1% to 2% solution). Epidural: bolus 10 to 25 mL (2% to 3% solution), approximately 1.5 to 2 mL for each segment to be anesthetized. Repeat doses at 40 to 60 min intervals. Infusion: 30 mL/hr (0.5% solution). Caudal: 10 to 25 mL (2% to 3% solution). Children: 0.4 to 0.7 mL/kg (L2 to T10 level of anesthesia). Repeat doses at 40 to 60 min intervals.

Onset and Duration

Rate of onset and potency of local anesthetic action may be enhanced by carbonation. Onset: Infiltration/epidural: 6 to 12 min. Peak effect: Infiltration/epidural: 10 to 20 min. Duration: Infiltration/epidural: 30 to 60 min (prolonged with epinephrine).

Adverse Effects

Hypotension, arrhythmias, bradycardia, respiratory depression, arrest, seizures, tinnitus, tremors, urticaria, pruritus, angioneurotic edema. High spinal: backache, loss of perianal sensation and sexual function, permanent motor, sensory, autonomic (sphincter control) deficit in lower segments, slowing of labor.

Precautions and Contraindications

Caution in patients with severe disturbances of cardiac rhythm, shock, heart block, or impaired hepatic function. Inflammation or infection at injection site. Elderly, pregnant are most at risk. Contraindicated in patients with hypersensitivity to local anesthetics, para-aminobenzoic acid/parabens. **Do not use for spinal anesthesia.**

Anesthetic Considerations

Reduce doses in obstetric, elderly, hypovolemic, high-risk patients, and those with increased intraabdominal pressure. **Do not use for spinal anesthesia.**

Name

Cimetidine (Tagamet)

Classification

Histamine (H_2) antagonist

Indications

Treatment of duodenal or gastric ulcers, gastroesophageal reflux disease. Prophylaxis of aspiration pneumonitis in patients at high risk during surgery.

Dose

Prophylaxis of aspiration pneumonitis: Adults: 300 to 400 mg P.O. 1.5 to 2 hr before induction of anesthesia with or without a similar dose the preceding evening. When a more rapid onset of effect is needed, I.V.: dilute 300 to 400 mg in D_5W or normal saline to a volume of at least 20 mL, and inject over a period not less than 5 min. A slower infusion, over 15 to 30 min, may be preferable owing to association of occasional severe bradycardia and hypotension with rapid infusion. Children younger than 12 years of age use not indicated. Dosage forms: Tablets: 300 mg, 400 mg. Parenteral injection: 150 mg/mL.

Onset and Duration

Onset: 15 to 45 min. Peak plasma levels: 1 to 2 hr P.O. Duration: 2 to 4 hr. Elimination $t_{1/2}$: 2 hr. Plasma cimetidine levels that suppress gastric acid secretion by 50% were maintained 4 to 5 hr following I.V. injection.

Adverse Effects

Mental status changes such as delirium, confusion, depression primarily in elderly or hepatic or renal-impaired patients. Leukopenia, thrombocytopenia, and gynecomastia reported rarely (1%). Hypotension and severe bradycardia are associated with rapid I.V. infusion. Serum creatinine and liver enzymes may rise during treatment, although hepatotoxicity and renal dysfunction are usually reversible.

Precautions and Contraindications

Caution suggested in renal or hepatic insufficiency. Microsomal metabolism of many drugs may be inhibited. Contraindicated in patients allergic to cimetidine or other H_2 antagonists.

Anesthetic Considerations

Cimetidine inhibits the hepatic mixed-function oxidase system; therefore it may prolong the half-life of many drugs, including diazepam, midazolam, metaprolol, propranolol, theophylline, lidocaine, and other amide local anesthetics. Ranitidine may be the drug of choice in patients receiving lidocaine local or regional anesthesia.

Name

Clonidine (Catapres, Dixarit) *Epidural Clonidine (Catapres, Duraclon)*

Classification

Central-acting α_2-adrenergic agonist; reduces sympathetic outflow by directly stimulating α receptors in the medulla vasomotor center.

Epidural action produces dose-dependent analgesia by preventing pain signal transmission at presynaptic and postjunctional α_2 adrenoceptors in the spinal cord.

Indications

Hypertension; epidural and spinal anesthesia; symptomatic control of alcohol, opiate, nicotine, and benzodiazepine withdrawal; diagnosis of pheochromocytoma; growth hormone stimulation test; cancer pain; Tourette's syndrome; attention deficit disorder; migraines. The use of epidural clonidine in combination with epidural opiate agonists results in a decreased opiate requirement that treats neuropathic pain more effectively than visceral pain.

Dose

Maintenance: 0.2 to 0.6 mg/day P.O. in two divided doses. Hypertensive emergencies: 0.15 mg I.V. over 5 min. Transdermal patch: every 7 days (maximum dose: 2.4 mg/day). Same doses for renal impairment.

Epidural: must be preservative-free. Post-operative pain: epidural clonidine combined with an opiate analgesic—150 g if added to fentanyl, 450 g/day if added to morphine. Neuropathic pain: continuous epidural infusion combined with an opiate analgesic is 30 g/hr. Plain clonidine epidural infusion is from 100 to 900 g per dose; Children: start at 0.5 g/kg/hr.

All dosages must be titrated to pain relief and incidence of side effects.

Onset and Duration

Onset: I.V. or P.O.: 30 to 60 min. Peak effect: 2 to 4 hr. May take too long for true HTN crisis. Duration: antihypertensive: 6 to 10 hr, dose dependent.

Adverse Effects

Rebound hypertension, atrioventricular block, bradycardia, congestive heart failure, orthostatic hypotension, sedation, nightmares, constipation, dry mouth, pruritus, urinary retention, contact dermatitis. The most common noncardiovascular adverse reactions to epidural clonidine include anxiety, asthenia, chest pain, confusion, diaphoresis, dizziness, drowsiness, dyspnea, fever, nausea/vomiting, and xerostomia.

Precautions and Contraindications

Avoid in conduction or sinoatrial disorders, hypersensitivity to clonidine, pregnancy, severe renal or hepatic disease. Concomitant administration of tricyclic antidepressants may increase dose.
- If dose held or changing to transdermal application, watch for rapid increase in blood pressure from unopposed α stimulation.
- Crosses the placenta easily. Should be discontinued 8 to 12 hr prior to delivery.

Epidural clonidine is *not recommended* for intrathecal administration or as an analgesic during labor and delivery, post-partum or peri-operative analgesia due to the risks of hemodynamic instability. Antagonist: Yohimbine, an α_2-adrenoreceptor antagonist will partially reverse the sedative and analgesic epidural effects. Clonidine is not antagonized by opiate agonists when used epidurally.

Anesthetic Considerations

Severe rebound hypertension from abrupt withdrawal with neurological sequelae and myocardial infarction. Labetalol has been successfully used in treatment of hypertensive crisis. Continue on day of surgery.
• Hepatic elimination 50%.
• Reduces perioperative requirements of narcotics and volatile agents.

Females and lower-weight patients have an increased risk to the hypotensive effects of epidural clonidine (use cautiously in patients with severe cardiac disease or hemodynamic instability). More profound decreases in blood pressure may be seen when administered into the upper thoracic spinal segments.

Name

Cocaine HCl (Cocaine)

Classification

Topical anesthetic and vasoconstrictor, ester-type local anesthetic

Indications

Used for topical anesthesia and vasoconstriction of mucous membranes (oral, laryngeal, and nasal).

Dose

Topical: 1.5 mg/kg (1% to 4% solution). Nasal: 1 to 2 mL each nostril (1% to 10% solution). Concentrations greater than 4% increase potential for systemic toxic reactions. Maximum safe dose: 1.5 mg/kg.

Onset and Duration

Onset: less than 1 min. Peak effect: 2 to 5 min. Duration: 30 to 120 min. Rapidly absorbed from all areas of application.

Adverse Effects

Seizures, sloughing of nasal mucosa, arrhythmias, tachycardia, hypertension; increases maximum allowable concentration of inhalation anesthetics

Precautions and Contraindications

Topical use only; not for intraocular or I.V. use. Potentiates other sympathomimetics; therefore use reduced doses (if any at all) in patients receiving pressors or ketamine. Use with caution in patients with nasal trauma.

Anesthetic Considerations

Hypertension, bradyarrhythmias, tachyarrhythmias, ventricular fibrillation, tachypnea, respiratory failure, euphoria, excitement, seizures, sloughing of corneal epithelium. Use with caution in patients with a history of drug sensitivities or drug abuse (high addiction potential) and pregnancy. Prolonged use can cause ischemic damage to nasal mucosa. Contraindicated for intraocular or I.V. use. Sensitizes the heart to catecholamines (epinephrine and monoamine oxidase inhibitors may increase cardiac arrhythmias, ventricular fibrillation, hypertensive episodes). Potentiates arrhythmogenic effects of sympathomimetics. High addiction potential.

Name

Codeine

Classification

Opioid agonist

Indications

Preoperative and postoperative analgesia

Dose

P.O.: 15 to 60 mg every 4 hr; I.M./S.C.: 15 to 60 mg every 4 hr.

Onset and Duration

Onset: P.O.: 30 to 60 min; I.M./SQ: 20 to 60 min. Duration: P.O.: 2 to 4 hr; I.M./SQ: 2 to 3 hr.

Adverse Effects

Sedation, clouded sensorium, euphoria, dizziness, seizures with large doses, hypotension, bradycardia, nausea, vomiting, constipation, dry mouth, ileus, urinary retention, pruritus, flushing

Precautions and Contraindications

Use with caution in head injury, increased intracranial pressure, increased cerebrospinal fluid pressure, hepatic or renal disease, hypothyroidism, Addison's disease, acute alcoholism, seizures, severe central nervous system depression, bronchial asthma, chronic obstructive pulmonary disease, respiratory depression, shock. Use with caution in patients with known hypersensitivity to the drug and the elderly.

Anesthetic Considerations

General anesthetics, other narcotic analgesics, tranquilizers, sedatives, hypnotics, alcohol, tricyclic antidepressants, or monoamine oxidase inhibitors increase central nervous system depression.

Name

Cyclosporine (Sandimmune)

Classification

Immunosuppressant

Indications

Prevent rejection of organ/tissue (kidney, liver, heart, allograft) in combination with steroid therapy.

Dose

Initial: P.O.: 15 mg/kg as a single dose 4 to 24 hr prior to transplantation, continue for 1 to 2 wk. Taper to maintenance dose: 5 to 10 mg/kg/day. I.V.: 0.5 to 6 mg/kg as single dose 4 to 12 hr prior to transplantation, continue until the patient is able to take oral medication.

Onset and Duration

Onset: 1 to 6 hr (variable). Duration: 1 to 4 days after. After oral administration, onset is variable. Elimination $t_{1/2}$: 10 to 27 hr.

Adverse Effects

Hypertension, hirsutism, tremor, acne, gum hyperplasia, headache, blurred vision, diarrhea, nausea, paresthesia, mild nephrotoxicity or hepatotoxicity

Precautions and Contraindications

History of hypersensitivity to cyclosporine or polyoxyethylated castor oil. Use with caution in patients with impaired hepatic, renal, cardiac function, malabsorption syndrome, and in those that are pregnant.

Anesthetic Considerations

Altered laboratory values: May elevate blood urea nitrogen, serum creatinine, serum bilirubin, SGOT(AST), SGPT(ALT), and LDH. May prolong the duration of neuromuscular blockade by nondepolarizing muscle relaxants.

Name

Dantrolene sodium (Dantrium)

Classification

Skeletal muscle relaxant

Indications

Treatment of malignant hyperthermia (MHT). Prophylaxis of malignant hyperthermia in patients with a family history. Control of spasticity secondary to multiple sclerosis, spinal cord injury, cerebral palsy, or stroke.

Dose

Adults: Malignant hyperthermia: 1 mg/kg rapid I.V. bolus. Repeat every 5 to 10 min until symptoms are controlled. The dose may be repeated to a cumulative dose of 10 mg/kg. Oral doses of 4 to 8 mg/kg per day for 1 to 3 days may be administered in three or four divided doses to prevent recurrence of the manifestations. Prophylaxis of MHT: 2.5 mg/kg I.V. bolus 10 to 30 min preinduction, then 1.25 mg/kg I.V. bolus 6 hr later. Dosage forms: Capsules: 25, 50, 100 mg. Parenteral injection: 20 mg. Administration: Reconstitute by adding 60 mL preservative-free sterile water for injection to each 20-mg vial and shake vial until clear. Avoid diluent that contains a bacteriostatic agent.

Protect from light and use within 6 hr. For direct I.V. injection. Avoid extravasation.

Onset and Duration

Effective blood concentrations: 100 to 600 ng/mL. I.V. blood concentrations of the drug remain at approximately steady-state levels for 3 or more hours after infusion is completed. Mean $t_{1/2}$: 5 to 9 hr. Onset: P.O.: 1 to 2 hr; I.V.: less than 5 min. Duration 8 to 12 hrs.

Adverse Effects

Hepatotoxicity (hepatitis) 0.5%, with mortality reported as high as 10%. Muscle weakness, tachycardia, erratic blood pressure, fatigue, central nervous system (CNS) depression, visual and auditory hallucinations, bowel obstruction, hematuria, crystalluria, urinary frequency, phlebitis, pericarditis, pleural effusion, postpartum uterine atony, myalgias.

Precautions and Contraindications

Monitor liver function at the beginning of therapy. Observe for hepatotoxicity, hepatitis. Owing to increased risk of hepatotoxicity, use with caution with severely impaired cardiac or pulmonary function and in women or patients over 35. Contraindicated in active hepatic disease such as hepatitis or cirrhosis (when spasticity is used to maintain motor function) and in lactation.

Anesthetic Considerations

Enhanced CNS and respiratory depression with other CNS depressants. Avoid concomitant use of calcium channel blockers, which can precipitate hyperkalemia and cardiovascular collapse.

Name

Desflurane (Suprane)

Classification

Inhalation anesthetic

Indications

General anesthesia

Dose

Titrate to effect for induction or maintenance of anesthesia. Minimum alveolar concentration (MAC): 6%. Dosage forms: Volatile liquid.

Onset and Duration

Onset: Loss of eyelid reflex 1 to 2 min; Duration: Emergence time 8 to 9 min.

Adverse Effects

Hypotension, arrhythmia, respiratory depression, apnea, dizziness, euphoria, increased cerebral blood flow and intracranial pressure, nausea, vomiting, ileus, hepatic dysfunction, malignant hyperthermia

Precautions and Contraindications

Contraindicated in patients with known or suspected genetic suscepti-bility to malignant hyperthermia. Changes in mental function may persist beyond the period of anesthetic administration and the imme-diate postoperative period.

Anesthetic Considerations

Abrupt onset of malignant hyperthermia may be triggered by desflu-rane; early signs include muscle rigidity, especially in the jaw muscles, and tachycardia and tachypnea unresponsive to increased depth of anesthesia. Crosses the placental barrier.

Name

Desmopressin (DDAVP)

Classification

Synthetic vasopressin analogue

Indications

Treatment of neurogenic diabetes insipidus, nocturnal enuresis, and in hemophilia A or von Willebrand's disease to increase Factor VIII activ-ity. Reduction of perioperative blood loss following cardiac surgery.

Dose

Preoperative: 30 min prior. Diabetes insipidus: 2 to 4 µg I.V. or SQ daily in two divided doses; Intranasal: 10 to 40 µg (0.1 to 0.4 mL) in one to three doses.

Pediatrics: 3 mos to 12 yr: hemophilia A or von Willebrand's dis-ease: 0.3 µg/kg I.V. diluted in saline and infused over 15 to 30 min. In children greater than 10 kg use 50 mL diluent, and in children less than 10 kg use 10 mL diluent. Repeated doses in less than 48 hr may increase the possibility of tachyphylaxis.

Intranasal: 0.05 to 0.3 mL daily in single or divided doses. Doses should start at 0.05 mL or less and be individualized since an extreme decrease in plasma osmolarity in the very young may produce convul-sions.

Dosage forms: Desmopressin acetate for injection should be stored at 4° C.

Nasal: 10 to 40 µg. May be divided into 3 doses. Supplied as 10 µg per 0.1 mL or 100 µg/mL.

Injection: 4 µg/mL.

Onset and Duration

Onset: Intranasal: 1 hr; I.V.: 30 min. Duration: 8 to 20 hr. Elimination $t_{1/2}$: 3.6 hr.

Adverse Effects

Hypotension, hypertension, transient headache (with higher doses), psychosis, seizures, water retention, hyponatremia, abdominal cramps, nasal congestion, rhinitis, facial flushing, hypersensitivity reactions

Precautions and Contraindications

Contraindicated in hypersensitivity to desmopressin acetate and in children under 3 months of age. Patients with type IIB von Willebrand's disease should not receive desmopressin since platelet aggregation may be reduced. Owing to an increased risk of thrombosis, use with caution in patients with coronary artery disease. Fluid intake should be decreased in those who do not need the antidiuretic effects of desmopressin. Seizure activity may be related to rapid decreases in serum sodium concentrations secondary to desmopressin. Avoid over hydration, post operative abdominal cramping may occur.

Anesthetic Considerations

None

Name

Dexamethasone (Decadron)

Classification

Long-acting corticosteroid

Indications

Croup, septic shock, cerebral edema, respiratory distress syndrome including status asthmaticus, acute exacerbations of chronic allergic disorders, corticosteroid-responsive bronchospastic states, allergic or inflammatory nasal conditions and nasal polyps

Dose

Initial: 0.5 to 9 mg I.M. or I.V. daily, depending on the disease being treated. In less severe diseases, doses lower than 0.5 mg I.M. or I.V. may suffice, whereas in others, doses higher than 9 mg may be required. Cerebral edema: 10 mg I.V. initially followed by 4 mg I.M. every 6 hr. Reduce dose after 2 to 4 days, then taper over 5 to 7 days. Corticosteroid-responsive bronchospastic states: Respihaler: three inhalations 3 to 4 times daily (maximum 12 inhalations daily). Nasal conditions: Turbinaire: two sprays each nostril 2 to 3 times daily (maximum 12 sprays/24 hr). Children: I.M. or I.V. push 6 to 40 µg/kg or 0.235 to 1.25 mg/m^2 given one or two times daily. Must be given slowly over 3 to 5 minutes I.V. push. Dosage forms: Respihaler inhalation: 0.1 mg/spray dexamethasone phosphate. Turbinaire intranasal: 0.1 mg/spray. Solution for injection: 4, 10, 24 mg/mL. Tablets: 0.25, 0.5, 0.75, 1, 1.5, 2, 4, 6 mg.

Onset and Duration

Onset: I.V., I.M.: within 8 hr; Inhalation: within 20 min. Elimination t$_{1/2}$: 200 min, however, metabolic effects at the tissue level persist for up to 72 hr.

PART 3 **Drugs**

Adverse Effects

Cushing's syndrome, adrenal suppression, hyperglycemia, hyperthyroidism, hypercalcemia, peptic ulcer, gastrointestinal hemorrhage, increased intraocular pressure, glaucoma, irritability, psychosis, osteoporosis

Precautions and Contraindications

Contraindicated in patients with peptic ulcer, osteoporosis, psychosis or psychoneurosis, acute bacterial infections, herpes zoster, herpes simplex ulceration of the eye, and other viral infections. Use with caution in diabetes mellitus, chronic renal failure, infectious disease, and the elderly. Corticosteroids may increase the risk of developing tuberculosis in patients with a positive purified protein derivative test. May increase the risk of development of serious or fatal infection in individuals exposed to viral illnesses such as chicken pox.

Anesthetic Considerations

Acute administration of I.V. or inhalation steroids may be helpful in shock and asthma. Toxicity following acute dosing is minimal.

Name

Diazepam (Valium)

Classification

Central nervous system agent; benzodiazepine; anticonvulsant and anxiolytic

Indications

Anxiety, alcohol withdrawal, status epilepticus, preoperative sedation, sedation for cardioversion. Used adjunctively for relief of skeletal muscle spasm associated with cerebral palsy, paraplegia, athetosis, stiff-man syndrome, tetanus.

Dose

Status epilepticus: Adults: I.M./I.V.: 5 to 10 mg; repeat if needed at 10 to 15 min intervals up to 30 mg, repeat if needed in 2 to 4 hr; Children: I.M./I.V.: less than 5 yr: 0.2 to 0.5 mg slowly 2 to 5 min up to 5 mg, total dose. Children greater than 5 year: 1 mg slowly 2 to 5 min up to 10 mg; repeat if needed in 2 to 4 hr.

Adults: Anxiety, muscle spasm convulsions, alcohol withdrawal: P.O.: 2 to 10 mg b.i.d. to q.i.d.; I.M./I.V.: 2 to 10 mg; repeat if needed in 3 to 4 hr; Children: P.O.: greater than 6 mos: 1 to 2.5 mg b.i.d. or t.i.d.

Dosage forms: Tablets: 2, 5, 10 mg; Capsules: (sustained release) 15 mg; Oral solution: 5 mg/5 mL and 5 mg/mL; Injection: 5 mg/mL.

Onset and Duration

Onset: P.O.: 30 to 60 min; I.M.: 15 to 30 min; I.V.: 1 to 5 min. Peak effect: 1 to 2 hr P.O. Duration: 15 min to 1 hr I.V.; up to 3 hr P.O.:

Elimination $t_{1/2}$: 20 to 50 hr; excreted primarily in urine. Metabolized in liver to active metabolites.

Adverse Effects

Drowsiness, fatigue, ataxia, confusion, paradoxical dizziness, vertigo, amnesia, vivid dreams, headache, slurred speech, tremor, muscle weakness, electroencephalogram changes, tardive dyskinesia, hypotension, tachycardia, edema, cardiovascular collapse, blurred vision, diplopia, nystagmus, xerostomia, nausea, constipation, incontinence, urinary retention, changes in libido

Precautions and Contraindications

Contraindicated in acute narrow-angle glaucoma, untreated open-angle glaucoma, during or within 14 days of monoamine oxidase inhibitor therapy. Safe use during pregnancy (category D) and lactation not established.

Anesthetic Considerations

Reduces requirements for volatile anesthetics, potential thrombophlebitis with I.V. administration. Decreased clearance and dosage requirements in old age. Effects antagonized by flumazenil. May cause neonatal hypothermia.

Name

Digoxin (Lanoxin)

Classification

Inotropic agent

Indications

Treatment of supraventricular arrhythmias, heart failure, atrial fibrillation, flutter

Dose

Adults: Loading: I.V./P.O.: 0.5 to 1 mg in divided doses (give 50% of loading dose as first dose, then 25% fractions at 4 to 8 hr intervals until adequate therapeutic response is noted, toxic effects occur, or the total digitalizing dose has been administered). Monitor clinical response before each additional dose. Maintenance: I.V./P.O.: 0.0625 to 0.25 mg; dosages should be individualized. Elderly adults (greater than 65 yr): P.O.: 0.125 mg or less daily as maintenance dose. Small patients may require less.

Children (greater than 2 yr): Loading: P.O.: 0.02 to 0.06 mg/kg divided every 8 hr for 24 hr; I.V.: 0.015 to 0.035 mg/kg divided every 8 hr for 24 hr. Maintenance: P.O.: 25% to 35% of digitalizing dose daily, divided into 2 doses.

Children 1 mo to 2 yr: Loading: P.O.: 0.035 to 0.060 mg/kg in 3 divided doses over 24 hr; I.V.: 0.02 to 0.05 mg/kg; Maintenance: P.O.: 25% to 35% of digitalizing dose daily divided every 12 hr.

Neonates under 1 mo: Loading: P.O.: 0.025 to 0.035 mg/kg

divided every 8 hr over 24 hr; I.V.: 0.015 to 0.025 mg/kg. Maintenance: P.O. 25% to 35% of digitalizing dose daily divided every 12 hr.

Premature infants: Loading: I.V.: 0.015 to 0.025 mg/kg in 3 divided doses over 24 hr. Maintenance: I.V.: 0.01 mg/kg daily divided every 12 hr.

Dosage forms: Tablets: 0.125, 0.25, 0.5 mg; Capsules: (Lanoxicaps) 0.05, 0.1, 0.2 mg; Oral solution: 0.05 mg/mL; Injection: 0.1 mg/mL, 1-mL ampule (100 mg); 0.25 mg/mL, 2-mL ampule (500 mg).

Onset and Duration

Onset: I.V.: 5 to 30 min; P.O.: 30 min to 2 hr. Duration: I.V./P.O.: 3 to 4 days.

Adverse Effects

Enhanced toxicity in hypokalemia, hypomagnesemia, hypercalcemia. Wild range of arrhythmias, atrioventricular block, headache, psychosis, confusion, nausea, vomiting, diarrhea, gynecomastia. Overdosage may cause complete heart block, atrioventricular dissociation, tachycardia, fibrillation.

Precautions and Contraindication

Contraindicated in ventricular fibrillation.

Anesthetic Considerations

Decrease dosage in patients with impaired renal function and the elderly. Monitor serum potassium, calcium, and digoxin levels. Use of synchronized cardioversion in patients with digitalis toxicity should be avoided since it may initiate ventricular fibrillation.

Increased serum levels with calcium channel blockers (e.g., verapamil, diltiazem, nifedipine), esmolol, flecainide, captopril, quinidine, amiodarone, benzodiazapines, anticholinergics, oral aminoglycosides, erythromycin. Succinylcholine may cause arrhythmias in digitalized patients. Additive bradycardia may occur with cardiac depressant anesthetics.

Name

Diltiazem (Cardizem)

Classification

Calcium channel blocker

Indications

Angina pectoris; supraventricular tachycardia

Dose

Bolus I.V.: 0.25 mg/kg over 2 min. If needed, follow after 15 min with 0.35 mg/kg over 2 min. Maintenance infusion of 5 to 15 mg/hr. Adults: P.O.: 30 mg t.i.d. or q.i.d. before meals and at bedtime. Dosage may be gradually increased to a maximum 360 mg/day in divided doses.

Sustained release capsules: 90 mg P.O.: b.i.d. titrate dosage to effect (maximum recommended dosage: 360 mg/day). Dosage forms: P.O.: 30, 60, 90, 120 mg; sustained release: 60, 90, 120, 180, 240, 300 mg; I.V.: 5 mg/mL, 5-mL and 10-mL vials.

Onset and Duration

Onset: P.O.: 30 min; I.V.: 1 to 3 min. Elimination $t_{1/2}$: 3 to 5 hr. Duration: 4 to 6 hr.

Adverse Effects

Hypotension, flushing, atrioventricular block, constipation, pruritus, bradycardia, edema, nausea, vomiting, diarrhea, depression, headache, fatigue, dizziness

Precautions and Contraindications

Hypotension, coadministration with digoxin, β-blockers, cimetidine. Potentiates cardiovascular depressant effects of volatile, injectable anesthetic agents.

Anesthetic Considerations

I.V. infusions of diltriazem are useful for intraoperative treatment of atrial tachyarrhythmias.

Name

Diphenhydramine (Benadryl)

Classification

Histamine (H_1) antagonist, ethanolamine class

Indications

Adjuvant with epinephrine in the treatment of anaphylactic shock and severe allergic reactions. Treatment of drug-induced extrapyramidal effects, motion sickness. Antiemetic.

Dose

Antihistamine or antiemetic: 10 to 50 mg I.M. or I.V. every 2 to 3 hr (maximum dosage: 400 mg/day).

Bennett et al. (1987) recommend increasing the dosing interval to every 6 to 12 hr in patients with moderate renal failure (glomerular filtration rate 10 to 50 mL/min).

Children: 1 to 2 mg/kg up to 150 mg/m^2 per day in up to 4 divided doses by slow I.V. push (3 to 5 min).

Dosage forms: Injection: 10 mg/mL, 50 mg/1 mL steridose syringe or ampule. Capsules: 25, 50 mg. Elixir and syrup: 12.5 mg/15 mL.

Onset and Duration

Onset: P.O.: 1 hr. Duration: 4 to 6 hr. Elimination $t_{1/2}$: 4 to 8 hr.

PART 3 Drugs

Adverse Effects

Most frequent is sedation. Dizziness, tinnitus, tremors, euphoria, blurred vision, nervousness, palpitations, hypotension, psychotic reactions, hypersensitivity. Other side effects are probably related to the antimuscarinic actions of diphenhydramine and include dry mouth, cough, urinary retention.

Precautions and Contraindications

Diphenhydramine is contraindicated in patients with a hypersensitivity to it and other antihistamines of a similar chemical structure. Antihistamines are contraindicated in patients on monoamine oxidase-inhibitor therapy. Avoid in patients with narrow-angle glaucoma.

Anesthetic Considerations

Concurrent central nervous system depressants may produce an additive effect with diphenhydramine.

Name

Dobutamine HCl (Dobutrex)

Classification

β_1 adrenergic agonist; also mild β_2- and α_1-receptor agonist

Indications

Vasopressor; positive inotrope

Dose

Infusion: 0.5 to 30 μg/kg per min. *Note:* Must be diluted and an I.V. pump (syringe pump in pediatric patients) must be used.

Onset and Duration

Onset: 1 to 2 min. Duration: less than 10 min.

Adverse Effects

Hypertension, bradycardia, arrhythmias, angina, shortness of breath, headache, phlebitis at injection site

Precautions and Contraindications

Arrhythmias and hypertension at high doses; increased risk of dangerous arrhythmias while using volatile agents. Use with caution in patients with idiopathic hypertrophic subaortic stenosis. Do not mix with sodium bicarbonate, furosemide, or other alkaline solution; correct hypovolemia before or during treatment.

Anesthetic Considerations

Useful for short-term intraoperative therapy for shock and congestive heart failure. Arterial line monitoring is highly recommended.

Name

Dopamine HCl (Intropin)

Classification

Naturally occurring catecholamine

Indications

Vasopressor; positive inotrope

Dose

Infusion: 1 to 5 μg/kg low dose for urinary support; pressor dose range: 5 to 20 μg/kg, greater than 20 μg/kg for extreme cases. *Note:* Must be diluted and an I.V. pump must be used.

Onset and Duration

Onset: 2 to 4 min. Duration: less than 10 min.

Adverse Effects

Nausea, vomiting, tachycardia, angina, arrhythmias, dyspnea, headache, anxiety

Precautions and Contraindications

Correct hypovolemia as quickly as possible before or during treatment.

Anesthetic Considerations

Avoid or use at greatly reduced dose if patient has received a monamine oxidase inhibitor. Infuse into a large vein; extravasation may cause sloughing. Treat extravasation by local infiltration of phentolamine (approximately 1 mg in 10 mL normal saline).

Name

Doxacurium chloride (Nuromax)

Classification

Nondepolarizing skeletal muscle relaxant

Indications

Adjunct to general anesthesia; skeletal muscle relaxation during surgery

Dose

Paralyzing: I.V.: 0.05 to 0.08 mg/kg. Pretreatment/maintenance: 0.005 to 0.01 mg/kg. Dosage form: 1 mg/mL injection.

Onset and Duration

Onset: less than 4 min. Duration: 30 to 160 min. Elimination: Renal.

Adverse Effects

Hypotension, flushing, ventricular fibrillation, myocardial infarction, bronchospasm, hypoventilation, apnea, depression, anuria, rash, urticaria, inadequate block, prolonged block

Precautions and Contraindications

Airway and oxygenation must be ensured before administration. Contraindicated in patients with epilepsy, convulsive disorders, mechanical disorders of ventilation, head injuries, cerebrovascular accident, known hypersensitivity to the drug, significant cardiovascular impairment.

Anesthetic Considerations

Monitor response with peripheral nerve stimulator. Reverse effects with anticholinesterase. Pretreatment may cause hypoventilation in some patients.

Name

Doxapram HCl (Dopram)

Classification

Central nervous system agent; respiratory and cerebral stimulant (analeptic)

Indications

Postanesthesia and drug-induced respiratory depression and to hasten arousal and return of pharyngeal and laryngeal reflexes. Chronic pulmonary disease associated with acute hypercapnia.

Dose

Slow I.V.: 0.5 to 1.5 mg/kg, repeat at 5 min (maximum dose: 2 mg/kg). Infusion: 5 mg/min until satisfactory respiratory response is obtained, then 1 to 3 mg/min (maximum total dose: 4 mg/kg, including bolus and infusion).

Onset and Duration

Onset: 20 to 40 sec. Peak effect: 1 to 2 min. Duration: 5 to 12 min.

Adverse Effects

Hypertension, chest pain, tachycardia, bradycardia, arrhythmias, cough, laryngospasm, bronchospasm, hiccups, seizures, hyperactivity, headaches, urinary retention, spontaneous voiding, nausea, vomiting, desire to defecate, decreased hemoglobin/hematocrit levels and red blood cell count, leukopenia. Delay administration for at least 10 min after discontinuation of volatile anesthetics because of sensitization of catecholamines. Concomitant use of monoamine oxidase inhibitors or other sympathomimetics may potentiate adverse cardiovascular effects.

Precautions and Contraindications

Head trauma, epilepsy or other seizure disorders, mechanical disorders of ventilation, cerebrovascular accident, significant cardiovascular impairment, severe hypertension, or known hypersensitivity to the drug. Use cautiously in patients with history of severe tachycardia or cardiac arrhythmia, increased cerebrospinal fluid pressure or cerebral edema, pheochromocytoma, or hyperthyroidism or hypermetabolic states.

Anesthetic Considerations

Respiratory depression may reoccur after doxaprams effects are terminated. Due to the low therapeutic index, repeat dosing is discouraged.

Name

Edrophonium chloride (Enlon, Reversol, Tensilon)

Classification

Anticholinesterase agent

Indications

Reversal of neuromuscular blockade; diagnostic assessment of myasthenia gravis and supraventricular tachycardia.

Dose

Reversal: slow I.V.: 0.5 to 1.0 mg/kg (maximum dose: 40 mg); with atropine (0.007 to 0.015 mg/kg), administer prior to the endrophonium.

Assessment of myasthenia/cholinergic crisis: slow I.V.: 1 mg every 1 to 2 min until change in symptoms (maximum dose: 10 mg). I.M.: 10 mg.

Onset and Duration

Onset: I.V.: 30 to 60 sec; I.M.: 2 to 10 min. Duration: I.V.: 5 to 20 min; I.M.: 10 to 40 min.

Adverse Effects

Bradycardia, tachycardia, atrioventricular block, nodal rhythm, hypotension. Increased oral, pharyngeal, bronchial secretions, bronchospasm, respiratory depression, seizures, dysarthria, headaches, lacrimation, miosis, visual changes, nausea, emesis, flatulence, increased peristalsis, rash, urticaria, allergic reactions, anaphylaxis

Precautions and Contraindications

Use with caution in patients with bradycardia, bronchial asthma, cardiac arrhythmias, peptic ulcer, peritonitis, or mechanical obstruction of the intestines or urinary tract.

Overdosage may induce a cholinergic crisis characterized by nausea, vomiting, bradycardia or tachycardia, excessive salivation and sweating, bronchospasm, weakness and paralysis.

Treatment with discontinuation of edrophonium and administration of atropine 10 μg/kg I.V. every 10 min until muscarinic symptoms disappear.

Owing to the brief duration of action of edrophonium, neostigmine or pyridostigmine is generally preferred for reversal of the effects of nondepolarizing muscle relaxants.

PART 3 Drugs

Anesthetic Considerations

Administer with anticholinergic to avoid cholinergic side effects (e.g., bronchoconstriction, bradycardia). Excellent alternative for intraoperative hypertension, especially in patients taking angiotensin-converting enzyme inhibitors.

Name

Enalaprilat (Vasotec IV)

Classification

Angiotensin converting enzyme (ACE) inhibitor

Indications

Hypertension

Dose

I.V.: 0.625 to 1.25 mg over 5 min every 6 hr. Dosage forms: 1.25 mg/mL, 1-ml and 2-mL vials.

Onset and Duration

Onset: 10 to 15 min. Duration: approximately 6 hr.

Adverse Effects

Cough, hypotension, renal impairment, angiodema

Precautions and Contraindications

Patients on diuretics may have to adjust dose while on ACE inhibitors. Contraindicated during pregnancy.

Anesthetic Considerations

Useful addition to antihypertensive drug choices for perioperative use.

Name

Enflurane (Ethrane)

Classification

Inhalation anesthetic

Indications

General anesthesia

Dose

Titrate to effect for induction or maintenance of anesthesia. Minimum alveolar concentration: 1.7% in 100% oxygen and 0.6% in 70% nitrous oxide. Dosage form: Volatile liquid: 125, 250 mL.

Onset and Duration

Onset: loss of eyelid reflex 2 to 3 min. Duration: emergence 15 min.

Adverse Effects

Hypotension, arrhythmia, respiratory depression, apnea, seizures, dizziness, euphoria, increased cerebral blood flow and intracranial pressure, nausea, vomiting, hepatic dysfunction, renal dysfunction, malignant hyperthermia, glucose elevation

Precautions and Contraindications

Anesthetic requirements decrease with age. Changes in mental function may persist beyond the period of anesthetic administration and the immediate postoperative period. Contraindicated in patients with seizure disorders and those with known or suspected genetic susceptibility to malignant hyperthermia.

Anesthetic Considerations

Abrupt onset of malignant hyperthermia may be triggered by enflurane. Early premonitory signs include muscle rigidity (especially of the jaw muscles), tachycardia, and tachypnea unresponsive to increased depth of anesthesia. Enflurane crosses the placental barrier.

Name

Enoxaparin (Lovenox, Low-molecular weight heparin [LMWH])

Classification

Anticoagulant (antithrombotic); inhibiting Factors Xa and IIa and only slightly affecting clotting times.

Indications

To prevent postoperative pulmonary embolism (PE) and/or deep-vein thrombosis (DVT). To reduce ischemic complications with cardiovascular patients having unstable angina and non-Q-wave myocardial infarctions.

Dose

Immediately after surgery: 30 mg or 40 mg SQ q 12 hr to prevent DVT or PE. 1 mg/kg SQ q 12 hr with 100 to 325 mg oral aspirin daily to treat unstable angina/non-Q-wave MI patients.

Onset and Duration

SQ onset: 20 to 60 min; peaks 3 to 5 hr. Duration: 12 hr. Elimination $t_{1/2}$: 3 to 4.5 hr.

Adverse Effects

Hemorrhage, epidural/subarachnoid or injection site hematomas, thrombocytopenia, increased AST, ALT liver enzymes, chills, fever, urticaria

Precautions and Contraindications

Avoid I.M. injections. Use with caution in pregnant patients and those with a history of coagulopathies or GI bleeding. Enoxaparin is absolutely contraindicated in patients with active bleeding, thrombocytopenia, history of heparin-induced thrombocytopenia, and pork or heparin sensitivities.

Anesthetic Considerations

Central axis blocks or removal of indwelling catheters should not occur at least 12 hr before or after the last administration of enoxaparin, or conservatively, not within the last 24 hr. Coagulation tests do not need to be routinely ordered while the patient is taking enoxaparin. However, if coagulation tests are abnormal or bleeding occurs, anti-Factor Xa is the most sensitive test to indicate therapeutic anticoagulation levels. Treat overdose with protamine sulfate. Each mg of protamine will neutralize 1 mg of enoxaparin.

Name

Ephedrine sulfate

Classification

Noncatecholamine sympathomimetic with mixed direct and indirect actions

Indications

Hypotension, bradycardia

Dose

I.V.: 5 to 25 mg × 2 (100 to 300 μg/kg); I.M.: 26 to 50 mg; P.O.: 25 to 50 mg every 3 hr.

Onset and Duration

Onset: I.V. almost immediate; I.M.: a few minutes. Duration: I.V.: 10 to 60 min.

Adverse Effects

Hypertension, tachycardia, arrhythmias, pulmonary edema, anxiety, tremors, hyperglycemia, transient hyperkalemia and then hypokalemia, necrosis at the site of injection. Tolerance may develop.

Precautions and Contraindications

Use cautiously in patients with hypertension and ischemic heart disease; unpredictable effect in patients in whom endogenous catecholamines are depleted; may produce an unacceptable degree of central nervous system stimulation, resulting in insomnia.

Anesthetic Considerations

Increased risk of arrhythmias with volatile anesthetic agents; potentiated by tricyclic antidepressants; increases the maximum allowable concentration of the volatile anesthetics.

Name

Epinephrine HCl (adrenaline chloride)

Classification
Endogenous catecholamine

Indications
Inotropic support; treatment of anaphylaxis; increase duration of action of local anesthetic; hemostasis; cardiac arrest; bronchodilation

Dose
Cardiac arrest: 0.5 to 1.0 mg I.V. bolus every 5 min as necessary. Inotropic support: 2 to 20 µg/min (0.1 to 1.0 µg/kg per min).

Onset and Duration
Onset: I.V.: immediate. Duration: I.V.: 5 to 10 min.

Adverse Effects
Restlessness, fear, throbbing headache, tachycardia, tachydysrhythmias, premature ventricular contractions, ventricular tachycardia, ventricular fibrillation, severe hypertension, angina, extension of myocardial infarction, pulmonary edema.

Precautions and Contraindications
Use with caution in patients with coronary artery disease, hypertension, diabetes mellitus, or hyperthyroidism, and in patients taking monoamine oxidase inhibitors.

Anesthetic Considerations
May be administered through the endotracheal tube.

Name
Esmolol (Brevibloc)

Classification
Cardioselective β-blocker

Indications
Supraventricular tachycardia (SVT); perioperative hypertension

Dose
SVT: Loading: 50 to 200 µg/kg/min for 1 min. Follow by infusion of 50 µg/kg/min for 4 min. If desired effect is not achieved, repeat loading dose and increase infusion to 100 µg/kg/min. May repeat process up to maximum of 300 µg/kg/min. Dosage forms: 10 mg/mL in 10-mL vial for direct I.V. injection. 250 mg/mL in 10-mL ampule for I.V. infusion. **USE ONLY AFTER DILUTION IN LARGE-VOLUME PARENTERAL FLUID TO PREPARE INFUSION.**

Onset and Duration
Onset: 1 to 2 min. Duration: 10 to 20 min. Peak effect: 5 to 6 min. Not to be infused for more than 48 hr.

PART 3 Drugs

Precautions and Contraindications

During pregnancy, monitor K^+ levels. Use with caution in patients with atrioventricular heart block or cardiac failure not caused by tachycardia, obstructive pulmonary disease, or diabetes.

Adverse Effects

Hypotension, bradycardia, congestive heart failure, bronchospasm, confusion, depression, urinary retention, nausea and vomiting, erythema

Anesthetic Considerations

May have additive cardiovascular depressant effects when coupled with volatile, injectable anesthetic agents. May enhance actions of non-depolarizing neuromuscular blocking agents such as tubocurarine, rocuronium, and pancuronium.

Name

Ethacrynic acid (Edecrin)

Classification

Loop diuretic

Indications

Edema of cardiac, hepatic, or renal origin. Hypertension, pulmonary edema. Usually reserved for patients who do not respond to thiazide diuretics or in whom a rapid onset of diuresis is desired.

Dose

0.5 to 1 mg/kg slowly over several minutes up to a maximum of 100 mg in a single dose. The usual average dose is 50 mg. Children: 1 mg/kg over 20 to 30 min. Dosage forms: 50-mg vial, powder for injection. Reconstitute by adding 50 mL D_5W or normal saline. Tablets: 25, 50 mg.

Onset and Duration

Onset: I.V.: 5 to 15 min. Duration: I.V.: 2 hr, but may last 6 to 7 hr. Elimination $t_{1/2}$: 1 to 4 hr.

Adverse Effects

Fluid electrolyte imbalance, including hypomagnesemia, hypocalcemia, hypokalemia, hypochloremia, metabolic alkalosis, hyperuricemia. Hypoglycemia and hyperglycemia, thrombocytopenia, agranulocytopenia, vertigo, ototoxicity (associated with rapid I.V. injection), pancreatitis, gastrointestinal hemorrhage, hepatotoxicity, hypotension, diarrhea.

Precautions and Contraindications

Avoid rapid I.V. injection. Use with extreme caution in patients with impaired renal or hepatic function. Contraindicated for use in patients once anuric renal failure is established. Also contraindicated in patients with hypotension, dehydration with low serum sodium or metabolic alkalosis with hypokalemia, nursing mothers, and infants and severe watery diarrhea.

Anesthetic Considerations

Loop diuretics have been reported to increase the neuromuscular blocking effect of tubocurarine, probably because of their potassium-depleting effects.

Name

Etidocaine HCl (Duranest)

Classification

Amide-type local anesthetic

Indications

Regional anesthesia: Infiltration, peripheral nerve block, epidural, caudal

Dose

Infiltration/peripheral nerve block: 50 to 400 mg (1% solution); Epidural: 100 to 300 mg (1% or 1.5% solution); Caudal: 100 to 300 mg (10 to 30 mL of 1% solution). Children: 0.4 to 0.7 ml/kg (for L2 to T10 level of anesthesia). (Maximum dose: 3 mg/kg without epinephrine, 4 mg/kg with epinephrine.)

Onset and Duration

Onset: Infiltration: 3 to 5 min; epidural: 5 to 15 min. Peak effect: Infiltration: 5 to 15 min; epidural 15 to 20 min. Duration: Infiltration: 2 to 3 hr, 3 to 7 hr with epinephrine; epidural: 3 to 5 hr.

Adverse Effects

Myocardial depression, arrhythmias, cardiac arrest, hypotension, respiratory depression, anxiety, apprehension, euphoria, tinnitus, seizures, urticaria, edema, nausea, vomiting. High spinal: Loss of bladder and bowel control.

Precautions and ContraIndications

Use cautiously in debilitated, elderly, or acutely ill patients, severe shock, heart block, pregnancy. Contraindicated in patients with hypersensitivity to amide-type local anesthetics.

Anesthetic Considerations

Do not use for spinal anesthesia. Owing to profound motor blockade, not recommended for epidural anesthesia for delivery. Benzodiazepines increase seizure threshold.

Name

Etomidate (Amidate)

PART 3 **Drugs**

Classification

Central nervous system agent; nonbarbiturate hypnotic without analgesic activity

Indications

Induction of general anesthesia

Dose

Adult: I.V.: 0.2 to 0.6 (usual 0.3) mg/kg over 30 to 60 sec. Dosage forms: Injection: 2 mg/mL, ampules and prefilled syringe.

Onset and Duration

Onset: 1 min. Duration: 3 to 10 min. Metabolized in liver, $t_{1/2}$ 75 min; excreted primarily in the urine.

Adverse Effects

Myoclonus, tonic movements, eye movements, hypertension, hypotension, tachycardia, bradycardia, and other arrhythmias, postoperative nausea and vomiting, hypoventilation, hyperventilation, transient apnea, laryngospasm, hiccups, snoring, adrenocortical suppression

Precautions and ContraIndications

Cautious use in immunosuppression. Contraindicated during labor and delivery. Safety during pregnancy, in nursing women, and in children under 4 years has not been established.

Anesthetic Considerations

Use with caution in patients with focal epilepsy. Use large veins. Myoclonus reduced by premedication with benzodiazepine or opioid.

Name

Famotidine (Pepcid)

Classification

Histamine (H2) antagonist

Indications

Duodenal or gastric ulcers and gastroesophageal reflux. Prophylaxis of aspiration pneumonitis in patients at high risk during surgery.

Dose

Prophylaxis of aspiration pneumonitis: Adults: 20 to 40 mg P.O. the evening before surgery and/or the morning of surgery before induction of anesthesia. If a more rapid onset is desired, 2 mL of I.V. famotidine (10 mg/mL) may be diluted to a concentration of 5 to 10 mL with D_5W, normal saline, or lactated Ringer's solution and given over at least 2 min prior to induction. Dosage forms: Tablets: 20, 40 mg. Parenteral injection: 10 mg/mL in 2-mL or 4-mL vials.

Onset and Duration

Onset: 20 to 45 min. Peak serum levels occur 1 to 3 hr P.O. Duration: Plasma famotidine concentrations that suppress gastric acid secretion by 50% are maintained for 12 hr following an oral dose of 40 mg, and 7 to 9 hr after a 20-mg dose.

Adverse Effects

Headache (2% to 4.5%), constipation (1.4%), and drowsiness are the most frequently reported. Mental confusion occurs occasionally in the elderly. Potential bradydysrhythmias and hypotension may be associated with rapid infusion. Reversible hepatitis and hepatotoxicity are infrequent. Reversible leukopenia, thrombocytopenia, granulocytopenia and aplastic anemia are rare.

Precautions and Contraindications

Caution suggested in hepatic or renal dysfunction (possible dose reductions required). Contraindicated in patients with known hypersensitivity to famotidine or other histamine2 antagonists.

Anesthetic Considerations

Use with caution when administering halothane anesthesia (arrhythmogenic). Maximum dose for prolongation of local anesthetics: 250 µg. Safe alternative to gastric prophylaxis preoperatively.

Name

Fenoldopam (Corlopam)

Classification

Antihypertensive (dopamine DA-1-receptor agonist)

Indications

A potent vasodilator that stimulates the postsynaptic dopamine DA-receptors, thereby lowering blood pressure, peripheral vascular resistance, renal vascular resistance, and increasing cardiac hemodynamics. Used short term (up to 48 hrs) for patients with severe hypertension/malignant hypertension.

Dose

Administer fenoldopam as a continuous infusion; no loading dose is needed. The infusion range is 0.04 to 0.8 µg/kg/min, titrate slowly for blood pressure reduction. Lower initial doses below 0.1 µg/kg/min are marginally antihypertensive but have less reflex tachycardia. Initial doses above 0.3 µg/kg/min or more have been associated with reflex tachycardia.

Onset and Duration

Onset: 5 min. Peak effect: 15 min. Rapidly metabolized, $t_{1/2}$ is 5 min.

Adverse Effects

Reflex tachycardia with a higher initial dosing regimen may increase intraocular pressure, hypotension, hypokalemia (infusion time greater than 6 hr can cause potassium to fall below 3 m Eq), headache, flushing, nausea

Precautions and ContraIndications

Fenoldopam has no absolute contraindications. Use with caution in cerebrovascular accident (CVA) patients secondary to hypertension. Contains metabisulfite compound, so do not use in patients sensitive to sulfites (especially asthmatics) since allergic reaction may result. Concomitant use of other antihypertensive agents (calcium channel blockers, nitrates, β_1-blockers, and α_2-blockers) may result in unexpected hypotension.

Anesthetic Considerations

Titrate drug slowly to prevent reflex tachycardia. Check potassium level if titrating long-term infusion (greater than 6 hr). Review for sulfite allergies, especially asthmatics. Use caution with open globe injuries and glaucoma patients since fenoldopam may increase intraocular pressure.

Name

Fentanyl (Sublimaze)

Classification

Opioid agonist

Indications

Produces analgesia and anesthesia

Dose

Analgesia: I.V.: 1 to 2 μg/kg.
Induction: 30 μg/kg. Infusion: 0.2 μg/kg per min; Epidural bolus: 1 to 2 μg/kg. Infusion: 2 to 60 μg/hr; Spinal bolus: 0.1 to 0.4 μg/kg. Dosage form: Injection: 0.05 mg/mL. Transdermal patch: 100 μg/hr. In conjunction with epidural administration: 1 to 2 μg/kg. For infusion with epidural: 2 to 60 μg/hr. In conjunction with spinal anesthesia: bolus dose of 0.1 to 0.4 μg/kg.

Onset and Duration

Onset: I.V.: within 30 sec; I.M.: less than 8 min; epidural/spinal: 4 to 10 min. Duration: I.V.: 30 to 60 min; I.M.: 1 to 2 hr; epidural/spinal; 4 to 8 hr.

Adverse Effects

Hypotension, bradycardia, respiratory depression, apnea, dizziness, blurred vision, seizures, nausea, emesis, delayed gastric emptying, biliary tract spasm, muscle rigidity

Precautions and ContraIndications

Reduce doses in elderly, hypovolemic, high-risk patients, and with concomitant use of sedatives and other narcotics. Crosses the placental barrier; may produce depression of respiration in the neonate. Prolonged depression may occur after cessation of transdermal patch use.

Anesthetic Considerations

Narcotic effects reversed by naloxone (0.2 to 0.4 mg I.V.). Circulatory and ventilatory depressant effects potentiated by narcotics, sedatives, volatile anesthetics, nitrous oxide; ventilatory depressant effects potentiated by amphetamines, monoamine oxidase inhibitors, phenothiazine, tricyclic antidepressants; analgesia enhanced by α_2-agonists. Muscle rigidity in higher dose range sufficient to interfere with ventilation.

Name

Flumazenil (Romazicon)

Classification

Benzodiazepine-receptor antagonist

Indications

Reversal of benzodiazepine-receptor agonist

Dose

I.V.: 0.2 to 1 mg (4 to 20 µg/kg), titrate to patient response, may repeat at 20-min intervals (maximum single dose: 1 mg, maximum total dose: 3 mg in any 1 hr). Dosage form: Injection: 0.1 mg/mL.

Onset and Duration

Onset: 1 to 2 min. Duration: 45 to 90 min (depends on plasma concentration of benzodiazepine.)

Adverse Effects

Arrhythmia, tachycardia, bradycardia, hypertension, angina, flushing, reversal of sedation, seizures, agitation, emotional lability, nausea, vomiting, pain at injection site, thrombophlebitis

Precautions and ContraIndications

Institute measures to secure airway, ventilation, and I.V. access prior to administering flumazenil. Resedation may occur and is more common with large doses of benzodiazepine.

Anesthetic Considerations

Do not use until the effects of neuromuscular blockade have been fully reversed. Administer in a large vein to minimize pain at the injection site. Monitor for resedation.

Name

Furosemide (Lasix)

PART 3 **Drugs**

Classification

Loop diuretic

Indications

Edema of cardiac, hepatic, or renal origin. Hypertension, pulmonary edema. Usually reserved for patients who do not respond to thiazide diuretics or in whom a rapid onset of diuresis is desired.

Dose

Diuresis: Adult: I.M. or I.V. 20 to 40 mg as a single dose. IV doses should be injected slowly over 1 to 2 min. Additional doses of 20 mg greater than the previous dose may be given every 2 hr until desired response is obtained. For I.V. bolus injections do not exceed 1 g/day given over 30 min. Acute pulmonary edema: 40 mg I.V. initially, may repeat in 1 hr with 80 mg if necessary. Children: I.M. or I.V. 1 mg/kg single dose initially, increasing by 1 mg/kg every 2 hr or more until desired response is obtained or to a maximum of 6 mg/kg/day. Dosage forms: Tablets: 20, 40, 80 mg; Injection: 10 mg/mL. Oral solutions: 10 mg/mL and 40 mg/5 mL.

Onset and Duration

Onset: onset of diuresis usually occurs 5 min I.V. Duration: 2 hr. Elimination $t_{1/2}$: widely variable; normal is $^1/_2$ to 1 hr but 11 to 20 hr has been reported in patients with hepatic or renal insufficiency.

Adverse Effects

Dehydration, hypotension, hypochloremic alkalosis, hypokalemia, hypomagnesemia, hyperglycemia, hyperuricemia. Ototoxicity has been reported with too rapid I.V. injection of large doses. Rarely reported are thrombocytopenia, neutropenia, jaundice, pancreatitis, and a variety of skin reactions.

Precautions and ContraIndications

Contraindicated in anuria (except for a single dose in acute anuria) and pregnancy. Use with caution in patients with severe or progressive renal disease and hepatic disease. Discontinue if renal function worsens. Caution should be used in patients allergic to sulfonamides and patients with severe electrolyte imbalance.

Anesthetic Considerations

Monitor electrolytes and fluid balance. Administer carefully in patients taking digitalis. May be associated with enhancement of nondepolarizing neuromuscular blocking drugs.

Name

Glucagon

Classification

Hormone; antidiabetic agent (antihypoglycemic); diagnostic agent

Indications

Treatment of hypoglycemia or beta-blocker overdose; inotropic agent used to relax smooth muscle of gastrointestinal tract for radiologic studies

Dose

Diagnostic aid for radiologic examination: I.V./I.M. 0.25 to 2 mg before initiation of radiologic procedure. Hypoglycemia: I.V./I.M. SQ: 0.5 to 1 mg.

Onset and Duration

Onset: less than 5 min. Peak effect: 5 to 20 min. Duration: 10 to 30 min.

Adverse effects

Hypertension, hypotension, respiratory distress, dizziness, lightheadedness, nausea, vomiting, urticaria, hypoglycemia, hyperglycemia

Precautions and Contraindications

Hypersensitivity to drug (due to its protein nature). Use cautiously in patients with history of insulinoma or pheochromocytoma. Safe use during pregnancy and in nursing women has not been established.

Anesthetic Considerations

Rapid I.V. administration may cause decrease in blood pressure. Potentiates hypoprothrombinemic effects of anticoagulants. Parenteral glucose must be given because release of insulin may subsequently cause hypoglycemia.

Name

Glycopyrrolate (Robinul)

Classification

Competitive acetylcholine antagonist at muscarinic receptor

Indications

Vagolytic premedication to block bradycardia during surgery from stimulation of the carotid sinus, traction on abdominal viscera, or extraocular muscles. Blockade of muscarinic effects of anticholinesterases. Adjunctive therapy in the treatment of bronchspasm and peptic ulcer disease. Compared with atropine, glycoprrolate has two times more potent antisialogogue activity, less tachycardia, and no clinically significant increases in intraocular pressure at doses used preoperatively. It has no sedative effects.

Dose

Adults: Premedication/vagolysis: I.V., I.M., SQ: 0.1 to 2 mg (4 to 6 μg/kg) adminstratered 30 to 60 min preinduction. May repeat in 2 to 3 min intervals for vagolysis up to 1.0 mg total. Blockade of muscarinic effects of anticholinestrease: 0.2 mg for each 1 mg of neostigmine or 5 mg of pyridostigmine. Bronchospasm: inhalation 0.4 to 0.8 mg every

8 hr. Dilute injectate solution in 2 to 3 mL normal saline and deliver by compressed air nebulizer. Children: Preoperative 2 yrs or older: 4 μg/kg. For oral administration, use injectable solution and dilute in 3 to 5 mL juice or carbonated cola beverage. Oral absorption is erratic. Intraoperative vagolysis: 0.01 mg/kg I.V. not to exceed 0.1 mg, may repeat in 2 to 3 min. Dosage forms: Injection: 0.2 mg/mL. Tablets: 1, 2 mg.

Onset and Duration

Onset: P.O.: 1 hr I.M./S.Q.: 15 to 30 min; Inhalation: 3 to 5 min; I.V. administration: less than 1 min respectively. Duration: duration of antisialogogue effect is 7 to 12 hr depending on route of administration and dose. Duration of vagal blockade is 2 to 3 hr I.V.; 8 to 12 hr P.O.

Adverse Effects

Tachycardia (high doses), bradycardia (low doses), headache, urinary hesitancy, retention, mydriasis, blurred vision, increased intraocular pressure, decreased sweating, excitement, agitation, drowsiness, confusion, dry nose and mouth, allergic reactions, constipation

Precautions and Contraindications

Avoid where tachycardia would be harmful, i.e., thyrotoxicosis, pheochromocytoma, coronary artery disease. Avoid in hyperpyrexial states because it inhibits sweating. Use with caution for patients with hepatic or renal disease, congestive heart failure, chronic pulmonary disease (since a reduction in bronchial secretions may lead to formation of bronchial plugs), hiatal hernia, gastroesophageal reflux, gastrointestinal infections, ulcerative colitis. Contraindicated in acute-angle glaucoma, obstructive disease of the gastrointestinal tract, obstructive uropathy, paralytic ileus, intestinal atony, and acute hemorrhage where cardiovascular status is unstable.

Anesthetic Considerations

Additive anticholinergic effects may occur with meperidine, some antihistamines, phenothiazines, tricyclic antidepressants, and antiarrhythmic drugs that possess anticholinergic activity (e.g., quinidine, disopyramide, procainamide).

Name

Granisetron (Kytril)

Classification

Selective serotonin receptor antagonist

Indications

Effective single agent used to control nausea and vomiting induced by cisplatin and other cytotoxic agents

Dose

Prophylaxis of chemotherapy-induced nausea and vomiting: 40 µg/kg or 3 mg as a single I.V. infusion over 5 min to 1 hr completed 30 min before chemotherapy is implemented. Breakthrough nausea and vomiting during the first 24 hrs following therapy: 2 to 3 repeat I.V. infusions of 40 µg/kg over 5 min with each separated by at least 10 min. Dilute with 20 to 50 mL 5% dextrose or 0.9% sodium chloride. P.O.: 1 mg twice daily. Pediatric: 10 µg/kg in children 2 to 16 yr of age. Granisetron has not been studied in children younger than 2 yr of age.

Onset and Duration

Onset: Peak plasma concentrations demonstrate wide interindividual variation. After a 40 µg/kg dose, nausea and vomiting subside within several minutes. Duration: Serum levels decline to less than 10 ng/mL at 24 hr following a single 40 µg/kg infusion. Antiemetic effects last up to 24 hr following I.V. infusion of 40 µg/kg. Elimination $t_{1/2}$: 10 to 11 hr.

Adverse Effects

Headache and constipation are most common. Also reported are somnolence, dizziness, diarrhea, flushing, and transient elevation of liver enzymes.

Precautions and Contraindications

Previous hypersensitivity to granisetron, liver disease (due to the noted elevation of liver enzymes after repeat administration of granisetron), pregnancy, breastfeeding

Anesthetic Considerations

Owing to the elevation of liver enzymes after repeat doses of granisetron, careful preoperative evaluation of liver function tests is necessary to aid in determining if anesthetic agents excreted hepatically should be avoided.

Injection should not be mixed in solution with other drugs. No specific antidote for overdose; give symptomatic treatment. Inducers or inhibitors of cytochrome P 450 drug-metabolizing enzymes may change the clearance and duration of granisetron.

Name

Halothane (Fluothane)

Classification

Potent inhalation anesthetic agent

Indications

Induction and maintenance of general anesthesia

Dose

Induction: 1% to 4%. Maintenance: 0.5% to 1.5%. Supplied: Glass bottle, volatile liquid.

Onset and Duration

Onset: 5 to 10 min to achieve surgical anesthesia. Duration: up to 1 hr after discontinuation. Dose-dependent; rapid, pleasant induction and smooth.

Adverse Effects

Hypotension, shallow and rapid respiration, arrhythmia (when sympathomimetic agents are used), vomiting, hypoxia, respiratory difficulty, postoperative shivering, liver damage, bradycardia, increased intracranial pressure, malignant hyperthermia

Precautions and Contraindications

Arrhythmia may be produced by the combination of halothane and catecholamines. May potentiate effects of nondepolarizing muscle relaxants. Avoid second-time use in individuals who show evidence of liver damage. Halothane has been associated with liver dysfunction (hepatitis, jaundice), especially in persons with prior hepatic disease or previous exposure to halothane. Changes in mental function may persist beyond the period of anesthetic administration and the immediate postoperative period.

Anesthetic Considerations

Use cautiously in patients with severe cardiac disease and during pregnancy (drug is a potent uterine relaxant). Have drugs available to treat bradycardia and hypotension. Keep patient warm postoperatively to minimize shivering.

Name

Heparin (Liquaemin Sodium, Panheparin)

Classification

Anticoagulant; accelerates the rate at which antithrombin III neutralizes thrombin and factors VII, IX, X, and XI.

Indications

Prophylaxis and treatment of deep venous thrombosis (DVT) and pulmonary thromboembolism (PE). Acute arterial occlusion, intracardiac mural thrombosis, following myocardial infarction after I.V. thrombolytic treatment, disseminated intravascular coagulation (DIC) with gross thrombosis, anticoagulation during cardiopulmonary bypass (CPB), prophylaxis of thromboembolism in patients with mitral valve disease or atrial fibrillation. Maintain patency of indwelling venipuncture devices (lock flush). Value in cerebral embolism secondary to transient ischemic attacks (TIAs) has not been established.

Dose

Dosage is highly individualized and based on daily activated partial thromboplastin time (aPTT) compared with 6 hr after each dosage change. Obtain baseline aPTT and adjust dose according to clinical state. For prophylaxis (i.e., hip surgery, atrial fibrillation, valve disease):

the ratio of aPTT to baseline aPTT should be 1.2 to 1.5; for prosthetic heart valves, DVT, PE, recurrent embolism: 1.5 to 2.0. For CPB monitor activated clotting time (ACT) and maintain ACT of 400 to 480 sec. Baseline ACT values are 80 to 150 sec. ACT should be determined 5 min after heparin administration. Adequate heparinization must be ensured prior to initiation of CPB.

Dosing guidelines: CPB: prior to induction of anesthesia. 300 units/kg of heparin should be prepared in case emergency initiation of CPB is necessary. I.V. bolus: 350 to 400 units/kg. Up to 500 units/kg may be required to maintain ACT greater than 400 sec in heparin-resistant patients. Additional heparin will be needed for prolonged CPB. A 100 unit/kg hourly reinforcement dose is given starting 2 hr after the initial dose. Prophylactic or low-dose subcutaneous therapy: 5000 units SQ every 8 to 12 hr. Baseline aPTT is obtained since bleeding complications are occasionally discovered, but routine PTT monitoring is not necessary. For surgical prophylaxis, ideally started 2 hr preoperatively. Full-dose continuous I.V. infusion for treatment of DVT or PE is based on ideal body weight: I.V. bolus loading dose: 70 units/kg (3000 to 10,000 units); I.V. maintenance dose: continuous infusion 13 to 16 units/kg/hr (750 to 1300 units/hr). For continuous I.V. infusion, 25,000 units heparin may be mixed in 500 mL D_5W or normal saline. The resulting solution is 50 units/mL. Dosage forms: Injection: 1000, 2500, 5000, 7500, 10,000, 20,000, and 40,000 units/mL. Lock flush solution: 10, 100 units/mL. Premixed infusion in dextrose: 50 units/mL. Premixed infusion in normal saline: 50, 100 units/mL.

Onset and Duration

Onset: I.V.: immediate; SQ: 20 to 30 min. Elimination $t_{1/2}$: 1 to 2 hr in healthy adults. Duration: half-life and duration increase with increasing doses; prolonged in liver and renal disease.

Adverse Effects

Hemorrhage, thrombocytopenia, white-clot syndrome (rare paradoxical thrombosis), necrotizing skin lesions, elevated liver enzymes, osteoporosis, priapism, hypersensitivity

Precautions and Contraindications

Avoid I.M. injections. Contraindicated in patients with hemophilia, thrombocytopenia, acute bleeding, peptic ulcer, esophagitis, diverticulitis, esophageal varices, arterial aneurysm, gastrointestinal or urinary tract malignancy, vascular retinopathy, recent liver or renal biopsy, acute pericarditis, threatened abortion, infective endocarditis, recent regional anesthesia, severe hypertension, recent cerebrovascular accident, recent surgery, recent surgery or trauma to brain, eye, or spinal cord.

Platelet counts, hematocrit, and occult blood in stool and urine should be monitored during entire course of therapy. Increased risk of bleeding with concomitant aspirin, nonsteroidal antiinflammatory drugs, dipyridamole, thrombolytic agents, dextran, dihydroergotamine, warfarin. I.V. nitroglycerin may antagonize the effects of heparin

PART 3 Drugs

and should be administered via a separate line if possible. Digoxin, nicotine, propranolol, antihistamines, and tetracycline may reduce heparin's effects.

Bleeding and heparin overdosage may be treated with protamine sulfate. 1 mg protamine neutralizes 100 units heparin.

Anesthetic Considerations

Regional anesthesia is contraindicated. Heparin continuous I.V. infusion should be discontinued 4 to 6 hr preoperatively and aPTT checked to ensure return to baseline.

Name

Hetastarch (Hespan)

Classification

Plasma expander

Indications

Adjunct for plasma volume expansion in shock due to hemorrhage, burns, sepsis, surgery, or other trauma.

Dose

Plasma volume expansion from 500 to 1000 mL. Total dosage does not usually exceed 1500 mL/day (20 mL/kg/day). In acute hemorrhagic shock, rates approaching 20 mL/kg/hr have been used. Dosage forms: 6% solution in 0.9% sodium chloride, 500-mL I.V. infusion bottle.

Onset and Duration

Onset: 15 to 30 min. Duration: 24 to 48 hr. Average $t_{1/2}$: 17 days.

Adverse Effects

Anaphylactic reactions (periorbital edema, urticaria, wheezing) have been reported. Peripheral edema of the lower extremities, chills, mild temperature elevation, muscle pain. Large volumes may alter coagulation times and result in transient prolongation of prothrombin time, partial thromboplastin time, bleeding, decreased hematocrit, excessive dilution of plasma proteins.

Precautions and Contraindications

Contraindicated in patients with severe bleeding disorders, severe cardiac failure, renal failure with oliguria or anuria. Hetastarch does not have oxygen carrying capacity, nor does it contain plasma proteins such as coagulation factors. Therefore it is not a substitute for blood or plasma.

Anesthetic Considerations

Infuse slowly to avoid volume overload. Check coagulation profile.

Name

Hyaluronidase (Wydase)

Classification

Enzyme

Indications

Adjunct to increase absorption and dispersion of other injected drugs; hypodermoclysis; subcutaneous urography

Dose

Adjunct: 150 units to injection medium containing other medication. Hypodermoclysis (adults and children greater than 3 yr of age): 150 units injected SQ before clysis or injected into clysis tubing near needle for each 1000-mL clysis solution. Subcutaneous urography (patient prone): 75 units SQ over each scapula, followed by injection of contrast medium at same sites.

Onset and Duration

Onset: immediate. Duration: 30 to 60 min.

Adverse Effects

Rash, urticaria, local irritation

Precautions and Contraindications

Use with caution in patients with blood-clotting abnormalities or severe hepatic or renal disease. Avoid injecting into diseased areas in order to prevent spread of infection.

Anesthetic Considerations

Useful to prevent thrombus formation during vascular procedures as well as volumbe expansion.

Name

Hydralazine (Apresoline)

Classification

Direct-acting arterial vasodilator

Indications

Antihypertensive; treatment of congestive heart failure

Dose

I.V. and I.M.: 2.5 to 40 mg (0.1 to 0.2 mg/kg); P.O.: 10 to 100 mg q.i.d. Dosage forms: Injection: 20 mg/mL; Tablets: 10, 25, 50, and 100 mg

Onset and Duration

Onset: I.V.: 5 to 20 min; I.M.: 10 to 30 min; P.O.: 30 to 120 min. Duration: I.V.: 2 to 4 hr; I.M./P.O.: 2 to 8 hr.

Adverse Effects

Hypotension, paradoxical pressor response, tachycardia, palpitations, angina, dyspnea, nasal congestion, peripheral neuritis, depression,

PART 3 Drugs

anxiety, headache, dizziness, nausea, vomiting, diarrhea, lupus-like syndrome, rash, urticaria, eosinophilia, hypersensitivity, leukopenia, splenomegaly, agranulocytosis

Precautions and Contraindications

Use cautiously in patients with coronary artery disease, mitral valvular rheumatic heart disease, and patients receiving monoamine oxidase inhibitors.

Anesthetic Considerations

May see reduced response to epinephrine. Enhanced hypotensive effects in patients receiving diuretics, monoamine oxidase inhibitors, diazoxide, and other antihypertensives.

Name

Hydrocortisone sodium succinate (A-Hydrocort, Solu-Cortef)

Classification

Corticosteroid (glucocorticoid and mineralocorticoid properties)

Indications

Treatment of choice for steroid-replacement therapy. Also used as anti-inflammatory and immunosuppressive; however, glucocorticoids (prednisone) are preferred for this use. Adjunctive therapy in anaphylaxis to prevent prolonged antigen-antibody reactions. Adjunctive treatment of ulcerative colitis (enema).

Dose

Adults: Shock: 500 mg to 2 g (succinate) I.V. every 2 to 6 hr until condition stabilized. Not recommended beyond 48 to 72 hr. Adjunctive therapy in anaphylaxis: hydrocortisone phosphate or succinate I.V. 5 mg/kg initially, then 2.5 mg/kg every 6 hr. Adrenal insufficiency: acute adrenal insufficiency—precipitated trauma or surgical stress: If adrenocorticotropic hormone testing is not being performed, 200 to 300 mg I.V. hydrocortisone succinate over several minutes, then 100 mg I.V. every 6 hr for 24 hr. If the patient is stable, dosage tapering may begin on the second day. Consider steroid replacement in any patient who has received corticosteroid therapy for at least 1 month in the past 6 to 12 months, with 50 to 100 mg I.V. (succinate) before, during, and after surgery. For intraarticular, soft tissue, and intrasynovial injections, use acetate only (acetate is not for I.V. use) 10 to 50 mg combined with local anesthetic such as procaine. Injections may be repeated every 3 to 5 days (for bursae) to once every 1 to 4 weeks (for joints). Children: 0.16 to 1 mg/kg or 6 to 30 mg/m^2 (phosphate or succinate) I.M. or I.V. 1 or 2 times daily. Dose depends on the disease being treated.

Onset and Duration

Onset: I.V. or I.M.: 5 min. Duration: approximates duration of hypothalamus-pituitary-adrenal axis suppression (i.e., 30 to 36 hr); after a single oral dose of hydrocortisone this is 1.25 to 1.5 days. Elimination: Plasma $t_{1/2}$: 1.5 hr.

Adverse Effects

Glaucoma and cataracts with long-term therapy. Muscle weakness, sodium retention, edema, hypokalemic alkalosis, hyperglycemia, Cushing's syndrome, peptic ulcer, increased appetite, delayed wound healing, psychotic behavior, congestive heart failure, hypertension, growth suppression, pancreatitis.

Acute adrenal insufficiency may occur with abrupt withdrawal after long-term therapy. Withdrawal symptoms include rebound inflammation, fatigue, weakness, arthralgia, fever, dizziness, lethargy, depression, orthostatic hypotension, dyspnea, anorexia, hypoglycemia.

Precautions and Contraindications

Contraindicated in systemic fungal infections. May mask or exacerbate infections. Use with caution in patients with ocular herpes simplex or history of peptic ulcer disease. In patients with myasthenia gravis, hydrocortisone interacts with anticholinesterase agents to produce severe weakness.

Anesthetic Considerations

Barbiturates may increase glucocorticoid metabolism, and a hydrocortisone dosage increase may be indicated.

Hypotension from stress of anesthesia and surgery may occur if regular doses of steroids were taken within 2 months preceding surgery. Supplemental steroids are indicated commencing with preoperative dose and continuing for 3 days if major surgery, for 24 hours if minor surgery, and 1 dose for a very brief procedure, then taper to normal therapy.

Owing to adrenal suppression, etomidate should be avoided in patients with adrenal insufficiency.

Name

Ibutilide Fumarate (Corvert)

Classification

Class III antiarrhythmic; cardiac action potential prolongation

Indications

Rapid conversion of atrial fibrillation/flutter of acute onset (less than 90 days) to sinus rhythm.

Dose

Adults greater than 60 kg: 1 vial (1 mg) infused over 10 min (may be repeated once in 10 min after completion of first dose). Adults less than 60 kg: 0.01 mL/kg infused over 10 min (may be repeated once in 10 min after completion of first dose). Not recommended for pediatric patients.

Onset and Duration

Onset: For antiarrhythmic properties given I.V. and immediate. The drug peaks in 10 min. $t_{1/2}$ is 6 hr. Atrial arrhythmias usually convert within 30 min after ibutilide therapy begins. Duration: 10 to 30 min.

Adverse Effects

Ventricular arrhythmias (often sustained torsades de pointes), heart block, CHF, bradycardia, tachycardia, hypotension, nausea, headache

Precautions and Contraindications

Contraindicated with patients sensitive to ibutilide, second- or third-degree A-V heart blocks, prolonged Q-T interval, and during pregnancy.

Anesthetic Considerations

Increased risk of proarrhythmias/polymorphic ventricular tachycardia when ibutilide is used with other drugs that prolong Q-T interval (phenothiazines, procainamide, quinidine, antihistamines). Mandatory ECG monitoring for 4 hr post-drug therapy since arrhythmias (PVCs, VT, tachycardia, bradycardia, varying degrees of heart blocks) can take place. Have emergency equipment available to perform overdrive pacing, defibrillate, or cardiovert the patient. Monitor serum potassium and magnesium since deficiencies in these electrolytes can precipitate polymorphic ventricular tachycardia.

Name

Insulin regular (rapid-acting) (Humulin R, Novolin R, Regular Iletin II)

Classification

Antidiabetic agent

Indications

Diabetic ketoacidosis, treatment of diabetes mellitus, hyperkalemia

Dose

Diabetes mellitus: in general therapy is initiated with regular insulin SQ 5 to 10 units in adults and 2 to 4 units in children 15 to 30 min before meals and at bedtime. Dose and frequency are carefully individualized, based on every 4 to 6 hr blood sugar monitoring. After satisfactory control is achieved, an intermediate form of insulin may be substituted; this is given before breakfast in a dose approximately two thirds to three fourths that of the previous total daily dose established for regular insulin.

Perioperative management of insulin-dependent diabetics: half the usual NPH-isophane insulin dose the morning of the day of surgery. It is critical for the patient who is receiving nothing orally and receiving insulin also to receive an I.V. infusion of dextrose 5 to 10 g/hr (equal to 100 to 200 mL of a 5% dextrose solution) to prevent hypoglycemia.

Postoperative: sliding scale every 4 to 6 hr. Individualize to patient.

Blood Sugar	Insulin Regular
less than 200 mg/dL	0 units
200 to 250 mg/dL	5 units SQ
250 to 300 mg/dL	10 units SQ
300 to 350 mg/dL	15 units SQ

If blood sugar is greater than 350 mg/dL, give Insulin regular 15 units SQ plus I.V. 1 to 2 units/hr. Monitor blood glucose hourly. Correct electrolyte imbalances (hypokalemia, hypophosphatemia) and acidosis.

Diabetic ketoacidosis: requires insulin by continuous infusion, hourly blood sugar determination, and correction of acidosis, dehydration, and electrolyte imbalances. After renal function is established, potassium replacement therapy may be needed.

Dosage form: Injection: 100 units/mL. U500 Insulin (500 units/mL) is available but should be used only to fill implanted insulin pumps. It should never be stocked outside the pharmacy.

Onset and Duration

	Onset (hr)	Peak (hr)	Duration (hr)
Regular (rapid) insulin	0.5 to 1	1 to 5	5 to 8
Intermediate insulins	1 to 4	4 to 12	24 to 28

Onset: $t_{1/2}$ regular insulin: 4 to 5 min I.V.

Adverse Effects

Dose-related hypoglycemia. Local allergic reactions, lipoatrophy, and resistance may be overcome by switching to more highly purified sources. In general, human insulin is least antigenic and pork is less antigenic than beef–pork or pure beef. Anaphylaxis. Hyperglycemia (rebound or Somogyi effect).

Precautions and Contraindications

Diabetic ketoacidosis is a life-threatening condition requiring prompt diagnosis and treatment.

Change in purity, strength, brand, type, or species source may result in the need for a change in dosage.

Treat hypoglycemia with 0.6 mL/kg 50% dextrose I.V.

Hypersensitivity may occur.

Insulin requirements may increase dramatically with stress, sepsis, trauma, or pregnancy.

Only Regular Insulins (clear insulins) may be administered through I.V. Intermediate insulins may only be given SQ.

Hypoglycemic action increased by concomitant administration of alcohol, β-blockers, monoamine oxidase inhibitors, salicylates, sulfonyl ureas.

Hypoglycemic action decreased by thyroid hormones, corticosteroids, dobutamine, epinephrine, furosemide, phenytoin.

Anesthetic Considerations

Blood sugar levels of 120 to 180 mg/dL should be sought and blood

PART 3 Drugs

sugar should be monitored frequently intraoperatively. If it is necessary to administer insulin intraoperatively, continuous I.V. infusion may be the best method. If given subcutaneously, variability of skin blood flow during anesthesia may cause unpredictable results.

Large I.V. boluses of insulin can put the patient at risk for dysrhythmias caused by intracellular shifts of potassium, phosphorus, and magnesium.

Name

Ipratropium Bromide (Atrovent, Itrop)

Classification

Anticholinergic, bronchodilator (parasympatholytic) preventing build-up of cyclic guanosine monophosphate (cyclic GMP)

Indications

Treatment and prevention of bronchospasm due to Chronic obstructive pulmonary disease (COPD), including emphysema and chronic bronchitis

Dose

Metered dose inhaler:
Adults: 2 to 4 sprays (initially, 18 g/spray), then 2 sprays every 4 hr. (maximum dose: 216 g or 12 sprays/day).
Currently not recommended for children under 12 years.
Oral nebulizer:
Adults: 500 g w/2.5 cc NS mixed via oral nebulization every 6 to 8 hr. May mix with albuterol in nebulizer if used within 1 hr of mixing.

Onset and Duration

Onset: within 15 to 30 min. Peak: 1 to 2 hr. Duration: 4 to 5 hr.

Adverse Effects:

Includes local or systemic anticholinergic effects, angina, blurred vision, headache, dizziness. May exacerbate bronchospasm.

Precautions and Contraindications

Use cautiously for patients with narrow-angle glaucoma, bladder obstruction, and benign prostatic hypertrophy. Classified as a pregnancy category B drug (well-controlled studies have not been conducted in pregnancy). Contraindicated in patients hypersensitive to soya lecithin or related food products such as soybean and peanut. Also contraindicated in patients hypersensitive to ipratropium bromide, atropine and its derivatives.

Pediatric safety and effectiveness not established below the age of 12 years.

Anesthetic Considerations

Do not use for relief of bronchospasm in acute COPD exacerbation as first-line drug. Use drugs with faster onset.

Name
Isoflurane (Forane)

Classification
Inhalation anesthetic

Indications
General anesthesia

Dose
Titrate to effect for induction or maintenance of anesthesia. Minimum alveolar concentration (MAC): 1.14%. Dosage form: volatile liquid: 100 mL.

Onset and Duration
Onset: few minutes, dose-dependent. Duration: emergence time: 15 min.

Adverse Effects
Hypotension, tachycardia, arrhythmia, coronary-artery steal, respiratory depression, apnea, dizziness, euphoria, increased cerebral blood flow and intracranial pressure, nausea, vomiting, ileus, hepatic dysfunction, malignant hyperthermia, glucose elevation

Precautions and Contraindications
Contraindicated in patients with known or suspected genetic susceptibility to malignant hyperthermia. Changes in mental function may persist beyond the period of anesthetic administration and the immediate postoperative period.

Anesthetic Considerations
Anesthetic requirements decrease with age. Crosses the placental barrier. Abrupt onset of malignant hyperthermia may be triggered by isoflurane; early signs include muscle rigidity, especially of the jaw muscles, tachycardia and tachypnea unresponsive to increased depth of anesthesia caused by digitalis intoxication. Arrhythmias with concomitant use of volatile anesthetics and other sympathomimetics.

Name
Isoproterenol HCl (Isuprel)

Classification
Synthetic sympathomimetic, almost exclusively β

Dose
I.M./SQ: 0.2 mg; I.V.: 0.02 to 0.06 mg; Infusion: 2 to 20 μg/min; Sublingual: 10 mg; 10 to 50 mg p.r.n.

Onset and Duration
Onset: I.V.: immediately; sublingual: 15 to 30 min. Duration: I.V.: 1 to 5 min; sublingual: 1 to 2 hr.

Adverse Effects

Tachyarrhythmias, hypertension, angina, paradoxical precipitation of Adams-Stokes attacks, pulmonary edema, headache, dizziness, tremors, nausea, vomiting, anorexia; may exacerbate ischemia and/or hypertension when used for chronotropic support.

Precautions and Contraindications

In patients with tachyarrhythmias, tachycardia, or heart block

Anesthetic Considerations

Useful as I.V. infusion for the treatment of refractory bradycardic states. Bronchodilating effect is better achieved with more specific β_2 agonists.

Name

Ketamine HCl (Ketalar)

Classification

Central nervous system agent; general anesthetic

Indications

Sole anesthetic agent for diagnostic and surgical procedures for short duration. Induction of anesthesia before administration of other general anesthetics.

Dose

Induction: Adult: I.V.: 1 to 4.5 mg/kg slowly over 60 sec. I.M.: 6 to 12 mg/kg. Half of initial dose may be repeated as needed. Dosage form: Injection: 10, 50, 100 mg/mL.

Onset and Duration

Onset: I.V.: 30 sec; I. M. 3 to 8 min. Duration: I. V.: 5 to 10 min.; I. M.: 12 to 25 min.

Adverse Effects

Hypertension, tachycardia, hypotension, arrhythmia, bradycardia, respiratory depression, apnea, laryngospasm, tonic or clonic movements, emergence delirium, hypersalivation, nausea, vomiting, diplopia, nystagmus, slight elevation in intraocular tension. Serious emergence reactions.

Precautions and Contraindications

Contraindicated in hypertension, coronary heart disease or cardiac hypertension, increased intracranial pressure, history of cerebrovascular accident, increased intraocular pressure, psychiatric disorders. Contraindicated for surgery or diagnostic procedures of pharynx, larynx, and bronchial tree. Safe use during pregnancy, including obstetrics, is not established. Cautious use in convulsive disorders.

Anesthetic Considerations

Do not mix with barbiturates in same syringe. Emergence reactions are common in adults with high doses and are reduced by premedication with

benzodiazepine. Catecholamine-depleted patients may respond to ketamine with unexpected reductions in blood pressure and cardiac output.

Name

Ketorolac tromethamine (Toradol)

Classification

Nonsteroidal anti-inflammatory

Indications

Short-term (less than 5 days) management of moderately severe, acute
pain that requires analgesia. Generally used in a postoperative setting.
Patients should be switched to alternative analgesics as soon as possible. Ketorolac therapy is not to exceed 5 days because of the potential
for increased frequency and severity of adverse reactions. The combined duration of use of Ketorolac I.V./I.M. and P.O. is not to exceed
5 days. Ketorolac P.O. is indicated only as continuation therapy to
Ketorolac I.V./I.M.

Dose

I.M. (give slowly and deeply into the muscle): Patients less than 65 yr:
One dose of 60 mg; Patients greater than 65 yr, renal-impaired, and/or
less than 50 kg: One dose of 30 mg.

I.V. (I.V. bolus over no less than 15 sec): Patients less than 65 yr:
One dose of 30 mg; Patients greater than 65 yr, renalimpaired, and/or
less than 50 kg: One dose of 15 mg.

Multipledose treatment (I.V. or SQ): Patients less than 65 yr:
30 mg every 6 hr, not to exceed 120 mg per day;

Patients greater than 65 yr, renal-impaired, and/or less than 50:
15 mg every 6 hr, not to exceed 60 mg per day.

Onset and Duration

Onset: I.V. or I. M.: 30 min with maximum effect in 1 to 2 hr. Duration:
4 to 6 hr.

Adverse Effects

Gastrointestinal: peptic ulcers, gastrointestinal bleeding, and/or perforation. Renal: ketorolac and its metabolites are eliminated primarily by
the kidneys, which, in patients with reduced creatinine clearance, will
result in diminished clearance of the drug. Renal toxicity with ketorolac has been seen in patients with conditions leading to a reduction in
blood volume and/or renal blood flow, where renal prostaglandins
have a supportive role in the maintenance of renal perfusion. In these
patients, administration of ketorolac may cause a dose-dependent
reduction in renal prostaglandin formation and may precipitate acute
renal failure. Risk of bleeding: ketorolac inhibits platelet function.
Hypersensitivity reactions ranging from bronchospasm to anaphylactic shock have occurred, and appropriate counteractive measures must
be available when administering the first dose.

Precautions and Contraindications

Fluid retention, edema, retention of sodium, oliguria, elevations of serum urea nitrogen and creatinine have been reported. Therefore ketorolac should be used only with caution in patients with cardiac decompensation, hypertension, or similar conditions. Ketorolac is contraindicated in patients with active peptic ulcer disease, recent gastrointestinal bleeding or perforation, or in patients with a history of peptic ulcer disease or gastrointestinal bleeding. Ketorolac is also contraindicated in patients with advanced renal impairment and in patients at risk for renal failure due to volume depletion. It is contraindicated in patients with suspected or confirmed cerebrovascular bleeding, patients with hemorrhagic diathesis, incomplete hemostasis, and those with a high risk of bleeding. It is contraindicated as a prophylactic analgesic before any major surgery and is contraindicated intraoperatively when hemostasis is critical. Ketorolac is also contraindicated in patients with previously demonstrated hypersensitivity to ketorolac tromethamine or allergic manifestations to aspirin (ASA) or other nonsteroidal anti-inflammatory drugs (NSAIDs). It is contraindicated for patients currently receiving ASA or NSAIDs because of the cumulative risk of inducing serious NSAID-related side effects. Ketorolac is contraindicated for intrathecal or epidural administration owing to its alcohol content. It is contraindicated in labor and delivery because it may adversely affect fetal circulation and inhibit uterine contractions. Because of the potential adverse effects of prostaglandin-inhibiting drugs on neonates, ketorolac is contraindicated in nursing mothers.

Anesthetic Considerations

Do not use as prophylactic analgesia before any major surgery or intraoperatively when hemostasis is critical; in patients with suspected or confirmed cerebrovascular bleeding, hemorrhagic diathesis, incomplete hemostasis, and at high risk of bleeding; in patients currently receiving ASA or NSAIDs; for epidural or intrathecal administration; or concomitantly with probenecid.

Use of ketorolac is not recommended in children.

Ketorolac reduced the diuretic response to furosemide in normovolemic healthy subjects by approximately 20%. Hypovolemia should be corrected before treatment with ketorolac is initiated. Ketorolac possesses no sedative or anxiolytic properties. Concomitant use with opiate-agonist analgesics can result in reduced opiate analgesic requirements. Ketorolac is highly bound to human plasma protein (99.2%).

Name

Labetalol (Normodyne, Trandate)

Classification

Adrenergic antagonist

Indications

Hypertension

Dose

I.V. bolus: 0.15 to 0.25 mg/kg given over 2 min, may repeat every 10 min up to 300 mg. Continuous infusion: 2 mg/min; Titrate to effect P.O.: 100 mg b.i.d. alone or with diuretic. May increase to 200 mg b.i.d. after 2 days. Further dose increase may be made every 1 to 3 days to maximal response. Maintenance dose: 200 to 400 mg b.i.d.

Onset and Duration

Onset: I.V.: 1 to 3 min; P.O.: 20 to 40 min. Duration: I.V.: 0.25 to 2 hr; P.O.: 4 to 12 hr.

Adverse Effects

Hypotension, bradycardia, ventricular arrhythmias, congestive heart failure, chest pain, bronchospasm, headache, diarrhea, systemic lupus erythematosus

Precautions and Contraindications

Cautious use in chronic bronchitis, emphysema, preexisting peripheral vascular disease, pheochromocytoma, and diabetes. Contraindicated in bronchial asthma, overt heart failure, greater than first-degree heart block, and hepatic failure.

Anesthetic Considerations

Inhalation anesthetics may enhance hypotensive effects.

Name

Lansoprazole (Prevacid)

Classification

Proton pump inhibitor

Indications

Ulcers and acid reflux

Dose

P.O.: 15 to 60 mg q.d. before meals

Onset and Duration

Onset: within 1 hr. Maximum effect: at 2 hr. Duration; greater than 24 hr.

Adverse Effects

Abdominal pain, nausea, diarrhea

Precautions and Contraindications

Slows gastric emptying of solids. Reduce doses in hepatic disease. Safety and effectiveness not established for patients less than 18 years of age. Contraindicated for patients hypersensitive to lansoprazole or similar proton pump inhibitors.

Anesthetic Considerations

Highly protein bound. Undergoes liver elimination.

Name

Levobupivacaine (Chirocaine)

Classification

Amide-type local anesthetic

Indications

Regional anesthesia

Dose

For infiltration/peripheral nerve block: 0.25%, 0.5%, 0.75%. Dosing similar to bupivacaine.

Onset and Duration

Onset: infiltration: 2 to 10 min; epidural: 4 to 7 min; spinal: less than 1 min. Peak effect: Infiltration and epidural: 30 to 45 mn; spinal: 15 min. Duration: Infiltration/spinal/epidural: 200 to 400 min (prolonged with epinephrine).

Adverse Effects

Hypotension, arrhythmias, cardiac arrest, respiratory impairment, arrest, seizures, tinnitus, blurred vision, urticaria, anaphylactoid symptoms. High spinal: urinary retention, lower extremity weakness and paralysis, loss of sphincter control, backache, palsies, slowing of labor.

Precautions and Contraindications

Use with caution in patients with hypovolemia, severe congestive heart failure, shock, and all forms of heart block. Contraindicated in patients with hypersensitivity to amide-type local anesthetics.

Anesthetic Considerations

I.V. access is essential during major regional block. Toxic plasma levels of bupivacaine may cause seizures and cardiopulmonary collapse.

Name

Lidocaine HCl (Xylocaine, Xylocaine jelly, Xylocaine viscous oral solution)

Classification

Amide-type local anesthetic; topical anesthetic; antiarrhythmic agent

Indications

Regional anesthesia, topical anesthesia, treatment of ventricular arrhythmias, attenuation of sympathetic response to laryngoscopy/intubation

Dose

Caudal or epidural: 20 to 30 mL 1% solution (200 to 300 mg); may also use 1.5% and 2.0% solutions. (Maximum dose: 200 to 300 mg/hr [4.5 mg/kg].) With epinephrine for anesthesia other than spinal, maximum safe dose is 500 mg (7 mg/kg.)

Spinal: 1.5 to 2 mL 5% solution with 7.5% dextrose (75 to 100 mg).

Antiarrhythmic: Slow I.V. bolus: 1 mg/kg (1% to 2% solution) followed by 0.5 mg/kg every 2 to 5 min (to maximum dose of 3 mg/kg/hr); Infusion (0.1% solution): 1 to 4 mg/min (20 to 50 μg/kg/min). Use only preservative-free forms for I.V.

Local anesthesia: Topical: 0.6 to 3 mg/kg (2% to 4% solution); infiltration/peripheral nerve block: 0.5 to 5 mg/kg (0.5% to 2% solution); transtracheal: 80 to 120 mg (2 to 3 mL of 4% solution); superior laryngeal nerve: 40 to 60 mg (2 to 3 mL of 2% solution on each side); stellate ganglion: 50 mg (5 mL of 1% solution); I.V. (regional): upper extremity: 200 to 250 mg (40 to 50 mL of 0.5% solution), lower extremity: 250 to 300 mg (100 to 120 mL of 0.25% solution).

Onset and Duration

Onset: I.V. (antiarrhythmic effects): 45 to 90 sec; infiltration: 0.5 to 1 min; epidural: 5 to 15 min. Peak effects: I.V. (antiarrhythmic effects): 1 to 2 min; infiltration and epidural: less than 30 min. Duration: I.V. (antiarrhythmic effects): 10 to 20 min; Infiltration: 0.5 to 1 hr, with epinephrine: 2 to 6 hr; epidural: 1 to 3 hr (prolonged with epinephrine).

Adverse Effects

Hypotension, bradycardia, arrhythmias, heart block, respiratory depression, arrest, anxiety, tinnitus, seizures, postspinal headache, palsies, urticaria, pruritus. High spinal: loss of bladder and bowel control, permanent motor, sensory autonomic (sphincter control), deficit of lower segments.

Precautions and Contraindications

Use with caution in patients with hypovolemia, severe congestive heart failure, shock, all forms of heart block, pregnancy. Contraindicated in patients with hypersensitivity to amide-type local anesthetics, supraventricular arrhythmias.

Anesthetic Considerations

Dosage should be reduced for elderly, debilitated, acutely ill patients. Anesthetic solutions containing epinephrine should be used with caution in peripheral or hypertensive vascular disease. Benzodiazepines increase seizure threshold. Do not use preparations containing preservatives for spinal or epidural anesthesia or for I.V. administration. Do not inject solutions containing epinephrine I.V.

Name

Lorazepam (Ativan)

Classification

Benzodiazepine; antianxiety agent; hypnotic; sedative

Indications

Premedication; induction agent; amnesia; temporary relief of insomnia

Dose

I.V., deep I.M.: 1 to 2 mg (0.05 mg/kg) (maximum dose: 4 mg). Dilute with equal volume D_5W or normal saline solution. P.O.: 1 to 2 mg, 2 to 3 times/day.

Preoperative medication: 0.05 mg/kg 2 hr before procedure (maximum dosage: 4 mg).

Dosage forms: Tablets: 0.5, 1, 2 mg; injection: 2 mg/mL, 4 mg/mL.

Onset and Duration

Onset: I.V.: 1 to 5 min; I.M.: 15 to 30 min; P.O.: 1 to 6 hr. Duration: 6 to 24 hr. Eliminaton $t_{1/2}$: 10 to 15 hr. Metabolized to inactive compounds.

Adverse Effects

Hypotension, hypertension, bradycardia, tachycardia, respiratory depression, dizziness, weakness, depression, agitation, amnesia, hysteria, urticaria, visual disturbances, blurred vision, diplopia, nausea, vomiting, abdominal discomfort, anorexia

Precautions and Contraindications

Intraarterial injection may cause arteriospasm; treat with local infiltration of phentolamine (5 to 20 mg in 10 mL normal saline). Use with caution in elderly and debilitated patients. Contraindicated for patients with known hypersensitivity to benzodiazepines and narrow-angle glaucoma.

Anesthetic Considerations

Unexpected hypotension and respiratory depression may occur when combined with opioids. Use with caution in elderly patients and patients with limited pulmonary reserve. Not for use in children less than 12 years old. Treat overdose with flumazenil. Decreased requirements for volatile anesthetics.

Name

Magnesium sulfate

Classification

Replacement agents; anticonvulsant

Indications

Prevention and control of seizures in toxemia/eclampsia of pregnancy, epilepsy, nephritis, and hypomagnesemia; treatment of acute magnesium deficiency; tocolytic therapy; adjunctive therapy of acute myocardial infarction, torsades de pointes ventricular tachycardia, and hypokalemiarelated arrhythmias; laxative

Dose

Preeclampsia/eclampsia: I.V.: 4 g in 250 mL D_5W or NS infused slowly, followed by 2 to 3 g/hr by continuous infusion. Blood level should not exceed 7 mEq/L. Hypomagnesemic seizures: Mild: 1 g given I.V./I.M. every 6 hr for 4 doses. Total parenteral nutrition: I.V.: 8 to 24 mEq/day.

Onset and Duration

Onset: I.V.: immediate; I.M.: less than 1 hr; P.O.: 1 to 2 hr. Peak effects: I.V.: few minutes; I.M.: 1 to 3 hr. Duration: I.V.: 30 min; I.M.: 3 to 4 hr.

Adverse Effects

Hypotension, circulatory collapse, heart block, respiratory paralysis, flaccid paralysis, depressed reflexes, hypocalcemia, flushing, sweating, hypothermia

Precautions and Contraindications

Not for use in patients with heart block or extensive myocardial damage. Use with caution in patients with impaired renal function, in digitalized patients, and with concomitant use of other central nervous system depressants or neuromuscular blocking agents. I.V. administration contraindicated during the 2 hr preceding delivery. P.O. administration contraindicated in patients with abdominal pain, nausea, vomiting, fecal impaction, or intestinal irritation, obstruction, or perforation.

Anesthetic Considerations

Magnesium sulfate potentiates both depolarizing and nondepolarizing muscle relaxants. Periodic monitoring of serum magnesium concentrations is essential during magnesium therapy. Maintain urine output at a minimum of 100 mL every 4 hours. Monitor deep tendon reflexes during magnesium therapy. Stop therapy as soon as desired effect is reached. Monitor respiratory function.

Name

Mannitol (Osmitrol, Resectisol irrigation)

Classification

Osmotic diuretic

Indications

Reduction of intracranial pressure and intraocular pressure; protection of renal function during periods of hypoperfusion (shock, burn, open-heart surgery, kidney transplants, abdominal aortic aneurysm repair); transurethral prostate resection (TURP) irrigation (minimizes hemolytic effects of water and promotes rapid excretion of absorbed irrigants)

Dose

Adults: Reduction of intracranial/intraocular pressure: 1.5 to 2 g/kg of 15% to 25% solution over 30 to 60 min. When used preoperatively, give 1 to 1.5 hr preoperatively for maximum pressure reduction. Test dose: Marked oliguria or suspected inadequate renal function: 0.2 g/kg or 12.5 g over 3 to 5 min. If satisfactory response not obtained, may repeat. If response still not obtained, *do not use mannitol.* Prevention of oliguric renal failure: 50 to 100 g I.V. over 2 hr. TURP: 2.5% to 5% irrigation instilled into bladder.

Children: 2 g/kg or 60 g/m2 as 15% to 20% solution over 2 to 6 hr to treat edema and ascites; over 30 to 60 min to treat cerebral or ocular edema. Dosage forms: Parenteral injection: 5%, 10%, 15%, 20%, 25%. Urogenital irrigation solution: 2.5% to 5%.

Onset and Duration

Onset: Diuresis in 1 to 3 hr; reduction of intracranial and intraocular pressure in 15 to 30 min. Duration: 3 to 8 hr.

Adverse Effects

Most serious are fluid imbalance and electrolyte loss. Less serious are pulmonary edema, hypertension, water intoxication, congestive heart failure, and skin necrosis with extravasation.

Precautions and Contraindications

Monitor serum osmolarity and electrolytes closely. Discontinue mannitol if there is low urine output. Mannitol may crystallize at low temperatures. Do not use a solution containing crystals—resolubilize in hot water with periodic shaking. Use of mannitol is contraindicated in patients with pulmonary edema, congestive heart failure, severe dehydration, impaired renal function not responsive to test dose, edema associated with capillary fragility, or acute intracranial bleeding (except during craniotomy).

Anesthetic Considerations

Mannitol disrupts the blood-brain barrier, enhancing penetration of other drugs into the central nervous system.

Name

Meperidine HCl (Demerol)

Classification

Synthetic opioid agonist

Indications

Analgesia

Dose

I.V./I.M.: 25 to 100 mg; I.V.: infusion 1 to 20 mg/hr for short duration, then titrate to patient's need.

Onset and Duration

Onset: P.O.: 1 to 45 min; I.M.: 1 to 5 min. Duration: P.O./I.V./I.M.: 2 to 4 hr.

Adverse Effects

Hypotension, cardiac arrest, respiratory depression or arrest, laryngospasm, euphoria, dysphoria, sedation, seizures, psychic dependence, constipation, biliary tract spasm, chest-wall rigidity, urticaria, pruritus

Precautions and Contraindications

Reduce the dose in elderly, hypovolemic, high-risk surgical patients, and with concomitant use of sedatives and other narcotics. Severe and occasionally fatal reactions can occur in patients who are receiving or have just received monoamine oxidase inhibitors; treat these patients with hydrocortisone. Not for long-term use. The toxic metabolite of meperidine HCl (normeperidine) is very hazardous, especially in the elderly.

Use with caution in patients with asthma, chronic obstructive pulmonary disease, increased intracranial pressure, or supraventricular tachycardia.

Meperidine crosses the placental barrier. Use during labor may produce depression of respiration in the neonate. If used resuscitation of the neonate may be required; therefore have naloxone available.

Cerebral irritation and seizures can occur when used in large doses. Meperidine potentiates the central nervous system and cardiovascular depression of narcotics, sedative-hypnotics, volatile anesthetics, and tricyclic antidepressants. There is a severe and sometimes fatal reaction with monoamine oxidase inhibitors. Analgesia is enhanced by α_2 agonists. Meperidine aggravates adverse effects of isoniazid. It is chemically incompatible with barbiturates.

Anesthetic Considerations

Use with caution when administering halothane because of increased arrhythmogenic potential.

Name

Mephentermine sulfate (Wyamine sulfate)

Classification

Synthetic noncatecholamine that stimulates α- and β- receptors, both directly and indirectly

Indications

Hypotension

Dose

I.V./I.M.: 10 to 45 mg (0.4 mg/kg); Infusion: 0.25 to 5 mg/min.

Onset and Duration

Onset: I.V.: 1 to 5 min; I.M.: 5 to 15 min. Duration: I.V.: 15 to 30 min; I.M.: 1 to 2 hr.

Adverse Effects

Hypertension, arrhythmias, anxiety, seizures, euphoria, paranoid psychosis

Precautions and Contraindications

Use with caution in patients with severe hypertension or

hyperthyroidism. There is also an increased risk of arrhythmias with use of volatile agents. Mephenterminse sulfate may increase uterine contractions, especially during the third trimester of pregnancy. It is not recommended for use in pregnant women.

Anesthetic Considerations

Use with caution in patients receiving monoamine oxidase inhibitors or tricyclic antidepressants.

Name

Mepivacaine HCl (Carbocaine, Isocaine, Polocaine)

Classification

Amide-type local anesthetic

Indications

Regional anesthesia: infiltration, brachial plexus block, epidural, caudal

Dose

Infiltration: 50 to 400 mg (0.5% to 1.5% solution). Brachial plexus block: 300 to 400 mg (30 to 40 mL of 1% solution). Epidural: 150 to 400 mg (15 to 20 mL of 1% to 2% solution). Caudal: 150 to 400 mg (15 to 20 mL of 1% to 2% solution). Children: 0.4 to 0.7 mL/kg (maximum safe dosage: 7 mg/kg with epinephrine).

Onset and Duration

Onset: Infiltration: 3 to 5 min. Epidural: 5 to 15 min. Peak effects: Infiltration/epidural: 15 to 45 min. Duration: Infiltration: 0.75 to 1.5 hr, 2 to 6 hr with epinephrine; Epidural: 3 to 5 hr (prolonged with epinephrine).

Adverse Effects

Myocardial depression, arrhythmias, cardiac arrest, respiratory depression or arrest, anxiety, apprehension, tinnitus, seizures, loss of hearing, urticaria, pruritus. High spinal: loss of bladder and bowel control and permanent motor, sensory, and autonomic (sphincter control) deficit of lower segments.

Precautions and Contraindications

Use with caution in debilitated, elderly, or acutely ill patients, especially if there is severe disturbance in cardiac rhythm or heart block. Use with caution in pregnant patients. Mepiracaine is contraindicated in patients with hypersensitivity to amide-type local anesthetics.

Anesthetic Considerations

Do not use solutions with preservatives for caudal or epidural block. Mepivacaine is not for use as spinal or obstetric anesthesia. Blood concentration may be reduced by rifampin and withdrawal symptoms may occur. There may be a severe reaction with monoamine oxidase inhibitors, with withdrawal symptoms precipitated by pentazocine in heroin addicts on methadone therapy. Mepivacaine potentiates central nervous system and cardiovascular depressant effects of other narcotic analgesics, volatile anesthetics, phenothiazines, sedative hypnotics, alcohol, and tricyclic antidepressants. Analgesia is enhanced by α_2 agonists.

Name
Metaraminol bitartrate (Aramine)

Classification
Synthetic noncatecholamine

Indications
Hypertension; stimulates α- and β-receptors, both directly and indirectly

Dose
I.M./SQ: 2 to 10 mg; I.V.: 0.5 to 5 mg.

Onset and Duration
Onset: I.V.: 1 to 5 min; I.M./SQ: 5 to 15 min. Duration: I.V.: 10 to 15 min; I.M./SQ: 1 to 2 hr.

Adverse Effects
Apprehension, restlessness, dizziness, headache, tremor, weakness, seizures, hypertension, hypotension, precordial pain, palpitations, arrhythmias, bradycardia, premature ventricular contractions, atrioventricular dissociation, nausea, vomiting, decreased urine output, hyperglycemia, flushing, pallor, sweating

Precautions and Contraindications
Use with caution in patients with hypertension, thyroid disease, diabetes, or cirrhosis, or in those receiving digoxin. Contraindicated in patients with peripheral or mesenteric thrombosis, pulmonary edema, hypercarbia, or acidosis.

Anesthetic Considerations
Increased risk of adverse cardiac effects with the use of general anesthetics.

Name
Methadone HCl (Dolophine HCl)

Classification
Synthetic narcotic

Indications
Analgesia; opiate recovery program

Dose
Analgesia: SQ/I.M./P.O.: 2.5 to 10 mg (0.1 mg/kg) every 4 hr; Epidural bolus: 1 to 5 mg. Narcotic abstinence syndrome: P.O.: 20 to 120 mg/day.

Onset and Duration

Onset: I.V.: several minutes; I.M.: 3 to 60 min; P.O.: 30 to 60 min; Epidural: 5 to 10 min. Duration: I.V./I.M./P.O.: about 6 hr; Epidural: 6 to 10 hr.

Adverse Effects

Hypotension, circulatory depression, bradycardia, syncope, respiratory depression, euphoria, dysphoria, disorientation, urinary retention, biliary tract spasm, constipation, anorexia, rash, pruritus, urticaria

Precautions and Contraindications

Reduce dose in the elderly, hypovolemic, or high-risk surgical patient or with use of narcotics and sedative hypnotics.

Anesthetic Considerations

Do not give pentazocine to heroin addicts on methadone. Ineffective for relief of general anxiety. Use with caution in patients with asthma, chronic obstructive pulmonary disease, or increased intracranial pressure. Methadone can produce the drug effects of morphine.

Name

Methohexital sodium (Brevital sodium)

Classification

Ultra short-acting barbiturate

Indications

General anesthetic for short surgical procedures; induction of hypnosis; supplementation of other anesthetics

Dose

I.V.: Induction: 50 to 120 mg (average 70 mg), 1 to 1.5 mg/kg usual dose in adults. Dosage forms: Powder for injection: 500, 2.5, and 5.0 mg.

Onset and Duration

Onset: few seconds. Duration: 5 to 8 min.

Adverse Effects

Circulatory depression, thrombophlebitis, myocardial depression, cardiac arrhythmia, respiratory depression, central nervous system disturbances, seizures, nausea and vomiting, abdominal pain, rectal irritation (rectal administration), pain at injection site

Precautions and Contraindications

Use with caution in patients with severe cardiovascular disease, hypotension, shock, Addison's disease, hepatic or renal dysfunction, myxedema, increased intracranial pressure, asthma, or myasthenia gravis. Methohexital sodium 13 contraindicated in patients with variegate porphyria or acute intermittent porphyria or in those with hypersensitivity to barbiturates.

Anesthetic Considerations

Consider reducing the dose when used in conjunction with narcotics. Overdosage may occur from too rapid or repeated injections. Do not mix with atropine sulfate, tubocurarine, or succinylcholine. Methonhexial sodium is incompatible with silicone. Use only if clear and colorless. Methohexital sodium is not compatible with lactated Ringer's.

Name

Methoxamine HCl (Vasoxyl)

Classification

α-Receptor agonist

Indications

Hypotension

Dose

I.V.: 1 to 5 mg, given slowly; I.M.: 5 to 15 mg (0.25 mg/kg).

Onset and Duration

Onset: I.V.: almost immediately; I.M.: 15 to 20 min. Duration: I.V.: 15 to 60 min; I.M. 60 to 90 min.

Adverse Effects

Reflex bradycardia, hypertension, hypotension, respiratory difficulty, tremors, dizziness, seizures, cerebral hemorrhage, headache, projectile vomiting, desire to void

Precautions and Contraindications

Use with extreme caution in elderly patients and in patients with bradycardia, partial heart block, myocardial disease, or severe arteriosclerosis. Methoxamine contains sulfites and thus may cause allergic-type reactions.

Anesthetic Considerations

Infuse into large veins to prevent extravasation. Treat extravasation with local infiltration of phentolamine (5 to 10 mg in 10 mL normal saline solution) or with sympathetic block.

Name

Methylene blue (Urolene Blue)

Classification

Antidote; diagnostic agent

Indications

Treatment of idiopathic and drug-induced methemoglobinemia; dye effect for tissue staining; urinary antiseptic (oral route). Antidote to cyanide poisoning.

Dose

I.V.: 1 to 2 mg/kg (inject over several min); P.O.: 65 to 130 mg t.i.d. with water.

Onset and Duration

Onset: I.V.: almost immediate. Peak effects: I.V.: less than 1 hr. Duration: I.V./P.O.: varies.

Adverse Effects

Tachycardia, hypertension, precordial pain, cyanosis, confusion, headache, nausea, vomiting, diarrhea, abdominal pain, bladder irritation, hemolytic anemia, methemoglobinemia, hyperbilirubinemia, stains skin blue

Precautions and Contraindications

Safe use during pregnancy is not established. Methylene blue is contraindicated in patients with renal insufficiency, hypersensitivity to methylene blue, G6PD deficiency (hemolysis), or intraspinal injection.

Anesthetic Considerations

Causes discoloration of urine and feces. Inject slowly to prevent local high concentration from producing additional methemoglobinemia. Monitor intake, output, and hemoglobin.

Name

Methylergonovine (Methergine)

Classification

Oxytocic (ergot alkaloid); adrenergic antagonist; sympatholytic

Indications

Prevention and treatment of postpartum hemorrhage caused by uterine atony or subinvolution

Dose

I.M.: 0.2 mg every 2 to 5 hr (maximum 5 doses); I.V.: 0.2 mg/mL (over 1 min while monitoring blood pressure and uterine contractions); P.O.: 0.2 to 0.4 mg every 6 to 12 hr for 2 to 7 days.

Onset and Duration

Onset: I.V.: immediate; I.M.: 2 to 5 min; P.O.: 5 to 15 min. Peak effects: 3 hr. Duration: I.V.: 45 min; I.M.: 3 hr; P.O.: 3 or more hr.

Adverse Effects

Hypertension, chest pain, palpitations, dyspnea, headache, nausea, vomiting, tinnitus. High doses can produce signs of ergotism.

Precautions and Contraindications

Use with caution in patients with hypertension, sepsis, obliterative vascular disease, hepatic, renal, or cardiac disease. Methylergonivine

is contraindicated in patients with hypersensitivity to ergot preparations, in pregnant patients, and in those with toxemia or untreated
hypocalcemia.

Anesthetic Considerations

Monitor for hypertension or other adverse effects. Parenteral sympathomimetics or other ergot alkaloids add to pressor effect and may lead
to hypertension. I.V. administration is not routine, as it can produce
sudden hypertension and CVAs.

Name

Metoclopramide (Reglan)

Classification

Dopamine-receptor antagonist; antiemetic; stimulant of upper gastrointestinal motility

Indications

Diabetic and postsurgical gastric stasis; prevention of chemotherapy-
induced emesis; facilitation of small-bowel intubation; gastroesophageal reflux; prevention of postoperative nausea and vomiting

Dose

Adults: 10 mg I.V. slowly over 1 to 2 min as a single dose. May repeat
once. Children: 6 to 14 yr: I.V.: 2.5 to 5 mg; children under 6 yr:
0.1 mg/kg. Dosage forms: 5 mg/mL in 2 and 10 mL vials. P.O.: tablets:
5 mg and 10 mg; syrup: 5 mg/5 mL.

Onset and Duration

Onset: 1 to 3 min. Duration: 2 to 3 hr. Elimination $t_{1/2}$: 2.5 to 5 hr in
patients with normal renal function.

Adverse Effects

Anxiety, restlessness, mental depression, gastrointestinal upset,
urticaria, allergic reactions, diarrhea. Drowsiness occurs frequently.
Extrapyramidal side effects such as opisthotonos, clonic convulsions,
oculogyric crisis, facial grimacing, involuntary movement of limbs,
and rarely stridor and dyspnea (possibly due to laryngospasm) occur
with 0.2% or less frequency in above doses but are more common in
children. Diphenhydramine may readily reverse extrapyramidal
effects. Butyrophenones and phenothiazines may potentiate
extrapyramidal side effects.

Precautions and Contraindications

Use with caution in pregnant patients. Metoclopramide may exacerbate Parkinson's disease and hypertension and may increase pressure
on suture lines following gut anastomosis or closure. Patients should
be cautioned that metoclopramide may impair their ability to perform
activities requiring mental alertness, including driving or operating
machinery. Alcohol and other central nervous system depressants may

PART 3 Drugs

enhance these effects.

Do not use metoclopramide with monoamine oxidase inhibitors, tricyclic antidepressants, or sympathomimetics. Metoclopramide should not be used in patients with pheochromocytoma, history of seizure disorder, or gastrointestinal hemorrhage, obstruction or perforation.

Anesthetic Considerations

Metoclopramide may increase the neuromuscular blocking effects of succinylcholine by inhibiting plasma cholinesterase.

Name

Midazolam (Versed)

Classification

Benzodiazepine; hypnotic; sedative

Indications

Preoperative sedation; induction of anesthesia; long-term sedation in intensive care unit; sedation prior to short diagnostic and endoscopic procedures

Dose

Should be individualized based on the patient's age, underlying pathology, and concurrent indications. Adolescents (under 12 years): I.V.: 0.5 mg; can be repeated every 5 min until desired effect is achieved. Adults: Preoperative sedation: I.M.: 0.07 to 0.08 mg/kg 30 to 60 min before surgery; usual dose: approximately 5 mg. I.V.: Initial 0.5 to 2 mg slow I.V. over 2 min. Usual total dose: 2.0 to 5 mg; decrease dose in elderly patients. Reduce dose by 30% if other central nervous system depressants are administered concomitantly. Dosage form: Injection: 1, 5 mg/mL.

Onset and Duration

Onset I.V.: 1 to 5 min; I.M.: 15 min; P.O./rectal: less than 10 min. Duration: 2 to 6 hr. Elimination $t_{1/2}$: 14 hr; excreted in urine.

Adverse Effects

Tachycardia, hypotension, bronchospasm, laryngospasm, apnea, hypoventilation, vasovagal episodes, euphoria, prolonged emergence, agitation, hyperactivity, pruritus, rash

Precautions and Contraindications

Midazolan is not for intraarterial injection. Its safe use in pregnancy, labor and delivery, by nursing mothers, or by children is not established. Midazolan is contraindicated in patients with intolerance to benzodiazepines and in those with acute narrow-angle glaucoma, shock, coma, or acute alcohol intoxication.

Anesthetic Considerations

Use with caution in elderly patients and in patients with chronic obstructive pulmonary disease, chronic renal failure, or congestive heart failure. Reduce doses in hypovolemia and with concomitant use of other sedatives or narcotics. Hypotension and respiratory depression may occur when given with opioids; consider smaller doses. Treat overdose with flumazenil.

Name
Milrinone (Primacor)

Classification
Inotropic agent

Indications
Chronic therapy for congestive heart failure; cardiac bypass procedures and heart transplants

Dose
I.V.: Loading dose: 50 µg/kg over 10 min; Maintenance dose: 0.375 µg/kg per min, 0.5 µg/kg per min, or 0.75 µg/kg per min. Dosage form: I.V.: 1 mg/mL.

Onset and Duration
Onset: I.V.: 2 min; P.O. 1 to 1.5 hr. Duration: 2 hr.

Adverse Effects
Thrombocytopenia, arrhythmia, angina, hypotension, headache, hyperthermia

Precautions and Contraindications
Use with caution in patients with renal insufficiency and in those with aortic or pulmonic valvular disease. Milrinone is contraindicated in patients with hypersensitivity to milrinone or amrinone.

Anesthetic Considerations
Milrinone is an attractive alternative to conventional inotropics. It may be useful if both an inotropic effect and vasodilation are desirable.

Name
Mivacurium (Mivacron)

Classification
Nondepolarizing skeletal muscle relaxant

Indications
Adjunct to general anesthesia; skeletal muscle relaxation during surgery

Dose
I.V.: Paralyzing: 0.07 to 0.25 mg/kg. Children: 0.1 to 0.2 mg/kg over 5 to 15 sec. Dosage forms: 0.5 mg/mL in 5% dextrose; 0.5 mg/mL.

PART 3 Drugs

Onset and Duration

Onset: 2 min. Duration: 6 to 10 min.

Adverse Effects

Hypotension, vasodilation, tachycardia, bradycardia, hypoventilation, apnea, bronchospasm, laryngospasm, dyspnea, rash, inadequate block, prolonged block

Precautions and Contraindications

Mivacurium is contraindicated in patients with hypersensitivity to the drug.

Anesthetic Considerations

Use with caution in patients with sensitivity to the release of histamine. Prolonged neuromuscular blockade may occur in patients with low plasma pseudocholinesterase; reverse the effects with anticholinesterase. Monitor the patient's response with peripheral nerve stimulator.

Name

Morphine sulfate (Astramorph, Duramorph, Morphine, MS Contin)

Classification

Opioid agonist

Indications

Premedication; analgesia; anesthesia; treatment of pain associated with myocardial ischemia and dyspnea associated with left ventricular failure and pulmonary edema

Dose

Analgesia: I.V.: 2.5 to 15 mg; I.M./SQ: 2.5 to 20 mg; P.O.: 15 to 30 mg every 4 hr as needed; P.O. extended release: 30 mg every 12 hr; Rectal: 5 to 20 mg every 4 hr. Anesthesia induction: I.V.: 1 mg/kg; Epidural bolus: 2 to 5 mg; Epidural infusion: 0.1 to 1 mg/hr; Spinal (preservative-free solution only): 0.2 to 1 mg. Children: I.V.: 0.05 to 0.2 mg/kg; I.M./SQ: 0.1 to 0.2 mg/kg.

Onset and Duration

Onset: I.V.: almost immediate; I.M.: 1 to 5 min; P.O.: less than 60 min; Epidural and spinal: 1 to 60 min. Duration: I.V./I.M./SQ: 2 to 7 hr; Epidural and spinal: 24 hr.

Adverse Effects

Hypotension, hypertension, bradycardia, arrhythmias, chest-wall rigidity, bronchospasm, laryngospasm, blurred vision, syncope, euphoria, dysphoria, urinary retention, antidiuretic effect, ureteral spasm, biliary tract spasm, constipation, anorexia, nausea, vomiting, pruritus, urticaria

Precautions and Contraindications

Reduce the dose in elderly, hypovolemic, or high-risk surgical patients and with concomitant use of sedatives and other narcotics. Morphine sulfate crosses the placental barrier; so usage in labor may produce depression of respiration in the neonate. Resuscitation of the neonate may be required; therefore have naloxone available.

Anesthetic Considerations

Central nervous system and cardiovascular depressant effects are potentiated by alcohol, sedatives, antihistamines, phenothiazines, butyrophenones, monoamine oxidase inhibitors, and tricyclic antidepressants. Morphine sulfate may decrease the effects of diuretics in patients with congestive heart failure. Analgesia is enhanced by or α_2 agonists.

Name

Nalmefene HCl (Revex)

Classification

Opiate antagonist

Indications

Complete or partial reversal of drug effects, respiratory depression, and overdose associated with either natural and synthetic opioids

Dose

Reversal of opiate depression: titrate to the desired response at increments of 0.25 µg/kg every 2 to 5 min. Doses greater than 1 mg/kg give no additional therapeutic effects. Titrated at a dose of 0.1 µg/kg every 2 to 5 min in patients with increased cardiovascular risk. Suspected opiate overdose: First dose 0.5 mg/70 kg; second dose 1.0 mg/70 kg if required 2 to 5 min later. Doses greater than 1.5 mg/70 kg do not provide increased therapeutic effects. Suspicion of opiate dependency: Uses a challenge dose of 0.1 mg/70 kg. If signs of withdrawal do not appear within 2 minutes, the recommended dosage guidelines should be followed.

Onset and Duration

Onset: I.V.: within 2 min; I.M. SQ: 5 to 15 min; I.V.: Administration of a 1 mg dose of nalmefene will block 80% of brain opiate receptors within 5 min. The duration of action and opiate receptor occupancy of nalmefene was shown to be significantly greater than that of naloxone, which has t1/2 of 1.1 hr. Duration: Equals that of most opioids. This provides the patient with added protection against possible renarcotization. Elimination $t_{1/2}$: 10.8 hr. Metabolized in liver via glucuronide conjugation; excreted in the urine. Plasma clearance is reported to be 0.8 L/hr per kg; plasma-protein binding: 45%.

Adverse Effects

Pulmonary edema, hypotension, hypertension, ventricular arrhythmias, bradycardia, dizziness, depression, agitation, nervousness, tremor, confusion, myoclonus, withdrawal syndrome, nausea, vomiting, diarrhea, dry mouth, headache, chills, pruritus, pharyngitis. A higher occurrence of adverse effects is reported with amounts exceeding recommended dosages.

Precautions and Contraindications

Nalmefene causes decreased plasma clearance in patients with liver or renal disease. The dose of nalmefene should be delivered over 60 seconds in patients with renal failure to minimize associated hypertension and dizziness. Dosage need not be adjusted for one-time administration. Recurrence of respiratory depression is possible even after a positive response to initial administration. Use with caution in patients at increased cardiovascular risk. Acute withdrawal symptoms are associated with administration to opiate-dependent patients. There is incomplete reversal of buprenorphine-induced depression. Use only in emergencies during pregnancy; use with caution in nursing women. Animal studies have shown a potential for seizure induction. Potential risk of seizure increases with the coadministration of nalmefene and flumazenil. Nalmefene is contraindicated in persons who display an allergic response related to the drug's administration. Safety and effectiveness of nalmefene for neonates and children has not been established.

Anesthetic Considerations

No adverse reactions were noted in studies where nalmefene was administered after benzodiazepines, volatile anesthetics, muscle relaxants, or their reversals.

Name

Naloxone HCl (Narcan)

Classification

Opioid antagonist

Indications

Opiate reversal

Dose

I.V./I.M./SQ: 0.1 to 2 mg titrated to patient response; may repeat at 2- to 3-min intervals; response should occur with a maximum dose of 10 mg. Children: 5 to 10 μg/kg every 2 to 3 min as needed.

Onset and Duration

Onset: I.V.: 1 to 2 min; I.M./SQ: 2 to 5 min. Duration: I.V./I.M./SQ: 1 to 4 hr.

Adverse Effects

Tachycardia, hypertension, hypotension, arrhythmias, pulmonary edema, nausea, and vomiting related to dose and speed of injection.

Precautions and Contraindications

Use with caution in patients with preexisting cardiac disease.

Anesthetic Considerations

Titrate slowly to effect results. Patients who have received naloxone should be carefully monitored because the duration of action of some opiates may exceed that of this drug.

Name

Naltrexone HCl (ReVia, Trexan)

Classification

Opiate receptor antagonist

Indications

Reversal of toxic effects of opioid drugs; treatment of opiate and alcohol addiction, Tourette's syndrome, tardive dyskinesia, Lesch-Nyhan disease, and dyskinesia associated with Huntington's disease

Dose

P.O.: 25 mg tablet followed by 25 mg in 1 hr if no signs of withdrawal present (withdrawal will begin 5 min after P.O. dose and may last up to 48 hr). Dosage form: Tablet: 25, 50 mg.

Onset and Duration

Onset: within 5 min; peak effects seen within 1 hr. Duration: 24 to 72 hr.

Adverse Effects

Headache, nervousness, confusion, restlessness, hallucinations, paranoia, nightmares, nausea, vomiting, diarrhea, abdominal pain and cramping, phlebitis, epistaxis, tachycardia, hypertension, edema, hepatotoxicity, joint muscle pain, and severe narcotic withdrawal

Precautions and Contraindications

Patients addicted to heroin or other opiates should be drug free for 10 days before initiation of therapy to avoid precipitation of withdrawal syndrome. Naltrexone contraindication is absolute in patients dependent on narcotics, in patients in acute withdrawal, and in those with liver disease or acute hepatitis. Serious overdose may occur after attempts to overcome the blocking effects of naltrexone.

Anesthetic Considerations

Baseline liver function studies should be performed. Primary active metabolite is subject to glucuronide conjugation. Aspartate transaminase levels may be temporarily elevated after initiation of therapy. Patients taking naltrexone may not respond to opiates administered during anesthesia. Blockade of naltrexone may be overcome by large (fatal) doses of opiates.

Name

Neostigmine methylsulfate (Prostigmin)

Classification
Anticholinesterase agent

Indications
Reversal of nondepolarizing muscle relaxants; myasthenia gravis

Dose
Reversal: Slow I.V.: 0.06 mg/kg (maximum dose: 6 mg), with atropine (0.015 mg/kg) or glycopyrrolate (0.01 mg/kg). Myasthenia gravis: P.O.: 15 to 375 mg daily (3 divided doses); I.M./Slow I.V.: 0.5 to 2 mg (dose must be individualized).

Onset and Duration
Onset: Reversal: I.V.: less than 3 min. Myasthenia gravis: I.M.: less than 20 min; P.O.: 45 to 75 min. Duration: 45 to 60 min.

Adverse Effects
Bradycardia, tachycardia, atrioventricular block, nodal rhythm, hypotension, bronchospasm, respiratory depression, seizures, dysarthria, headaches, nausea, emesis, flatulence, increased peristalsis, urinary frequency, rash, urticaria, allergic reactions, anaphylaxis, increased oral, pharyngeal, and bronchial secretions,

Precautions and Contraindications
Use with caution in patients with bradycardia, bronchial asthma, epilepsy, cardiac arrhythmias, peptic ulcer, peritonitis, or mechanical obstruction of the intestines or urinary tract. Overdosage may induce a cholinergic crisis characterized by nausea, vomiting, bradycardia or tachycardia, excessive salivation and sweating, bronchospasm, weakness, and paralysis; treatment includes discontinuation of neostigmine use and administration of atropine (10 mg/kg I.V. every 3 to 10 min until muscarinic symptoms disappear).

Anesthetic Considerations
May increase postoperative nausea and vomiting.

Name
Nicardipine (Cardene)

Classification
Calcium channel blocker

Indications
Hypertension; chronic stable angina; vasospastic angina

Dose
Angina: initially 20 mg P.O. t.i.d., titrate dosage according to patient response; usual dosage 20 to 40 mg P.O. t.i.d. Hypertension: initially 20 to 40 mg P.O. t.i.d., increase dosage according to patient response; I.V.: 5 mg/hr, increased by 2.5 mg/hr increments every 15 min, up to 15 mg/hr.

Onset and Duration

Onset: I.V.: 1 min; P.O.: 30 min to 2 hr; sustained release 1 to 4 hr. Duration: I.V./P.O.: 3 hr.

Adverse Effects

Edema, dizziness, headache, flushing, hypotension

Precautions and Contraindications

Use with caution in patients with hypersensitivity to nicardipine, other dihydropyridines, or other calcium channel antagonists, and those with symptomatic hypotension or advanced aortic stenosis.

Anesthetic Considerations

Nicardipine is an intravenous calcium channel blocker. It may be useful in controlling perioperative hypertension.

Name

Nifedipine (Adalat, Procardia)

Classification

Calcium channel blocker

Indications

Hypertension; chronic stable angina; vasospastic angina

Dose

10 to 30 mg t.i.d. up to 180 mg/day; Unlabeled route: sublingual

Onset and Duration

Onset: P.O.: 20 min; Sublingual: 5 to 20 min. Duration: P.O./sublingual: 12 hr.

Adverse Effects

Hypotension, palpitations, peripheral edema, bronchospasm, shortness of breath, nasal and chest congestion, headache, dizziness, nervousness, nausea, diarrhea, constipation, inflammation, joint stiffness, peripheral edema, pruritus, urticaria, fevers, chills, sweating

Precautions and Contraindications

Monitor blood pressure carefully during initial administration and titration. Use with caution in hypovolemic patients, the elderly, and those with acute myocardial infarction and unstable angina.

Anesthetic Considerations

Nifedipine potentiates the effects of depolarizing and nondepolarizing muscle relaxants and provides additive cardiovascular depressant effects with the use of volatile anesthetics or other antihypertensives. Nifedipine increases the toxicity of digoxin, carbamazepine, and oral hypoglycemics. It may bring about cardiac failure, atrioventricular conduction disturbances, and sinus bradycardia with concurrent use

PART 3 **Drugs**

of β-blockers; severe hypotension and bradycardia may occur with bupivacaine. Concomitant use of I.V. verapamil and dantrolene may result in cardiovascular collapse.

Name

Nitroglycerin (Nitro-Bid, Nitro-Dur, Nitrogard, Nitrostat, Nitrol, Tridil, Nitrocine, Transderm-Nitro, Nitroglyn, Nitrodisc)

Classification

Peripheral vasodilator

Indications

Antianginal; controlled hypotension, treatment of pulmonary edema and congestive heart failure associated with acute myocardial infarction

Dose

Initially, titrate 5 µg/min to 20 µg/min; thereafter titrate by 10 µg/min steps. I.V. infusion: 5 mg/min. Tablets: 0.15 to 0.6 mg every 5 min as needed to maximum of 3 doses in 15 min (sustained releasebuccal 1 to 2 mg every 3 to 5 hr); place tablet between lip and gum above incisors. Dosage forms: Injection: 0.5 mg/mL and 5 mg/mL: Tablets: sublingual: 0.15 mg, 0.3 mg, 0.4 mg, 0.6 mg. Sustained release-buccal: 1, 2, 3 mg.; P.O.: 2.5, 2.6, 6.5, 9 mg. Capsules: 2.5, 6.5, 9 mg. Aerosol translingual: 0.4 mg/metered dose. Transdermal systems: 2.5, 5, 7.5, 10, 15 mg/24 hr. Ointment: 2% (1 inch contains 15 mg nitroglycerine). Dilution for infusion: 8 mg diluted in 250 mL D_5W or normal saline (32 µg/mL), 50 mg in 250 mL, 100 mg in 250 mL (400 µg/mL).

Onset and Duration

Onset: I.V.: 1 to 2 min; sublingual: 1 to 3 min; P.O. sustained release: 20 to 45 min; Transdermal: 40 to 60 min. Duration: 30 min to 2 hr depending on route.

Adverse Effects

Orthostatic hypotension, tachycardia, flushing, palpitations, fainting, headache, dizziness, weakness, nausea, vomiting

Precautions and Contraindications

Use with caution in patients with hypotension, uncorrected hypovolemia, inadequate cerebral circulation, increased intracranial pressure, head trauma, cerebral hemorrhage, or severe anemia. Nytroglyserin is contraindicated in patients with compensatory hypertension such as with arteriovenous shunts, coarctation of the aorta, and inadequate cerebral circulation.

Anesthetic Considerations

The hypotensive effects of nitroglycerin are potentiated by alcohol, phenothiazines, calcium channel blockers, β-blockers, other nitrates, and antihypertensives. Nitroglycerin may the antagonize the anticoagulant effect of heparin. Methemoglobinemia may occur at high doses.

Because of light sensitivity, wrap the I.V. solution container in foil. Monitor plasma thiocyanate concentrations in patients receiving infusions for greater than 48 hours.

Attenuation of hypoxic pulmonary vasoconstriction may occur with nitroglycerin. Infusion rates of greater than 3 mg/kg/min may result in decreased platelet aggregation. The hypotensive effects of nitroglyceine are potentiated by volatile anesthetics, ganglionic blocking agents, other antihypertensives, and circulatory depressants. Elevated mixed venous PO_2 may also occur.

Name
Nitroprusside sodium (Nipride, Nitropress)

Classification
Peripheral vasodilator

Indications
Hypertension; controlled hypotension; treatment of cardiogenic pulmonary edema; treatment of cardiogenic shock

Dose
Infusion: 10 to 300 µg/min (0.25 to 10 µg/kg/min); Maximum dose: 10 µg/kg/min for 10 min or chronic infusion of 0.5 µg/kg/min.

Onset and Duration
Onset: 30 to 60 sec. Duration: 1 to 10 min.

Adverse Effects
May cause reflex tachycardia; cyanide toxicity may occur even in low doses. Treatment: Immediately discontinue nitroprusside use, administer oxygen, treat acidosis with bicarbonate, start sodium nitrate 3% solution 4 to 6 mg/kg over 3 min, to produce 10% methemoglobin, which will reversibly bind free cyanide ion. Follow with infusion of sodium thiosulfate (vitamin B_{12}), 150 to 200 mg/kg.

Precautions and Contraindications
Use with caution in patients with renal or hepatic failure, which may lead to increased risk of cyanide toxicity. There is a potential for fetal cyanide toxicity in pregnant patients.

Anesthetic Considerations
Titrate carefully for short periods of deliberate hypotension. Monitor for cyanide toxicity.

Name
Nitrous oxide (N_2O)

Classification
Inhalation anesthetic

PART 3 Drugs

Indications

Component of balanced obstetric anesthesia or dental analgesia

Dose

Induction: 70% in an oxygen mixture. Maintenance: 70% in oxygen. Analgesia: 20% to 30%. Supplied in steel cylinders (blue) as a colorless liquid under pressure.

Onset and Duration

Onset: 1 to 5 min. Duration: 5 to 10 min after cessation of continuous inhalation.

Adverse Effects

Primarily caused by lack of oxygen from improper administration technique. Confusion, cyanosis, convulsions, possible bone marrow depression and malignant hyperthermia.

Precautions and Contraindications

Caution patient not to drive or operate other machinery until the effects of the drug have completely disappeared. Inform the patient that confusion, vivid dreams, dizziness, and hallucinations may occur on termination. Inspired oxygen concentrations of at least 30% should be given.

Anesthetic Considerations

Nitrous oxide is nonflammable but will support combustion. There is a noticeable second-gas effect that initially hastens the uptake of other agents when high concentrations are used. Nitrous oxide diffuses into air-containing cavities 34 times faster than nitrogen can leave. This can cause a potentially dangerous pressure accumulation (i.e., middle-ear perforation, bowel obstruction, pneumothorax). Check the endotracheal tube cuff volume and pressure periodically during general anesthesia.

Name

Nizatidine (Axid)

Classification

H_2-receptor antagonist

Indications

Treatment of duodenal or gastric ulcers and gastroesophageal reflux disease; prophylaxis of aspiration pneumonitis in patients at high risk during surgery.

Dose

For prophylaxis of aspiration pneumonitis in adults: 150 mg P.O. 2 hr prior to the induction of anesthesia; may be given with or without a similar dose the preceding evening. For patients with impaired renal function as evidenced by serum creatinine level greater than 2.5 mg% a single dose only is needed. Dosage form: 150 mg capsule

Onset and Duration

Onset: Peak plasma levels occurred 1 to 3 hr after oral administration and were below detectable limits in healthy patients 12 hr later. Elimination $t_{1/2}$: 1 to 2.8 hr.

Adverse Effects

Headache is the most common side effect, followed by gastrointestinal effects and dizziness (4.5%). Rarely, thrombocytopenia, leukopenia, and anemia occur. Somnolence (2%) and mental confusion can occur in the elderly. Incidence of hepatitis is 0.04% to 0.15%.

Precautions and Contraindications

Caution is suggested in patients with hepatic or renal dysfunction. Nizatidine is contraindicated for patients with known hypersensitivity to nizatidine or other H_2 antagonists.

Anesthetic Considerations

Nizatidine is safe for use during anesthesia.

Name

Norepinephrine bitartrate (Levophed)

Classification

Catecholamine.

Indications

Vasoconstrictor; inotrope. Potent peripheral vasoconstrictor of arterial and venous beds. Potent inotropic stimulator of the heart (β_1-adrenergic action) but to a lesser degree than epinephrine or isoproterenol. Does not stimulate β_2-adrenergic receptors of the bronchi or peripheral blood vessels. Increases systolic and diastolic blood pressures and coronary artery blood flow. Cardiac output varies reflexly with systemic hypertension but is usually increased in hypotensive subjects when blood pressure is raised to an optimal level. On other occasions, increased baroreceptor activity reflexly decreases the heart rate. Reduces renal, hepatic, cerebral, and muscle blood flow.

Dose

Infusion: 8 to 12 mg/min. Use lowest effective dose.

Onset and Duration

Onset: 1 min. Duration: 2 to 10 min.

Adverse Effects

Bradycardia, tachyarrhythmias, hypertension, decreased cardiac output, headache, plasma volume depletion. Administer into large vein to minimize extravasation. Treat extravasation with local infiltration of phentolamine (10 mg in 10 mL normal saline) or sympathetic block.

Precautions and Contraindications

Norepinephrine bitartrate is contraindicated in patients with mesenteric or peripheral vascular thrombosis.

Anesthetic Considerations

Norepinephrine bitartrate causes an increased risk of arrhythmias with use of volatile anesthetics or bretylium, or in patients with profound hypoxia or hypercarbia. The pressor effect is potentiated in patients receiving monoamine oxidase inhibitors, tricyclic antidepressants, guanethidine, or oxytocics. Norepinephrine bitartrate may cause necrosis or gangrene with extravasation.

Name

Omeprazole (Prilosec, Losec, Omid)

Classification

Proton pump inhibitor

Indications

Gastro-esphageal reflux disease

Dose

P.O.: 10 to 40 mg q.d. before meals.

Onset and Duration

Onset: within 1 hr (Maximum effect: 2 hr). Duration: up to 72 hr.

Adverse Effects

Headache, diarrhea, abdominal pain, nausea, vomiting, rash, constipation, dizziness

Precautions and Contraindications

Omeprazole is contraindicated in patients with hypersensitivity to omeprazole or other similar proton pump inhibitors.

Anesthetic Considerations

Omeprazoile is highly protein bound. Undergoes liver and renal elimination. Omeprazole may prolong the elimination of drugs metabolized by oxidation in the liver (i.e. diazepam, warfarin, phenytoin).

Name

Ondansetron HCl (Zofran)

Classification

Gastrointestinal agent; serotonin (5HT3) receptor antagonist; antiemetic

Indications

Prevention of nausea and vomiting associated with cancer chemotherapy; postoperative nausea and vomiting.

Dose

With chemotherapy: I.V.: 3 doses—0.15 mg/kg first dose 30 min before chemotherapy, then 4 to 8 hr after first dose (may give as 8 mg bolus, then 1 mg/hr continuous infusion with maximum dose of 32 mg/day). Perioperative nausea and vomiting: 2 to 4 mg.

Onset and Duration

Onset: Variable. Most effective if therapy begins before emetogenic chemotherapy. Peak effects: 1 to 1.5 hr. Duration: 12 to 24 hr.

Adverse Effects

Tachycardia, angina, dizziness, lightheadedness, headache, sedation, diarrhea, constipation, dry mouth, rash, bronchospasm, hypersensitivity reactions.

Precautions and Contraindications

Use with caution in pregnant or nursing women and in children younger than 3 years old. Ondansetron is contraindicated in patients with hypersensitivity to the drug.

Anesthetic Considerations

Monitor cardiovascular status, especially in patients with a history of coronary artery disease.

Name

Oxytocin (Pitocin, Syntocinon)

Classification

Oxytocic; lactation stimulant

Indications

Initiates or improves uterine contraction at term after dilation of cervix and delivery of fetus; stimulates letdown reflex in nursing mothers to relieve pain from breast engorgement.

Dose

Administration of oxytocin is always via continuous I.V. infusion. Augmentation of labor: 10 IU (1 mL) diluted in 1000 mL of infusate. Infusion rates vary from 1 to 10 mU/min. Minimize of postpartum bleeding: 20 to 100 mU/min. Effects appear within 3 min, are maximal at about 20 min, and disappear within 15 to 20 min. after discontinuing the infusion. In practical terms, 20 to 40 IU is usually added to 1000 mL of fluid and administered to effect. Promotion of milk ejection: Nasal: 1 spray or drop in one or both nostrils 2 to 3 min before nursing or pumping breasts.

Onset and Duration

Onset: I.V.: immediate; Nasal: few mins; I.M.: 3 to 5 min. Peak effects: I.V.: less than 20 min; I.M.: 40 min. Duration: IV: 20 min to 1 hr; Nasal: 20 min; I.M.: 2 to 3 hr.

Adverse Effects

Hypersensitivity leading to uterine hypertonicity, tetanic contractions, uterine rupture, cardiac arrhythmias, nausea, vomiting, hypertension, subarachnoid hemorrhage, seizures from water intoxication, hyponatremia

Precautions and Contraindications

Use with caution with other vasoactive drugs. Oxytocin is contraindicated in patients with hypersensitivity to the drug. Oxytocin is also contraindicated in complications of pregnancy: significant cephalopelvic disproportion, fetal distress in which delivery is not imminent, prematurity, placenta previa, or past history of uterine sepsis or of traumatic delivery. Nasal preparation is contraindicated during pregnancy.

Anesthetic Considerations

Administration should follow delivery of fetus. Oxytocin may increase the pressor effects of sympathomimetics. Prolonged I.V. infusion of oxytocin with excessive fluid volume may cause severe water intoxication with seizures, coma, and death. Infuse oxytocin by I.V. only after dilution in large volume, parenteral with an infusion pump.

Name

Pancuronium (Pavulon)

Classification

Nondepolarizing skeletal muscle relaxant

Indications

Adjunct to general anesthesia; skeletal muscle relaxation during surgery

Dose

I.V. paralyzing: 0.04 to 0.1 mg/kg; Pretreatment/maintenance: 0.01 to 0.02 mg/kg. Dosage forms: Injection: 1 mg/mL in 10-mL vial; Ampule: 2 mg/mL.

Onset and Duration

Onset: 1 to 3 min. Duration: 40 to 65 min.

Adverse Effects

Tachycardia, hypertension, hypoventilation, apnea, bronchospasm, salivation, flushing, anaphylactoid reactions, inadequate block, prolonged block

Precautions and Contraindications

Pancuronium is contraindicated in patients with myasthenia gravis, bromide hypersensitivity, severe coronary artery disease, or in those with conditions in which tachycardia is undesirable.

Anesthetic Considerations

Pretreatment doses may cause hypoventilation in some patients. Monitor patient response with peripheral nerve stimulator. Reverse the effects with anticholinesterase.

Name
Phentolamine (Regitine)

Classification
α-adrenergic blocker

Indications
Controlled hypotension; treatment of perioperative hypertensive crisis that may accompany pheochromocytomectomy; prevention or treatment of dermal necrosis or sloughing after I.V. administration or extravasation of barbiturate or sympathomimetic

Dose
Antihypertensive: I.V./I.M.: 2.5 to 5 mg. Antisloughing infiltration: 5 to 10 mg (maximum dose: 10 mg); dilute in 10 mL normal saline. Dosage forms: Injection: 5 mg/mL; dilution for infusion 200 mg in 100 mL D_5W or normal saline.

Onset and Duration
Onset: I.V.: 1 to 2 min; I.M.: 5 to 20 min. Duration: I.V.: 10 to 15 min; I.M.: 30 to 45 min.

Adverse Effects
Hypotension, tachycardia, arrhythmias, myocardial infarction, dizziness, cerebrovascular spasm and occlusion, flushing, diarrhea, nausea, vomiting

Precautions and Contraindications
Use with caution in patients with ischemic heart disease. Phentolamine-induced α-receptor blockade will potentiate β_2-adrenergic vasodilation of epinephrine, ephedrine, dobutamine, or isoproterenol.

Anesthetic Considerations
Use with epinephrine, ephedrine, dobutamine, or isoproterenol. Phentolamine may cause a paradoxical fall in blood pressure.

Name
Phenylephrine (Neo-Synephrine)

Classification
Synthetic noncatecholamine that stimulates α_1-adrenergic receptors

Indications
Vasoconstriction; treatment of hypotension, shock, supraventricular tachyarrhythmias; prolongation of duration of local anesthetics

Dose
I.V.: 50 to 100 µg; do not exceed 0.5 mg initial dose or repeat sooner

PART 3 Drugs

than 15 minutes. I.V. infusion: 20 to 50 µg/min; titrate to effect.

Onset and Duration

Onset: almost immediate. Duration: 15 to 20 min.

Adverse Effects

Reflex bradycardia, arrhythmias, hypertension, headache, restlessness, reflex vagal action

Precautions and Contraindications

Use with extreme caution in elderly patients and patients with hyperthyroidism, bradycardia, partial heart block, or severe arteriosclerosis.

Anesthetic Considerations

Infuse phenylephrine into a large vein; treat extravasation with phentolamine (5 to 10 mg in 10 mL normal saline and/or sympathetic block). Volatile agents used with phenylephrine may increase the risk of arrhythmias.

Name

Phenytoin (Dilantin)

Classification

Anticonvulsant

Indications

Anticonvulsant; treatment of cardiac arrhythmias from digitalis intoxication, ventricular tachycardia, and paroxysmal atrial tachycardia resistant to conventional methods; treatment of migraine or trigeminal neuralgia

Dose

Anticonvulsant: I.V.: 10 to 15 mg/kg in 50 to 100 mL normal saline at a rate not exceeding 50 mg/min or 1.5 g/24 hr.

Maintenance: I.V./P.O.: 100 mg every 6 to 8 hr or 300 to 400 mg once a day.

Antiarrhythmic: I.V.: 1.5 mg/kg slow push every 5 min until arrhythmia is suppressed or undesirable effects appear (maximum dosage: 10 to 15 mg/kg per day).

Children: Anticonvulsant: loading dose 10 to 15 mg/kg 1 gram intravenous piggyback in normal saline up to 20 mg/kg in 24 hours.

P.O. maintenance: 4 to 8 mg/kg daily in 2 to 3 equally divided doses.

Dosage forms: Injection: 50 mg/mL; Capsules and extended-release capsules: 30, 100 mg; Chewable tablets: 50 mg; Oral suspension: 30 mg/5 mL, 125 mg/5 mL.

Onset and Duration

Onset: I.V.: 3 to 5 min Therapeutic levels: 10 to 20 mg/mL; can be attained in 1 to 2 hr after appropriate loading. Elimination $t_{1/2}$: highly variable; increases as plasma levels increase; ranges from 8 to 60 hr (average 22 hr). Patients with liver disease may have highly variable clearance due to saturation kinetics. Duration: 8 to 24 hr depending on dose.

Adverse Effects

Adverse effects are often dose-related. Nausea, vomiting, gum hyperplasia, megaloblastic anemia (due to folate deficiency), osteomalacia (with chronic therapy), thrombocytopenia, granulocytopenia, toxic hepatitis, rarely exfoliative dermatitis, Stevens-Johnson syndrome, lupus erythematosus (SLE). Nystagmus (blood level greater than 20 mg/mL), ataxia (blood level greater than 30 mg/mL), and somnolence (blood level greater than 40 mg/mL). At rates exceeding 50 mg/min, hypotension, cardiovascular collapse, and central nervous system depression may occur.

Precautions and Contraindications

If a rash occurs during therapy, the drug should be discontinued; if the rash is exfoliative, purpuric, or bullous or if SLE or Stevens-Johnson syndrome is suspected, phenytoin should not be restarted.

Phenytoin will precipitate in all solutions other than normal saline. Flush the line before and after administration. Do not mix phenytoin with other drugs. Phenytoin must be administered with an in-line 0.22 micron I.V. filter and must be administered within 1 hr of mixing, owing to short stability.

Plasma levels should be monitored during therapy after a steady state is achieved and whenever toxicity is suspected.

Phenytoin should be administered by I.V. only with extreme caution in patients with respiratory depression or myocardial depression. I.V. use is contraindicated in patients with sinus bradycardia, sinoatrial block, second- or third-degree atrioventricular block or Adams-Stokes syndrome. Phenytoin is not useful in infantile febrile seizures, and safe use during pregnancy has not been established.

Abrupt withdrawal in patients with epilepsy may precipitate status epilepticus.

Phenytoin is highly protein-bound and has multiple drug interactions. Serum levels may be increased by diazepam, theophylline, warfarin, cimetidine, acute alcohol intake, and halothane. Serum levels are decreased by chronic alcoholism.

Anesthetic Considerations

Phenytoin treatment may increase the dose requirements for all nondepolarizing muscle relaxants except atracurium. Dose-response curves are shifted to the right and the duration is markedly reduced.

Further confusion is generated by the observation that acute administration of phenytoin to a patient receiving vecuronium will augment the blockade. Phenytoin follows Michaelis-Menten kinetics. A small incremental dose can radically increase free drug levels at equilibrium.

Name

Physostigmine salicylate (Antilirium)

PART 3 Drugs

Classification

Anticholinesterase agent

Indications

Reversal of prolonged somnolence and anticholinergic poisoning

Dose

I.V./I.M.: 0.5 to 2 mg (10 to 20 µg/kg) at rate of 1 mg/min, repeat dosing at intervals of 10 to 30 min.

Onset and Duration

Onset: I.V./I.M.: 3 to 8 min. Duration: I.V./I.M.: 30 min to 5 hr.

Adverse Effects

Bradycardia, bronchospasm, dyspnea, respiratory paralysis, seizures, salivation, nausea, vomiting, miosis

Precautions and Contraindications

High doses may cause tremors, ataxia, muscle fasciculations, and ultimately a depolarization block. Use with caution in patients with epilepsy, parkinsonian syndrome, or bradycardia. Do not use in the presence of asthma, diabetes, mechanical obstruction of the intestine or urogenital tract, or in patients receiving choline esters or depolarizing muscle relaxants.

Anesthetic Considerations

Rapid I.V. administration may cause bradycardia and hypersalivation, leading to respiratory problems or possibly seizures. Treatment of cholinergic crisis includes mechanical ventilation with repeated bronchial aspiration and I.V. administration of atropine 2 to 4 mg every 3 to 10 min until control of muscarinic symptoms is achieved or until signs of atropine overdose appear.

Name

Pipecuronium bromide (Arduan)

Classification

Nondepolarizing skeletal muscle relaxant

Indications

Adjunct to general anesthesia; skeletal muscle relaxation during surgery

Dose

I.V. paralyzing: 0.07 to 0.10 mg/kg; Pretreatment and maintenance: 0.01 to 0.015 mg/kg; Children: (3 mo to 1 yr) adult dosage on a mg/kg basis; Dosage forms: Powder for injection: 10 mg (10 mL).

Onset and Duration

Onset: less than 3 min. Duration: 45 to 120 min. Elimination: renal.

Adverse Effects

Hypotension, hypertension, bradycardia, myocardial infarction, hypoventilation, apnea, depression, anuria, urticaria, rash, inadequate block, prolonged block, hypoglycemia, hyperkalemia, increased creatinine. Pipecronium bromide enhanced neuromuscular blockade in patients with myasthenia gravis.

Precautions and Contradications

Patients may exhibit allergy to drug. Due to long duration of action, post-operative ventilation is likely to be required.

Anesthetic Considerations

Reverse any effects with anticholinesterase. Monitor patient response with a peripheral nerve stimulator. Pretreatment doses may cause hypoventilation in some patients. Pipecuronium bromide is recommended only for procedures anticipated to last 90 minutes or longer.

Name

Prilocaine HCl (Citanest)

Classification

Amide-type local anesthetic

Indications

Regional anesthesia: infiltration/peripheral nerve block, topical, epidural, I.V. regional

Dose

Infiltration/peripheral nerve block: 0.5 to 6 mg/kg (0.5% to 2% solution); Topical: 0.6 to 3 mg/kg (2% to 4% solution); Epidural: 200 to 300 mg (1% to 2% solution); (Maximum safe dosage: 6 mg/kg without epinephrine; 9 mg/kg with epinephrine 1:200,000).

Onset and Duration

Onset: Infiltration: 1 to 2 min; Epidural: 5 to 15 min; Peak effects: Infiltration/epidural: less than 30 min. Duration: Infiltration: 0.5 to 1.5 hr without epinephrine, 2 to 6 hr with epinephrine; Epidural: 1 to 3 hr (prolonged with epinephrine).

Adverse Effects

Hypotension, arrhythmia, collapse, respiratory depression, paralysis, seizures, tinnitus, blurred vision, urticaria, anaphylactoid reactions, methemoglobinemia. High spinal: urinary retention, lower-extremity weakness and paralysis, loss of sphincter control, headache, backache, slowing of labor.

Precautions and Contraindications

Use with caution in patients with hypovolemia, severe congestive heart failure, shock, all forms of heart block, or pregnancy. Prilocaine is contraindicated in patients with hypersensitivity to amide-type local

PART 3 Drugs

anesthetics and in infants under 6 mo old (low dose may cause methemoglobinemia).

Anesthetic Considerations

Treat methemoglobinemia with methylene blue (1 to 2 mg/kg injected over 5 min). In I.V. regional blocks, deflate the cuff after 40 min and not before 20 min.

Name

Procainamide (Procan SR, Pronestyl)

Classification

Class la antiarrhythmic

Indications

Treatment of lidocaine-resistant ventricular arrhythmias; arrhythmia control in malignant hyperthermia; treatment of atrial fibrillation or paroxysmal atrial tachycardia.

Dose

Loading: slow I.V. push 100 mg every 5 min (maximum: 500 mg)—do not exceed 50 mg/min (Children: 3 to 6 mg/kg given over 5 min). Dilute 1000 mg in 50 mL D_5W. I.M.: 100 to 500 mg in doses divided every 3 or 6 hr. Maintenance: Infusion: 2 to 6 mg/min (Children: 0.02 to 0.08 mg/kg/min). Therapeutic level: 3 to 10 mg/mL. Dosage form: Injection: 100 mg/mL, 500 mg/mL. Dilution for infusion: 2 g in 500 mL D_5W (4 mg/mL).

Onset and Duration

Onset: I.V.: immediate; I.M. 10 to 30 min. Duration: 2.5 to 5 hr.

Adverse Effects

Hypotension, heart block, arrhythmias, seizures, confusion, depression, psychosis, anorexia, nausea, vomiting, diarrhea, systemic lupus erythematosus (SLE), pruritus, fever, chills

Precautions and Contraindications

Use with caution in patients with first-degree heart block or arrhythmias associated with digitalis toxicity. Reduce doses in patients with congestive heart failure or renal failure. Procainamide is contraindicated in patients with complete heart block, torsades de pointes, or SLE.

Anesthetic Considerations

Procainamide requires periodic monitoring of patient plasma levels, vital signs, and electrocardiogram (QRS widening greater than 25% may signify overdosage). Procainamide potentiates the effect of both nondepolarizing and depolarizing muscle relaxants.

Name

Procaine HCl (Novocain)

Classification

Ester-type local anesthetic

Indications

Local anesthetic: infiltration, peripheral nerve block, sympathetic nerve block, regional anesthesia

Dose

Infiltration: less than 500 mg (0.5 to 2% solution); Epidural: less than 500 mg (1 to 2% solution). Spinal: 50 to 200 mg (10% solution with glucose 5%). Solutions with preservatives may not be used for epidural or spinal block.

Onset and Duration

Onset: Infiltration/spinal: 2 to 5 min, Epidural: 5 to 25 min. Peak effects: Infiltration/epidural/spinal: less than 30 min. Duration: Infiltration: 0.25 to 0.5 hr (without epinephrine), 0.5 to 1.5 hr (with epinephrine), epidural/spinal: 0.5 to 1.5 hr (prolonged with epinephrine).

Adverse Effects

Hypotension, bradycardia, arrhythmias, heart block, respiratory depression or arrest, tinnitus, seizures, dizziness, restlessness, loss of hearing, euphoria, postspinal headache, palsies, urticaria, pruritus, angioneurotic edema. Additionally with use as high spinal: loss of bladder and bowel control and permanent motor, sensory, and autonomic (sphincter control) deficits of lower segments.

Precautions and Contraindications

Use with caution in patients with severe cardiac disturbances (heart block, arrhythmias) or inflammation/sepsis at injection site. Procaine is contraindicated in patients with hypersensitivity to local anesthetics, paraaminobenzoic acid (PABA)/parabens, or ester-type anesthetics.

Anesthetic Considerations

Central nervous system effects are generally dose-dependent and of short duration. Vasopressors and oxytocics may cause hypertension. Preparations containing preservatives should not be used for epidural and spinal anesthesia. Reduce doses for spinal anesthesia in obstetric, elderly, hypovolemic, and high-risk patients, as well as in patients with increased intra-abdominal pressure.

Name

Prochlorperazine Maleate (Compazine)

Classification

Gastrointestinal agent; antiemetic; psychotherapeutic; phenothiazine antipsychotic

Indications

Antiemetic used to control nausea and vomiting; antipsychotic used in the management of manifestations of psychotic disorders of excessive anxiety, tension, and agitation

Dose

Antiemetic: P.O.: 5 to 10 mg t.i.d. or q.i.d; rectal: 25 mg b.i.d; I.V./I.M.: 5 to 10 mg (5 mg/mL per min). Do not administer SQ because of local irritation. Maximum dose: 40 mg/day.

Onset and Duration

Onset: I.V.: a few minutes; I.M.: 10 to 20 min. P.O.: 30 to 40 min; Rectal: 60 min. Peak effects: I.V./I.M./P.O.: 15 to 30 min. Duration: I.V./I.M./P.O./Rectal: 3 to 4 hr.

Adverse Effects

Extrapyramidal reactions, dystonia, central nervous system depression, hypotension

Precautions and Contraindications

Prochlorperazine maleate is contraindicated in pediatric patients and in patients with parkinsonian disease.

Anesthetic Considerations

Prochlorperazine maleate may produce an additive central nervous system depression when used with anesthetics. Avoid using Prochlorperazine maleate with droperidol or metoclopramide because of extrapyramidal effects.

Name

Promethazine HCl (Phenergan, Pentazine, Phenazine, Prothazine)

Classification

Phenothiazine: Gastrointestinal agent, antiemetic, antivertigo agent, antihistamine (H_1-receptor antagonist), sedative or adjunct to analgesics

Indications

Motion sickness or nausea; rhinitis; allergy symptoms; sedation; routine preoperative or postoperative sedation; adjunct to analgesics

Dose

I.V:. Administer cautiously because of hazard of phlebitis, necrosis, and gangrene of extremities—must dilute with equal volume of compatible diluent and administer slowly. For children, administer no larger dose than 0.5 mg/kg.) I.M., P.O., rectal: 12.5 to 50 mg. DO NOT administer SQ or intra-arterially due to risk of necrosis and gangrene of extremities. Dosage forms: Tablet: 12.5 mg, 25 mg, and 50 mg, Syrup: 6.25 mg/5 mL and 25 mg/5 mL. Suppositories: 12.5 mg, 25 mg, 50 mg. Injection: 25 mg/mL and 50 mg/mL.

Onset and Duration

Onset: I.V.: 150 sec; I.M., P.O., rectal: 15 to 30 min. Duration: I.V., I.M.,

P.O., rectal: 2 to 5 hr.

Adverse Effects

Hypotension, bradycardia, bronchospasm, drowsiness, sedation, dizziness, confusion, extrapyramidal reactions, agranulocytosis, and thrombocytopenia may occur.

Precautions and Contraindications

Use with caution, as the central nervous system and circulatory depressant actions of alcohol, sedative-hypnotics, and anesthetics are potentiated. Promethazine is contraindicated in patients with Parkinson's disease and in those receiving MAO inhibitors.

Anesthetic Considerations

Anesthetic recovery may be prolonged. Do not use in children under 2 years of age.

Name

Propofol (Diprivan)

Classification

Anesthesia induction agent

Indications

Anesthesia induction and maintenance; I.V. sedation; prolonged sedation in critical care

Dose

I.V. bolus: 1.0 to 2.5 mg/kg. Dilute in suitable I.V. fluid, preferably D_5W. DO NOT dilute the final solution to less than 2 mg/mL in order to protect suspension. DO NOT use any filter with a pore size smaller than 5 mm. Infusion: 25 to 200 µg/kg/min. Dosage form: 10 mg/mL in 20-mL ampules and 50-mL and 100-mL vials

Onset and Duration

Onset: Immediate. Duration: 5 to 20 min, depending on dose.

Adverse Effects

Hypotension, bradycardia, respiratory depression, prolonged somnolence, vivid dreams, burning on injection, hiccups, disinhibition, and arrhythmias may occur.

Precautions and Contraindications

Reduce the dose or avoid in patients with cardiac compromise, in elderly patients, and in those with respiratory disease, hypotension, or increased intracranial pressure. Watch for respiratory and cardiac depression when coadministering other central nervous system or cardiac depressant drugs. Strict aseptic technique must be used when handling to avoid bacterial growth in the emulsion vehicle. Propofol is contraindicated in patients with an egg or soybean allergy.

Anesthetic Considerations

Minimize pain on injection by giving a small dose of plain lidocaine (1%) before injection. Both convulsant and anticonvulsant effects have been reported, so do not use in patients with a history of seizures. The antiemetic properties of propofol may be an advantage in patients at risk for postoperative nausea and vomiting.

Name

Propranolol (Inderal, Ipran, others)

Classification

Nonselective β-adrenergic receptor antagonist

Indications

Hypertension; angina; ventricular and supraventricular arrhythmias; hyperthyroidism; migraines

Dose

I.V.: 0.25 mg increments, up to 3 mg; P.O.: 10 to 80 mg every 6 to 8 hr or 80 to 240 mg/day sustained release. Dosage forms: Injection: 1 mg/mL (1 mL); Tablet: 10 mg, 20 mg, 40 mg, 60 mg, 80 mg, 90 mg.

Onset and Duration

Onset: I.V.: less than 2 min; P.O.: 30 to 60 min. Duration: I.V.: 1 to 4 hr; P.O.: up to 24 hr sustained release.

Adverse Effects

Bradycardia, hypotension, atrioventricular block, bronchospasm, hypoglycemia, claudication, diarrhea, nausea, vomiting, constipation, nightmares, mental depression. Insomnia may occur. Propranolol may increase plasma triglycerides and decrease high-density lipoproteins.

Precautions and Contraindications

Propranolol is contraindicated in asthmatic patients and in patients with reduced myocardial reserve, peripheral vascular disease, diabetes, congestive heart failure, or shock. If the drug is discontinued abruptly, withdrawal may be manifested as increased nervousness, increased heart rate, increased intensity of angina, or increased blood pressure (related to up regulation). The effects of propranolol may be potentiated by inhalational anesthetics and other cardiodepressant drugs.

Anesthetic Considerations

Esmolol is preferred over propranolol for intraoperative use, due to more controllable duration. Propranolol may be useful as an antiarrhythmic because of its membrane-stabilizing properties.

Name

Protamine sulfate

Classification

Heparin antagonist

Indications

Treatment of heparin overdosage; heparin neutralization after extracorporeal circulation in arterial and cardiovascular surgery

Dose

Dosage is based on blood coagulation studies, usually 1 mg protamine for every 100 U of heparin remaining in the patient, given slowly by I.V. over 10 minutes in doses not to exceed 50 mg.

Because heparin blood concentrations decrease rapidly, the required dose of protamine sulfate decreases based on the elapsed time. One half of the usual dose of protamine should be given if 30 minutes have elapsed since heparin administration, and one fourth of the usual dose should be given if 2 hours or more have elapsed.

Dosage forms: Parenteral injection for I.V. use only: 10 mg/mL, 5-mL ampule or vial. Reconstitute a 50-mg vial by adding 5 mL sterile water or bacteriostatic water containing 0.9% benzyl alcohol. The resultant solution contains 10 mg/mL. A protamine solution is intended for I.V. bolus use and not for further dilution. If further dilution is desired, however, 5% dextrose or 0.9% NaCl I.V.P.B. may be used and given over 30 min.

Children: Injections preserved with benzyl alcohol may cause toxicity in the neonate.

Onset and Duration

Onset: Neutralization of heparin occurs within 5 min. Duration: Neutralization of heparin persists approximately 2 hr.

Adverse Effects

Rapid I.V. injection of protamine is associated with hypotension, bradycardia, and flushing. Other possible effects of protamine include hypersensitivity, anaphylaxis, dyspnea, noncardiac pulmonary edema, circulatory collapse, pulmonary hypertension, and "heparin rebound" (after the use of protamine in cardiopulmonary bypass). A paradoxical anticoagulant effect may occur with total doses greater than 100 mg.

Precautions and Contraindications

Monitor the activated partial thromboplastin time or the activated coagulation time at least 5 to 15 minutes after protamine administration to determine its effect. Have equipment readily available to treat shock. Patients with a sensitivity to fish, vasectomized or infertile males, and patients who have previously received either protamine or insulins containing protamine are considered at higher risk for hypersensitivity. If protamine is used in these patients, pretreatment with a corticosteroid or antihistamine should be considered. Protamine is contraindicated in patients with a history of allergy to the drug.

PART 3 Drugs

Anesthetic Considerations
None

Name
Pyridostigmine bromide (Mestinon, Regonol)

Classification
Anticholinesterase agent

Indications
For reversal of nondepolarizing muscle relaxants

Dose
Reversal: I.V.: 10 to 30 mg (0.1 to 0.25 mg/kg), preceded by atropine (0.015 mg/kg) or glycopyrrolate (0.01 mg/kg) I.V. Myasthenia gravis: P.O.: 60 to 1500 mg/day. S.R.: 180 to 540 mg daily or twice daily. To supplement oral dosage preoperatively and postoperatively, during labor and post partum, during myasthenic crisis, or when oral therapy is impractical: give 1/30 the oral dose I.M. or very slowly I.V.

Neonates of myasthenic mothers: 0.05 to 0.15 mg/kg I.M. Differentiate between cholinergic and myasthenic crisis in neonates. Administration 1 hr before completion of the second stage of labor enables patients to have adequate strength during labor and provides protection to infants in the intermediate postnatal stage.

Onset and Duration
Onset: Reversal: I.V.: 2 to 5 min; Myasthenia: I.M.: less than 15 min; P.O.: 20 to 30 min. Duration: Reversal: I.V.: 90 min; Myasthenia: P.O.: 3 to 6 hr; I.M.: 2 to 4 hr.

Adverse Effects
Bradycardia, atrioventricular block, nodal rhythm, hypotension, increased bronchial secretions, bronchospasm, respiratory depression, nausea, vomiting, diarrhea, abdominal cramps, increased peristalsis, increased salivation, muscle cramps, fasciculations, weakness, miosis, diaphoresis

Precautions and Contraindications
Use with caution in patients with bradycardia, bronchial asthma, cardiac arrhythmias, or peptic ulcer and in patients with peritonitis or mechanical obstruction of the intestines or urinary tract.

Anesthetic Considerations
Overdosage of pyridostigmine may induce a cholinergic crisis characterized by nausea, vomiting, bradycardia or tachycardia, excessive salivation and sweating, bronchospasm, weakness, and paralysis. Treatment of a cholinergic crisis includes discontinuation of pyridostigmine and administration of atropine (10 mg/kg I.V. every 3 to 10 minutes until muscarinic symptoms subside).

Name

Ranitidine (Zantac)

Classification

H_2-receptor antagonist

Indications

Treatment of duodenal or gastric ulcers and gastroesophageal reflux; prophylaxis of aspiration pneumonitis in patients at high risk during surgery

Dose

For patients with normal renal function: 50 mg I.V.P.B. diluted in at least 25 mL D_5W, NS, or suitable diluent, given over 15 to 20 min at least 1 hr before induction of anesthesia. The drug may be given with or without a similar dose the preceding evening. For patients with impaired renal function, as evidenced by creatinine clearance less than 50 mL/min: single dose only is needed 1 to 4 hr before induction of anesthesia.

Alternatively, 150 mg ranitidine orally may be substituted for 50 mg I.V.P.B. When given orally, however, it is recommended to be given 2 hr preinduction.

Children 2 to 18 years: 0.1 to 0.8 mg/kg/dose I.V.P.B. at least 1 hr before induction infused over at least 5 min. Dilute to concentration of 0.5 to 2.5 mg/mL.

Dosage forms: 150-mg tablets; Parenteral injection: 25 mg/mL in 2-mL or 10-mL multidose vials.

Onset and Duration

Onset: Mean gastric acid concentration significantly decreases 1 hr after I.V. infusion. Duration: Gastric acid inhibitory effects persist 8 to 12 hr. Elimination $t_{1/2}$: 2 to 3 hr.

Adverse Effects

Headache (1.8%), fatigue, dizziness, and mild gastrointestinal disturbances are the most frequent: Reversible hepatitis and potential hepatotoxicity have been reported infrequently. Reversible leukopenia, thrombocytopenia, granulocytopenia, and aplastic anemia have been reported rarely. Bradydysrhythmias and hypotension may be associated with rapid I.V. infusion.

Precautions and Contraindications

Use with caution in patients with hypersensitivity to ranitidine or other H_2-receptor antagonists. Caution is suggested in patients with hepatic insufficiency.

Anesthetic Considerations

Useful for gastric preparation in high-risk aspiration-prone patients. Do not use in non–high-risk patients.

PART 3 **Drugs**

Name

Rapacuronium (Raplon)

Classification

Nondepolarizing neuromuscular blocking agent

Indications

Tracheal intubation and intraoperative skeletal muscle relaxation; in critical care to facilitate mechanical ventilation.

Dose

Adults: 1.5 mg/kg for intubation. Children: 2 to 5 mg/kg for intubation.

Onset and Duration

Onset: 45 to 90 sec. Duration: 15 to 30 min.

Adverse Effects

Adverse effects may include hypotension, tachycardia, and prolongation in patients with renal disease. Dose-related histamine release.

Precautions and Contraindications

Use is contraindicated in patients known to have hypersensitivity to rapacuronium. Proper airway maintenance capabilities must be ensured before administration.

Anesthetic Considerations

Considered the most rapid-acting nondepolarizing muscle relaxant. Useful for rapid sequence induction in adults and children. Dose-related tachycardia and histamine release occur in a small number of patients.

Name

Remifentanil (Ultiva)

Classification

Opiate analgesic, μ-receptor agonist

Indications

Perioperative analgesia

Dose

Infusion only: Induction: 0.5 to 1 μg/kg/min; Maintenance: 0.05 to 0.8 μg/kg/min; Postoperative constipation in postanesthesia care unit: 0.025 to 0.2 μg/kg/min.

Dosage forms: 1 mg powder in 3-mL vial; 2 mg powder in 5-mL vial; 5 mg powder in 10-mL vial.

Supplemental bolus of 0.05 μg/kg may be given during induction and maintenance. Supplemental bolus is not recommended postoperatively because of risk of apnea or significant respiratory depression. Changes in infusion rate take 2 to 5 min for clinical response to change.

Onset and Duration

Onset: 1 to 5 min. Duration: Continuous infusion effect ceases 5 to 15 min after infusion is stopped.

Adverse Effects

Adverse effects are similar to those of other opiate agonists and include nausea, vomiting, hypotension, bradycardia, respiratory depression, apnea, muscle rigidity, and pruritus.

Precautions and Contraindications

Oxygen saturation should be continuously monitored throughout administration. Resuscitative and airway management equipment must be immediately available. Remifentanil should not be mixed with lactated Ringer's injection or lactated Ringer's 15% dextrose but can be coadministered with these solutions in a freely running I.V. line. Do not run remifentanil in the same line with blood, because this drug is metabolized by esterase enzymes. The I.V. line should be cleared after discontinuation to prevent inadvertent administration. Remifentanil is contraindicated for epidural or intrathecal administration due to glycine in the vehicle formulation.

Anesthetic Considerations

The effects of remifentanil rapidly dissipate after discontinuation of the infusion, so preparation for postoperative care may include longer-acting opiates or nonsteroidal anti-inflammatory agents. Because remifentanil is metabolized by nonspecific esterases, no change in kinetics has been noted in patients with cholinesterase deficiencies or renal or hepatic disease. Normal kinetics were noted in pediatric, geriatric, and obese patients.

Name

Ritodrine HCl (Yutopar)

Classification

β_2-adrenergic agonist, tocolytic agent, sympathomimetic

Indications

Management of preterm labor (tocolysis)

Dose

Infusion: Prepare in D_5W if clinically appropriate or in NaCl 0.9% I.V. solution of 0.3 mg/mL. Start at 0.1 mg/min (20 mL/hr at this concentration) and slowly increase by 0.05 mg/min every 10 to 15 min, up to 0.35 mg/min. Continue infusion for at least 12 hr after cessation of uterine contractions at maximum rate achieved.

P.O.: Start before discontinuation of the I.V. infusion at 10 mg every 2 hr for 24 hr, then 10 to 20 mg every 4 to 6 hr (maximum dose: 120 mg/d).

PART 3 Drugs

Dosage forms: Tablet: 10 mg; Injection: 10 mg/mL in 5-mL ampules and vials; Injection: 15 mg/mL in 10-mL vials and 10-mL pre-filled syringe; Solution for I.V. infusion: 150 mg in D_5W 500 mL (0.3 mg/mL).

Onset and Duration

Onset: I.V.: immediate; P.O.: 40 to 60 min. Duration: I.V.: 3 to 6 hr.

Adverse Effects

β_1 agonist effects are common and include tachycardia, arrhythmias, hypertension, hyperventilation, pulmonary edema, tremors, headache, anxiety, nausea, vomiting and diarrhea, and hyperglycemia. Reactive hypoglycemia may occur in the postpartum infant.

Precautions and Contraindications

Pulmonary edema is common with overhydration, so fluid intake should be closely monitored, especially in patients taking corticosteroids. Monitor glucose and electrolyte levels. Ritodrine is contraindicated before 20 weeks of pregnancy and in preeclampsia, eclampsia, intrauterine fetal death or fetal distress, uncontrolled maternal diabetes, maternal hyperthyroidism and hypertension, and placental detachment. Concern surrounds the clinical benefits related to perinatal morbidity and mortality.

Anesthetic Considerations

Patients may experience wide swings in vital signs secondary to β-receptor stimulation. Bradycardia and hypotension may occur after cessation of therapy. Glucose, insulin, and potassium levels are commonly altered during therapy and should be evaluated. Mild hypokalemia is usually not treated. Additive hypertension and tachycardia occur when ritodrine is given with other sympathomimetics. Adverse effects may be antagonized by β-blocking agents.

Name

Rocuronium (Zemuron)

Classification

Nondepolarizing neuromuscular blocking agent

Indications

Tracheal intubation and intraoperative skeletal muscle relaxation; in critical care to facilitate mechanical ventilation

Dose

Adults and children: intubation: 0.6 mg/kg. Maintenance: Adults: 0.1 to 0.2 mg/kg; Children: 0.08 to 0.12 mg/kg I.V.

Onset and Duration

Onset: 60 to 90 seconds with intubating doses of 3 to 5 times ED_{95} (0.9 to 1.5 mg/kg); $ED_{95} = 0.3$ mg/kg. Duration: 30 to 120 min, depending on dose.

Adverse Effects

Adverse reactions are rare. A prolonged effect occurs in patients with hepatic disease.

Precautions and Contraindications

Rocuronium is contraindicated in patients known to have hypersensitivity to rocuronium. Proper airway maintenance capabilities must be ensured before administration.

Anesthetic Considerations

Use of inhalation agents, antibiotics, and magnesium may prolong the duration of action. Many clinicians consider it the agent of choice for nondepolarizing rapid sequence induction and when intubating doses are used. No significant cardiac or histamine-releasing effects occur with clinical doses of rocuronium.

Name

Ropivacaine HCl (Naropin)

Classification

Amide-type local anesthetic

Indications

Regional anesthesia: epidural, peripheral nerve block. Local infiltration.

Dose

Epidural: 75 to 250 mg (0.2% to 0.5% solution); Obstetrics: less than 150 mg (0.5% solution). Infiltration: less than 200 mg (0.2% to 0.5% solution). Peripheral nerve block: less than 275 mg (0.5% solution). Spinal doses have not been established. Do not exceed 770 mg in 24 hours.

Onset and Duration

Onset: Epidural: 5 to 13 min, Obstetrics: 11 to 26 min. Infiltration: 1 to 5 min. Peripheral nerve block: 10 to 45 min. Duration: Epidural: 3 to 5 hr, Obstetrics: 1.7 to 3.2 hr. Infiltration: 2 to 6 hrs. Peripheral nerve block: 3.7 to 8.7 hr.

Adverse Effects

Hypotension, nausea, vomiting, bradycardia, parasthesia, fetal bradycardia, back pain, chills, fever, headache, pain, dizziness, pruritis, urinary retention, arrhythmias, seizures, high spinal

Precautions and Contraindications

Reduce doses in debilitated, elderly, or acutely ill patients, and in children. Use with caution in patients with hypotension, hypovolemia, or heart block. Ropivacaine is not recommended for children under

12 years of age. It is not for use in paracervical/retrobulbar/intravenous regional/subarachnoid blocks. Ropivacaine contraindicated in patients with known hypersensitivity to amide-type local anesthetics.

Anesthetic Considerations

Considerations are similar to bupivacaine but with less depth and duration of the motor blockade. Use with epinephrine has no effect on onset, duration or systemic absorption. Undergoes liver and renal elimination.

Name

Salmeterol Xinafoate (Serevent)

Classification

β_2-adrenergic agonist, antiasthmatic, bronchodilator

Indications

Maintenance treatment of asthma and COPD; prevention of bronchospasm

Dose

Powder: one inhalation (50 μg) b.i.d. (morning and evening 12 hr apart); Aerosol: two inhalations (42 μg) b.i.d. (morning and evening 12 hr apart).

Onset and Duration

Asthma maintenance: Onset to produce bronchodilation: 10 to 20 min. Duration: 12 hr.

COPD: Onset to bronchodilation: within 30 min. Duration: up to 12 hr.

Adverse Effects

Paradoxical bronchospasm, sympathomimetic cardiovascular effects, ventricular arrhythmias, ECG changes (flattening of the T wave, prolonged QT interval, ST depression), laryngospasm, stridor, excitement, aggravation of diabetes mellitus and ketoacidosis

Precautions and Contraindications

Use with caution in patients with hypersensitivity to salmeterol, acute deteriorating asthma, coronary insufficiency, arrhythmias, hypertension, convulsive disorders, or thryrotoxicosis. Safety of salmeterol during pregnancy and in children has not been established. Use with extreme caution in patients taking MAOIs or tricyclics—cardiovascular sympathomimetic effects may be potentiated under these circumstances.

Anesthetic Considerations

Use of β-antagonists may block effects and predispose patients to bronchospasm. Dosing intervals of less than 12 hr may induce bronchospasm.

Name

Scopolamine (Transderm Scop)

Classification

Competitive acetylcholine antagonist at muscarinic receptor

Indications

Prevention and treatment of nausea and vomiting induced by motion (motion sickness), premedication, amnesia, sedation, or vagolysis. Greater sedation, amnesia, antisialogogue and ocular effects than atropine with lesser effects on heart, bronchial smooth muscle, and gastrointestinal tract. Widely used premedicant for cardiac patients in combination with morphine and a major tranquilizer.

Dose

P.O.: 0.4 to 1.2 mg; Usual adult I.M., I.V., or SQ dose: 0.3 to 0.65 mg 30 to 80 min before induction. Transderm patch: 1.5 mg/2.5 cm^2; delivers 0.5 mg/72 hr; apply to postauricular skin.

Children: 0.006 mg/kg or 0.2 mg/m^2 I.M. or I.V. Maximum dose: 0.3 mg.

Dosage forms: 0.3, 0.4, 0.86, 1 mg/mL parenteral injection; Transderm patch: 1.5 mg/2.5 cm^2.

Onset and Duration

Onset: After I.V. administration: almost immediate; After P.O. or I.M. administration: about 30 min. Duration: After I.V. administration: 30 to 60 min; After I.M. administration: 4 to 6 hr. Transdermal systems are designed to provide an antiemetic effect within 4 hr of application with a duration of up to 72 hr.

Adverse Effects

Hallucinations, delirium, and coma may occur in central anticholinergic syndrome. Treatment is with pyridostigmine, 15 to 60 mg/kg. Other effects include paradoxical bradycardia in low doses, mydriasis, blurred vision, tachycardia, drowsiness, restlessness, confusion, anaphylaxis, dry nose and mouth, constipation, urinary hesitancy, retention, increased intraocular pressure, decreased sweating. Children and elderly are more susceptible to adverse effects.

Precautions and Contraindications

Use with caution when tachycardia would be harmful (i.e., thyrotoxicosis, pheochromocytoma, coronary artery disease). Avoid using scopolomine in patients in hyperpyrexial states because it inhibits sweating. Use with caution in patients with hepatic or renal disease, congestive heart failure, chronic pulmonary disease (because a reduction in bronchial secretions may lead to formation of bronchial plugs), hiatal hernia, gastroesophageal reflux, gastrointestinal infections, or ulcerative colitis. Scopolamine is contraindicated in patients with acute-angle glaucoma, obstructive disease of the gastrointestinal tract, obstructive uropathy, intestinal atony, or acute hemorrhage when cardiovascular status is unstable.

Anesthetic Considerations

Scopolamine potentiates the sedative effects of narcotics, benzodi-azepines, anticholinergics, antihistamines, and volatile anesthetics.

Name

Sodium Citrate (Bicitra)

Classification

Nonparticulate neutralizing buffer

Indications

Prophylaxis of aspiration pneumonitis during anesthesia; metabolizes to sodium bicarbonate and thus acts as systemic alkalinizer. When given within 60 minutes of surgery, sodium citrate is effective in raising the gastric pH above 2.5 in most patients. Theoretically, this decreases the risk of pulmonary damage secondary to aspiration of gastric contents; however, this remains controversial.

Dose

Adults: 15 mL diluted in 15 mL water as a single dose; Children: 5 to 15 mL diluted in 5 to 15 mL water as a single dose, or 1 mEq/kg as a single dose.

Dosage forms: Sodium citrate dihydrate 500 mg (321.5 mg of citrate) per 5 mL and citric acid monohydrate 334 mg per 5 mL. Each 1 mL contains 1 mEq sodium and 1 mEq citrate.

Onset and Duration

Onset: 2 to 10 min. Duration 60 to 90 min. Maximally effective when given less than 60 min preoperatively.

Adverse Effects

Saline laxative effect results when sodium citrate is given orally; metabolic alkalosis occurs in large doses in patients with renal dysfunction.

Precautions and Contraindications

Sodium citrate is contraindicated in patients with severe renal impairment with oliguria, azotemia, or anuria. It is also contraindicated in patients with Addison's disease, heat cramps, acute dehydration, adynamic episodica hereditaria, or severe myocardial disease.

Anesthetic Considerations

Useful for patients at a high risk for aspirations.

Name

Somatostatin (Zecnil)

Classification

Synthetic somatostatin; growth hormone release-inhibiting factor; also inhibits glucagon, insulin, secretin, gastrin, and thyroid-stimulating hormone

Indications

Prophylaxis in preoperative management of patients with carcinoid syndrome and treatment of hypotensive episodes associated with surgical manipulation of carcinoid tumor, gastrointestinal bleeding, malignant diarrhea, enterocutaneous and pancreatic fistulas, and short bowel syndrome; epidural somatostatin is effective in treating postoperative pain; intrathecal and intraventricular somatostatin were employed for terminal cancer pain in limited studies.

Dose

Adults: Continuous infusion required to sustain therapeutic effects; Usual infusion rate; 250 µg/hr, with or without initial 250-µg bolus. Dilute 3 mg somatostatin in 50 mL D_5W or NS and infuse continuously over 12 hr (250 µg/hr) on a syringe pump. (Octreotide [Sandostatin], a long-acting analogue of somatostatin, may also be used. Initial dose is 50 µg S.Q., but I.V. injection can be used during emergency.) Dosage forms: Somatostatin (Zecnil): 3 mg lyophilized ampules; Octreotide (Sandostatin): 0.1, 0.05, 0.5 mg/mL injection.

Somatostatin is currently designated an "orphan drug" by the Food and Drug Administration.

Onset and Duration

Onset: 5 to 10 min after initiation of infusion. Duration: effects decrease rapidly after discontinuance of infusion to baseline in 1 hr; Plasma $t_{1/2}$: 1 to 3 min. (Half-life of octreotide: After I.V.: 45; After S.Q.: 80 min).

Adverse Effects

Nausea, vomiting, diarrhea, and abdominal cramps may occur during infusion. Glucose intolerance in nondiabetic patients and reduced insulin requirements in insulin-dependent diabetics have been noted. Less frequent effects include arrhythmias and hyponatremia.

Precautions and Contraindications

Use with caution in patients with diabetes. Rebound hypersecretion of growth hormone and other hormones usually occurs after infusion is discontinued. Monitor blood glucose levels during therapy. Rebound fistula output is also noted in patients with enterocutaneous fistulas. Somatostatin is contraindicated in patients with previous hypersensitivity to the drug or with octreotide.

Anesthetic Considerations

None

Name

Sotalol Hydrochloride (Betapace, Sotagard)

Classification

Antiarrhythmic, non-selective β-adrenergic blocking agent

PART 3 **Drugs**

Indications

Life-threatening ventricular arrhythmias (i.e. sustained ventricular tachycardia); Torsade de pointes or VT/VF from NSVT or SVT arrhythmias; atrial fibrillation

Dose

Treatment of sustained V-Tach: Adults: Initially, 80 mg P.O. b.i.d. (maximum dose: 320 mg per day, given in two divided doses.

Conversion and maintenance of sinus rhythm in patients with atrial fibrillation: Adults: 80 to 160 mg P.O. b.i.d.; **Children: Safety and efficacy have not been established.**

Onset and Duration

Onset of action following oral administration: approximately 1 hr; peaks in 2.5 to 4 hr. Low lipid solubility; does not cross the blood-brain barrier. Duration: 4 to 6 hr.

Adverse Effects

Fatigue, bradycardia, dyspnea, angina, palpitations, dizziness, nausea and vomiting, asthenia, light headedness, elevated LFT's.

Overdosage rarely results in death. Treat by hemodialysis due to low protein binding.

Precautions and Contraindications

Patients with impaired renal function require dosage reductions. Sotalol is contraindicated in patients with bronchial asthma, bronchitis, sinus bradycardia, second- and third-degree AV block (may use if patient has functioning pacemaker), uncontrolled CHF, or cardiogenic shock.

Safety and efficacy has not been established in children.

Adequate evaluation for use during pregnancy has not been established.

Anesthetic Considerations

Use with caution when using Lidocaine or calcium-channel blockers because the additive electrophysiologic effect may cause a proarrhythmic event.

Name

Succinylcholine (Anectine, Quelicin, others)

Classification

Depolarizing skeletal muscle relaxant

Indications

Surgical muscle relaxation for short procedures; facilitates endotracheal intubation

Dose

Aduts: I.V.: 1 to 1.5 mg/kg (maximum: 150 total dose). Children: I.V.:

1.0 to 2.0 mg/kg; I.M.: 2 to 4 mg/kg. Pretreat with atropine due to incidence of bradycardia. Dosage form: Injection: 20 mg/mL; Powder for infusion: 500 mg (mix in 500 mL for 1 mg/mL solution).

Onset and Duration
Onset: immediate. Duration: 5 to 10 min.

Adverse Effects
Numerous side effects have been reported that relate to the skeletal muscle depolarizing action of the drug, including hyperkalemia, postoperative muscle pain, increased gastric pressure, and increased intraocular pressure. Numerous cardiac arrhythmias have been reported, including sudden cardiac arrest and bradycardia with repeat dosing or with any dose in children. Prolonged paralysis and inadequate recovery may occur with infusion doses. Masseter muscle spasm may be a premonitory sign of malignant hyperthermia along with sudden unexplained tachycardia or an abrupt increase in carbon dioxide elimination. (See Appendix 10 for malignant hyperthermia protocol.)

Precautions and Contraindications; Anesthetic Considerations
Succinylcholine should not be used for routine intubation in children younger than 12 years of age due to reports of sudden cardiac arrest in children with undiagnosed Duchenne's muscular dystrophy and with muscle disorders. Succinylcholine is contraindicated in patients with malignant hyperthermia; genetic variants of plasma cholinesterase or cholinesterase deficiencies; myopathies associated with elevated creatine phosphokinase values; muscle disorders or muscular dystrophies; acute narrow-angle glaucoma; severe muscle trauma or muscle wasting; neurologic injury (ie: paraplegia, quadriplegia, spinal cord injury, or cerebrovascular accident); hyperkalemia; severe sepsis; electrolyte imbalances; or third degree burns over more than 25% total body surface;. Repeated doses at short intervals (less than 5 min) are associated with bradycardia.

Name
Sufentanil Citrate (Sufenta)

Classification
Opioid agonist; produces analgesia and anesthesia

Indications
Perioperative analgesia

Dose
Analgesia: I.V./I.M.: 0.2 to 0.6 µg/kg. Induction: I.V.: 2 to 10 µg/kg. Infusion: 0.01 to 0.05 µg/kg/min. Epidural: bolus: 0.2 to 0.6 µg/kg; Infusion: 5 to 30 µg/hr (0.2 to 0.6 µg/kg/hr). Spinal: 0.02 to 0.08 µg/kg.

Onset and Duration
Onset: I.V.: immediate; epidural and spinal: 4 to 10 min. Duration: I.V.:

20 to 45 min; I.M.: 2 to 4 hr; Epidural and spinal: 4 to 8 hr.

Adverse Effects

Possible effects include: hypotension, bradycardia, respiratory depression, apnea, dizziness, sedation, euphoria, dysphoria, anxiety, nausea, vomiting, delayed gastric emptying, biliary tract spasm, muscle rigidity

Precautions and Contraindications

Reduce dose in elderly, hypovolemic, or high-risk patients and in patients taking sedatives or other narcotics. Sufentanil crosses the placental barrier; if used during labor depression of respiration in the neonate may result.

Anesthetic Considerations

The narcotic effect of sufentanil is reversed with naloxone (I.V.: 0.2 to 0.4 mg). Duration of reversal may be shorter than the duration of the narcotic effect. The circulatory and ventilatory depressant effects of sufentanil are potentiated by other narcotics, sedatives, nitrus oxide, and volatile anesthetics; its ventilatory depressant effects are potientiated by monoamine oxidase inhibitors, phenothiazines and tricyclic antidepressants. Analgesia is enhanced by α_2 agonists. The skeletal muscle rigidity associated with higher doses of sufentanil is sufficient to interfere with ventilation. Increased incidences of bradycardia occur with the additional use of vecuronium.

Name

Terbutaline sulfate (Brethine, Brethaire, Bricanyl)

Classification

β_2-adrenergic agonist, bronchodilator

Indications

Bronchodilator for treatment of asthma

Dose

Bronchodilator: SQ: 0.25 mg (may repeat in 15 to 30 min. Maximum dose: 0.5 mg in 4 to 6 hr). Inhalation: 2 breaths separated by 60 sec every 4 to 6 hr; P.O.: 5 mg t.i.d. (2.5 to 5 mg, every 6 hr; maximum dose: 15 mg/day.) Children less than 12 years old: P.O.: 0.05 mg/kg/dose t.i.d. (maximum dose: 0.15 mg/kg/dose or 5 mg day); S.Q.: 5 to 10 µg/kg/dose every 20 min for 3 doses. Dosage forms: Injection: 1 mg/mL (1 mL); Tablet: 2.5 mg, 5 mg.

Onset and Duration

Onset: SQ: 30 to 60 min; P.O.: 2 to 3 hr; Inhalation: 1 to 2 hr. Duration: SQ: 1 to 4 hr; P.O.: 4 to 8 hr; Inhalation: 2 to 6 hr.

Adverse Effects

Adverse effects are similar to those of other β-agonists and include hypertension, tachycardia, arrhythmias, tremors, dizziness, headache, nausea, vomiting, gastrointestinal upset, hypokalemia, and hyperglycemia.

Precautions and Contraindications

Use with caution in patients with hypertension, ischemic heart disease, arrhythmias, congestive heart failure, diabetes mellitus, hyperthyroidism, or seizures. Action of terbutaline is antagonized by β-adrenergic blocking agents. Tolerance to terbutaline develops with repeated use.

Anesthetic Considerations

Patients may experience wide swings in vital signs secondary to β-receptor stimulation. Bradycardia and hypotension may occur after cessation of therapy. Glucose, insulin, and potassium levels are commonly altered during therapy and should be evaluated. Mild hypokalemia is usually not treated. Additive hypertension and tachycardia occur when terbutaline is given with other sympathomimetics. Adverse effects of terbutaline may be antagonized by β-blocking agents.

Name

Tetracaine HCl (Pontocaine)

Classification

Ester-type local anesthetic

Indications

Local, spinal, and topical anesthesia

Dose

Spinal: 2 to 20 mg adjusted to height (rarely greater than 15 mg). Decrease usual dose in pregnant women. Dilute with equal volume of sterile dextrose 10% (hyperbaric) to more easily control height. Apply topical spray 2% solution in short spurts of less than 2 sec. Maximum safe dose: 1.5 mg/kg. Inject slowly—not greater than 1 mL/5 sec. Pediatric doses have not been established. Dosage forms: Injection: 1% (2 mL) for spinal anesthesia; Ointment (ophthalmic): 0.5% (3.5 g); Solution (ophthalmic): 0.5% (15 mL); Topical: 2% (30 mL, 118 mL).

Onset and Duration

Onset: Spinal: 5 to 10 min; Fixing time: 20 to 30 min. Duration: 1 to 3 hr, possibly longer if 10 to 20 mg of epinephrine is added to spinal bolus.

Adverse Effects

With spinal use: hypotension, bradycardia, respiratory depression or apnea, high or total spinal with paralysis, infection secondary to spinal needle placement, headache

Precautions and Contraindications

Avoid the use of tetracaine in patients allergic to ester-type local anesthetics (ie: procaine, chloroprocaine, and cocaine). Tetracaine contains *para*-aminobenzoic acid (PABA), so avoid its use in patients with an allergy to this sunscreen. Tetracaine is reserved for spinal or topical anesthesia only because other local anesthetic drugs are safer for injection or infiltration. Seizures may occur with toxic doses. Monitor vital signs carefully during the initial administration. Tetracaine is not for ocular use.

Anesthetic Considerations

Tetracaine is a long-standing agent for spinal anesthesia. Use amide local anesthetics such as lidocaine or bupivacaine if an allergy to tetracaine is suspected. Watch for high spinal level in patients during use of this drug. Produces a stronger motor block and more relaxation than bupivacaine. Adequate hydration during use will minimize hypotension. Reduce the dose in morbidly obese, obstetric, or elderly patients as well as in patients with increased abdominal pressure.

Name

Thiamylal (Surital)

Classification

Barbiturate; ultra short-acting intravenous sedative-hypnotic; anesthesia-inducing agent

Indications

Induction agent for general anesthesia; sole anesthetic for short surgical procedures.

Dose

Induction: 3 to 5 mg/kg of 2.5% solution intravenously. Dosage form: Injection: Powder: dilute to 10 mg/mL.

Onset and Duration

Onset: immediate. Duration: 10 to 30 min depending on dose.

Adverse Effects

Possible effects include: hypotension, respiratory depression, apnea, laryngospasm, bradycardia

Precautions and Contraindications

Do not use thiamylal in patients with allergies to any barbiturate or with a history of porphyria. Reduce the dose or possibly avoid using thiamylal in elderly patients and in patients with severe cardiovascular disease, shock, or asthma.

Anesthetic Considerations

Actions of thiamylal are nearly identical to those of thiopental. Use with caution in patients with cardiorespiratory compromise or moderate to severe multiorgan failure. Reduce the dose in elderly patients.

Name
Thiopental sodium (Pentothal)

Classification
Ultra short-acting barbiturate

Indications
Induction of anesthesia or hypnosis; treatment of seizures caused by inhalation or local anesthetics

Dose
Induction: I.V.: 3 to 5 mg/kg. Maintenance: I.V.: 50 to 100 mg whenever patient moves. Seizures: 75 to 125 mg (3 to 5 mL of 2.5% solution) for seizures following anesthesia; 125 to 250 mg over a 10-min period for seizures due to a local anesthetic. Dosage forms: Injection: 250-mg, 400-mg, 500-mg syringes; also supplied in vials with diluent, 500 mg, 1 g; also supplied in kits with 1, 2.5, 5 g. Rectal suspension: 400 mg/g.

Onset and Duration
Onset: 5 to 20 sec. Duration: 20 to 30 min; Plasma $t_{1/2}$: 3 min; Elimination $t_{1/2}$: 9 hr.

Adverse Effects
Inadequate doses may increase sensitivity to pain. Profound dose-dependent depression of respiration. Extravascular injection may cause severe pain and tissue necrosis.

Precautions and Contraindications
Use with caution in patients that are lactating; in asthmatic patients, or in patients with hypersensitivity to barbiturates. Thiopental is contraindicated in variegate porphyria and acute intermittent porphyria.

Anesthetic Considerations
Thiopental solutions should be freshly prepared; discard then after 24 hours or if a precipitate is present. The effect of thiopental is potentiated by the injection of contrast media. The use of thiopental reduces the maximum allowable concentration of inhalation anesthetics. Do not mix thiopental with other drugs.

Name
Torsemide (Demadex, Presaril)

Classification
Loop diuretic

Indications
Treatment of edema as a result of cardiac, hepatic, or renal dysfunction; hypertension

Dose

Congestive heart failure: 10 to 20 mg oral or IV once daily; may titrate to therapeutic effect. Safety has not been established for doses exceeding 200 mg per day.

Renal dysfunction: 20 mg oral or IV once daily; may titrate to effect. Safety has not been established in does exceeding 200 mg per day.

Hypertension: 5 mg once daily; increase to 10 mg as needed, then add another antihypertensive medication if desired effect has not been achieved.

Onset and Duration

Onset: IV: 10 min; peaks within 1 to 2 hr. Duration: diuresis for all routes lasts 6 to 8 hr.

Adverse Effects

Dizziness, headache, nausea, vomiting, hyperglycemia, and polyuria. Additional effects include: hyperuricemia, electrolyte/volume depletions, esophageal bleeding, salycylate toxicity, arrhythmias, dyspepsia

Precautions and Contraindications

Use with caution in patients with hypersensitivity to this drug or in patients with sulfonylureas, anuria, and hepatic dysfunction. Torsemide can reduce lithium elimination. Safety is not established during pregnancy or in children.

Anesthetic Considerations

Patient electrolyte/volume status should be monitored carefully. Electrolyte imbalances may predispose patients on digitalis to toxicity.

Name

Trimethaphan (Arfonad)

Classification

Autonomic ganglion blocking agent; antihypertensive

Indications

Controlled hypotension during surgery; used during neurologic procedures and abdominal aneurysm repair

Dose

1% solution (500 mg in 500 mL); Infuse 0.3 to 2 mg/min and adjust to effect.

Onset and Duration

Onset: immediate. Duration: 5 to 30 min depending on duration of infusion.

Adverse Effects

Hypotension, tachycardia, histamine release, mydriasis, urinary retention, dry mouth

Precautions and Contraindications

Avoid using trimethaphan in asthmatic patients because of frequent histamine release. Excessive hypotension and tachycardia may occur, especially in hypovolemic patients. Avoid using trimethaphan in patients with deficiencies of plasma cholinesterase.

Anesthetic Considerations

Trimethaphan should be used as a supplement for deliberate hypotensive techniques. Tachyphylaxis develops frequently and is minimized by infusing slowly for brief periods. Nitroprusside and nitroglycerin are more commonly used.

Name

Tubocurarine chloride

Classification

Nondepolarizing skeletal muscle relaxer

Indications

Adjunct to general anesthetics to provide adequate muscle relaxation

Dose

Neonates under 1 month: 0.3 mg/kg single dose; Maintenance: 0.15 mg/kg as needed. Children and adults: 0.2 to 0.4 mg/kg single dose; Maintenance: 0.04 to 0.2 mg/kg. Dosage forms: Injection: 3 mg/mL.

Onset and Duration

Onset: less than 2 min. Duration: 25 to 90 min; Elimination: renal, hepatic.

Adverse Effects

Hypotension, bradycardia, arrhythmia, respiratory depression, apnea, inadequate block, prolonged block, rash, urticaria

Precautions and Contraindications

Use with caution in asthmatic patients. Tubocurarine is contraindicated in patients in whom release of histamine is a hazard and in patients with hyperthermia, myasthenia gravis, electrolyte imbalance, or acidosis.

Anesthetic Considerations

Patient response should be monitored with a peripheral nerve stimulator. The effects of tubocurarine can be reversed with anticholinesterase. Pretreatment doses may induce a degree of neuromuscular blockade and cause hyperventilation in some patients.

Name

Vancomycin (Vancocin)

Classification

Antimicrobial agent

PART 3 Drugs

Indications

Treatment of documented or suspected methicillin-resistant *Staphylococcus aureus* or β-lactam–resistant coagulase-negative *Streptococcus*. Treatment of documented or suspected staphylococcal or streptococcal infections in penicillin- or cephalosporin-allergic patients.

Prophylaxis of bacterial endocarditis in high-risk patients (rheumatic heart disease, mitral valve prolapse, valvular heart dysfunction, bioprosthetic and allograft valves) undergoing dental, oral, or upper respiratory procedures and are penicillin or cephalosporin allergic. Prophylaxis in penicillin-allergic patients undergoing gastrointestinal, biliary, or genitourinary tract surgery or instrumentation and are at risk of developing enterococcal endocarditis.

Prophylactic therapy for potential infections related to ventricular-peritoneal shunt, vascular graft, or open-heart surgery in penicillin-allergic patients.

Because vancomycin is not absorbed orally, the only indication for oral vancomycin is pseudomembranous colitis.

Dose

Initial I.V. dosage recommendation: Adults: initial I.V. dose 15 mg/kg, followed by 10 mg/kg every 12 hr in patients with normal renal function. Maximum dose: 3 g/day. Patients with mild renal failure (creatinine clearance less than or equal to 50 mL/min) should receive vancomycin every 24 to 72 hr; patients with moderate renal failure (creatinine clearance of 10 to 50 mL/min) should receive vancomycin every 72 to 240 hr; patients with severe renal failure (creatinine clearance less than 10 mL/min) should receive vancomycin every 240 hr.

Children: Children heavier than 5 kg and older than 7 days postnatal age and younger than 13 years of age: 10 mg/kg every 6 hr. Children older than 13 years of age: dosed as adults.

Peak and trough serum levels should be monitored if therapy extends beyond 24 hr perioperative prophylaxis. Dosage and dosage interval should be adjusted to produce peak levels of 25 to 40 mg/mL and trough levels of 5 to 10 µg/mL.

Dosage forms: Parenteral injection for I.V. use: 500-mg or 1-g vials. Reconstitute sterile powder by adding 10 mL or 20 mL sterile water to 500-mg or 1-g vials, respectively. Reconstituted solution containing 500 mg or 1 g must be further diluted with at least 100 mL or at least 250 mL D_5W or NS, respectively. Infuse I.V.P.B. over 1 to 1.5 h.

Onset and Duration

Onset: 15 to 30 min. Duration: 8 to 12 hr. Half-life varies: 4 to 6 hr reported in patients with normal renal function. Usually given 1 hr before procedure for prophylaxis of endocarditis. Some clinicians suggest the dose should be repeated 8 to 12 hr later in patients with normal renal function, however, the American Heart Association, American Academy of Pediatrics, and the American Dental Association state that a second dose is unnecessary.

Adverse Effects

Red-man syndrome (erythema, pruritus, and rash involving face, neck, upper trunk, and arms), hypertension, and tachycardia are associated with rapid infusion. Ototoxity is associated with prolonged serum concentrations greater than 40 mg/mL. Other effects include chills, fever, neutropenia, thrombocytopenia, agranulocytosis, and phlebitis.

Precautions and Contraindications

Monitor renal-function tests frequently during therapy. Use with caution in patients with renal impairment or in patients receiving other nephrotoxic or ototoxic drugs. Vancomycin is contraindicated in patients with hypersensitivity to the drug. Avoid using vancomycin use in patients with previous hearing loss.

Anesthetic Considerations

Vancomycin potentiation of succinylcholine-induced neuromuscular blockage during vancomycin use has been reported. The drug may increase neuromuscular blockade by nondepolarizing muscle relaxants, whose dose should be titrated.

Name

Vasopressin (Pitressin)

Classification

Antidiuretic hormone

Indications

Treatment of diabetes insipidus; treatment of bleeding esophageal varices and other types of upper gastrointestinal bleeding; control of refractory operative bleeding in intrauterine procedures

Dose

Diabetes insipidus or treatment of abdominal distention in postoperative patients: 5 to 10 U 3 to 4 times daily as needed.
Gastrointestinal hemorrhage: 0.2 to 1 U/min infused I.V. After 12 hr of hemorrhage control, decrease the dose by half and then stop within the next 12 to 24 hr. I.V. nitroglycerin should be infused concomitantly to control side effects.

Locally to operative site: 20 U in 30 mL NS as a gauze soak.

Children: For diabetes insipidus: I.M. or SQ: 2.5 to 5 U every 6 to 8 hr; titrate based on response.

I.V.: 1 to 3 mU/kg/hr

Gastrointestinal bleeding: 0.01 U/kg/min.

Dosage forms: 20 pressor U/mL aqueous injection; must be diluted for I.V. infusion in D_5W or NS to a concentration of 100 to 1000 U/L.

Onset and Duration

Onset: 15 to 30 min. Duration: Antidiuretic action: I.M. or SQ: 2 to 8 hr administration; the pressor effects last 30 to 60 min after I.V. injection. Elimination $t_{1/2}$: 10 to 35 min.

PART 3 Drugs

Adverse Effects

Tremor, sweating, vertigo, water intoxication, hyponatremia, metabolic acidosis, abdominal cramps, nausea, vomiting, urticaria, and anaphylaxis; angina in patients with pre-existing cardiovascular impairment

Precautions and Contraindications

Use with extreme caution in patients who cannot tolerate rapid retention of extracellular water or who have coronary artery disease. Use a central vein, preferably with I.V. infusion, due to the possibility of tissue necrosis with extravasation. Monitor patients with epilepsy, migraine, asthma, or heart failure closely. I.V. administration should be used only for emergency treatment of gastrointestinal hemorrhage. Vasopressin is contraindicated in patients with anaphylaxis or hypersensitivity to the drug and in those with chronic nephritis with nitrogen retention, until reasonable nitrogen blood levels are attained.

Anesthetic Considerations

Patient should be watched carefully following injection for abrupt cardiac changes. Urine monitoring is manditory.

Name

Vecuronium (Norcuron)

Classification

Nondepolarizing muscle relaxant

Indications

Intraoperative muscle relaxation; endotracheal intubation; facilitation of mechanical ventilation in critical care

Dose

I.V.: 0.05 to 0.2 mg/kg for paralysis. Dosage form: Powder for injection 10 mg (5 mL, 10 mL).

Onset and Duration

Onset: 1 to 3 min. Duration: 30 to 90 min.

Adverse Effects

Prolonged paralysis occurs in patients with hepatic disease. Apnea ensues immediately on administration, so appropriate airway management and resuscitative equipment must be immediately available. No significant cardiac effects are noted.

Precautions and Contraindications

Airway equipment must be on hand for intubation and controlled ventilation in conjunction with the use of this drug. Drug duration of action may be prolonged in patients with liver disease.

Anesthetic Considerations

Monitor response with a nerve stimulator to avoid excessive dosing. Long-term infusions in critical care may result in prolonged recovery and an inability to reverse due to active metabolites. Corticosteroid therapy in patients with multiorgan failure may exacerbate this effect.

Name

Verapamil (Isoptin, Calan, others)

Classification

Calcium-channel blocker

Indications

Supraventricular arrhythmias; hypertension; angina

Dose

I.V.: 2.5 to 10 mg slowly; may repeat in 30 to 60 min. P.O.: 120 to 480 mg/day in divided doses. Dosage forms: Injection: 2.5 mg/mL (2 mL); Tablet: 40 mg, 80 mg, 120 mg; Tablet, sustained release: 120 mg, 180 mg, 240 mg.

Onset and Duration

Onset: I.V.: 2 to 5 min; P.O.: 30 to 60 min. Duration: I.V.: 30 min to 2 hr; P.O.: 4 to 12 hr.

Adverse Effects

Hypotension, heart block, tachycardia, or bradycardia; ankle edema and constipation with chronic oral use.

Precautions and Contraindications

Significant hypotension may occur in patients with poor left ventricular function. Verapamil may exacerbate atrioventricular block or Wolff-Parkinson-White syndrome. Additive depression occurs with concomitant use of other cardiac depressants.

Anesthetic Considerations

Titrate slowly, due to significant cardiac depressant effects, which are additive with anesthetics. Diltiazem infusion may be a better option for the treatment of intraoperative atrial arrhythmias. β-blockers are superior for the treatment of sinus tachycardia.

Name

Vitamin K, Phytonadione (Aquamephyton, Mephyton)

Classification

Water-soluble vitamin

Indications

Prevention and treatment of hypoprothrombinemia caused by drug- or anticoagulant-induced vitamin K deficiency or hemorrhagic diseases of the newborn

PART 3 **Drugs**

Dose

I.V. route should be used for emergencies only. Inject slow I.V. only, not greater than 1 mg/min.

Newborn hemorrhage: I.M., SQ prophylaxis: 0.5 to 1 mg within 1 hr of birth. Treat with 1 to 2 mg/day.

Anticoagulant reversal: Infants: 1 to 2 mg every 4 to 8 hr. Adult P.O., I.V., I.M., SQ: 2.5 to 10 mg, may repeat I.V., SQ, I.M. dose every 6 to 8 hr and oral dose in 12 to 48 hr. Dosage forms: Tablet: 5 mg; Injection: 2 mg/mL in 0.5-mL ampule and 10 mg/mL in 1-mL ampule and 2.5- mL, 5-mL vials.

Onset and Duration

Onset: I.V., I.M., SQ: 1 to 3 hr. P.O.: 4 to 12 hr. Duration: 6 to 48 hr depending on dose and route of administration.

Adverse Effects

Severe anaphylaxis may occur with I.V. use. Severe hemolytic anemia has been reported in neonates given large doses (greater than 20 mg).

Precautions and Contraindications

Use intravenous route in emergencies only, due to possibility of severe anaphylaxis. Vitamin K is ineffective in hereditary hypoprothrombinemia or hypoprothrombinemia secondary to severe liver disease.

Anesthetic Considerations

Prothrombin time must be monitored. Transfusion of blood or fresh-frozen plasma may be necessary in severe hemorrhagic states.

Name

Warfarin (Coumadin)

Classification

Anticoagulant; depresses formation of vitamin K–dependent clotting factors (II, VII, IX, X) in the liver

Indications

Treatment or prophylaxis of deep-vein thrombosis or pulmonary thromboembolism; prophylaxis of thromboembolism in patients with atrial fibrillation, undergoing cardioversion of atrial fibrillation, with prosthetic heart valves, after major surgery requiring prolonged immobilization (total knee or hip replacements), and after myocardial infarction in patients who are at high risk of embolism (those with congestive heart failure, atrial fibrillation, previous myocardial infarction, or history of thromboembolism).

Dose

Warfarin dosing is adjusted according to PT. Standardization of PT results among laboratories is accomplished with the use of an International Normalized Ratio equation:

$$INR = (PT_{patient}/PT_{Reference})^{ISI}$$

where ISI is the International Sensitivity Index.

The typical goal INR is 2 to 3, except for patients with prosthetic valves, for whom 2.5 to 3.5 is the desired goal. Commonly, doses of 5 to 10 mg/day are tapered to 2 to 10 mg/day, as indicated by the PT. Consult the pharmacy for institutional guidelines. Multiple drug interactions may increase or decrease response.

Dosage forms: 2-, 2.5-, 5-, 7.5-, 10-mg tabs; 50 mg for parenteral injection with 2-mL diluent.

Onset and Duration

Onset: Antithrombogenic effects may not occur for up to 5 to 7 days after initiation of therapy. Many clinicians recommend that heparin be administered concurrently for 3 to 7 days until the desired PT is achieved. Duration: Single oral dose: 2 to 5 days. Elimination $t_{1/2}$: 0.5 to 3 days.

Adverse Effects

Dose-dependent bleeding, ranging from minor local bleeding or ecchymosis (2% to 10%) to major hemorrhagic complications occasionally resulting in death. Major hemorrhage usually involves gastrointestinal or genitourinary tract, but may involve hepatic, cerebral, or pericardial sites. Minor bleeding can be treated with vitamin K I.M. or I.V. 5 to 10 mg up to 50 mg. Frank bleeding should be treated with administration of fresh whole blood or fresh-frozen plasma (15 mL/kg). Additional effects include: agranulocytosis, leukopenia, thrombocytopenia, necrosis of skin, purple-toe syndrome, neuropathy.

Precautions and Contraindications

Numerous drugs may affect patient response to warfarin, especially hepatic-enzyme inducing or reducing drugs and highly protein-bound drugs; consultation with a pharmacist or physician regarding all drugs is recommended. Use with extreme caution in patients with protein C deficiency, congestive heart failure, carcinoma, liver disease, or poor nutritional state. Warfarin is contraindicated in bleeding patients or in patients with hemorrhagic blood dyscrasias, aneurysms, pericarditis or pericardial effusions, uncontrolled hypertension, recent or contemplated surgery of the eye, brain or spinal cord or any traumatic surgery resulting in large open surfaces, recent or cerebrovascular accident. Renal and hepatic function in these patients should be monitored periodically. PT should be monitored daily initially. After PT is stabilized, these patients should be monitored every 4 to 6 weeks. Warfarin is teratogenic and is contraindicated in pregnancy. Risks of hemorrhage may increase with concomitant use of aspirin, nonsteroidal anti-inflammatory drugs, cimetidine, amiodarone, steroids, chloral hydrate, metronidizole, streptokinase, urokinase, antibiotics, and heparin. Discontinue warfarin promptly in patients with purple-toe syndrome or skin necrosis. Further dosing with warfarin is contraindicated in these patients.

PART 3 Drugs

Anesthetic Considerations

Regional anesthesia is contraindicated. If possible, barbiturates should be avoided as they may decrease warfarin's effect. When emergency surgery is necessary in patients receiving warfarin, fresh-frozen plasma (15 mL/kg) or whole blood can restore coagulation to normal.

Generic Name	Trade Name
adenosine	Adenocard
adrenaline (epinephrine)	
albuterol	Proventil, Ventolin
alfentanil	Alfenta
alprostadil (prostaglandin E_1)	Prostin VR Pediatric
aminocaproic acid	Amicar
aminophylline	Elixophyllin, Theodur, Theolair
amiodarone	Cordarone
amrinone	Inocor
atracurium	Tracrium
atropine	Atropine sulfate, others
bretylium	Bretylol
bumetanide	Bumex
bupivicaine	Marcaine HCl, Sensorcaine
chloroprocaine	Nesacaine
cimetidine	Tagamet
clonidine	Catapres
cocaine	
codeine	
coumarin (warfarin)	Coumadin
cyclosporine	Optimmune, Sandimmune
tubocurarine chloride	Tubocurarine
dantrolene sodium	Dantrium
dexamethasone	Decadron, Hexadrol
desflurane	Suprane
desmopressin	DDAVP
diazepam	Valium
digoxin	Lanoxin
diltiazem	Cardizem
diphenhydramine	Benadryl
dobutamine	Dobutrex
dolasetron	Anzemet
dopamine	Intropin
doxacurium	Nuromax
doxapram	Dopram
edrophonium	Enlon, Tensilon
enalapril	Vasotec IV
enflurane	Ethrane
enoxaparin	Lovenox
ephedrine	
epinephrine (adrenaline)	
esmolol	Brevibloc
ethacrynic acid	Edecrin
etidocaine	Duranest
etomidate	Amidate
famotidine	Pepcid
fenoldopam	Corlopam
fentanyl	Duragesic, Oralet, Sublimaze
flumazenil	Romazicon
furosemide	Lasix
glucagon	
glycopyrrolate	Robinul
granisetron	Kytril
halothane	Fluothane
heparin	

Generic Name	Trade Name
hetastarch	Hespan
hyaluronidase	Wydase
hydralazine	Apresoline
hydrocortisone	Hydrocort, Solu-Cortef
Ibutilide	Covert
insulin	Humulin, Novolin
ipratropium	Atrovent
isoflurane	Forane
isoproterenol	Isuprel
ketamine	Ketalar
ketorolac	Toradol
labetalol	Normodyne, Trandate
lansoprazole	Prevacid
lidocaine	Xylocaine
lorazepam	Ativan
magnesium sulfate	
mannitol	
meperidine	Demerol
mephenteramine	Wyamine Sulfate
mepivacaine	Carbocaine, Polocaine
metaraminol	Aramine
methadone	Dolophine HCl
methohexital	Brevital Sodium
methoxamine	Vasoxyl
methylene blue	Urolene Blue
methylergonovine	Methergine
metoclopramide	Reglan
midazolam	Versed
milrinone	Primacor
mivacurium	Mivacron
morphine	Astramorph PF, Duramorph, Morphine, MS Contin
nalmefene	Revex
naloxone	Narcan
naltrexone	ReVia
neostigmine	Prostigmin
nicardipine	Cardene
nifedipine	Adalat, Procardia
nitroglycerin	Nitro-Bid, Nitro-Dur, Nitrogard, Nitrostat, Nitrol, Nitrocine, Nitroglyn, Nitrodisc, Transderm-Nitro, Tridil
nitroprusside	Nipride
nitrous oxide	
nizatidine	Axid
norepinephrine	Levophed
ondansetron	Zofran
oxytocin	Pitocin, Syntocinon
pancuronium	Pavulon
phentolamine	Regitine
phenylephrine	Neo-Synephrine
phenytoin	Dilantin
physostigmine	Antilirium
pipecuronium	Arduan
prilocaine	Citanest

Generic Name	Trade Name
procainamide	Procan SR, Pronestyl
procaine	Novocain
prochlorperazine	Compazine
promethazine	Phenergan
propofol	Diprivan
propranolol	Inderal
prostaglandin E_1 (alprostadil)	Prostin VR Pediatric
protamine	
pyridostigmine	Mestinon, Regonol
ranitidine	Zantac
rapacuronium	Raplon
remifentanil	Ultiva
ritodrine	Yutopar
ropivacaine	Naropin
rocuronium	Zemuron
salmeterol	Serevent
scopolamine	
sevoflurane	Ultane
sodium citrate	Bicitra, Shohl solution
somatostatin	
sotalol	Betapace
succinylcholine	Anectine, Quelicin
sufentanil	Sufenta
terbutaline	Brethaire, Bricanyl
tetracaine	Pontocaine
thiamylal	Surital
thiopental sodium	Pentothal
torsemide	Demadex
trimethaphan	Arfonad
tropisetron	Novoban
vancomycin	Vancocin
vasopressin	Pitressin Synthetic
vasopressin tannate	Pitressin Tannate
vecuronium	Norcuron
verapamil	Calan, Isoptin
vitamin K (phytonadione)	AquaMEPHYTON, Konakion
warfarin (coumarin)	Coumadin

Pediatric Drug Doses

Drug	Route	Dose
Emergency (Resuscitation) Drugs		
Atropine	IV	0.02 mg/kg per dose (minimum 0.1 mg/dose; maximum 1.0 mg)
Adenosine	IV	100 µg/kg rapid IV bolus, incremental doses 100 µg/kg every 2 min to a maximum of 300 µg/kg or 12 mg in older children
Calcium chloride	IV	10 to 20 mg/kg
Calcium gluconate	IV	50 to 100 mg/kg
Epinephrine	IV	0.01 mg/kg (0.1 mg/kg via ETT)
Lidocaine	IV	1 mg/kg
Sodium bicarbonate	IV	1 mEq/kg per dose
		0.3 × kg × base deficit
Opiates		
Codeine	IM/PO	0.5 to 1 mg/kg
Meperidine	IV	0.2 to 1 mg/kg
	IM	1 to 2 mg/kg
Midazolam	IV	0.05 to 0.1 mg/kg
	IM	0.2 to 0.3 mg/kg
	PO	0.5 to 0.75 mg/kg
Morphine	IV	0.05 to 0.2 mg/kg
	IM/SQ	0.1 to 0.2 mg/kg
Remifentanil	Infusion	0.5 to 1 µg/kg/min (induction)
		0.05 to 0.08 µg/kg/min (maintenance)
Sufentanil	IV	0.1 to 0.5 µg/kg with nitrous oxide; 5 to 10 µg/kg alone
Fentanyl	IV	1 to 5 µg/kg
Induction Agents		
Propofol	IV	2 to 3 mg/kg
Ketamine	IV	1 to 2 mg/kg
	IM	5 to 10 mg/kg
Methohexital	IV	1 to 2 mg/kg
Thiopental	IV	3 to 6 mg/kg
Muscle Relaxants		
Atracurium	IV	0.2 to 0.5 mg/kg
Cisatracurium	IV	0.1 mg/kg
Mivacurium	IV	0.1 to 0.2 mg/kg
Pancuronium	IV	0.04 to 0.15 mg/kg
Succinylcholine	IV	1 to 2 mg/kg
	IM	2.5 to 4 mg/kg
Rocuronium	IV	0.6 to 1 mg/kg (intubation)
		0.08 to 0.12 mg/kg (maintenance)
Rapacuronium	IV	1 to 3 mg/kg
Vecuronium	IV	0.04 to 0.2 mg/kg
Reversal Agents		
Edrophonium	IV	0.5 to 1 mg/kg
Neostigmine	IV	0.05 to 0.07 mg/kg
Pyridostigmine	IV	0.2 mg/kg
Naloxone	IV/IM/SQ	5 to 10 µg/kg
Nalmephene	IV	0.25 µg/kg

NPO Deficit = 2 cc/kg/hr that the patient is NPO prior to surgery

50% of this deficit is replaced within the first hour of surgery with the remaining 50% being replaced over the next 2 hours.

NPO deficits are usually replaced over the first 3 hours of surgery.

Example: What is the NPO deficit for a 50-kg patient who was NPO for 10 hours prior to surgery?

2 cc/kg/hr = $2 \times 50 \times 10 = 1000$ cc
@1st hr, 500 cc will be replaced
  2nd hr, 250 cc will be replaced
  3rd hr, 250 cc will be replaced

Subtract any IVF replacement from the NPO deficit total.

Total fluid maintenance requirements =
Insensible loss + 3rd space loss requirements

Insensible loss = 1 to 2 cc/kg/hr
3rd space loss requirements depend on the type of tissue trauma related to the surgical procedure that is being performed.

Degree of tissue trauma	Fluid requirements
Minimal tissue trauma	
(eg, eye cases, laparscopic cholecystectomy)	1 to 2 cc/kg/hr
Low tissue trauma	
(eg, arthroscopies, ENT)	3 to 4 cc/kg/hr
Moderate tissue trauma	
(eg, total joint replacements)	5 to 6 cc/kg/hr
Severe tissue trauma	
(eg, bowel resection, total hip replacement)	7 to 8 cc/kg/hr
Trauma cases may require	10 to 15 cc/kg/hr

Example: A 50-kg patient is scheduled for a laparoscopic cholecystectomy. What are the maintenance fluid requirements for this patient during surgery?

Insensible loss = 2 cc/kg/hr
3rd space loss = 2 cc/kg/hr
Total fluid replacement requirements = insensible loss + 3rd space loss
                                requirements
                              = 2 cc/kg/hr + 2 cc/kg/hr
                              = 4 cc/kg/hr $\times$ 50 kg
                              = 200 cc/hr

Estimating maintenance fluid requirements for children

Weight (kg)	Fluid requirements
For the first 10 kg	4 cc/kg/hr
For the next 10 kg	add 2 cc/kg/hr
For each kg > 20 kg total	add 1 cc/kg/hr

Example: What are the maintenance fluid requirements for a 25-kg child?

10 kg = 4 cc/kg/hr = 40 cc/hr
10 kg = 2 cc/kg/hr = 20 cc/hr
 5 kg = 5 cc/kg/hr = 5 cc/hr
_____
25 kg   = 65 cc/hr

Composition of Crystalloid Solutions

Solution	Tonicity	Na+ (meq/L)	Cl- (meq/L)	K+ (meq/L)	Ca²⁺ (meq/L)	Mg²⁺ (meq/L)	Glucose (g/L)	Lactate (meq/L)	HCO₃⁻ (meq/L)	Acetate (meq/L)	Plasmalyte (meq/L)
D₅W	Hypo (253)						50				
0.9 NS	Iso (308)	154	154								
D₅ ¼ NS	Iso (355)	38.5	38.5				50				
D₅ ½ NS	Hyper (432)	77	77				50				
D₅ NS	Hyper (586)	154	154				50				
LR	Iso (273)	130	109	4	3			28			
D₅ LR	Hyper (525)	130	109	4	3		50				
3% NS	Hyper (1026)	513	513								
5% NS	Hyper (1710)	855	855								
7.5% NaHCO₃	Hyper (1786)	893							893		
Plasmalyte	Iso (294)	140	98	5		3				27	23

Colloid Solutions

Albumin

Natural blood colloid

Available as a 5% or 25% solution
  5% is used w/hypovolemic
  25% is used w/fluid restricted

Derived from pooled human blood serum or plasma, and pasteurized

No antibody, blood group, or Rh concerns

Allergic reactions are usually mild
  Urticaria, chills, fever, decreased BP

Doesn't alter blood coaguability

Not filtered by the kidneys

Hespan

Synthetic colloid

Available as a 6% solution

Average molecular weight = 450,000
  small molecules are eliminated by the kidney
  and large molecules must be first broken down
  by amylase

Duration = 24 to 36 hr

Dose: 500 cc/day, not to exceed 1500 cc/day or
  20 cc/kg

Doses > 20 cc/kg Hespan, hemostasis is a
  concern

Contraindicated in patients w/pre-existing bleeding
  problems

No antibody, blood group, or Rh concerns

Allergic reactions are rare

Dextran

Synthetic colloid

2 types:

- Dextran-40 (Rheomacrodex)
  low molecular weight = 40,000
  greater H_2O binding excreted
  at a more rapid rate
    50% is excreted in 3 hr
    60% is excreted in 6 hr
    75% is excreted in 24 hr

- Dextran-70
  high molecular weight = 70,000
  less H_2O binding excreted slowly
    50% is excreted after 24 hr

Contraindicated in renal and heart patients

Anaphylactic reactions are more
  common w/Dextran-70

Promit is used for pre-treatment

0.3 cc/kg of 15 g/dL IVP over 1 min
  15 min before the transfusion starts

Action: binds IgG sites that react to
  Dextran; stabilizes masts cells and
  basophils that decrease histamine release

Notify blood bank if used, may interfere
  w/crossmatch

Decreases blood viscosity, platelet aggregation,
  and coagulation factors VIII, X, and IX

Blood Therapy

Average Blood Volumes

Age	Blood Volume
Premature neonate	95 cc/kg
Full-term neonate	85 cc/kg
Infants 3 to 12 months	80 cc/kg
Over 12 months	70 cc/kg
Adult male	75 cc/kg
Adult female	65 cc/kg

Estimation of Blood Loss Requirements

Before surgery is to take place, calculate: patient's estimated blood volume (EBV)
20% and 30% blood loss
allowable blood loss (ABL)

EBV = average blood volume $\times$ wt (kg)

Example: calculate the EBV of a 50-kg adult female
65 cc $\times$ 50 kg = 3250 cc

20% blood loss = 0.2 $\times$ EBV
30% blood loss = 0.3 $\times$ EBV

Example: calculate 20% and 30% blood loss for a 50-kg female
0.2 $\times$ 3250 = 650 cc blood loss
0.3 $\times$ 3250 = 975 cc blood loss

ABL is the amount blood that is lost before replacement is needed.

$$ABL = \frac{EBV \times (Hi - Hf)}{Hi}$$

Hi: initial Hct (%)
Hf: final lowest acceptable
= Hi $-$ (30% $\times$ Hi)

Example: calculate the ABL for a 50 kg female w/Hct of 45%

$$ABL = \frac{3250 \times (45 - [45 - \{0.3 \times 45\}])}{45}$$

$$= \frac{3250 \times (45 - [45 - 14])}{45}$$

$$= \frac{3250 \times (45 - 31)}{45}$$

$$= \frac{3250 \times 14}{45}$$

$$= 1011 \text{ cc}$$

Fluid Replacement Requirements

Replace 1 cc EBL with:
   3 cc **crystalloid**
   1 cc **colloid**
   1 cc **whole blood**
   1 cc **PRBC's**

For each unit of PRBC's transfused, Hgb increases by 1gm/dL and the Hct increases by 3%.

Estimating Blood Loss

During surgery, blood loss is estimated by visualization and measurement of numerous sites.

1. **Suction containers**
   Measure the total amount of all suction containers and subtract the total irrigation fluid used

2. **Dry sponges (saturated w/blood)**
   4 × 4 holds ~ 10 cc blood
   Ray-techs ~ 10 to 20 cc blood
   Lap sponges ~ 100 cc blood
   Wet sponges, (those saturated w/saline before use), hold ~ 20 to 30% of the dry sponge value.

3. **Surgical field**

4. **Weight**
   If weighing sponges, 1 gm weight = 1cc blood.

Compatibility Testing

The indication for administering PRBC's is to increase the O_2 carrying capacity and not to increase blood pressure.

1. **Type and screen**
   99.8% compatible
   ABO-Rh typing only
   Recipient is screened only to look for antibodies
   Serum is screened for antibodies, antibodies are identified if present
   Takes ~ 1 hr
   No blood is allocated
   No donor blood is involved

2. **Type and crossmatch**
   99.95% compatible
   Blood donor and recipient blood are mixed
   Blood is mixed to check for incompatibilities
   Indirect antiglobulin test detects antibodies or complements on the donor cells
   Involves type, screen, and crossmatch; cannot perform crossmatch w/out
      a type and screen
   Takes ~ 1 hr

3. **Type specific**
   99.94% compatible
   Emergencies only
   Provides ABO type only
   Blood is released
   Crossmatch is continued after the blood is released

4. **Universal blood**
   Indicated in dire emergency only
   Must draw blood from the recipient before blood is administered for type and
      crossmatch; this will make it possible to identify the patient's blood type and
      crossmatch before the recipient's blood is contaminated
   Type O: "universal donor" (lacks both A and B antigens)
   Type AB: "universal recipients" (lack both anti-A and anti-B antibodies)

Blood Component Therapy

1. **Whole blood (500 cc)**
   Used primarily in hemorrhagic shock
   Contains RBC, WBC, platelets (non-functioning after 2 hr), and plasma
   Increases both RBC and plasma volumes
   Does not contain factors VII and X

2. **PRBCs (250 cc)**
   Contains RBC, WBC, platelets, but has a decreased plasma volume
   Increases RBC
   Raises Hgb 1gm/dL and Hct by 3%

3. **Platelets (single donor bag = 10 to 25 cc or multiple donor bag = 50 to 70 cc)**
   Indicated for bleeding from thrombocytopenia
   Pooled from random donors
   40 cc platelets per unit of PRBCs
   Each unit increases platelet count by 5000 to 10,000

4. **Fresh Frozen Plasma (FFP) (220 to 250 cc/bag)**
   Indicated for the treatment of some coagulation disorders and when PT/PTT
      are > 1.5 times the normal
   Contains all coagulation factors but no platelets
   Need ABO prior to FFP transfusion
   Needs ~ 30 minutes to thaw

5. **Cryoprecipitate (10 to 20 cc)**
   Indicated for deficiency of factors VIII, XIII, von Willebrand's disesase,
      or hemophilia
   Contains factors VIII, XIII, and von Willebrand's disease

Complications of Blood Therapy

1. **Immune/Non-hemolytic**
   A. Febrile
      Most common
      Due to recipient antibodies against donor WBC's and platelets
   B. Allergic
      Occurs in about 3% of all transfusions
      Caused by immunoglobulin antibodies against substances in the
         donor plasma w/activation of mast cells and histamine release
      Most commonly present w/abrupt onset of pruitic erythema or urticaria
         on arms and trunk
   C. Anaphylaxis
      Occurs in IgA-deficient patients who have developed an anti-IgA
      Immune complex activates mast cells, basophils, etc..., which results
         in hypotension, dyspnea, laryngeal edema, and wheezing
2. **Immune/Hemolytic**
   A. Acute hemolytic transfusion reaction
      Occurs in 1:10,000; 20% to 60% mortality
      Usually due to donor blood ABO incompatiblity
      Complement activation leads to hemolysis and may result in DIC, H/A,
         chills, N/V, hypotension, dyspnea, bleeding, and hemoglobinuria;
         acute renal failure may occur

Transfusion Reaction Treatment
1. Stop blood transfusion.
2. Optimize circulation w/ 0.9 NS fluid boluses to flood out system.
3. Monitor SaO_2 carefully; tiny clots in the lungs may be present as the lungs are
   one of the first organs to be affected which causes VQ mismatch; 100% O_2 via
   mask or intubate if necessary based on assessment.
4. Administer bronchodilators.
5. Induce diuresis w/Lasix or Mannitol.
6. Alkanalize urine w/mEq/kg HCO_3; this is done only if urine pH is < 7 or 8 because
   if the pH is low, free Hgb will obstruct the collecting ducts and block up the kidneys
   causing renal failure; the theory is that if the pH is increased, the free Hgb will be
   flushed out.
7. Use available sources (call pathologist from blood bank).

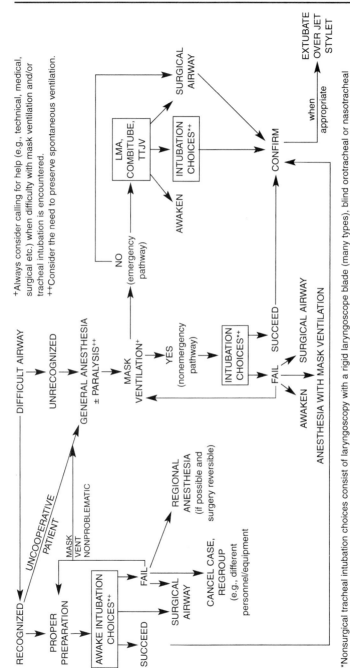

Figure 19-4 Difficult airway algorithm. (From Benumof JL. Laryngeal mask airway and the ASA difficult airway algorithm. *Anesthesiology 1996;84(3):687.*)

Universal Algorithm for Adult Emergency Cardiac Care (EEC)

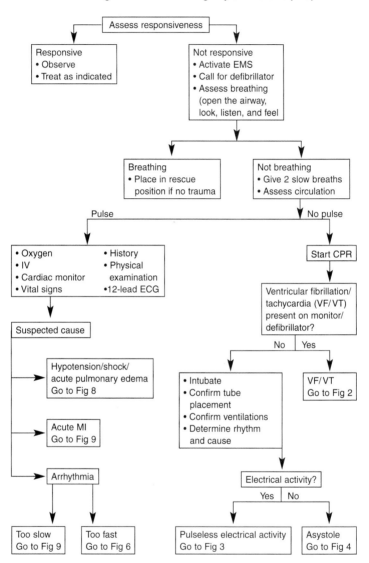

Algorithm for Ventricular Fibrillation and Pulseless Ventricular Tachycardia (VF/VT)

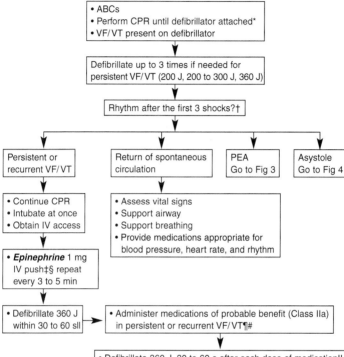

```
┌─────────────────────────────────────────────┐
│ • ABCs                                        │
│ • Perform CPR until defibrillator attached*   │
│ • VF/VT present on defibrillator              │
└─────────────────────────────────────────────┘
                      │
┌─────────────────────────────────────────────┐
│ Defibrillate up to 3 times if needed for      │
│ persistent VF/VT (200 J, 200 to 300 J, 360 J) │
└─────────────────────────────────────────────┘
                      │
┌─────────────────────────────────────────────┐
│ Rhythm after the first 3 shocks?†             │
└─────────────────────────────────────────────┘
```

Persistent or recurrent VF/VT	Return of spontaneous circulation	PEA Go to Fig 3	Asystole Go to Fig 4

• Continue CPR • Intubate at once • Obtain IV access	• Assess vital signs • Support airway • Support breathing • Provide medications appropriate for blood pressure, heart rate, and rhythm

• ***Epinephrine*** 1 mg IV push‡§ repeat every 3 to 5 min

• Defibrillate 360 J within 30 to 60 sll   • Administer medications of probable benefit (Class IIa) in persistent or recurrent VF/VT¶#

• Defibrillate 360 J, 30 to 60 s after each dose of medicationII
• Pattern should be drug-shock, drug-shock

Class I: definitely helpful
Class IIa: acceptable, probably helpful
Class IIb: acceptable, possibly helpful
Class III: not indicated, may be harmful
* Precordial thump is a Class IIb action in witnessed arrest, no pulse, and no defibrillator immediately available.
† Hypothermic cardiac arrest is treated differently after this point. See section on hypothermia.
‡ The recommended dose of **epinephrine** is 1 mg IV push every 3 to 5 min. If this approach fails, several Class IIb dosing regimens can be considered:
  • Intermediate: **epinephrine** 2 to 5 mg IV push, every 3 to 5 min
  • Escalating: **epinephrine** 1 mg-3 mg-5 mg IV push (3 min apart)
  • High: **epinephrine** 0.1 mg/kg IV push, every 3 to 5 min
§ ***Sodium bicarbonate*** (1 mEq/kg) is Class I if patient has known preexisting hyperkalemia
II Multiple sequenced shocks (200 J, 200 to 300 J, 360 J) are acceptable here (Class I), especially when medications are delayed

¶ • ***Lidocaine*** 1.5 mg/kg IV push. Repeat in 3 to 5 min to total loading dose of 3 mg/kg; then use
  • ***Bretylium*** 5 mg/kg IV push. Repeat in 5 min at 10 mg/kg
  * ***Magnesium sulfate*** 1 to 2 g IV in torsades de pointes or suspected hypomagnesemic state or severe refractory VF
  • ***Procainamide*** 30 mg/min in refractory VF (maximum total 17 mg/kg)
• ***Sodium bicarbonate*** (1 mEq/kg IV): Class IIa
  • if known preexisting bicarbonate-responsive acidosis
  • if overdose with tricyclic antidepressants
  • to alkalinize the urine in drug overdoses
Class IIb
  • if intubated and continued long arrest interval
  • upon return of spontaneous circulation after long arrest interval
Class III
  • hypoxic lactic acidosis

Algorithm for Pulseless Electrical Activity (PEA)

PEA includes
- Electromechanical dissociation (EMD)
- Pseudo-EMD
- Idioventricular rhythms
- Ventricular escape rhythms
- Bradyasystolic rhythms
- Postdefibrillation idioventricular rhythms

- Continue CPR
- Intubate at once
- Obtain IV access
- Assess blood flow using Doppler ultrasound

Consider possible causes
(Parentheses = possible therapies and treatments
- Hypovolemia (volume infusion)
- Hypoxia (ventilation)
- Cardiac tamponade (pericardiocentesis)
- Tension pneumothorax (needle decompression)
- Hypothermia
- Massive pulmonary embolism (surgery, ***thrombolytics***)
- Drug overdoses such as tricyclics, digitalis, β-blockers, calcium channel blockers
- Hyperkalemia*
- Acidosis†
- Massive acute myocardial infarction (go to Fig 9)

- ***Epinephrine*** 1 mg IV push,*‡ repeat every 3 to 5 min

- If absolute bradycardia (< 60 beats/min) or relative bradycardia, give ***atropine*** 1 mg IV
- Repeat every 3 to 5 min up to a total of 0.04 mg/kg§

Class I: definitely helpful
Class IIa: acceptable, probably helpful
Class IIb: acceptable, possibly helpful
Class III: not indicated, may be harmful
- ***Sodium bicarbonate*** 1 mEq/kg is Class I if patient has known preexisting hyperkalemia
† ***Sodium bicarbonate*** 1 mEq/kg:
  Class IIa
  - if known preexisting bicarbonate-responsive acidosis
  - if overdose with tricyclic antidepressants
  - to alkalinize the urine in drug overdoses
  Class IIb
  - if intubated and long arrest interval
  - upon return of spontaneous circulation after long arrest interval
  Class III
  - hypoxic lactic acidosis
‡ The recommended dose of ***epinephrine*** is 1 mg IV push every 3 to 5 min.
  If this approach fails, several Class IIb dosing regimens can be considered.
  - Intermediate: ***epinephrine*** 2 to 5 mg IV push, every 3 to 5 min
  - Escalating: ***epinephrine*** 1 mg-3 mg-5 mg IV push (3 min apart)
  - High: ***epinephrine*** 0.1 mg/kg IV push, every 3 to 5 min
§ Shorter ***atropine*** dosing intervals are possibly helpful in cardiac arrest (Class IIb).

Asystole Treatment Algorithm

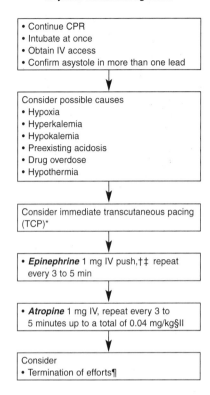

- Continue CPR
- Intubate at once
- Obtain IV access
- Confirm asystole in more than one lead

Consider possible causes
- Hypoxia
- Hyperkalemia
- Hypokalemia
- Preexisting acidosis
- Drug overdose
- Hypothermia

Consider immediate transcutaneous pacing (TCP)*

- **_Epinephrine_** 1 mg IV push,†‡ repeat every 3 to 5 min

- **_Atropine_** 1 mg IV, repeat every 3 to 5 minutes up to a total of 0.04 mg/kg§ǁ

Consider
- Termination of efforts¶

Class I: definitely helpful
Class IIa: acceptable, probably helpful
Class IIb: acceptable, possibly helpful
Class III: not indicated, may be harmful
- TCP is a Class IIb intervention. Lack of success may be due to delay in pacing. To be effective, TCP must be performed early, simultaneously with drugs. Evidence does not support routine use of TCP for asystole.
† The recommended dose of **_epinephrine_** is 1 mg IV push every 3 to 5 min. If this approach fails, several Class IIb dosing regimens can be considered:
  - Intermediate: **_epinephrine_** 2 to 5 mg IV push, every 3 to 5 min
  - Escalating: **_epinephrine_** 1 mg-3 mg-5 mg IV push (3 min apart)
  - High: **_epinephrine_** 0.1 mg/kg IV push, every 3 to 5 min
‡ **_Sodium bicarbonate_** 1 mEq/kg is Class I if patient has known preexisting hyperkalemia.

§ Shorter **_atropine_** dosing intervals are Class IIb in asystolic arrest.
ǁ **_Sodium bicarbonate_** 1 mEq/kg: Class IIa
  - if known preexisting bicarbonate-responsive acidosis
  - if overdose with tricyclic antidepressants
  - to alkalinize the urine in drug overdose
Class IIb
  - if intubated and continued long arrest interval
  - upon return of spontaneous circulation after long arrest interval
Class III
  - hypoxic lactic acidosis
¶ If patient remains in asystole or other agonal rhythms after successful intubation and initial medication and no reversible causes are identified, consider termination of resuscitative efforts by a physician. Consider interval since arrest.

Bradycardia Algorithms (with the Patient Not in Cardiac Arrest)

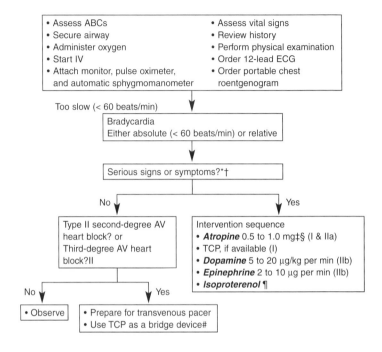

* Serious signs or symptoms must be related to the slow rate.
  Clinical manifestations include:
  symptoms (chest pain, shortness of breath, decreased level of consciousness) and
  signs (low BP, shock, pulmonary congestion, CHF, acute MI).
† Do not delay TCP while awaiting IV access or for *atropine* to take effect if patient
  is symptomatic.
‡ Denervated transplanted hearts will not respond to *atropine*. Go at once to pacing,
  catecholamine infusion, or both.
§ *Atropine* should be given in repeat doses in 3 to 5 min up to a total of 0.04 mg/kg.
  Consider shorter dosing intervals in severe clinical conditions. It has been
  suggested that atropine should be used with caution in atrioventricular (AV) block
  at the His-Purkinje level (type II AV block and new third-degree block with wide
  QRS complexes) (Class IIb).
II Never treat third-degree heart block plus ventricular escape beats with *lidocaine*.
¶ *Isoproterenol* should be used, if at all, with extreme caution. At low doses it is
  Class IIb (possibly helpful); at higher doses it is Class III (harmful).
Verify patient tolerance and mechanical capture. Use analgesia and sedation as
  needed.

Tachycardia Algorithm

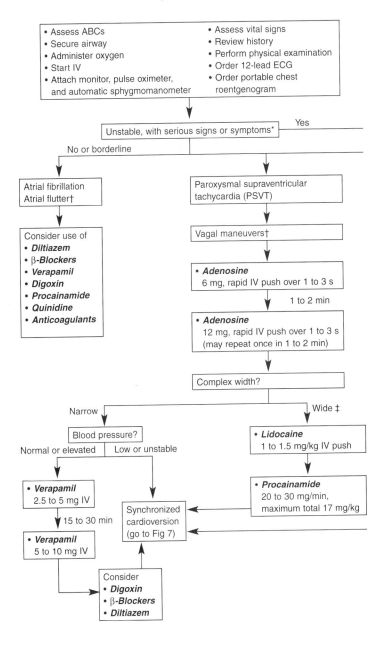

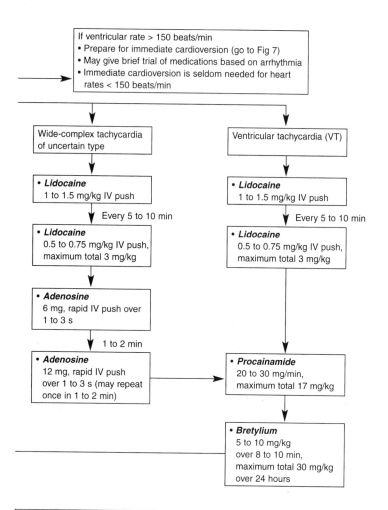

If ventricular rate > 150 beats/min
- Prepare for immediate cardioversion (go to Fig 7)
- May give brief trial of medications based on arrhythmia
- Immediate cardioversion is seldom needed for heart rates < 150 beats/min

Wide-complex tachycardia of uncertain type

- **Lidocaine** 1 to 1.5 mg/kg IV push

Every 5 to 10 min

- **Lidocaine** 0.5 to 0.75 mg/kg IV push, maximum total 3 mg/kg

- **Adenosine** 6 mg, rapid IV push over 1 to 3 s

1 to 2 min

- **Adenosine** 12 mg, rapid IV push over 1 to 3 s (may repeat once in 1 to 2 min)

Ventricular tachycardia (VT)

- **Lidocaine** 1 to 1.5 mg/kg IV push

Every 5 to 10 min

- **Lidocaine** 0.5 to 0.75 mg/kg IV push, maximum total 3 mg/kg

- **Procainamide** 20 to 30 mg/min, maximum total 17 mg/kg

- **Bretylium** 5 to 10 mg/kg over 8 to 10 min, maximum total 30 mg/kg over 24 hours

* Unstable condition must be related to the tachycardia. Signs and symptoms may include chest pain, shortness of breath, decreased level of consciousness, low blood pressure (BP), shock, pulmonary congestion, congestive heart failure, acute myocardial infarction.
† Carotid sinus pressure is contraindicated in patients with carotid bruits; avoid ice water immersion in patients with ischemic heart disease.
‡ If the wide-complex tachycardia is known with certainty to be PSVT and BP is normal/elevated, sequence can include **verapamil**.

Electrical Cardioversion Algorithm (with the Patient Not in Cardiac Arrest)

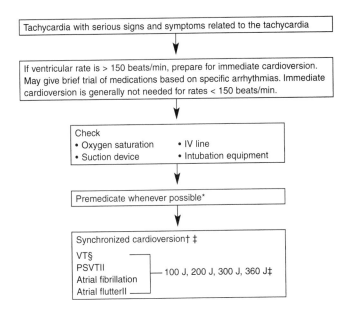

Tachycardia with serious signs and symptoms related to the tachycardia

If ventricular rate is > 150 beats/min, prepare for immediate cardioversion. May give brief trial of medications based on specific arrhythmias. Immediate cardioversion is generally not needed for rates < 150 beats/min.

Check
- Oxygen saturation
- Suction device
- IV line
- Intubation equipment

Premedicate whenever possible*

Synchronized cardioversion† ‡

VT§
PSVTII
Atrial fibrillation
Atrial flutterII
— 100 J, 200 J, 300 J, 360 J‡

---

* Effective regimens have included a sedative (e.g., ***diazepam, midazolam, barbiturates, etomidate, ketamine, methohexital***) with or without an analgesic agent (e.g., ***fentanyl, morphine, meperidine***). Many experts recommend anesthesia if service is readily available.
† Note possible need to resynchronize after each cardioversion.
‡ If delays in synchronization occur and clinical conditions are critical, go to immediate unsynchronized shocks.
§ Treat polymorphic VT (irregular form and rate) like VF:
  200 J, 200 to 300 J, 360 J
II PSVT and atrial flutter often respond to lower energy levels (start with 50 J).

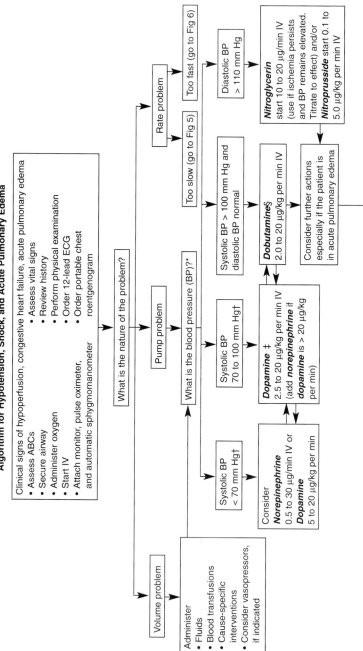

Algorithm for Hypotension, Shock, and Acute Pulmonary Edema

Clinical signs of hypoperfusion, congestive heart failure, acute pulmonary edema

- Assess ABCs
- Secure airway
- Administer oxygen
- Start IV
- Attach monitor, pulse oximeter, and automatic sphygmomanometer
- Assess vital signs
- Review history
- Perform physical examination
- Order 12-lead ECG
- Order portable chest roentgenogram

What is the nature of the problem?

Volume problem

Administer
- Fluids
- Blood transfusions
- Cause-specific interventions
- Consider vasopressors, if indicated

Pump problem

What is the blood pressure (BP)?*

Systolic BP < 70 mm Hg†

Consider
Norepinephrine
0.5 to 30 µg/min IV or
Dopamine
5 to 20 µg/kg per min

Systolic BP 70 to 100 mm Hg†

Dopamine ‡
2.5 to 20 µg/kg per min IV
(add **norepinephrine** if **dopamine** is > 20 µg/kg per min)

Systolic BP > 100 mm Hg and diastolic BP normal

Dobutamine§
2.0 to 20 µg/kg per min IV

Consider further actions especially if the patient is in acute pulmonary edema

Rate problem

Too slow (go to Fig 5)

Too fast (go to Fig 6)

Diastolic BP > 110 mm Hg

Nitroglycerin
start 10 to 20 µg/min IV
(use if ischemia persists and BP remains elevated. Titrate to effect) and/or
Nitroprusside start 0.1 to 5.0 µg/kg per min IV

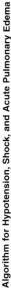

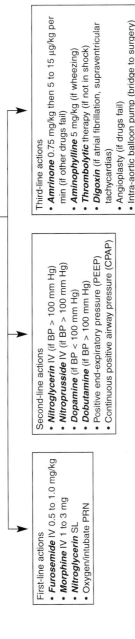

First-line actions
- *Furosemide* IV 0.5 to 1.0 mg/kg
- *Morphine* IV 1 to 3 mg
- *Nitroglycerin* SL
- Oxygen/intubate PRN

Second-line actions
- *Nitroglycerin* IV (if BP > 100 mm Hg)
- *Nitroprusside* IV (if BP > 100 mm Hg)
- *Dopamine* (if BP < 100 mm Hg)
- *Dobutamine* (if BP > 100 mm Hg)
- Positive end-expiratory pressure (PEEP)
- Continuous positive airway pressure (CPAP)

Third-line actions
- *Amrinone* 0.75 mg/kg then 5 to 15 µg/kg per min (if other drugs fail)
- *Aminophylline* 5 mg/kg (if wheezing)
- *Thrombolytic* therapy (if not in shock)
- *Digoxin* (if atrial fibrillation, supraventricular tachycardias)
- Angioplasty (if drugs fail)
- Intra-aortic balloon pump (bridge to surgery)
- Surgical interventions (valves, coronary artery bypass grafts, heart transplant)

* Base management after this point on invasive hemodynamic monitoring if possible.
† Fluid bolus of 250 to 500 mL normal saline should be tried. If no response, consider sympathomimetics.
‡ Move to *dopamine* and stop *norepinephrine* when BP improves.
§ Add *dopamine* when BP improves. Avoid *dobutamine* when systolic BP < 100 mm Hg.

Acute Myocardial Infarction Algorithm

Community
- Community emphasis on "call first/call fast, call 911"
- National Heart Attack Alert Program

EMS System
EMS system approach that should address
- Oxygen-IV-cardiac monitor-vital signs
- *Nitroglycerin*
- Pain relief with narcotics
- Notification of emergency department
- Rapid transport to emergency department
- Prehospital screening for *thrombolytic* therapy*
- 12-lead ECG, computer analysis, transmission to emergency department*
- Initiation of *thrombolytic* therapy*

Emergency Department
"Door-to-drug" team protocol approach
- Rapid triage of patients with chest pain
- Clinical decision maker established (emergency physician, cardiologist, or other)

Time interval in emergency department

Assessment
Immediate:
- Vital signs with automatic BP
- Oxygen saturation
- Start IV
- 12-lead ECG (MD review)
- Brief, targeted history and physical
- Decide on eligibility for *thrombolytic* therapy
Soon:
- Chest roentgenogram
- Blood studies (electrolytes, enzymes, coagulation studies)
- Consult as needed

Treatments to consider if there is evidence of coronary thrombosis plus no reasons for exclusion (some but not all may be appropriate)
- Oxygen at 4 L/min
- *Nitroglycerin* SL, paste or spray (if systolic BP > 90 mm Hg)
- *Morphine* IV
- *Aspirin* PO
- *Thrombolytic* agents
- *Nitroglycerin* IV (limit systolic BP drop to 10% if normotensive; 30% drop if hypertensive; never drop below 90 mm Hg systolic)
- β-*Blockers* IV
- *Heparin* IV
- Percutaneous transluminal coronary angioplasty
- Routine *lidocaine* administration is not recommended for all patients with AMI

*Optional guidelines

30 to 60 min to *thrombolytic* therapy

Parameter	Formula	Normal Range
CO	HR × SV	4.0 to 8.0 L/min
CI	CO ÷ BSA	2.5 to 4.0 L/min
CVP	cm H_2O = mm Hg × 1.34	2 to 6 mm Hg
PCWP	—	8 to 12 mm Hg
MAP	[(DBP × 2) + SBP] ÷ 3	70 to 105 mm Hg
SVR	[(MAP – CVP) ÷ CO] × 80	800 to 1200 dynes/cm/sec^{-5}
PVR	[(PAM – PCWP) ÷ CO] × 80	37 to 250 dynes/cm/sec^{-5}
SV	(CO × 1000) ÷ HR	60 to 100 mL/beat
SVI	SV ÷ BSA	33 to 47 mL/beat per m^2
LVSWI	[SVI × (MAP – PCWP)] × 0.0136	38 to 85 g • m^2/beat
RVSWI	[SVI × (PAM – PAD)] × 0.0136	7 to 12 g • m^2/beat
RVEDV	SV ÷ EF	100 to 160 mL
RVESV	EDV – SV	50 to 100 mL
RVSV	(CO × 1000) ÷ HR	60 to 100 mL
EF	(EDV – ESV) ÷ EDV or SV ÷ EDV	40% to 60%
CPP	MAP – CVP or MAP – ICP	70 to 80 mm Hg

CO, *cardiac output;* CI, *cardiac index;* CVP, *central venous pressure;*
PCWP, *pulmonary capillary wedge pressure;* MAP, *mean arterial pressure;*
SVR, *systemic vascular resistance;* PVR, *pulmonary vascular resistance;*
SV, *stroke volume;* SVI, *stroke volume index;* LVSWI, *left ventricular stroke
work index;* RVSWI, *right ventricular stroke work index;* RVEDV, *right ventricular
end-diastolic volume;* RVESV, *right ventricular end-systolic volume;* RVSV, *right
ventricular stroke volume;* EF, *ejection fracture;* CPP, *coronary perfusion pressure.*

APPENDIX 7 Pulmonary Function Test Values

Test	Normal Values
Vital capacity (VC)	60 to 70 mL/kg
Tidal volume (VT)	
(spontaneous ventilation)	6 to 8 mL/kg
Minute ventilation (VE)	80 mL/kg
Functional residual capacity (FRC)	28 to 32 mL/kg
Forced expiratory	
volume in 1 second (FEV_1)	> 75%
Forced vital capacity (FVC)	60 to 70 mL/kg
Dead space (VDS)	2 mL/kg
VDS/VT	33%
FEV_1/FVC	> 75%

Nomogram for the Determination of Body Surface Area of Children and Adults

To determine the surface area, find the height of the person and the weight on the appropriate scales, and then connect these points with a straight edge. The point at which this line intersects with the line of the surface area scale indicates the surface area of the patient in square meters. (From Boothby WM, Sandiford RB. *Boston Med Surg J.* 1921; 185:337, as shown in Rakel RE. *Conn's Current Therapy.* Philadelphia, PA: W.B. Saunders Co.; 1991.)

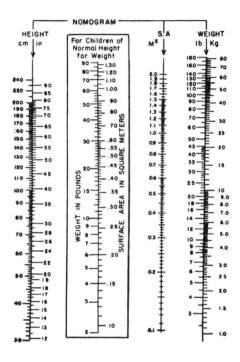

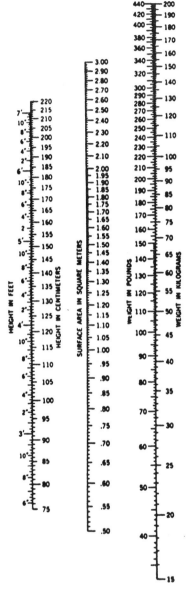

The surface area is estimated by a straight line connecting the height of the patient with his/her weight intersecting the surface area line. If the patient is of average size, the surface area can be estimated from weight alone (see boxed scale in diagram). (From Behrman, RE. *Nelson Textbook of Pediatrics*. 14th ed. Philadelphia, PA; W.B. Saunders Co.; 1992.)

Age	Weight (kg), 50th Percentile	Respiratory Rate (breaths/min)	Heart Rate (beats/min)	Systolic Blood Pressure (mm Hg)
Premature	< 3 kg	50 to 60/min	120 to 180	40 to 60
Newborn	3 to 4	35 to 40	100 to 180	50 to 70
1 mo	4	35 to 40	100 to 180	50 to 70
3 mo	5	24 to 30	100 to 180	60 to 110
6 mo	7	25 to 30	100 to 180	60 to 110
12 mo	10.0	20 to 25	90 to 150	65 to 115
2 y	12.0	16 to 22	90 to 150	75 to 125
3 y	15.0	16 to 22	90 to 150	75 to 125
5 y	20.0	14 to 20	60 to 140	80 to 120
7 y	30.0	14 to 20	60 to 140	90 to 120
10 y	40.0	12 to 20	60 to 100	90 to 120

Estimating Weight in Kilograms

< 1 y: (age [mo]) $\times$ 0.5 + 3.5
> 1 y: (age [y]) $\times$ 2 + 1

Estimating Endotracheal Tube (ETT) Size*

Age	ETT Size	Laryngoscope Blade	Distance (cm)
Premature	2.5	0 Miller	According to weight: 500 g @ 6 cm 1000 g @ 7 cm 2000 g @ 8 cm 3000 g @ 9 cm
Newborn	3.0 to 3.5	0 Miller	10
6 mo	3.5 to 4	1 Miller	10 to 11
1 y	4.0	1 to Miller/Mac	11
2 y	4.5 to 5.0	1 or 2 Miller/Mac	12.5

Over 20 mo: 4.0 + age (y) ÷ 4

Length of insertion (over 1 y: 12 + age ÷ 2)

* This is only a guide; prepare an ETT one size larger and one size smaller than the ETT size selected.

Estimated Blood Volume (EBV)

Age	Volume (mL/kg)
Premature	90
Full-term	90
0 to 2 y	80–
2+ y	70–

Maximum Allowable Blood Loss (MABL)

$$MABL = \frac{EBV \times (Initial\ Hct - Target\ Hct)}{Initial\ Hct}$$

NPO Time

Age (mo)	Clear liquids (h)	Milk/Solids (h)
0 to 6	2	4
6 to 36	2 to 4	4 to 6
> 36	2 to 44	6 to 8

Calculation of Maintenance Fluid Requirements

Weight (kg)	Requirement
0 to 10	4 mL/kg per h
10 to 20	40 mL + 2 mL/kg > 10
> 20	60 mL + 1 mL/kg > 20

NPO Deficit

NPO hours × Maintenance: Replace 50% the first hour, 25% the second hour, and 25% the third hour.

LOOK FOR: Elevated end-tidal CO_2, rigidity, tachycardia, hypercarbia, tachypnea, cardiac arrhythmias, respiratory and metabolic acidosis, fever, unstable/rising blood pressure, cyanosis/mottling, and myoglobinuria.

Acute Phase Treatment

1. **GET HELP, GET DANTROLENE.** Immediately discontinue all volatile inhalation anesthetics and succinylcholine. Hyperventilate with 100% oxygen at high gas flows for at least 10 L/min. The circle system and CO_2 absorbent need not be changed.

2. Administer dantrolene sodium 2.5 mg/kg bolus rapidly. Continue to administer dantrolene until signs of MH (e.g., tachycardia, rigidity, increased end-tidal CO_2, and temperature elevation) are controlled. Occasionally, a total dose greater than 10 mg/kg may be needed. Each vial of dantrolene contains 20 mg of dantrolene and 3 grams of mannitol. Each vial should be mixed with 60 mL of sterile water for injection USP without a bacteriostatic agent.

3. Administer bicarbonate to correct metabolic acidosis as guided by blood gas analysis. In the absence of blood gas analysis, 1 to 2 mEq/kg should be administered.

4. Simultaneous with the above, actively cool the hyperthermic patient. Use IV cold saline (not Ringer's lactate) 15 mL/kg q 15 min × 3.
   a. Lavage stomach, bladder, rectum, and open cavities with cold saline as appropriate.
   b. Surface cool with ice and hypothermia blanket.
   c. Monitor closely since overvigorous treatment may lead to hypothermia.

5. Arrhythmias will usually respond to treatment of acidosis and hyperkalemia. If they persist or are life threatening, standard antiarrhythmic agents may be used, with the exception of calcium channel blockers (may cause hyperkalemia and CV collapse).

6. Determine and monitor end-tidal CO_2, arterial, central, or femoral venous blood gases, serum potassium and other electrolytes, urine output, PT/PTT, and calcium for baseline values. Repeat as clinically indicated.

7. Hyperkalemia is common and should be treated with hyperventilation, bicarbonate, intravenous glucose, and insulin (10 units regular insulin in 50 mL 50% glucose titrated to potassium level or 0.15 U/kg regular insulin in 1 mL/kg 50% glucose). Life-threatening hyperkalemia may also be treated with calcium administration (e.g., 2 to 5 mg/kg of $CaCl_2$). Check blood glucose every 2 hours if insulin has been given.

8. Ensure urine output of greater than 2 mL/kg/hr by hydration and/or administration of mannitol or furosemide. Consider central venous or PA monitoring because of fluid shifts and hemodynamic instability that may occur.

9. **Sudden Unexpected Cardiac Arrest in Children:** Children less than about 10 years of age who experience sudden cardiac arrest after succinylcholine in the absence of hypoxemia and anesthetic overdose should be treated for acute hyperkalemia first. In this situation calcium chloride should be administered along with other means to reduce serum potassium. They should be presumed to have subclinical muscular dystrophy and a neurologist should be consulted.

---

* Names of on-call physicians available to consult in MH emergencies may be obtained 24 hours a day through the MH Emergency HOTLINE: 1-800-MH-HYPER (1-800-644-9737).

For nonemergency or patient referral calls: MHAUS, P. O. Box 1069, Sherburne, NY 13460-1069. Telephone: 1-800-986-4287. MH INFO-BY-FAX: 1-800-440-9990. Website: www.mhaus.org E-mail: mhaus@norwich.net

(From Emergency Therapy for Malignant Hyperthermia. Sherburne, NY: Malignant Hyperthermia Association of the United States; 1999.)

Post Acute Phase

A. Observe the patient in an ICU setting for at least 24 hours since recrudescence of MH may occur.
B. Administer dantrolene 1 mg/kg or more every 4 to 6 hours for 24 to 48 hours after the episode.
C. Follow ABG, CK, potassium, urine and serum myoglobin, clotting studies, and core body temperature until such time as they return to normal values. Central temperature (e.g., rectal, esophageal) should be continuously monitored until stable.
D. Counsel the patient and family regarding MH and further precautions. Refer the patient to MHAUS. Fill out an Adverse Metabolic Reaction to Anesthesia (AMRA) report available through MHAUS. A letter to the patient's primary care doctor is advised.

CAUTION: This protocol may not apply to every patient and may require alteration according to specific patient needs.

This checkout, or a reasonable equivalent, should be conducted before administration of anesthesia. These recommendations are only valid for an anesthesia system that conforms to the current and relevant standards and includes an ascending bellows ventilator and at least the following monitors; capnograph, pulse oximeter, oxygen analyser, respiratory volume and monitor (spirometer), and breathing system pressure monitor with high- and low-pressure alarms.

Emergency Ventilation Equipment
1. **Verify that backup ventilation equipment is available and functioning.**

High-Pressure System
2. **Check the oxygen cylinder supply.**
   a. Open the O_2 cylinder and verify that it is at least half full (about 1000 psi).
   b. Close the cylinder.
3. **Check the central pipeline supplies.**
   Check that the hoses are connected and that pipeline gauges read about 50 psi.

Low-Pressure System
4. **Check the initial status of the low-pressure system.**
   a. Close the flow control valves and turn off the vaporizers.
   b. Check the fill level and tighten the vaporizers' filler caps.
5. **Perform a leak check of machine low-pressure system.**
   a. Verify that the machine master switch and flow control valves are OFF.
   b. Attach a "suction bulb" to common (fresh) gas outlet.
   c. Squeeze the bulb repeatedly until fully collapsed.
   d. Verify that the bulb stays *fully* collapsed for at least 10 seconds.
   e. Open one vaporizer at a time and repeat 'c' and 'd' above.
   f. Remove the suction bulb and reconnect a fresh gas hose.
6. **Turn on the machine master switch** and all other necessary electrical equipment.
7. **Test the flowmeters.**
   a. Adjust the flow of all gases through their full range, checking for smooth operation of floats and undamaged flowtubes.
   b. Attempt to create an hypoxic O_2 / N_2O mixture and verify correct changes in the flow and/or alarm.

Scavenging System
8. **Adjust and check the scavenging system.**
   a. Ensure that proper connections between the scavenging system and both the adjustable pressure-limiting (APL) (pop-off) valve and the ventilator relief valve.
   b. Adjust the waste gas vacuum (if possible).
   c. Fully open the APL valve and occlude the Y-piece.
   d. With minimum O_2 flow, allow the scavenger reservoir bag to collapse completely and verify that the absorber pressure gauge reads about zero.
   e. With the O_2 flush activated, allow the scavenger reservoir bag to distend fully, and then verify that the absorber pressure gauge reads < 10 cm H_2O.

Breathing System
9. **Calibrate the O_2 monitor.**
   a. Ensure that the monitor reads 21% in room air.
   b. Verify that the low O_2 alarm is enabled and functioning.
   c. Reinstall sensor in circuit and flush the breathing system with O_2.
   d. Verify that the monitor now reads greater than 90%.

10. **Check the initial status of the breathing system.**
    a. Set the selector switch to "Bag" mode.
    b. Check that the breathing circuit is complete, undamaged, and unobstructed.
    c. Verify that CO_2 absorbent is adequate.
    d. Install the breathing circuit accessory equipment (e.g. humidifier, positive end-expiratory pressure . . . PEEP valve) to be used during the case.
11. **Perform a leak check of the breathing system.**
    a. Set all gas flows to zero (or minimum).
    b. Close the APL (pop-off) valve and occlude the Y-piece.
    c. Pressurize the breathing system to about 30 cm H_2O with O_2 flush.
    d. Ensure that the pressure remains fixed at least 10 seconds.
    e. Open the APL 9 (pop-off) valve and ensure that pressure decreases.

Manual and Automatic Ventilation Systems
12. **Test the ventilator systems and unidirectional valves.**
    a. Place a second breathing bag on the Y-piece.
    b. Set the appropriate ventilator parameters for the next patient.
    c. Switch to automatic ventilation (ventilator) mode.
    d. Turn the ventilator ON and fill the bellows and breathing bag with O_2 flush.
    e. Set the O_2 flow to minimum and the other gas flows to zero.
    f. Verify that during inspiration, the bellows delivers appropriate tidal volume and that during expiration the bellow fills completely.
    g. Set fresh gas flow to about 5 L/min.
    h. Verify that the ventilator bellows and simulated lungs fill and empty appropriately without sustained pressure at end expiration.
    i. Check for proper action of the unidirectional valves.
    j. Exercise the breathing circuit accessories to ensure proper function.
    k. Turn the ventilator OFF and switch to manual ventilation (Bag/APL) mode.
    l. Ventilate manually and ensure the inflation and deflation of artificial lungs and the appropriate feel of system resistance and compliance.
    m. Remove the second breathing bag from the Y-piece.

Monitors
13. **Check, calibrate, and/or set the alarm limits of all monitors.**
    Capnometer   Pulse oximeter
    Oxygen analyzer (spirometer)   Respiratory volume monitor
    Pressure monitor with high and low airway alarms

Final Position
14. **Check the final status of the machine.**
    a. Vaporizers off
    b. APL valve open
    c. Selector switch to "Bag"
    d. All flowmeters to zero
    e. Patient suction level adequate
    f. Breathing system ready to use

Test	Normal Serum Values
ACT	80 to 120 s
Albumin, total	6.6 to 7.9 g/dL
fractional	4.4 to 4.5 g/dL
Alkaline phosphatase	45 to 125 U/L
Ammonia	80 to 110 µg/dL
Amylase	20 to 110 U/L
Anion gap	8 to 14 mEq/L
ABG: pH	7.35 to 7.45
$PaCO_2$	35 to 45 mm Hg
PaO_2	80 to 100 mm Hg
HCO_3	22 to 26 Meq/L
Bilirubin, direct	0 to 0.4 mg/dL
indirect	0.1 to 1.2 mg/dL
BUN	8 to 20 mg/dL
Cr	0.2 to 1.5 mg/dL
Ca	4.5 to 5.5 mEq/L
Cl	100 to 108 mEq/L
CK, total	
female	15 to 57 U/L
male	24 to 100 U/L
MB	0 to 7 IU/L
MM	6 to 70 IU/L
Fibrinogen	195 to 365
FSP/FDP	< 3 µG/mL
Glucose, fasting	70 to 100 mg/dL
Hb, female	15 to 16 g/dL
male	14 to 18 g/dL
glycosylated	5.5% to 9%
HCT, female	37% to 47%
male	42% to 52%
INR	1
K	3.8 to 5.5 mg/dL
LDH, total	48 to 115 IU/L
LDH_1	17.5% to 28.3% of total LDH
LDH_2	30.4% to 36.4% of total LDH ($LDH_1 < LDH_2$)
Mg	1.5 to 2.5 mEq/L
Na	134 to 145 mEq/L
Phosphorus	1.8 to 2.6 mEq/L
Platelets	130,000 to 370,000/mm^3
Pseudocholinesterase	8 to 80 U/mL
PT	11 to 13.2 s
PTT	22.5 to 32.2 s
RBC, female	4.2 to 5.4 million/µL
male	4.7 to 6.2 million/µL
AST	8 to 20 U/L
ALT, female	9 to 24 U/L
male	10 to 32 U/L
T_3	90 to 230 ng/dL
T_4	5 to 13 µg/dL
TSH	0.406 µU/mL
WBC	4100 to 10,900/µL

Therapeutic drug level

Amitriptyline	160 to 240 ng/mL
Digoxin	0.8 to 2 ng/mL
Lidocaine	1 to 5µg/dL
Lithium	0.7 to 1.5 mEq/L
Phenobarbital	10 to 30 µg/mL
Phenytoin	10 to 20 µg/mL
Theophylline	5 to 20 µg/mL

APPENDIX 13 Standards for Nurse Anesthesia Practice*

I. Perform a thorough and complete preanesthesia assessment.

II. Obtain informed consent for the planned anesthetic intervention from the patient or legal guardian.

III. Formulate a patient-specific plan for anesthesia care.

IV. Implement and adjust the anesthesia care plan based on the patient's physiologic response.

V. Monitor the patient's physiologic condition as appropriate for the type of anesthesia and specific patient needs.

VI. There shall be complete, accurate, and timely documentation of pertinent information on the patient's medical record.

VII. Transfer the responsibility for care of the patient to other qualified providers in a manner that assures continuity of care and patient safety.

VIII. Adhere to appropriate safety precautions, as established within the institution, to minimize the risks of fire, explosion, electrical shock, and equipment malfunction. Document on the patient's medical record that the anesthesia machine and equipment were checked.

IX. Universal precautions shall be taken to minimize the risk of infection to the patient, the CRNA, and other staff.

X. Anesthesia care shall be assessed to assure its quality and contribution to positive patient outcomes.

XI. The CRNA shall respect and maintain the basic rights of patients.

* Adopted by the American Association of Nurse Anesthetists, June 1989. Revised 1992, 1996. ©, American Association of Nurse Anesthetists. Adapted with permission.

1. High-risk patients

Healthcare providers
Spina bifida patients/patients with congenital urologic abnormalities
Workers in rubber industry
Patients with a history of atopy and multiple allergies
Intolerance to latex-based products: balloons, rubber gloves, condom, etc.
Having multiple operations, particularly as a neonate
Chronic bladder catheterization

2. Latex free

Circuits
Latex free breathing bag (green)
Endotracheal tubes
LMA's (regular and reusable)
Airways—oral, nasal
Vinyl gloves
Silk tape
Pulse oximeter probes
  Nondisposable
  Disposable—D_{20}, D_{25}
          N-25 (neonatal)
          I-20 (infant)
Nylon tourniquet
Conmed V—lead dots
3M precordial stickers
ESOP. Stethescope
NIBP (latex free reusable) (grey)
Stop cocks for IV's
Hudson Hood type face mask (except elastic headstrap)
Skin temp—adhesive strip
Warming blankets, including adhesive strip

3. Contains latex

Nasal canula $ETCO_2$ (gray)
Regular breathing bag
Head straps
Laser trach ETTs (Sheridan)
Rubber bite blocks
Standard latex gloves
3M microprobe (plastic tape-clear)
Pulse oximeter probes—disposable except those listed as latex free
Latex tourniquet
3M ECG pads
Tegaderm dressing
Band-Aids®
Swan Ganz catheter (balloon)
Rubber tubing
Regular BP cuff tubing (wrap in stockinet or tape)
Rubber seal medication vials
Plungers in syringes
Foley catheters
Rubber IV injection ports all IVs (Level 1 included)
Elastic strap on hudson hood face mask

4. **Preoperative preparation**

   Assessment specific history of latex allergy or risk factors

   Consider allergy consultation

   First case of the day to decrease aerollergen concentration

   Display latex allergy signs inside and outside operating room

   Have latex allergy cart and latex-free products available

   Notify all members of health care team that no latex gloves or latex products should contact patient

5. **Intraoperative care**

   Remove all latex products from the operating room

   Substitute all items with non-latex alternatives as possible

   Sterile field table must be a latex-free set up

   Use a latex-free reservoir bag, airways, endotracheal tubes, and laryngeal mask airways

   Use a non-latex breathing circuit with plastic mask and bag

   Ventilator must have a non-latex bellows

   Place all monitoring devices, cords/tubes in stockinet and secure with tape to prevent direct skin contact

   Items sterilized in ethylene oxide must be rinsed before use

   Remove rubber stoppers from multidose vials

   Beware of latex intravenous injection ports, penrose-type tourniquets, and rubber band, use latex-free gloves as tourniquet, tape latex inject ports, or use silicone injection ports, or stopcocks

   Use latex-free ECG electrodes and bovie pads

   Wrap Webril around extremities if using a blood pressure cuff that contains latex

   Use neoprene or polymer gloves for patient contact

   Use latex-free or glass syringes

   Draw up medication immediately prior to the beginning of the case or their administration

   Use latex-free urinary catheters

6. **Treatment of anaphylactic reaction**

   Remove latex products

   Discontinue anesthetic agents as soon as possible

   Inform the surgical team to stop treatment/abort procedure

   Assess and sustain the ABCs of resuscitation

   Volume expansion

   Positive pressure ventilation with 100% oxygen

   Epinephrine 0.5 to 1 μg/kg bolus and escalate to higher doses, then 0.1 to 0.5 μg/min infusion

   Diphenhydramine 0.5 to 1 mg/kg IV

   Aminophylline 5 to 6 mg/kg slow IV over 20 minutes

   Hydrocortisone 0.25 to 1 mg/kg IV

   Ranitidine 0.5 to 2 mg/kg IV, maximum dose 150 mg

   Sodium bicarbonate 0.5 to 1 mEq/kg

7. **Postoperative care**

   Communicate with PACU/ICU nurses regarding patient's latex allergy

   Latex allergy cart going with patient to PACU/ICU

   Latex allergy signs on chart and patient's bed

   Continue patient care with latex-free technique

α-adrenergic antagonists, 68, 195, 267
α-agonists, 28, 320
abdominal aortic aneurysm, 31–33, 257–260
abortion, 328
acetaminophen, 191
acetazolamide, 118
acetylcholine, 63, 64, 65, 219
acetylsalicylic acid, 155, 302
acidemia, 90
acidosis, 329, 332. *See also specific types of acidosis*
acquired immunodeficiency syndrome (AIDS). *See* AIDS
acromegaly, 77, 81–82, 205
acute intermittent porphyria, 77
acute liver disease, 77, 89. *See also* chronic liver disease
acute mastoiditis, 49
acute renal failure, 96, 114. *See also* renal failure
Adalat. *See* nifedipine
Addison's disease, 75, 80–81
adenocarcinoma, 135, 145, 157, 230
Adenocard, 368. *See also* adenosine
adenoidectomy, 300–301, 338–339
adenoid hypertrophy, 300
adenosine, 8, 255, 368
adenosine triphosphate, 73
adenylate cyclase, 320
adrenalectomy, 157–159
adrenaline chloride. *See* epinephrine HCl
adrenocortical steroids, 38
Adriamycin, 152. *See also* doxorubicin
adult respiratory distress syndrome (ARDS), 51–52
    burns and, 359
    hepatic failure and, 90
    hip arthroplasty and, 274
    pancreatitis and, 135
    restrictive pulmonary disease and, 50
advanced cardiac life support algorithm, 500–510
A-Hydrocort. *See* hydrocortisone (hydrocortisone sodium succinate)
AICD. *See* automatic implantable cardioverter defibrillator (AICD)
AIDS, 105–106
    hemophilia and, 43, 105, 107
    immunosuppression and, 123
    tuberculosis and, 43
albumin
    aneurysms and, 259
    arteriovenous surgery and, 208
    cardioplegia and, 249

CPB and, 240
    craniotomy and, 196
    hemorrhagic shock and, 16
    hepatitis and, 86, 133
    liver transplant and, 132
    nephrectomy and, 167
    renal failure and, 186
albuterol (albuterol sulfate), 243, 368–369
aldosterone, 251
    Addison's disease and, 80
    hyperaldosteronism and, 85
    hypertension and, 11
    hypoaldosteronism and, 84
    hypothermia and, 121, 125
    infants and, 331
    spironolactone and, 158
Alfenta. *See* Alfentanil HCl
alfentanil HCl, 369
alkalosis, 134, 329. *See also* metabolic alkalosis; respiratory alkalosis
alopecia, 92, 104, 122, 246
Alport's syndrome, 168
alprostadil, 370
alveolar proteinosis, 50
amantadine, 59
amaurosis fugax, 56
amenorrhea, 205
Amicar, 255. *See also* aminocaproic acid
Amidate. *See* etomidate
aminocaproic acid, 191, 256, 370–371
aminophylline, 38, 222, 243, 371–372
amiodarone, 8, 9, 372–373
amphetamines, 117
amrinone (amrinone lactate), 25, 243, 373–374
amyloidosis, 186
anal fistulotomy/fistulectomy, 155–156
anastomosis, 137, 152, 235, 255
Anectine. *See* succinylcholine
anemia, 100–101
    AIDS and, 105, 106
    azathioprine and, 228
    bleeding ulcer and, 140
    cirrhosis and, 88
    hepatitis and, 340
    hypothyroidism and, 79
    iron deficiency, 92, 156
    kidney transplant and, 172
    laryngectomy and, 294
    leukemia and, 104
    lupus and, 122
    pernicious, 64
    portasystemic shunts and, 271
    pregnancy and, 317

renal failure and, 97
spinal instrumentation and, 184
anesthesia, checkout recommendations for, 519–520
anesthesia, for therapeutic/diagnostic procedures
CT scan/MRI, 350–351
nuclear medicine, 352–353
overall care plan for, 347–350
anesthesia, standards for practice, 347–350, 523
aneurysms. *See specific types of aneurysms*
angina
aneurysms and, 257, 265
aortic stenosis and, 19
bypass grafting and, 266
coronary-subclavian steal syndrome and, 31
in geriatrics, 125
IHD and, 2, 3
laparoscopy and, 323
mediastinoscopy and, 214
myocardial infarction and, 7
obesity and, 117
angina pectoris, 2, 3, 76, 78, 209
angiodysplasia, 145
angioplasty, 4, 7
angiotensin, 11, 251, 331
angiotensin-converting enzyme inhibitors, 12, 20, 84
aniridia, 117
anterior cervical diskectomy/fusion, 178–180
anterior pituitary dysfunction, 79
anthochromia, 191
antianginals, 258, 262
antiarrhythmic agents, 6, 10, 35, 74, 258, 262
antibiotics. *See also specific antibiotics*
aneurysms and, 191, 258
arteriovenous surgery and, 208
bacterial pharyngitis and, 49
bone fractures and, 280
bypass grafting and, 267
cor pulmonale and, 45
craniotomy and, 196
endoscopy and, 358
epiglottitis and, 49
ESWL and, 164
hip arthroplasty and, 272
hypertrophic cardiomyopathy and, 28
laminectomy and, 177
leukemia and, 104
Ludwig's edema and, 49
mitral regurgitation and, 23
nephrectomy and, 167
otitis media and, 49

pelvic exenteration and, 327
portasystemic shunts and, 271
prostatectomy and, 163
prostate resection and, 161
ptosis surgery and, 316
retropharyngeal infections and, 49
septic shock and, 17
sinusitis and, 49
thiomectomy and, 220
transplants and, 134, 169, 171
tricuspid regurgitation and, 24
anticholinergics, 69, 118, 209
anticholinesterase drugs, 63, 64, 65, 221
anticoagulants, 25, 28, 29, 258, 356
anticoagulation therapy, 22, 30, 44, 266, 280
anticonvulsant drugs, 55, 121, 198, 212
antiemetics
D & C and, 328
intraocular procedures and, 310
jaw wiring and, 299, 303, 304
maxillofacial surgery and, 300
open eye procedure and, 307
antiepileptic drugs, 55, 212
antifibrinolytic agents, 191, 244
antihyperfibrinolytic agents, 240
antihypertensives, 12, 85, 191, 196, 258, 262
anti-inflammatory agents, 38, 39, 122, 272, 277, 286
Antilirium. *See physostigmine salicylate*
antimalarial agents, 122
antimicrobial therapy, 42
antipsychotic drugs, 59, 121, 209
antipyretics, 191
antirheumatic agents, 272
antithrombotics, 4
antithyroid drugs, 78, 79, 288, 290
anxiolytics, 267, 280, 324, 325, 327. *See also specific anxiolytics*
aortic aneurysm, 164. *See also* abdominal aortic aneurysm; thoracic aortic aneurysm
aortic regurgitation, 19–20, 237–238, 246, 275
aortic resection, 33
aortic stenosis, 18–19, 236–237, 245
aortic valve disease, 24
aorto-bifemoral bypass grafting, 266–267
aorto-occlusive disease, 32
apnea, 350. *See also* sleep apnea
benzodiazepines and, 333
hydrocephalus and, 58
in infants, 345
obstructive, 302, 338
pregnancy and, 318
sedatives and, 40
appendectomy, 143–145

appendicitis, 143
appetite suppressants, 117
Apresoline. *See* hydralazine
aprotinin, 228, 244
Aquamephyton. *See* vitamin K
Aramine. *See* metaraminol bitartrate
ARDS. *See* adult respiratory distress
    syndrome (ARDS)
Arduan. *See* pipecuronium bromide
Arfonad. *See* trimethaphan
arrhythmias, 6
    ablation and, 357
    aortic stenosis and, 19
    bypass grafting and, 266
    cardiac, 2, 68, 71, 83, 95
    cardiomyopathies and, 25, 26, 29
    CHF and, 10, 11, 14
    chronic constrictive pericarditis and, 35
    drugs for, 8–9
    ESWL and, 164
    in geriatrics, 125
    hepatitis and, 86
    hypertension and, 13
    hypothermia and, 119
    intraocular procedures and, 309
    lupus and, 122
    malignant hyperthermia and, 73, 74
    mediastinoscopy and, 214
    myocardial infarction and, 7, 11
    pneumonia and, 41
    seizures and, 55
    thoracic aortic aneurysm and, 266
    thoracotomy and, 217
    ventricular, 355
Artane. *See* trihexyphenidyl hydrochloride
arteriovenous malformation neurosurgery,
    207–209
arthritis, 122, 126, 276. *See also*
    osteoarthritis; rheumatoid arthritis
arthroscopy, 286–287
ascites
    abdominal aortic aneurysm and, 257
    CHF and, 14
    chronic constrictive pericarditis and, 35
    cirrhosis and, 87, 88
    hepatic failure and, 92, 93
    hypothyroidism and, 79
    liver transplant and, 133
    portasystemic shunts and, 270
    restrictive pulmonary diseases and, 50
aspirin, 4, 44, 106, 122, 290
asthma, 37, 39–40, 115, 219, 351, 363. *See
    also* chronic obstructive pulmonary
    disease (COPD)
Astramorph. *See* morphine (morphine
    sulfate)

atelectasis
    anal fistulotomy and, 156
    autonomic dysreflexia and, 68
    bronchoscopy and, 221
    cholecystectomy and, 128
    cirrhosis and, 88
    CPB and, 253
    esophagectomy and, 154
    gastrectomy and, 141
    hepatic failure and, 90
    liver resection and, 131
    liver transplant and, 133
    lung biopsy and, 216
    pancreatitis and, 135
    portasystemic shunts and, 270
    pulmonary embolism and, 44
    small bowel resection and, 143
    splenectomy and, 140
atherosclerosis, 30, 56, 96, 125, 233, 264
atracurium, 5, 55, 170, 374–375. *See also*
    cisatracurium
atrial fibrillation
    AICD and, 357
    arrhythmias and, 8, 10
    cardiomyopathies and, 8, 25, 27, 28
    cardioversion and, 355
    mitral stenosis and, 21, 22, 238
    thyroid disease and, 78, 290
atrial pacing, 8, 10
atropine (atropine sulfate), 243, 350, 351,
    375–376
    arteriovenous surgery and, 208
    cardioversion and, 355
    heart denervation and, 228
    hernia repair and, 345
    hyperthermia caused by overdose, 121
    intra-abdominal procedures and, 341
    muscle relaxation reversal by, 5, 289
    myringotomy and, 337
    neck dissection and, 297
    ocular procedures and, 306, 308
    parasympathetic response, 158
    for pediatrics, 333
    strabismus repair and, 308
    tonsillectomy and, 338
    vagal-mediated reflexes and, 215
Atrovent. *See* ipratropium bromide
autoimmune disease, 62, 64, 65
automatic implantable cardioverter
    defibrillator (AICD), 356–357. *See also*
    cardioverter/defibrillator
autonomic dysreflexia, 67–68
autonomic hyperreflexia, 175, 188. *See also*
    autonomic dysreflexia
autonomic neuropathy, 98
Axid. *See* nizatidine

axiolysis, 167, 171
azathioprine, 225, 228
azidothymidine (AZT), 106
azotemia, 88, 96, 98
AZT. *See* azidothymidine (AZT)

baclofen, 62
bacteremia, 128
bacterial pharyngitis, 49
β_2-adrenergic agonists, 38, 320
β_2 agonist, 75
β-agonists, 28, 288
barbiturates. *See also specific barbiturates*
    cerebral aneurysm and, 193
    craniotomy and, 200
    hepatitis and, 87
    intracranial hypertension and, 66
    mitral regurgitation and, 239
    open eye procedure and, 307
    for pediatrics, 332
barotrauma, 222
β-blockers
    aneurysms and, 31, 192, 258
    arrhythmias and, 8, 9, 10
    CAD and, 234, 235
    cardiomyopathies and, 25, 26, 27, 28, 29
    CPB and, 255
    hypertension and, 12, 13
    IHD and, 4
    mitral stenosis and, 22
    peripheral vascular procedures and, 262
    pheochromocytoma and, 160
    thyroid disease and, 78, 288, 289, 290
Benadryl. *See* diphenhydramine
benzodiazepines, 245. *See also specific*
    benzodiazepines
    ARDS and, 52
    asthma and, 40
    burns and, 360
    chronic constrictive pericarditis and, 35
    craniotomy and, 198
    dilated cardiomyopathy and, 26
    epilepsy surgery and, 212
    hallucinations and, 333
    mitral regurgitation and, 239
    multiple sclerosis and, 62
    nephrectomy and, 167
    pregnancy and, 319, 321
    prostatectomy and, 163
    tonsillectomy and, 300
    transplants and, 134, 171
Betapace. *See* sotalol (sotalol
    hydrochloride)
Bicitra. *See* sodium citrate
bigeminy, 209
bilateral adrenalectomy, 80

bilateral salpingo-oophorectomy, 324
biliary atresia, 339
biliary tract disease, 113
bilirubin, 84, 87, 92
biplanar fluoroscopy, 95
bleomycin, 104, 138, 152, 231
blood replacement therapy, 16
bone grafting, 284
bone/joint disease, 43
bone marrow transplantation, 104, 334
bony ankylosis, 272
bowel ischemia, 265
brachytherapy, 354
bradycardia
    anesthesia level and, 246
    arrhythmias and, 10
    atropine treatment with, 245, 346
    autonomic dysreflexia and, 67
    electroconvulsive therapy and, 209
    ESWL and, 166
    glaucoma and, 118
    hydrocephalus and, 58
    hypertension and, 228
    hypothermia and, 119
    hypothyroidism and, 79
    IHD and, 5
    mediastinoscopy and, 214
    mitral regurgitation and, 239
    Norcuron and, 245
    ocular procedures and, 307, 308
    orbital fractures and, 311
    in pediatrics, 329, 333
    pregnancy and, 320, 322
    spinal cord transection and, 185
    sufentanil and, 245
bradykinesia, 59, 60
bradykinin, 114, 250
brain aneurysm, 57
breast biopsy, 229–230
Brethaire. *See* terbutaline (terbutaline
    sulfate)
Brethine. *See* terbutaline (terbutaline sulfate)
bretylium, 9, 376–377
Bretylol. *See* bretylium
Brevibloc. *See* esmolol
Brevital, 355
Brevital sodium. *See* methohexital
    (methohexital sodium)
Bricanyl. *See* terbutaline (terbutaline sulfate)
bromocriptine, 59, 82
bronchiectasis, 37, 219, 224. *See also* chronic
    obstructive pulmonary disease (COPD)
bronchiolar hyperreactivity, 39
bronchitis, 37, 38, 219, 257, 294. *See also*
    chronic obstructive pulmonary disease
    (COPD)

bronchoconstriction, 39, 320
bronchodilation, 115, 222, 258
bronchopulmonary lavage, 218–219
bronchoscopy, 153, 221–223, 365
Budd-Chiari syndrome, 90
bumetanide, 377–378
Bumex. *See* bumetanide
bupivacaine (bupivacaine HCl), 319, 322, 345, 346, 378. *See also* Marcaine
burns, 332, 359–361
butyrophenones, 60
bypass graft, 167, 266–267, 356

CABG, 7, 255
CAD. *See* coronary artery disease (CAD)
Calan. *See* verapamil
calcification, 18, 22
calcific disease, 18, 237
calcitonin, 114, 291
calcium, 73, 89, 250, 259
calcium antagonists, 8, 12, 191
calcium channel antagonists, 27
calcium channel blockers, 4, 74, 194, 199, 234, 249, 255, 258
calcium chloride, 253, 261, 333
captopril, 15
carbamazepine, 55, 212
Carbocaine. *See* mepivacaine HCl
carboxyhemoglobin, 243
carcinoid syndrome, 21, 114–115
Cardene. *See* nicardipine
cardiac glycosides, 47
cardiac ischemia, 13, 175
cardiac murmur, 27. *See also* systolic murmur
cardiac pacing, 9
cardiac radiofrequency ablation, 8, 10, 357
cardiac surgery, 119, 242–255
cardiac tamponade, 31, 35–36, 239–240, 254, 278, 293
cardiac valve fibrosis, 275
cardiomegaly, 97, 100, 104, 125, 159, 205
cardiomyopathy, 25–29
    AICD and, 356
    carcinoid syndrome and, 115
    chemotherapy and, 231
    CHF and, 13, 25, 26, 27, 88
    esophagectomy and, 152, 153
    liver transplant and, 133
    muscular dystrophy and, 182
    myasthenia gravis and, 63
    portasystemic shunts and, 270
    reversible, 79
cardioplegia, 249
cardiopulmonary bypass (CPB), 31, 33, 35, 226–227, 233, 248–252
cardiopulmonary disease, 41, 128, 240–241

cardiotomy, 240, 246
cardiovascular disease, 47, 195, 217
cardioversion, 28, 355
cardioverter/defibrillator, 10
Cardizem, 244. *See also* diltiazem
carotid endarterectomy, 268–269
carotid stenosis, 281
carpal tunnel syndrome, 82
Catapres. *See* clonidine
catecholamines
    ADH release by, 250
    CPB and, 246
    hypertension and, 11, 246
    hypotension and, 81
    inactivation of, 252
    intra-abdominal procedures and, 340
    ischemia and, 246
    kallikrein and, 115
    in pediatrics, 329
    pheochromocytoma and, 82, 83, 159, 160
    portsystemic shunts and, 270
    tachycardia and, 359
cefazolin, 225, 286
cellulitis, 48
cerebral aneurysm, 190–194
cerebral edema. *See under* edema
cerebral ischemia, 12
cerebral palsy, 308
cerebrovascular accident, 56–57
    in geriatrics, 159
    hypertension and, 12, 13
    pheochromocytoma and, 159
cerebrovascular disease, 56–57
    bypass grafting and, 266
    diabetes and, 56, 76
    hypertension and, 12, 56
cesarean section, 317–322
chemotherapy, 43, 103, 104, 138, 229, 363
CHF. *See* congestive heart failure (CHF)
Chirocaine. *See* levobupivacaine
chlordiazepoxide, 294
chloroprocaine HCl, 378–379
chlorpropamide, 77
cholangitis, 112–113
cholecystectomy, 113, 128–130
choledochojejunostomy, 137
cholinesterase inhibitors, 220
Christmas disease. *See* hemophilia B
chronic constrictive pericarditis, 34–35
chronic granulomatous disease. *See* tuberculosis
chronic liver disease, 77, 89, 132
chronic lung disease, 221
chronic lymphocytic leukemia. *See* leukemia
chronic myeloid leukemia. *See* leukemia

chronic obstructive pulmonary disease (COPD), 37–38
abdominal aortic aneurysm and, 257
bypass grafting and, 266
cor pulmonale and, 45, 46
electroconvulsive therapy and, 209
endarterectomy and, 268
esophagectomy and, 152
in geriatrics, 125
incidence/prevalence of, 37
laryngectomy and, 294
laser procedures and, 363
myasthenia gravis and, 64
neck dissection and, 296
pneumonia and, 41
pneumothorax/hemothorax and, 53
pulmonary hypertension and, 47
chronic peripheral arterio-occlusive disease, 30
chronic renal failure, 97–99, 268. *See also* renal failure
chronic renal insufficiency, 77
cimetidine, 379–380
cirrhosis, 87–89, 130, 270
cisatracurium, 5, 89, 94, 98, 168, 170, 236, 345
cisplatin, 139
Citanest. *See* prilocaine HCl
claudication, 30
Cleocin, 354
clindamycin, 17
clofibrate, 77
clonidine, 83, 380–382
coagulation cascade, 51
coagulation defects, 17, 164
coagulopathies, 93. *See also* disseminated intravascular coagulation; hemophilia A; hemophilia B; von Willebrand's disease
aneurysms and, 260, 266
ARDS and, 52
burns and, 359
cirrhosis and, 88
correction of, 87, 89
hip arthroplasty and, 274
hypothermia and, 119
laryngectomy and, 294
pancreatitis and, 136
portasystemic shunts and, 271
transplants and, 133, 134, 172
trauma and, 361
coarctation, 12
Cocaine (cocaine HCl), 197, 301, 382–383
codeine, 383
colectomy, 145
collagen vascular disease, 25
colloids
aneurysms and, 194, 259

bone fractures and, 281, 283
bypass grafting and, 167
craniotomy and, 199
hemorrhagic shock and, 16
in L-dopa therapy, 60
for pediatrics, 335
pheochromocytoma and, 84
spinal cord transection and, 185
colonoscopy, 150–151
Compazine. *See* prochlorperazine maleate
congestive heart failure (CHF), 13–15
acromegaly and, 205
aneurysms and, 257, 265
bypass grafting and, 266
cerebrovascular disease and, 56
cirrhosis and, 88
COPD and, 37
cor pulmonale and, 45
electroconvulsive therapy and, 209
esophagectomy and, 152, 153
in geriatrics, 122
hypertension and, 12, 13
hypothyroidism and, 79
IHD and, 2, 3, 13
intra-abdominal procedures and, 340
leukemia and, 104
lupus and, 122
malnutrition and, 124
muscular dystrophy and, 70
myocardial infarction and, 7, 11
obesity and, 116
pheochromocytoma and, 83
portasystemic shunts and, 270
renal failure and, 97
scoliosis and, 181
splenectomy and, 138
stenosis and, 19, 21
thyroid disease and, 78, 290
transsphenoidal resection and, 197
urolithiasis and, 95
Conn's syndrome. *See* hyperaldosteronism
constrictive pericarditis, 26, 239–240
continuous arteriovenous hemofiltration, 96
convulsions. *See* seizures
COPD. *See* chronic obstructive pulmonary disease (COPD)
Cordarone. *See* amiodarone
Corlopam. *See* fenoldopam
corneal transplant, 309
corneal ulceration, 289
coronary artery bypass, 4, 28, 31, 234–235
coronary artery disease (CAD), 7, 233–236
AICD and, 356
aneurysms and, 257, 265
cardiomyopathy and, 25

CHF and, 11
diabetes and, 76
IHD and, 2
laryngectomy and, 294
liver transplant and, 133
neck dissection and, 296
portasystemic shunts and, 270
transsphenoidal resection and, 197
coronary-subclavian steal syndrome, 31
cor pulmonale, 45–46, 50, 181, 304. *See also* pulmonary hypertension
corticosteroids. *See also specific corticosteroids*
adenoma and, 207
cerebral aneurysm and, 191
CPB and, 240
dilated cardiomyopathy and, 25
fat embolization and, 282
Guillain-Barré syndrome and, 61
hip arthroplasty and, 2274
hyperthermia and, 121
lupus and, 122
multiple sclerosis and, 62
myasthenia gravis and, 64
obesity and, 228
pericarditis and, 34
restrictive pulmonary diseases and, 50
Takayasu's arteritis and, 29
transsphenoidal resection and, 197
cortisol, 79, 80, 81, 85, 158
Corvert. *See* ibutilide (ibutilide fumarate)
Coumadin, 44. *See also* warfarin
CPB. *See* cardiopulmonary bypass (CPB)
craniofacial procedure, 334
cranioplasty, 203–204
craniotomy, 55, 195–196, 198–200
cricoarytenoid arthritis, 122
cricothyroidotomy, 69, 364
Crohn's disease, 143, 155
cromolyn sodium, 38, 40, 243
cryoprecipitate, 107, 108
cryosurgery, 325
cryptoglandular fistula, 155
crystalloids
aneurysms and, 32, 194, 259, 265
arteriovenous surgery and, 208
bone fractures and, 281, 283, 285
burns and, 360
bypass grafting and, 267
craniotomy and, 196, 199
Cushing's syndrome and, 158
hemorrhagic shock and, 16
hypotension and, 278
hysterectomy and, 324
in vitro fertilization and, 326
in L-dopa therapy, 60

pancreatitis and, 114, 135
for pediatrics, 335
peripheral vascular procedures and, 261
pheochromocytoma and, 84
polycythemia vera and, 102
spinal cord transection and, 185
transplants and, 169, 170, 225
trauma and, 362
curare, 73
Cushing's syndrome (disease), 12, 80, 157, 158, 205
cyanosis, 24, 53, 73, 115, 117, 215, 342
cyclocryotherapy, 117
cyclosporine, 123, 225, 228, 383–384
cystectomy, 173–174
cystic fibrosis, 37, 219, 224, 225. *See also* chronic obstructive pulmonary disease (COPD)
cystoscopy, 165, 174–175, 345
cytarabine, 138
cytochrome P450, 140
cytopenia, 139

dacryocystorhinostomy (DCR), 314–315
Dantrium. *See* dantrolene (dantrolene sodium)
dantrolene (dantrolene sodium), 62, 71, 74, 384–385
Daunorubicin, 104, 152
D & C. *See* dilatation and curettage (D & C)
DC cardioversion, 8, 9, 10
DCR. *See* dacryocystorhinostomy (DCR)
DDAVP. *See* desmopressin
Decadron, 364. *See also* dexamethasone
decongestants, 49
decubitus ulcer, 186
deep venous thrombosis (DVT), 44, 188, 273, 275, 280, 282, 284, 285
defibrillation, 10, 35
delirium tremens, 294
Demadex. *See* torsemide
Demerol, 333. *See also* meperidine HCl
depolarizing muscle relaxants, 65, 94, 220, 322, 334. *See also* nondepolarizing muscle relaxants (NDMRs)
deprenyl, 59
desflurane, 385–386
arteriovenous surgery and, 208
asthma and, 40
cranioplasty and, 204
craniotomy and, 196, 200
hepatic failure and, 94
myringotomy and, 337
pheochromocytoma and, 160
renal failure and, 98
UPPP and, 305

desmopressin, 77, 108, 386–387
dexamethasone, 80, 191, 387–388
dextran, 16, 44, 103, 262
dextrocardia, 342
dextrose, 167, 171, 196, 299, 344
DI. *See* diabetes insipidus (DI)
diabetes. *See also* diabetes insipidus (DI);
    diabetes mellitus
    acromegaly and, 205
    aneurysms and, 257
    bypass grafting and, 266
    endarterectomy and, 268
    in geriatrics, 125
    gestational, 318
    IHD and, 2
    impotence and, 175
    myocardial infarction and, 6, 75, 76
    renal failure and, 96
diabetes insipidus (DI), 76–77, 197, 290
diabetes mellitus, 75–76
    acromegaly and, 82
    aneurysms and, 31
    hypoaldosteronism and, 84
    myocardial infarction and, 233
    obesity and, 116
    pancreatitis and, 113
    renal failure and, 97
    transsphenoidal resection and, 197
diabetic glomerulonephropathy, 168
diabetic nephropathy, 97
diabetic retinopathy, 76
dialysis, 96, 97, 133, 169, 291
diaphoresis, 60, 83, 190
diaphragmatic hernia, 110, 341–343
diaphragmatic paralysis, 296, 298
diazepam, 55, 294, 388–389
difficult airway algorithm, 499
digitalis, 14, 45, 47, 79
digoxin, 389–390
    abdominal aortic aneurysm and, 258
    arrhythmias and, 8, 9
    cardiomyopathies and, 25, 27
    cardioversion and, 355
    CHF and, 14
    mitral regurgitation and, 23
    mitral stenosis and, 22
    peripheral vascular procedures and, 262
Dilantin, 212. *See also* phenytoin
dilatation and curettage (D & C), 328
diltiazem, 8, 10, 390–391
dimenhydrinate, 165
dinitrogen monoxide, 52
diphenhydramine, 254, 351, 391–392
diphenylhydantoin, 54
diplopia, 63, 220
Diprivan, 333. *See also* propofol

dipyridamole, 155, 242
disopyramide, 8, 9
dissecting aneurysm, 31, 56
disseminated intravascular coagulation, 74,
    108–109
diuretics
    arteriovenous surgery and, 208
    bypass grafting and, 267
    cardiomyopathies and, 25, 28
    CHF and, 15
    cor pulmonale and, 45
    craniotomy and, 195
    ESWL and, 166
    hypertension and, 12
    hypovolemia caused by, 193
    mitral regurgitation and, 23
    mitral stenosis and, 22
    obesity and, 117
    pulmonary hypertension and, 47
diverticulosis, 145
Dixarit. *See* clonidine
dobutamine (dobutamine HCl), 243, 392
    CHF and, 15, 242
    CPB and, 253
    hernia repair and, 343
    hypertrophic cardiomyopathy and, 28
    mitral stenosis and, 22
Dobutrex. *See* dobutamine (dobutamine
    HCl)
Dolophine HCl. *See* methadone HCl
dopamine (dopamine HCl), 243, 393
    aneurysms and, 192, 259, 260
    CHF and, 15
    CPB and, 250
    craniotomy and, 199
    hernia repair and, 342, 343
    hypertrophic cardiomyopathy and, 28
    mitral stenosis and, 122
    nephrectomy and, 167
    Parkinson's syndrome and, 59
    peripheral vascular procedures and, 261
    pheochromocytoma and, 159
    prostatectomy and, 163
    septic shock and, 17
    transplants and, 172, 226, 227
Dopram. *See* doxapram HCl
doxacurium (doxacurium chloride), 5,
    393–394
doxapram HCl, 394–395
doxorubicin, 104, 138, 231
droperidol, 202, 337, 339
d-tubocurarine, 40
Duraclon. *See* clonidine
Duramorph. *See* morphine (morphine sulfate)
Duranest. *See* etidocaine HCl
DVT. *See* deep venous thrombosis (DVT)

dysarthria, 63
dysmenorrhea, 324
dysphagia, 49, 63, 152, 190
dyspnea
    adenoma and, 205
    aortic regurgitation and, 20
    ARDS and, 52
    asthma and, 39
    CHF and, 14
    COPD and, 38
    cor pulmonale and, 45
    hernia and, 342
    IHD and, 2, 3
    kyphoscoliosis and, 72
    leukemia and, 104
    lupus and, 122
    mitral stenosis and, 21
    myocardial infarction and, 7
    obesity and, 116
    pneumonia and, 41
    pneumothorax/hemothorax and, 53
    pulmonary embolism and, 20
    pulmonary hypertension and, 47
    restrictive pulmonary diseases and, 50
    thoracic aortic aneurysm and, 265
    transsphenoidal resection and, 197
    tuberculosis and, 43
dysrhythmia
    abdominal aortic aneurysm and, 257
    ablation and, 357
    aortic stenosis and, 237
    autonomic hyperreflexia and, 188
    bronchoscopy and, 221, 223
    cardiac, 166, 307
    CPB and, 253
    in vitro fertilization and, 326
    liver transplant and, 133
    mediastinoscopy and, 214
    pheochromocytoma and, 159
    splenectomy and, 138
    vasoconstrictors and, 302
    ventricular, 297

Eaton-Lambert syndrome, 215, 216, 217.
    See also myasthenic syndrome
echothiophate, 118
eclampsia, 54, 55
eclamptic seizures, 55
Edecrin. *See* ethacrynic acid
edema. *See also* pulmonary edema
    arthroscopy and, 287
    burns and, 359
    cerebral, 93, 199, 208, 213, 299
    COPD and, 37
    laser procedures and, 363, 365
    from Ludwig's angina, 49

    pancreatic, 114
    periorbital, 303
    peripheral, 3, 7, 14, 45, 92
    perivascular, 238
    pneumonia and, 41
    radiation and, 294
    spinal cord injury and, 68
    subglottic, 150, 223
    tonsillectomy and, 339
    tracheostomy and, 295
edrophonium (edrophonium chloride), 63,
    333, 395–396
effusion, 50, 132. *See also* pericardial
    effusion; pleural effusion
Eisenmenger's syndrome, 224
electroconvulsive therapy, 209–210
embolectomy, 260–264
emphysema, 37, 38, 53, 224, 257, 293, 294,
    363. *See also* chronic obstructive
    pulmonary disease (COPD)
enalapril, 15
enalaprilat, 396
encephalitis, 59
endarterectomy, 56, 262, 268–269
endocardial biopsy, 25
endocarditis (infective)
    aortic regurgitation and, 19
    aortic stenosis and, 237
    hypertrophic cardiomyopathy and, 28
    lupus and, 122
    mitral regurgitation and, 22
    tricuspid regurgitation and, 24
endometriosis, 323, 324, 326
endoscopic sclerosis, 89
endoscopy, 358
enflurane, 55, 94, 99, 160, 396–397
Enlon. *See* edrophonium (edrophonium
    chloride)
enoxaparin, 397–398
enteral supplements, 124
enterocolitis, 339
eosinophil count, 39
eosinophilic granuloma, 50
ephedrine (ephedrine sulfate), 256, 398
    andrenalectomy and, 158
    arteriovenous surgery and, 208
    cardiomyopathies and, 26, 28
    endarterectomy and, 268
    hypotension and, 263
    pregnancy and, 319, 320, 321, 322
    thoracotomy and, 218
epidural clonidine. *See* clonidine
epiglottitis, 48, 49
epilepsy surgery, 211–213
epinephrine, 243, 256, 351
    bradycardia and, 346

carcinoid syndrome and, 115
COPD and, 38
CPB and, 251, 253, 254
DCR and, 314
glaucoma and, 117
heart/lung transplant and, 228
hemostasis and, 361
hernia repair and, 343, 345
laminectomy and, 178
with local anesthesia, 78
mitral stenosis and, 22
nasal surgery and, 301
for pediatrics, 333
peripheral vascular procedures and, 261
pheochromocytoma and, 159
rhytidectomy and, 312
thromboangitis obliterans and, 30
tonsillectomy and, 338
transsphenoidal resection and, 197
epinephrine HCl, 398–399
episiotomy, 322
esmolol, 256, 399–400
aneurysms and, 192, 265
arteriovenous surgery and, 208
bone fractures and, 281
endarterectomy and, 268, 269
hypertension and, 13
IHD and, 5
myocardial infarction and, 8
pheochromocytoma and, 84, 160
thyroidectomy and, 290
esophageal resection, 151–154
esophageal transection, 89
esophageal varices, 133
esophagectomy. See esophageal resection
esophagitis, 148
esophagogastroduodenoscopy, 149
esophagoscopy/gastroscopy, 149–150
esotropia, 307
ESWL. See extracorporeal shock wave
lithotripsy (ESWL)
ethacrynic acid, 400–401
ethambutol, 43
ethosuximide, 55, 212
Ethrane. See enflurane
etidocaine HCl, 401
etomidate, 401–402
Addison's disease and, 81
aortic stenosis and, 237
bypass grafting and, 267
CAD and, 236
cardiac tamponade and, 239
cranioplasty and, 203, 204
electroconvulsive therapy and, 210
glaucoma and, 118
heart/lung transplant and, 226

liver resection and, 131
mitral regurgitation and, 239
pancreatectomy and, 136
portasystemic shunts and, 271
seizures and, 54
thoracic aortic aneurysm and, 265
ventriculoperitoneal shunt and, 211
exotropia, 307
exstrophy, 340
external fixator placement, 278–279
extracorporeal circuit, 240
extracorporeal shock wave lithotripsy
(ESWL), 95, 147, 164–166

facelift. See rhytidectomy
famotidine, 402–403
fat embolization, 279, 281, 282, 286
febrile illness, 25
femoral hernia, 146
femoral neuropathy, 282
fenoldopam, 403–404
fentanyl
adenoma and, 206
aneurysms and, 192, 193, 265
aortic stenosis and, 237
arteriovenous surgery and, 208
bypass grafting and, 267
colonoscopy and, 151
CPB and, 252
craniotomy and, 195, 196, 199
cystoscopy and, 174
D & C and, 328
endoscopy and, 358
hysterectomy and, 325
IHD and, 5
intra-abdominal procedures and, 341
lithotripsy and, 148
for pediatrics, 333
pheochromocytoma and, 83
portasystemic shunts and, 271
pregnancy and, 321
stereotactic surgery and, 200
transplants and, 134, 226, 227
fetal distress, 317
fibrinolysis, 88, 121, 132, 133
flecainide, 8, 9
fluid management, guidelines for, 491–498
flumazenil, 405
Fluothane. See halothane
flutter. See atrial fibrillation
Forane, 337. See also isoflurane
4-aminopyridine, 65
furosemide, 405–406
aneurysms and, 259
calcium levels and, 291
CHF and, 15

CPB and, 250
craniotomy and, 199
intracranial hypertension and, 66
kidney transplant and, 170, 172
malignant hyperthermia and, 74
nephrectomy and, 167
oliguria and, 228
peripheral vascular procedures and, 261
fusiform aneurysm, 31

galactosemia, 90
gallbladder disease. *See* cholangitis
gallbladder lithotripsy, 147–149
gallstones, 112, 113, 128, 129
gamma globulin, 61
ganglionic blockers, 68
gangrene, 29, 260
gastrectomy, 140–141
gastric devascularization, 89
gastric reflux, 111, 152
gastric stapling, 116
gastrinoma, 135
gastroduodenostomy, 140
gastrojejunostomy, 137, 140
gastroplasty, 116
gastroschisis, 339
gastroscopy. *See* esophagoscopy/gastroscopy
gastrostomy, 141–142
genital herpes, 317
genitourinary abscesses, 43
gentamicin, 17
geriatrics, 125–126
glaucoma, 117–118, 209, 309
glomerulonephritis, 97, 122
glossectomy, 296
glucagon, 151, 406–407
glucocorticoids, 40, 171, 291
glucose, 196, 203
glycerin, 118
glycine, 162
glycopyrrolate, 350, 407–408
   genitourinary procedures and, 346
   hernia repair and, 345
   IHD and, 5
   intra-abdominal procedures and, 341
   laryngectomy and, 295
   open eye procedures and, 306
   tachycardia and, 209
   thoractomy and, 217
   thyroidectomy and, 289
goiter, 78
goniotomy, 117
grand mal seizures, 54–55, 209
granisetron, 408–409
granulocytopenia, 106
granulomatous colitis, 150

Graves' disease, 75, 78
Guillain-Barré syndrome, 60–61
gynecomastia, 92

halothane, 351, 409–410
   cirrhosis and, 89
   genitourinary procedures and, 346
   hepatic failure and, 90, 94
   hepatitis and, 86, 337
   hernia repair and, 345
   malignant hyperthermia and, 71, 73,
      308
   myringotomy and, 337
   for nuclear medicine, 353
   for pediatrics, 333
   pheochromocytoma and, 83
   tonsillectomy and, 338
headaches
   acromegaly and, 81
   autonomic dysreflexia and, 68
   cerebral aneurysm and, 191
   in geriatrics, 126
   hydrocephalus and, 58
   intracranial hypertension and, 65
   pheochromocytoma and, 83, 159,
      160
heart-lung machine, 240
heart transplant, 25, 224–228
HELLP syndrome, 318
hemaglobinuria, 251
hematoma
   hip pinning and, 284
   intracranial, 54
   neck dissection and, 298
   retroperitoneal, 282
   spinal instrumentation and, 183
   thyroidectomy and, 289
hematuria, 166, 173, 174
hemiparesis, 190
hemiplegia, 190, 282
hemisternotomy. *See* sternotomy
hemochromatosis, 87, 133
hemodialysis, 96, 97, 98, 167, 171
hemodilution, 182, 248, 251
hemodynamic oxidase inhibitors, 209
hemolysis, 100, 102, 318
hemophilia, 105
hemophilia A, 106–107
hemophilia B, 107
hemoptysis
   bronchoscopy and, 221
   mitral stenosis and, 21
   pneumonia and, 41
   pulmonary embolism and, 43
   thoracic aortic aneurysm and, 265
   tuberculosis and, 43

hemorrhage
  aneurysms and, 259, 266
  bypass grafting and, 267
  cerebrovascular disease and, 56, 188
  CPB and, 255
  craniotomy and, 196
  endarterectomy and, 269
  esophagectomy, 154
  in vitro fertilization and, 326
  intracerebral, 83, 209, 303
  intracranial, 54, 340
  intraventricular, 58
  knee arthroplasty and, 276
  nephrectomy and, 166
  pancreatectomy, 137
  pancreatitis and, 136
  thyroid storm mimicking of, 78
  tracheotomy, 293
  variceal, 87, 270
hemorrhagic cystitis, 173
hemorrhagic shock, 16
hemorrhoidectomy, 156–157
hemorrhoids, 156
hemothorax, 53, 154, 279
heparin, 244, 410–412
  aneurysms and, 32, 258, 259, 260
  bypass grafting and, 267
  coagulopathies and, 109
  coronary bypass and, 235
  CPB and, 240, 253, 255
  endarterectomy and, 268
  fat embolization and, 282
  hit arthroplasty and, 272
  nephrectomy and, 167
  peripheral vascular procedures and, 262,
    263
  pulmonary embolism and, 44
  transplants and, 104, 170
heparinization, 247
hepatectomy, 90, 132
hepatic artery thrombosis, 134
hepatic encephalopathy, 87, 88, 92
hepatic failure, 89–90, 92–94
hepatitis, 86–87, 90
  hemophilia and, 107
  liver resection and, 130
  liver transplant and, 133
  lupus and, 122
hepatomegaly, 14, 88, 115
hepatorenal syndrome, 87, 88, 92
hepatosplenomegaly, 35, 45, 104
hepatotoxicity, 228
hernia repair, 334, 341–345
herniorrhaphy, 146–147
herpes simplex, 90
Hespan. *See* hetastarch

hetastarch, 412
  aneurysms and, 32, 259
  arteriovenous surgery and, 208
  CPB and, 240
  craniotomy and, 196
  hemorrhagic shock and, 16
  nephrectomy and, 167
  prostatectomy and, 163
hiatal hernia, 111, 148
hip arthroplasty, 272–275
hip pinning, 282–284
hirsutism, 80
histamine
  release of, 40, 44, 115, 160, 245
  secretion of, 114
  septic shock and, 17
HIV. *See* human immunodeficiency virus (HIV)
HIV infection. *See* AIDS
Hodgkin's disease, 138
HTN. *See* hypertension (HTN)
human immunodeficiency virus (HIV), 105.
    See also AIDS
Humulin R. *See* insulin (regular)
hungry bone syndrome, 291
hyaluronidase, 412–413
hydralazine, 13, 15, 121, 256, 413–414
Hydrate. *See* dimenhydrinate
hydrocele, 176
hydrocephalus, 57–58
  craniotomy and, 195
  in infants, 340
  intracranial hypertension and, 65, 66
  strabismus repair and, 308
  ventriculoperitoneal shunt and, 210
hydrocortisone (hydrocortisone sodium
    succinate), 40, 84, 158, 277, 414–415
hydronephrosis, 166, 168
hydrothorax, 58
hyperadrenocorticism, 12, 158. *See also*
    Cushing's syndrome (disease)
hyperaldosteronism, 85, 88, 133, 157, 205
hypercalcemia, 77, 95, 290, 291
hypercalciuria, 95
hypercapnia
  craniotomy and, 198
  in geriatrics, 125
  hernia repair and, 343
  in vitro fertilization and, 326
  pulmonary embolism and, 44
  pulmonary hypertension and, 304
  spinal instrumentation and, 182
hypercarbia
  ARDS and, 51
  autonomic dysreflexia and, 68
  cerebral aneurysm and, 194
  cholecystectomy and, 129

craniotomy and, 200
esophagectomy and, 152
glaucoma and, 118
intracranial hypertension and, 66
malignant hyperthermia and, 73
mitral stenosis and, 238
in pediatrics, 329, 330, 331
pneumonia and, 41, 42
hypercholesterolemia, 116
hypercoagulation, 44
hypereosinophilic syndromes, 29
hyperglycemia
burns and, 359
carcinoid syndrome and, 115
craniotomy and, 199
Cushing's disease and, 80, 158, 205
diabetes and, 75, 76
malnutrition and, 124
pancreatectomy and, 137
pancreatitis and, 114
in pediatrics, 331
pheochromocytoma and, 159
pregnancy and, 321
hyperhidrosis, 82
hyperinflation, 37
hyperkalemia
Addison's disease and, 81
CPB and, 250
in geriatrics, 125
hypertension and, 12
hypoaldosteronism and, 84
malignant hyperthermia and, 73, 74
peripheral vascular procedures
and, 264
renal failure and, 97
seizures and, 55
spinal cord transection and, 187
hyperlipidemia, 2, 6, 113, 228
hypermagnesemia, 97
hypernatremia, 331
hyperoxaluria, 95
hyperparathyroidism, 95, 98, 113, 290
hyperphosphatemia, 97
hyperplasia, 63, 157, 290
hyperpnea, 330
hypersplenism, 92, 270
hypertension (HTN), 11–13. *See also*
pulmonary hypertension
acromegaly and, 205
adrenalectomy and, 157, 159
aneurysms and, 31, 257, 264, 265
arteriovenous surgery and, 208
autonomic dysreflexia and, 67, 68
bypass grafting and, 266
CAD and, 233
carcinoid syndrome and, 115

cardiomyopathies and, 25, 28
craniotomy and, 195, 199
Cushing's disease and, 80
cystoscopy and, 175
electroconvulsive therapy and, 209
endarterectomy and, 268, 269
essential, 11–12
in geriatrics, 125
hematoma and, 313
hydrocephalus and, 58
hyperaldosteronism and, 85
impotence and, 175
intracranial, 65–67, 198
intraocular procedures and, 309
kidney transplant and, 172
laryngectomy and, 294
mediastinoscopy and, 214
neck dissection and, 296
nephrectomy and, 166, 168
obesity and, 117
pregnancy and, 317, 318, 319
prostate resection and, 162
spinal cord transection and, 188
systemic and, 13, 97, 116, 196
thyroidectomy and, 289, 290
transsphenoidal resection and, 197
vasoconstrictors and, 302
hypertensive nephrosclerosis, 97
hyperthermia, 78, 90, 120–121, 252, 290
hyperthyroidism, 78, 288
hypertriglyceridemia, 115
hyperuricemia, 97
hyperventilation
anemia and, 101
arteriovenous surgery and, 208
asthma and, 39
CHF and, 14
cirrhosis and, 88
CPB and, 250
craniotomy and, 199
gastrectomy and, 141
hepatic failure and, 90
intracranial hypertension and, 66
liver transplant and, 133
malignant hyperthermia and, 74
in pediatrics, 329
renal failure and, 99
seizures and, 55, 213
septic shock and, 17
stereotactic surgery and, 202
hypervolemia, 133, 157, 161, 291
hypoadrenocorticism, 80, 159, 160. *See also*
Addison's disease
hypoalbuminemia, 88, 92, 97
hypoaldosteronism, 84
hypocalcemia, 97, 98, 124

hypocarbia
  asthma and, 39
  cerebral aneurysm and, 193
  cranioplasty, 204
  craniotomy and, 200
  glaucoma and, 118
  seizures and, 55
hypochloremia, 340
hypoglycemia
  Addison's disease and, 81
  adrenalectomy and, 159
  cirrhosis and, 88
  diabetes and, 76
  hepatic failure and, 92, 93
  in infants, 344
  liver resection and, 132
  malnutrition and, 124
  pancreatitis and, 136
  in pediatrics, 331, 334
  pheochromocytoma and, 160
  pregnancy and, 319
  prevention of, 87
hypokalemia
  adenoma and, 205
  adrenalectomy and, 157
  CHF and, 14, 15
  cirrhosis and, 88
  cor pulmonale and, 46
  CPB and, 254
  Cushing's disease and, 80, 157, 158
  diabetes insipidus and, 77
  heart/lung transplant and, 225
  hyperaldosteronism and, 85
  hypertension and, 12
  intra-abdominal procedures and, 340
  liver transplant and, 133
  malnutrition and, 124
hypomagnesemia, 9, 86, 124
hyponatremia
  cirrhosis and, 88
  dilutional, 79, 162
  hypoaldosteronism and, 84
  liver transplant and, 133
  prostate resection and, 161, 162
  renal failure and, 97
hypoparathyroidism, 289, 291
hypophosphatemia, 124
hypophysectomy, 77, 207
hypoplasia, 343
hypoproteinemia, 92
hyporeninemia, 84
hypospadia, 175, 345–346
hypotension
  Addison's disease and, 81
  anesthesia level and, 246
  aortic regurgitation and, 20

arteriovenous surgery and, 208
bone fractures and, 278, 281
bypass grafting and, 267
cardiac tamponade and, 36, 239
cardiomyopathies and, 26, 28
chronic constrictive pericarditis and, 35
cirrhosis and, 89
CPB and, 248
diskectomy and, 179
drug-induced, 27
electroconvulsive therapy and, 209
ESWL and, 166
in geriatrics, 126
hepatitis and, 87
hypertension and, 12, 13
hypervolemia and, 329
intraocular procedures and, 309
liver resection and, 131
malignant hyperthermia and, 73
methylmethacrylate and, 274
myocardial infarction and, 6
pancreatectomy and, 136
in pediatrics, 334
peripheral vascular procedures and, 261
pheochromocytoma and, 160
pneumothorax/hemothorax and, 53
pregnancy and, 317, 319, 321
prostate resection and, 162
pulmonary embolism and, 44–45
seizures and, 55
septic shock and, 17
spinal cord transection and, 187
spinal instrumentation and, 182,
  183–184
stenosis and, 19, 238
systemic, 318
thoractomy and, 218
thyroid disease and, 78
hypothalamic dysfunction, 79
hypothermia, 119–120
  anemia and, 100
  aneurysms and, 33
  arteriovenous surgery and, 208
  burns and, 360
  CPB and, 241, 248–249, 250, 251
  in geriatrics, 125
  glaucoma and, 118
  hydrocephalus and, 58
  ischemia and, 192
  liver resection and, 132
  pancreatitis and, 113
  in pediatrics, 332
  portasystemic shunts and, 271
  sickle cell disease and, 101
  spinal instrumentation and, 181, 184
  urolithiasis and, 95

hypothyroidism, 75, 79, 220
hypoventilation
    acidosis and, 291
    colectomy and, 145
    esophagectomy and, 154
    hydrocephalus and, 58
    hypoaldosteronism and, 84
    kyphoscoliosis and, 72
    mitral stenosis and, 22
    scoliosis and, 181
    sickle cell disease and, 102
hypovolemia
    anemia and, 174
    arteriovenous surgery and, 208
    bypass grafting and, 267
    CHF and, 15
    diabetes and, 75
    esophagectomy and, 152
    gastrotomy and, 142
    hyperaldosteronism and, 85
    hypertension and, 12, 13
    hypertrophic cardiomyopathy
        and, 28
    hypoaldosteronism and, 84
    hypothyroidism and, 79
    pancreatectomy and, 137
    in pediatrics, 329
    pheochromocytoma and, 83
    pneumothorax/hemothorax and, 53
    renal disease and, 168
    renal hypoperfusion and, 359
    tonsillectomy and, 339
hypoxemia
    ARDS and, 52
    asthma and, 39
    bone fractures and, 278, 279
    bronchoscopy and, 221
    cirrhosis and, 88
    diaphragmatic hernia and, 110
    esophagectomy and, 152, 154
    fat embolization and, 282
    gastrotomy and, 142
    heart/lung transplant and, 226, 227
    hepatic failure and, 90
    hip arthroplasty and, 274
    in infants, 344
    intra-abdominal procedures and, 340
    intracranial hypertension and, 66
    kyphoscoliosis and, 72
    laryngectomy and, 294
    lupus and, 122
    malignant hyperthermia and, 73
    mitral stenosis and, 22
    obesity and, 116
    OLV and, 229
    in pediatrics, 329

    pneumonia and, 41
    pneumothorax/hemothorax and, 53
    polycythemia and, 225
    portasystemic shunts and, 270
    pulmonary embolism and, 44
    pulmonary hypertension and, 47
    restrictive pulmonary diseases
        and, 50
    scoliosis and, 181
    spinal cord transection and, 185
    thoractomy and, 218
hypoxia
    appendicitis and, 143
    femoral prosthesis and, 274
    in geriatrics, 125
    heart/lung transplant and, 227, 228
    hydrocephalus and, 58
    hypertension from, 304
    in infants, 342, 343
    in vitro fertilization and, 326
    in pediatrics, 329, 330, 331
    valvular heart disease and, 238
hysterectomy, 323, 324–325

ibutilide (ibutilide fumarate), 8,
    415–416
IHD. *See* ischemic heart disease (IHD)
immunosuppressants, 134, 143, 151, 220
immunosuppression, 105, 123
immunosuppressive therapy, 62
incarcerated hernia, 339
Inderal. *See* propranolol
indigo carmine, 167, 172, 174
indomethacin, 84, 106
infarction, 102. *See also* myocardial
    infarction (MI)
infection
    after tonsillectomy, 301
    aneurysms and, 33
    bacterial, 87
    cardiac tamponade and, 36
    COPD and, 37
    C-section and, 317
    diabetes and, 75, 76
    gastrointestinal, 60
    heart/lung transplant and, 228
    intracranial, 48
    intracranial hypertension and, 65
    pericarditis and, 34
    postpartum, 56
    pulmonary, 72, 133, 292
    respiratory, 48–49, 60, 300, 336
    retropharyngeal, 48, 49
    seizures and, 54
infertility, 176
inflammatory bowel disease, 150

inguinal hernia, 146, 344
in vitro fertilization, 326
Inocor. *See* amrinone (amrinone lactate)
inotropes. *See also specific inotropes*
    Addison's disease and, 81
    bypass grafting and, 267
    CAD and, 234
    cardiac tamponade and, 36
    CHF and, 15
    craniotomy and, 195
    portasystemic shunts and, 271
    vasodilation and, 25
insulinoma, 135
insulin (regular), 74, 76, 98, 250, 254, 416–418
intercostal neuritis, 148
intermaxillary fixation, 298
internal fixation, 278–279, 282–286
interstitial fibrosis, 224
intervertebral hernia, 177, 178
intestinal atresia, 339
intestinal ischemia, 122
intraocular procedures, 309–310
Intropin. *See* dopamine (dopamine HCl)
iodine, 78, 79
ipodate, 290
Ipran. *See* propranolol
ipratropium bromide, 38, 39, 416
irradiation, 79, 138
ischemia, 27. *See also* myocardial ischemia
    aneurysms and, 31, 33, 194
    aortic stenosis and, 237
    azotemia and, 95
    bone fractures and, 283
    cerebrovascular disease and, 56
    CPB and, 246, 253, 254
    craniotomy and, 200
    intracranial hypertension and, 65
    lung biopsy and, 216
    mucosal, 251
    myocardial infarction and, 11
    reperfusion and, 241
    spinal cord injury and, 68
ischemic heart disease (IHD), 2–6
    acromegaly and, 205
    chronic peripheral arterio-occlusive disease and, 30
    hypertension and, 2, 4, 5, 12
    mitral dysfunction and, 23
ischemic optic neuropathy, 184
Isocaine. *See* mepivacaine HCl
isoflurane, 419
    arteriovenous surgery and, 208
    asthma and, 40
    bone fractures and, 281
    cranioplasty and, 204
    craniotomy and, 196, 200
    epilepsy surgery and, 212–213
    genitourinary procedures and, 346
    heart/lung transplant and, 226
    hepatic failure and, 94
    lung biopsy and, 216
    myringotomy and, 337
    for pediatrics, 333
    pheochromocytoma and, 160
    pregnancy and, 319
    renal failure and, 98
    stereotactic surgery and, 202
    tonsillectomy and, 338
    transsphenoidal resection and, 206
    UPPP and, 305
    vasodilation with, 236
isoniazid, 43, 90
isoproterenol (isoproterenol HCl), 9, 227, 228, 419–420
Isoptin. *See* verapamil
Isuprel. *See* isoproterenol (isoproterenol HCl)
Itrop. *See* ipratropium bromide
IVD, 45

jaw wiring, 116
jugular venous distention, 7, 14

kallikrein, 115, 250
Kaposi's sarcoma, 105
Ketalar. *See* ketamine (ketamine HCl)
ketamine (ketamine HCl), 350, 420–421
    abdominal aortic aneurysm and, 259
    burns and, 360
    CAD and, 236
    carcinoid syndrome and, 115
    cardiac tamponade and, 36, 239
    CHF and, 14
    hemorrhagic shock and, 16
    hypertrophic cardiomyopathy and, 28
    intraocular procedures and, 310
    laser procedures and, 364
    liver resection and, 131
    pancreatectomy and, 136
    Parkinson's syndrome and, 60
    for pediatrics, 333
    pheochromocytoma and, 160
    portasystemic shunts and, 271
    pregnancy and, 319, 320
    seizures and, 54, 55, 212
    spinal cord transection and, 187
    thyroid disease and, 78, 289
    trauma and, 362
ketoacidosis, 75, 76
ketorolac (ketorolac tromethamine), 176, 302, 421–422
kidney stones. *See* urolithiasis

kidney transplant, 168–173
knee arthroplasty, 275–276
kyphoscoliosis, 50, 70, 72–73
Kytril. *See* granisetron

labetalol, 13, 208, 256, 268, 422–423
lactated Ringer's
   adenoma and, 206
   anal fistulotomy and, 156
   arteriovenous surgery and, 208
   arthroplasty and, 275, 277
   cranioplasty and, 203
   DCR and, 314
   esophagectomy and, 153
   esophagoscopy and, 150
   facial trauma and, 303
   fractures and, 278, 311
   gallbladder lithotripsy and, 148
   gastrotomy and, 142
   genitourinary procedures and, 346
   hernia repair and, 344
   herniorrhaphy and, 147
   hypokalemia and, 99
   kidney transplant and, 171
   laryngectomy and, 295
   laser procedures and, 364
   liver resection and, 131
   lung biopsy and, 216
   maxillofacial surgery and, 299
   myringotomy and, 337
   nasal surgery and, 302
   neck dissection and, 296
   nephrectomy and, 167
   pancreatectomy and, 136
   ptosis surgery and, 315
   rhytidectomy and, 313
   splenectomy and, 139
   strabismus repair and, 308
   tonsillectomy and, 338, 339
   UPPP and, 305
lactulose, 87
Lanoxin. *See* digoxin
lansoprazole, 423–424
laparoscopy, 323, 324
laparotomy, 141, 142
laryngectomy, 293–296, 298
laser procedures for airway, 363–365
Lasix. *See* furosemide
latex allergy, 524–525
laudanosine, 55
L-dopa, 59
LEEP. *See* loop electrosurgical excision
   procedure (LEEP)
LeFort procedures, 303–304
left ventricular dysfunction, 2, 122, 257
left ventricular hypertrophy, 18, 27, 97, 239

leukemia, 103–104
leukocytosis, 41, 44, 113
leukopenia, 88, 92, 228
levobupivacaine, 424
Levophed, 243. *See also* norepinephrine
   (norepinephrine bitartrate)
lidocaine (lidocaine HCl), 424–425
   aneurysms and, 192, 265
   arrhythmias and, 9, 10, 158
   arteriovenous surgery and, 208
   asthma and, 40
   bronchoscopy and, 222
   bypass grafting and, 267
   cardioplegia and, 249
   cardioversion and, 355
   craniotomy and, 195, 196, 199, 200
   D & C and, 328
   DCR and, 314
   diskectomy and, 180
   endarterectomy and, 269
   hypertension and, 12
   IHD and, 5
   intracranial hypertension and, 67
   laser procedures and, 365
   myringotomy and, 337
   open eye procedure and, 306, 307
   orbital fractures and, 311
   for pediatrics, 333
   pheochromocytoma and, 83, 84, 160
   pregnancy and, 320, 322
   rhytidectomy and, 312
   strabismus repair and, 308
   thyroidectomy and, 289
   tonsillectomy and, 338
   UPPP and, 305
   ventricular defibrillation and, 253
Lioresal. *See* baclofen
Liquaemin Sodium. *See* heparin
lithium, 77, 209
lithotripsy, 357. *See also* extracorporeal
   shock wave lithotripsy (ESWL);
   gallbladder lithotripsy
liver dysfunction, 123
liver resection, 130–132
liver transplantation, 87, 88, 89, 93, 94,
   132–134
loop electrosurgical excision procedure
   (LEEP), 325–326
lorazepam, 245, 252
Losec. *See* omeprazole
Lovenox. *See* enoxaparin
low-molecular weight heparin (LMWH).
   See enoxaparin
Lown-Ganong Levine, 357
Ludwig's angina, 48, 49
lumbar laminectomy/fusion, 177–178

lumbar puncture, 60, 66, 191
lumboperitoneal shunt, 58
lung/heart transplantation, 224–228
lupus. *See* systemic lupus erythematosus
lupus nephritis, 168
lymphadenectomy, 296
lymphadenopathy, 105
lymphangioleiomyomatosis, 224
lymphocytosis, 86
lymphopenia, 105

magnesium sulfate, 9, 55, 321–322,
    426–427
malignant hyperthermia, 73–74. *See also*
    hyperthermia
    emergency therapy for, 517–518
    kyphoscoliosis and, 73
    muscular dystrophy and, 71, 182
    strabismus repair and, 308
    thyroid disease and, 78
malnutrition, 123–125
    gastrotomy and, 142
    laryngectomy and, 294
    neck dissection and, 296
mannitol, 427–428
    aneurysms and, 32, 192, 194, 259
    cardioplegia and, 249
    CPB and, 240, 250
    craniotomy and, 199
    glaucoma and, 118
    intracranial hypertension and, 66
    malignant hyperthermia and, 74
    oliguria and, 228
    peripheral vascular procedures and, 261
    transplants and, 133, 170, 172
Marcaine, 314, 325, 378
Marfan's syndrome, 31, 264
mastectomy, 231–232
maxillofacial trauma, 298–300
Meckel's diverticulum, 143
mediastinal shift, 53, 342
mediastinoscopy, 214–215
megacolon, 339
meningitis, 43, 299
meningomyelocele, 57
meperidine HCl, 428–429
meperidine (meperidine HCl), 428–429. *See
    also* normeperidine
    pancreatitis and, 114
    pregnancy and, 321
    renal failure and, 99
    stereotactic surgery and, 202
mephentermine sulfate, 429–430
Mephyton. *See* vitamin K
mepivacaine HCl, 430–431
mesodermal dysgenesis syndrome, 117

Mestinon. *See* pyridostigmine
    (pyridostigmine bromide)
metabolic acidosis
    adenoma and, 205
    arthroscopy and, 287
    cerebral aneurysm and, 193
    cor pulmonale and, 46
    diabetes and, 75
    hemorrhagic shock and, 16
    hepatic failure and, 90
    hyperaldosteronism and, 85
    hypothermia and, 120
    intraocular procedures and, 309
    malignant hyperthermia and, 73
    pneumonia and, 41
    renal failure and, 97
metabolic alkalosis, 133, 135, 137
metanephrine, 82
metaraminol bitartrate, 431
methadone HCl, 431–432
methemalbumin, 113
Methergine, 320. *See also* methylergonovine
methimazole, 288, 290
methionine, 92
methohexital (methohexital sodium), 349,
    432–433
    cardioversion and, 355
    electroconvulsive therapy and, 210
    for pediatrics, 333
methotrexate, 138, 139
methoxamine HCl, 433
methyldopa, 90
methylene blue, 167, 172, 174, 175, 433–434
methylergonovine, 434–435
methylmethacrylate cement, 274
methylprednisolone, 40, 186, 228, 351
metoclopramide, 435–436
    breast biopsy and, 230
    heart/lung transplant and, 225
    myringotomy and, 337
    portal hypertension and, 98
    renal failure and, 98
    scleroderma and, 126
    tonsillectomy and, 339
metrizamide, 55
mexiletine, 9
MG. *See* myasthenia gravis (MG)
MI. *See* myocardial infarction (MI)
midazolam, 245, 436–437
    amnesia and, 226
    cardioversion and, 355
    CHF and, 15
    colonoscopy and, 151
    craniotomy and, 196
    genitourinary procedures and, 345
    hernia repair and, 344

IHF and, 4
intra-abdominal procedures and, 340
intraocular procedures and, 309
LEEP and, 325
local anesthesia toxicity with, 55
myringotomy and, 337
portasystemic shunts and, 271
seizures and, 54
stereotactic surgery and, 202
strabismus repair and, 308
thoracic aortic aneurysm and, 265
tonsillectomy and, 338
Midazolam hydrochloride. *See* midazolam
milrinone, 25, 243, 437
miosis, 117
mithramycin, 291
mitral regurgitation (MR), 22–23, 238–239, 246
 cardiomyopathies and, 26, 27
 muscular dystrophy and, 70
mitral stenosis (MS), 21–22, 238, 245
mitral valve disease, 18, 24
Mivacron. *See* mivacurium
mivacurium, 98, 437–438
monoamine oxidase inhibitors, 209
mononucleosis, 105
monoparesis, 260
moricizine, 8
morphine (morphine sulfate), 99, 234, 332, 333, 438–439
MR. *See* mitral regurgitation (MR)
MS. *See* mitral stenosis (MS); multiple sclerosis (MS)
MS Contin. *See* morphine (morphine sulfate)
multiple endocrine neoplasia, 82
multiple sclerosis (MS), 61–62
muscle biopsy, 71, 73
muscle paralysis, 28
muscle relaxants. *See also* depolarizing muscle relaxants; nondepolarizing muscle relaxants (NDMRs)
 aortic stenosis and, 237
 ARDS and, 52
 arthroplasty and, 276, 277
 bypass grafting and, 267
 cranioplasty and, 204
 craniotomy and, 199
 hemorrhoidectomy and, 157
 herniorrhaphy and, 147
 hypothermia and, 120
 laparotomy and, 142
 laser procedures and, 365
 LeFort procedures and, 303
 maxillofacial surgery and, 299
 mediastinoscopy and, 215

myasthenia gravis and, 221
 pregnancy and, 321
 prostatectomy and, 163
 scrotal procedures and, 176
 spinal instrumentation and, 184
 thyroidectomy and, 289
 titration of, 78
 tonsillectomy and, 300, 338, 339
muscular dystrophy, 70–71, 73
myasthenia gravis (MG), 61, 63–64, 75, 219, 289
myasthenic syndrome, 65
mydriasis, 159, 191
myelination, 331
myocardial infarction (MI), 2, 6–7, 10–11, 22
 aneurysms and, 31, 260, 266
 bypass grafting and, 266
 CPB and, 254
 electroconvulsive therapy and, 209
 endarterectomy and, 269
 in geriatrics, 122
 hypertension and, 6, 12
 peripheral vascular procedures and, 261
 pheochromocytoma and, 83, 159
myocardial ischemia
 aneurysms and, 260, 265
 blood pressure decrease leads to, 12
 bypass grafting and, 267
 CHF and, 2
 hypertension and, 13
 mitral regurgitation and, 22
 pancreatitis and, 135
 pancuronium and, 5
 pneumonia and, 41
myocarditis, 122
myoglobinuria, 350
myomectomy, 28
myotomy, 28
myringotomy, 49, 336–337
myxedema coma. *See* hypothyroidism

nalmefene HCl, 439–440
naloxone HCl, 440–441
naltrexone HCl, 441
Narcan, 183, 333. *See also* naloxone HCl
narcotics. *See also specific narcotics*
 ARDS and, 52
 arthroscopy and, 286
 bone fractures and, 280, 281, 285
 breast biopsy and, 230
 bronchoscopy and, 222
 burns and, 361
 cholecystectomy and, 128, 129
 D & C and, 328
 epilepsy surgery and, 212
 heart/lung transplant and, 226

hernia repair and, 342
hip arthroplasty and, 272
hydrocephalus and, 58
IHD and, 4, 5
laryngectomy and, 295
maxillofacial surgery and, 300
open eye procedure and, 306
peripheral vascular procedures and, 262
pregnancy and, 319, 321
scrotal procedures and, 176
thoracotomy and, 217
thymectomy and, 220
thyroidectomy and, 289
trauma and, 363
UPPP and, 305
Naropin. *See* ropivacaine HCl
nasal surgery, 301–303
NDMRs. *See* nondepolarizing muscle
  relaxants (NDMRs)
neck dissection. *See* radical neck dissection
necrosis
  caseation, 42
  muscle, 71
  pancreatic, 114
  pneumonia and, 41
  tubular, 96, 359
neomycin, 87
neoplasia
  cardiac tamponade and, 36
  diabetes and, 77
  endocrine, 135, 159
  intraepithelial, 325
  nephrectomy and, 166
neostigmine (neostigmine methylsulfate), 5,
  64, 228, 289, 333, 341, 345, 441–442
Neo-Synephrine, 57, 235, 243, 245, 248, 250,
  269. *See also* phenylephrine
nephrectomy, 166–168
nephropathy, 76
nephrotic syndrome, 77
nephrotoxicity, 228
Nesacaine, 320. *See also* chloroprocaine
neuromuscular blocking agents, 55, 64, 66
neurosurgery, 119
neutropenia, 103
nicardipine, 442–443
nicotinic acid, 90
nifedipine, 256, 443–444
Nipride, 234, 261, 445. *See also* nitroprusside
  (nitroprusside sodium)
nitrates, 4, 258
Nitro-Bid. *See* nitroglycerin
Nitrocine. *See* nitroglycerin
Nitrodisc. *See* nitroglycerin
Nitro-Dur. *See* nitroglycerin
Nitrogard. *See* nitroglycerin

nitroglycerin, 243, 245, 256, 444–445
  adenoma and, 206
  aneurysms and, 32, 192, 193, 258, 260
  angina and, 27
  CAD and, 234, 235
  cardioplegia and, 249
  cerebrovascular disease and, 57
  CHF and, 15
  craniotomy and, 199
  endarterectomy and, 268
  heart/lung transplant and, 226
  hernia repair and, 343
  hypertension and, 13, 246
  hypertrophic cardiomyopathy and, 28
  IHD and, 3, 4
  myocardial infarction and, 7
  peripheral vascular procedures and, 261,
    262
  pheochromocytoma and, 160
  vasospasm prevention with, 247
Nitroglyn. *See* nitroglycerin
Nitrol. *See* nitroglycerin
nitroprusside (nitroprusside sodium), 256, 445.
  See also sodium nitroprusside
  aneurysms and, 32, 193
  autonomic dysreflexia and, 68
  CHF and, 15
  craniotomy and, 199
  hip arthroplasty and, 274
  hypertension and, 186
  IHD and, 5
  peripheral vascular procedures and, 262
  pheochromocytoma and, 83, 84, 160
  spinal cord transection and, 186
Nitrostat. *See* nitroglycerin
nitrous oxide, 351, 445–446
  adenoma and, 206
  bone fractures and, 285
  cardiomyopathies and, 26, 28
  cerebral aneurysm and, 192, 193
  cholecystectomy and, 130
  chronic constrictive pericarditis and, 35
  COPD and, 38
  craniotomy and, 196
  epilepsy surgery and, 212
  genitourinary procedures and, 346
  hepatic failure and, 94
  hernia repair and, 342, 345
  hypertension and, 13
  IHD and, 5
  intra-abdominal procedures and, 341
  intraocular procedures and, 310
  kyphoscoliosis and, 72
  leukemia and, 104
  lung biopsy and, 216
  malignant hyperthermia and, 73

myasthenia gravis and, 64
myringotomy and, 337
nephrectomy and, 168
nuclear medicine and, 353
pheochromocytoma and, 84
pneumothorax/hemothorax and, 53
pregnancy and, 321
pulmonary hypertension and, 47
thyroidectomy and, 289
tonsillectomy and, 338
tracheotomy and, 292
transplants and, 172, 227
nizatidine, 446–447
nondepolarizing muscle relaxants
  (NDMRs). *See also specific NDMRs*
  aneurysms and, 32, 192, 259
  arteriovenous surgery and, 208
  asthma and, 40
  bone fractures and, 281, 284
  burns and, 360
  cardiac tamponade and, 36
  cardiomyopathies and, 26, 28
  chronic constrictive pericarditis and, 35
  craniotomy and, 196
  Eaton-Lambert syndrome and, 215, 216
  endarterectomy and, 269
  glaucoma and, 118
  Guillain-Barré syndrome and, 61
  hepatic failure and, 94
  hysterectomy and, 324
  in vitro fertilization and, 326
  intraocular procedures and, 310
  kidney transplant and, 170, 172
  laparoscopy and, 323
  laryngectomy and, 295
  magnesium sulfate and, 322
  multiple sclerosis and, 62
  muscular dystrophy and, 71
  myasthenia gravis and, 63, 64, 220
  myasthenic syndrome and, 65
  neck dissection and, 297
  nephrectomy and, 168
  ocular procedures and, 307, 308
  parathyroidectomy and, 291
  for pediatrics, 334
  pelvic exenteration and, 327
  peripheral vascular procedures and, 263
  pheochromocytoma and, 83
  portasystemic shunts and, 271
  renal failure and, 98
  seizures and, 55
  stereotactic surgery and, 202
  tracheotomy and, 293
nonsteroidal anti-inflammatory drugs, 155,
  328, 339
Norcuron, 245. *See also* vecuronium

norepinephrine (norepinephrine bitartrate),
  256, 447–448
  CPB and, 251
  heart denervation and, 228
  hernia repair and, 343
  pheochromocytoma and, 82, 84, 159
normeperidine, 99, 168, 173
normetanephrine, 82
normocapnia, 99, 197
normocarbia, 211, 239, 327
Normodyne. *See* labetalol
normotension, 82, 83, 183, 247
normothermia, 183, 346
normovolemia, 26
Novocain. *See* procaine (procaine HCl)
Novolin R. *See* insulin (regular)
Nuromax. *See* doxacurium (doxacurium
  chloride)

obesity, 2, 116–117
  adenoma and, 205
  apnea and, 304
  cerebrovascular disease and, 56
  Cushing's disease and, 80
  diabetes and, 75, 76
  ESWL and, 164
  laser procedures and, 364
  restrictive pulmonary diseases and, 50
obstructive disease. *See* chronic obstructive
  pulmonary disease (COPD)
obstructive uropathy, 77, 168
occlusion, 29
octreotide, 115
oliguria, 14, 17, 88, 228
OLV. *See* one-lung ventilation (OLV)
omeprazole, 448
Omid. *See* omeprazole
omphalocele, 339
ondansetron (ondansetron HCl), 337, 339,
  448–449
one-lung ventilation (OLV), 228–229
open eye procedure, 306–307
open globe, 117
open lung biopsy, 216
open reduction, 278–279, 282–286
ophthalmic surgery, 118
opiates
  cardiomyopathies and, 26, 28
  esophagectomy and, 153, 154
  genitourinary procedures and, 346
  hysterectomy and, 325
  in vitro fertilization and, 326
  laparoscopy and, 323
  LEEP and, 325
  myringotomy and, 337
  orbital fractures and, 311

pancreatectomy and, 136–137
pelvic exenteration and, 327
stereotactic surgery and, 202
tonsillectomy and, 338, 339
opioids. *See also specific opioids*
arthroscopy and, 287
asthma and, 40
CAD and, 236
cerebral aneurysm and, 193
chronic constrictive pericarditis and, 35
cirrhosis and, 89
COPD and, 38
craniotomy and, 200
endarterectomy and, 269
hepatitis and, 87
hydrocephalus and, 58
hypertension and, 12, 13
IHD and, 5
kidney transplant and, 170, 173
lung biopsy and, 216
myasthenia gravis and, 64
nephrectomy and, 167
peripheral vascular procedures and, 263
pheochromocytoma and, 83
pulmonary hypertension and, 47
seizures and, 55
spinal instrumentation and, 184
thyroid disease and, 77, 289
oral contraceptives, 56, 121
orbital fractures, 310–311
orchiectomy, 176
orthopnea, 14, 20, 117
orthostasis, 278
orthostatic hypotension, 15, 83, 159, 272. *See also* hypotension
Osmitrol. *See* mannitol
osteoarthritis, 82, 116
osteodystrophy, 98
osteopenia, 158
osteoporosis, 80, 82, 186
otitis media, 48, 49
oxytocin, 319, 320, 449–450

pacemaker, 10, 14, 95
palmar erythema, 88, 92
pancreatectomy, 135–137
pancreatic transplant, 76
pancreatitis, 113–114, 135, 148
pancreatoduodenectomy, 137
pancuronium (pancuronium bromide), 245, 450–451
CAD and, 236
cardiac tamponade and, 36
cirrhosis and, 89
CPB and, 252
IHD and, 5

intra-abdominal procedures and, 341
peripheral vascular procedures and, 263
tachycardia and, 28
thyroid disease and, 78
Panheparin. *See* heparin
papilledema, 66, 190, 191
paralysis, 60, 82, 185, 190, 200, 314, 315
paralysis agitans. *See* Parkinson's syndrome (disease)
paraplegia, 31, 68, 69, 184, 185, 260
parathyroid carcinoma, 290
parathyroidectomy, 290–291
paresis, 62
paresthesias, 60
Parkinson's syndrome (disease), 59–60, 202
patent ductus arteriosis, 340, 341, 343
Pavulon, 245. *See also* pancuronium (pancuronium bromide)
pectus excavatum, 50
pediatrics
anatomy and physiology, 329–332
conversion factors for, 515–516
drug doses for, 490
equipment, 335–336
esophagogastroduodenoscopy, 149
fluids, 334–335
genitourinary procedures, 345–346
hernia repair, 341–345
intra-abdominal procedures, 339–341
myringotomy, 336–337
penile procedures, 175
pharmacology, 332–334
strabismus repair, 308
tonsillectomy and adenoidectomy, 300, 338–339
pelvic exenteration, 327–328
pelvic reconstruction, 279–282
pelvic relaxation syndrome, 324
penectomy/penile resection, 175
penicillin, 121
penile implant, 175
Pentazine. *See* promethazine HCl
pentolinium, 68
Pentothal, 328, 346, 362. *See also* thiopental (thiopental sodium)
Pepcid. *See* famotidine
pericardial effusion, 34, 79, 275
pericardial tamponade, 276
pericardiocentesis, 36, 239
pericardiotomy, 36, 247
pericarditis, 34, 122
peripheral neuropathy, 76, 98, 104, 139, 246
peripheral vascular disease, 12, 29, 76. *See also* aortic aneurysm
peripheral vascular procedures, 260–264

peritoneal dialysis, 96, 98
peritonitis, 43
peritonsillar abscess, 48, 49
peroneal nerve palsy, 276
petechiae, 274, 278, 282
phagocytosis, 71
pharyngitis, 48, 49
Phenazine. *See* promethazine HCl
Phenergan. *See* promethazine HCl
phenobarbital, 55
phenothiazine, 60, 73, 74
phenoxybenzamine, 68, 160
phentolamine, 68, 83, 84, 160, 451
phenylephrine, 256, 451–452
    adenoma and, 206
    aneurysms and, 192, 258, 260
    arteriovenous surgery and, 208
    cardiomyopathies, 26, 28
    craniotomy and, 199
    endarterectomy and, 268
    hernia repair, 343
    peripheral vascular procedures and, 261
    pheochromocytoma and, 84, 160
    thoractomy and, 218
    thyroid disease, 78
phenytoin, 9, 54, 55, 90, 452–453
pheochromocytoma, 82–84, 159–160
    adrenalectomy and, 157
    electroconvulsive therapy and, 209
    hypertension and, 12, 159, 160
    hyperthermia and, 120
phlebotomy, 103
phosphates, 291
phospholine iodine, 64
photophobia, 190
physostigmine salicylate, 453–454
phytonadione. *See* vitamin K
pilocarpine hydrochloride, 118
pipecuronium bromide, 5, 454–455
Pitocin, 328. *See also* oxytocin
Pitressin. *See* vasopressin
pituitary adenoma, 204
pituitary hypersecretion, 157
pituitary tumor, 204–107
placenta previa, 317, 318
plasma exchange, 61
plasmapheresis, 62, 64
pleural effusion
    left ventricular failure and, 14
    leukemia and, 104
    liver transplant and, 133
    lupus and, 122
    pancreatectomy and, 135
    pulmonary embolism and, 44
    rheumatoid arthritis and, 276
    splenectomy and, 138

    thoracic aortic aneurysm and, 265
    tuberculosis and, 43
pleurisy, 148
pneumonectomy, 218
pneumonia, 40–42
    asthma and, 39
    bacterial, 41
    bronchoscopy and, 221
    esophagectomy and, 152
    gallstones and, 148
    kyphoscoliosis and, 72
    laryngectomy and, 293
    liver resection and, 132
    lung biopsy and, 216
    lupus and, 122
    muscular dystrophy and, 70
    spinal cord transection and, 188
    thoractomy and, 217
    viral, 41
pneumonitis, 42, 50, 142, 149
pneumothorax
    andrenalectomy and, 159
    bone fractures and, 279
    COPD and, 38
    esophagoscopy and, 150
    hernia repair and, 342–343
    in vitro fertilization and, 326
    kidney transplant and, 170, 171
    laryngectomy and, 296
    laser procedures and, 364
    mastectomy and, 232
    maxillofacial trauma and, 298
    mediastinoscopy and, 215
    neck dissection and, 298
    nephrectomy and, 168
    pheochromocytoma and, 160
    restrictive pulmonary diseases and, 50
    spinal instrumentation and, 184
    tracheotomy and, 293
poikilothermia, 119, 332
Polocaine. *See* mepivacaine HCl
polycystic renal (kidney) disease, 97, 168, 190
polycythemia, 56, 157, 225
polycythemia vera, 102–103
polydipsia, 77
polyneuritis. *See* Guillain-Barré syndrome
polyuria, 77, 290
Pontocaine. *See* tetracaine HCl
portal hypertension, 87, 88, 132, 133, 270. *See also* cirrhosis
portal vein thrombosis, 134
portasystemic shunt, 270–271
potassium
    for arrhythmias, 9
    malignant hyperthermia and, 73

monitoring of, 12, 15
release of, 62, 71
potassium chloride, 10
potassium iodide, 288
prazosin, 15, 83, 160
prednisolone, 40, 64
pregnancy
appendectomy and, 143, 144
ESWL and, 164
gallstones and, 148
hernia and, 146
lupus and, 121
pancreatitis and, 113
restrictive pulmonary diseases and, 50
thyroid disease and, 77, 78
Presaril. *See* torsemide
Prevacid. *See* lansoprazole
prilocaine HCl, 455–456
Prilosec. *See* omeprazole
Primacor. *See* milrinone
primary adrenal insufficiency. *See* Addison's disease
primary aldosteronism, 12
primidone, 55, 212
Priscoline. *See* tolazoline
probenecid, 106
procainamide, 8, 9, 10, 25, 121, 456
procaine (procaine HCl), 249, 456–457
Procan SR. *See* procainamide
Procardia. *See* nifedipine
prochlorperazine maleate, 457–458
prognathism, 82
prolactinoma, 204, 205
promethazine HCl, 458–459
Pronestyl. *See* procainamide
propafenone, 8, 9
propofol, 351, 459–460
bone fractures and, 285
CAD and, 236
colonoscopy and, 151
cranioplasty and, 304
cystoscopy and, 174
D & C and, 328
endoscopy and, 358
epilepsy surgery and, 212
genitourinary procedures and, 346
intraocular procedures and, 310
lithotripsy and, 148
nuclear medicine and, 353
rhytidectomy and, 313
stereotactic surgery and, 202
trauma and, 362
propranolol, 249, 256, 290, 460
propylthiouracil, 288, 290
prostaglandins, 114, 343
prostatectomy. *See* radical prostatectomy

Prostigmin. *See* neostigmine (neostigmine methylsulfate)
Prostin VR$_R$. *See* Alprostadil
protamine (protamine sulfate), 256, 460–462
aneurysms and, 32, 259, 260
CPB and, 253
endarterectomy and, 268
heart/lung transplant and, 228
nephrectomy and, 167
peripheral vascular procedures and, 261
proteinosis, 219
proteinuria, 186
Prothazine. *See* promethazine HCl
Proventil. *See* albuterol (albuterol sulfate)
ptosis, 63, 220, 315–316
pulmonary disease, 43, 45, 65, 268, 294
pulmonary dysfunction, 42, 49, 71, 72
pulmonary edema
aortic regurgitation and, 238
ARDS and, 51
asthma and, 39
autonomic dysreflexia and, 68
CHF and, 13, 14
cystectomy and, 174
dilated cardiomyopathy and, 25
malignant hyperthermia and, 74
mitral regurgitation and, 23
mitral stenosis and, 21
nephrectomy and, 168
pregnancy and, 321
pulmonary embolism and, 44
renal failure and, 97, 98
restrictive pulmonary diseases and, 50
spinal cord transection and, 188
thoracotomy and, 218
tonsillectomy and, 338
transplants and, 171, 173, 227, 228
pulmonary effusion, 275
pulmonary embolism, 43–45
dilated cardiomyopathy and, 25, 26
Guillain-Barré syndrome and, 60
hip arthroplasty and, 273, 275
liver transplant and, 132
pulmonary fibrosis, 46, 50, 138, 149, 276, 294
pulmonary hypertension, 46–47, 224–228. *See also* hypertension (HTN)
asthma and, 39
CHF and, 13
cor pulmonale and, 45, 46
dilated cardiomyopathy and, 25
hypoxia and, 304
in infants, 343
irreversible, 224
kyphoscoliosis and, 72

liver transplant and, 132, 133
mitral stenosis and, 21, 22
obesity and, 116
in pediatrics, 321
pulmonary embolism and, 44
restrictive pulmonary diseases and, 50
scleroderma and, 126
scoliosis and, 181
tricuspid regurgitation and, 24
pulmonary hypoplasia, 110
pulmonary thromboembolism, 37
pulmonary vascular disease, 37, 224
pulmonary vasculature resistance, 46, 110, 120, 181, 329
pulmonic stenosis, 115
pulsus paradoxus, 35, 45
pyelonephritis, 148, 168
pyloric stenosis, 339
pyridostigmine (pyridostigmine bromide), 5, 64, 462

quadriplegia, 68, 184, 185
Quelicin. *See* succinylcholine
quinidine, 8, 9, 10, 25

radiation cystitis, 173
radical mastectomy. *See* mastectomy
radical neck dissection, 296–298
radical prostatectomy, 162–164
radiculopathy, 276
radiofrequency catheter ablation. *See* cardiac radiofrequency ablation
ranitidine, 225, 463
rapacuronium, 168, 170, 187, 464
Raplon. *See* rapacuronium
Raynaud's phenomenon, 30
Regitine. *See* phentolamine
Reglan. *See* metoclopramide
Regonol, 333. *See also* pyridostigmine (pyridostigmine bromide)
Regular Iletin II. *See* insulin (regular)
regurgitation, 61, 63, 71, 111, 152. *See also specific types of regurgitation*
remifentanil, 464–465
renal calculus, 148
renal disease, 12, 84, 125, 168
renal dysfunction, 12, 122, 123
renal failure. *See also* acute renal failure; chronic renal failure
aneurysms and, 33, 260, 266
bypass grafting and, 267
hypertension and, 12, 98, 133, 168
liver transplant and, 132, 134
lupus and, 122
malignant hyperthermia and, 74
myoglobinuria and, 359

portasystemic shunts and, 271
spinal cord transection and, 186
renal transplantation, 98, 113
renin, 11, 60, 251, 331
reperfusion, 241
Resectisol irrigation. *See* mannitol
respiratory acidosis, 72, 73, 90, 227
respiratory alkalosis
anemia and, 101
ARDS and, 51, 52
asthma and, 39
bone fractures and, 278
cirrhosis and, 88
COPD and, 37
fat embolization and, 282
hepatic failure and, 90
liver transplant and, 133
pneumonia and, 41
pregnancy and, 318
pulmonary embolism and, 44
renal failure and, 99
seizures and, 55
respiratory distress syndrome, 60. *See also* adult respiratory distress syndrome (ARDS)
restrictive pulmonary diseases, 49–51
kyphoscoliosis and, 72
leukemia and, 104
lupus and, 122
retinal detachment, 209
retinopathy, 117, 159. *See also* diabetic retinopathy
revascularization, 4, 25, 30, 132, 134, 240
reversible ischemic neurologic deficit, 56
Reversol. *See* edrophonium (edrophonium chloride)
Revex. *See* nalmefene HCl
ReVia. *See* naltrexone HCl
Reye's syndrome, 90
rheumatic disease, 18, 237
rheumatic fever, 19, 21, 22, 24
rheumatoid arthritis
arthroplasty and, 272, 275, 276, 277
chronic constrictive pericarditis and, 35
mitral stenosis and, 21
myasthenia gravis and, 64
spinal cord resection and, 185
rhinoplasty, 301
rhinorrhea, 303
rhytidectomy, 312–313
rifampin, 43
right ventricular hypertrophy, 37, 38, 47, 181, 216, 238. *See also* cor pulmonale
ritodrine (ritodrine HCl), 321, 465–466
Robinul, 333. *See also* glycopyrrolate
rocuronium, 168, 170, 187, 236, 466–467

Romazicon. *See* flumazenil
ropivacaine HCl, 467–468

saccular aneurysm, 31
saline
    adenoma and, 206
    arteriovenous surgery and, 208
    arthroplasty and, 275, 277
    bronchopulmonary lavage and, 219
    calcium levels and, 291
    craniotomy and, 196
    CSF removal and, 58
    DCR and, 314
    facial trauma and, 303
    fractures and, 278, 311
    genitourinary procedures and, 345
    hernia repair and, 344
    kidney transplant and, 171
    laryngectomy and, 295
    laser procedures and, 364
    lung biopsy and, 216
    maxillofacial surgery and, 299
    myringotomy and, 337
    nasal surgery and, 302
    neck dissection and, 297
    nephrectomy and, 167
    phenytoin and, 55
    prostate resection and, 162
    ptosis surgery and, 315
    rhytidectomy and, 312
    spinal instrumentation and, 182
    splenectomy and, 139
    strabismus repair and, 308
    tonsillectomy and, 338
    tracheotomy and, 293
    UPPP and, 305
salmeterol xinafoate, 468
Sandimmune. *See* cyclosporine
sarcoidosis, 25, 50, 77, 95
schizophrenia, 122
scleroderma, 126
scoliosis, 180, 181
scopolamine, 5, 469–470
sedatives
    arthroscopy and, 286
    bronchoscopy and, 222
    bypass grafting and, 267
    hip arthroplasty and, 272
    intracranial hypertension and, 66
    open eye procedure and, 306
    pancreatectomy and, 136
    peripheral vascular procedures and, 262
    scrotal procedures and, 176
    thymectomy and, 220
seizures, 54–55
    autonomic dysreflexia and, 68

    craniotomy and, 196
    epilepsy surgery for, 212
    hip arthroplasty and, 274
    in infants, 344
    intraocular procedures and, 309
    malignant hyperthermia and, 74
    multiple sclerosis and, 62
    vasoconstrictors and, 302
selegiline, 59
Sensorcaine. *See* bupivacaine (bupivacaine
    HCl)
sepsis
    Addison's disease and, 80
    ARDS and, 51, 52
    cirrhosis and, 88
    disseminated intravascular coagulation
        and, 108
    Guillain-Barré syndrome and, 60
    hepatic failure and, 93
    hyperthermia and, 120
    malnutrition and, 123
    pneumonia and, 41
    renal failure and, 96
    thyroid disease and, 78
    transplants and, 132, 224
septicemia, 114
septic shock, 17
septoplasty, 301
septorhinoplasty, 301
Serevent. *See* salmeterol xinafoate
serotonin, 114
sevoflurane, 333, 337, 338, 345, 346, 351, 353
shock
    Addison's disease and, 81
    ARDS and, 51
    hemorrhagic, 16
    pancreatitis and, 114
    pulmonary embolism and, 44
    septic, 17
    thyroid disease and, 78, 290
shoulder arthroplasty, 276–277
sickle cell disease, 77, 90, 101–102
sinusitis, 48, 49
sinus tachycardia. *See* tachycardia
sleep apnea, 71, 116, 304, 314, 338, 351. *See
    also* apnea
small bowel resection, 143
sodium, 22, 60, 84
sodium bicarbonate, 74, 97, 240, 259, 333
sodium citrate, 318, 470
sodium iodide, 290
sodium nitroprusside, 243
    arteriovenous surgery and, 208
    bone fractures and, 281
    cerebrovascular disease and, 57
    hypertension and, 13, 246

transurethral resection of the prostate, 161–162
trauma, 361–363
  aneurysms and, 31
  aortic regurgitation and, 19
  ARDS and, 51
  arthoplasty and, 276
  bone fractures and, 279, 280, 281, 282, 284
  cardiac tamponade and, 36
  maxillofacial, 298–300, 303
  mitral regurgitation and, 22
  pneumothorax/hemothorax and, 52, 53
  seizures and, 54
  tricuspid regurgitation and, 24
tremors, 59, 78, 290
Trexan. See Naltrexone HCl
tricuspid annuloplasty, 24
tricuspid regurgitation, 16, 24, 115, 224, 238
tricuspid valve murmurs, 45
Tridil. See nitroglycerin
trihexyphenidyl hydrochloride, 59
trimethaphan, 68, 478*479
trismus, 49
tubal disease, 326
tuberculosis, 42–43
tubocurarine chloride, 479. See also d-tubocurarine

ulcerative colitis, 145, 150
ulcers, 138, 140, 359
Ultiva. See remifentanil
UPPP. See uvulopalatopharyngoplasty (UPPP)
uremia, 113
uremic encephalopathy, 98
uremic neuropathy, 98
Urolene blue. See methylene blue
urolithiasis, 95
uvulopalatopharyngoplasty (UPPP), 304–305

vagal stimulation, 44
vaginal birth, 322
vaginal reconstruction, 327
vagolytics, 160
Valium. See benzodiazepines; diazepam
valporate, 212
valproic acid, 55, 90
valve replacement, 20, 24, 28
valvular heart disease, 18, 133, 266. See also aortic regurgitation; aortic stenosis; mitral regurgitation (MR); mitral stenosis (MS); tricuspid regurgitation
valvular inefficiency, 29
valvuloplasty, 19, 22

Vancocin. See vancomycin
vancomycin, 479–481
vanillyl-mandelic acid, 82, 159
vascular disease, 46. See also pulmonary vascular disease
vasoactive drugs, 69
vasoconstriction
  aneurysms and, 31
  autonomic dysreflexia and, 67
  CPB and, 254
  epinephrine and, 314
  hypothermia and, 119
  mitral stenosis and, 238
  nasal surgery and, 301
  in pediatrics, 329
  peripheral, 14, 60
  portasystemic shunts and, 270
  pregnancy and, 320
  pulmonary embolism and, 44
  pulmonary hypertension and, 47
  renal, 331
  restrictive pulmonary diseases and, 50
  sickle cell disease and, 102
vasoconstrictors, 22, 195, 271, 302, 312. See also specific vasoconstrictors
vasodilation
  autonomic dysreflexia and, 68
  autonomic hyperreflexia and, 188
  cerebral, 66
  hypothermia and, 119
  methylmethacrylate and, 274
  peripheral, 88, 283
  pregnancy and, 318
  promotion of, 239
  septic shock and, 17
vasodilators. See also specific vasodilators
  aortic regurgitation and, 20
  carcinoid syndrome and, 115
  cardiomyopathies and, 25, 28
  CHF and, 15
  craniotomy and, 195, 200
  ESWL and, 166
  hypertension and, 12, 168, 237
  mitral regurgitation and, 23
  myocardial infarction and, 7
  portasystemic shunts and, 271
  seizures and, 55
  spinal cord transection and, 188
  transplants and, 172, 226, 227
vasopressin, 89, 197, 251, 481–482
vasopressors. See also specific vasopressors
  aortic stenosis and, 237
  carcinoid syndrome and, 115
  esophagectomy and, 154
  ESWL and, 165
  hemorrhagic shock and, 16

hip arthroplasty and, 273
hypotension and, 178
laminectomy and, 177, 178
liver resection and, 131
peripheral vascular disease and, 33
peripheral vascular procedures and, 262
Vasotec IV. *See* enalaprilat
Vasoxyl. *See* methoxamine HCl
vecuronium, 482–483
    CAD and, 236
    cirrhosis and, 89
    craniotomy and, 196
    hepatic failure and, 94
    hernia repair and, 345
    IHD and, 5
    intra-abdominal procedures and, 341
    nephrectomy and, 168
    peripheral vascular procedures and, 263
    thoracic aortic aneurysm and, 265
    transplants and, 170, 226
venous telangiectasia, 115
Ventolin. *See* albuterol (albuterol sulfate)
ventricular dysfunction, 20, 340
ventricular dyskinesia, 3
ventricular fibrillation, 9, 71, 119, 237, 250,
    252, 253, 355, 356
ventricular hypertrophy, 116, 238
ventricular tachycardia, 10, 27, 237, 311, 355,
    356, 357. *See also* tachycardia
ventriculoatrial shunt, 58
ventriculoperitoneal shunt, 58, 210–211
ventriculopleural shunt, 58

ventriculostomy, 199
verapamil, 8, 10, 483
Versed, 174, 328, 333, 349, 351, 353, 358. *See
    also* midazolam
vinblastine, 139
visceromegaly, 82
vitamin K, 483–484
vitrectomy, 309
vocal cord dysfunction, 298
volvulus, 340
von Willebrand's disease, 108

warfarin, 258, 484–486
wedge resection of lung lesion. *See* open
    lung biopsy
Whipple's resection, 137–138
Wilm's tumor, 340
Wilson's disease, 87, 90, 133
Wolff-Parkinson-White syndrome, 8, 10, 357
Wyamine sulfate. *See* mephentermine sulfate
Wydase, 314. *See also* hyaluronidase

Xylocaine. *See* lidocaine (lidocaine HCl)

Yutopar. *See* ritodrine (ritodrine HCl)

Zantac. *See* ranitidine
Zecnil. *See* somatostatin
Zemuron, 245. *See also* rocuronium
zidovudine, 106
Zofran. *See* ondansetron (ondansetron HCl)
Zollinger-Ellison syndrome, 135